KU-533-221

Nursing Interventions
for Infants,
Children,
and Families

Martha Craft-Rosenberg

Janice Denehy

Editors

Sage Publications, Inc.
International Educational and Professional Publisher
Thousand Oaks ■ London ■ New Delhi

Copyright © 2001 by Sage Publications, Inc.

All rights reserved. No part of this book may be reproduced or utilized in any form or by any means, electronic or mechanical, including photocopying, recording, or by any information storage and retrieval system, without permission in writing from the publisher.

For information:

Sage Publications, Inc.
2455 Teller Road
Thousand Oaks, California 91320
E-mail: order@sagepub.com

Sage Publications Ltd.
6 Bonhill Street
London EC2A 4PU
United Kingdom

Sage Publications India Pvt. Ltd.
M-32 Market
Greater Kailash I
New Delhi 110 048 India

Printed in the United States of America

Library of Congress Cataloging-in-Publication Data

Main entry under title:

Nursing interventions for infants, children, and families / edited by
Martha Craft-Rosenberg and Janice Denehy.
    p. cm.
Rev. ed. of: Nursing interventions for infants & children. 1990.
Includes bibliographical references and index.
ISBN 0-7619-0725-4 (cloth)
  1. Pediatric nursing. I. Craft-Rosenberg, Martha. II. Denehy, Janice
Ann.
  RJ245 .N877 2000
  610.73′62—dc21
                                           00-008361

This book is printed on acid-free paper.

01 02 03 04 05 06 7 6 5 4 3 2 1

Acquisition Editor:	Rolf Janke
Editorial Assistant:	Heidi Van Middlesworth
Production Editor:	Sanford Robinson
Editorial Assistant:	Cindy Bear
Typesetter:	Danielle Dillahunt
Indexer:	Molly Hall
Cover Designer:	Ravi Balasuriya

LEEDS METROPOLITAN
UNIVERSITY
LEARNING CENTRE
1703546850
HK-BV
CC-31490
27-1-03   5.8.02
610.7362   NUR   2c

Contents

Introduction

In the past decade, health care has seen many sweeping changes—changes that not only influenced the care of children and families but also affected the manner in which care is delivered. There have also been many advances in science, and a better understanding of health promotion and disease prevention has been obtained. Simultaneously, nursing knowledge has grown through research and is beginning to provide a strong empirical base for nursing practice. The integration of research findings into practice is now an important part of nursing education and nursing practice as nurse scholars and leaders work to advance nursing science and improve nursing practice.

This book is the second edition of *Nursing Interventions for Infants and Children*. Feedback from nurses, educators, and editors on the first edition was used to make modifications to this edition. First, the scope of the book was expanded to include interventions for childbearing families. Second, more emphasis was placed on outcome measurement because of the increasing demand for nurses to demonstrate the efficacy of their interventions. In addition, nursing now has standardized language to identify and measure nurse-sensitive outcomes (Iowa Outcomes Project, 1997). Whereas the first edition included nursing diagnoses and interventions, this edition includes outcomes and illustrates how diagnoses, interventions, and outcomes can be linked in nursing practice. Although these linkages have not been tested, they are presented as hypotheses for further research and potential options for clinical practice. It is our intent that the discussion of assessment, diagnoses, interventions, and outcomes will enhance critical thinking and clinical decision making in nursing practice, education, and research.

Advanced practice nurses are becoming increasingly important for the health of children and families. This book will provide assistance in the selection and implementation of these interventions. Some advanced practice nurses may select interventions for specific populations, such as Athlete Health Promotion, Teen Pregnancy: Primary Prevention, and Adolescent Suicide Prevention. Others might select interventions on specific topics, such as Telephone Consultation, Substance Abuse Prevention, or Early Intervention. The contents of this book will complement medical interventions currently being used by advanced practice nurses to improve the health of children and families.

This book was compiled to synthesize the literature on selected nursing interventions, to illustrate how interventions are applied in practice, and to articulate the need for further research. The chapters in this book are designed to describe important interventions needed to restore, maintain, and promote the health of children and families in today's health care environment. Although the interventions in this volume are not exhaustive, they represent a cross section of interventions designed for childbearing and child-rearing families, interventions for children of different age groups, interventions appropriate for children with acute and chronic conditions, and interventions for well children in the ambulatory care, school, and community setting.

Nurses are now practicing in a cost-conscious environment in which there must be evidence that the nursing interventions they implement make a contribution to the health of children and families. Therefore, each chapter includes information on evaluating the outcomes of care, often using the outcome measures developed in *Nursing Outcomes Classification (NOC)* (Iowa Outcomes Project, 2000). Many of the interventions in this book are in *Nursing Interventions Classification (NIC)* (Iowa Intervention Project, 2000), and others have been developed specifically for chapters in this book. All practicing nurses and readers of this book are encouraged to identify and develop additional interventions needed in their practice areas. This is essential as nursing matures as a profession and all nurses take responsibility for developing the knowledge base needed to support and advance nursing practice.

As we begin the next century, we look back to our rich heritage in planning for the future. The nursing paradigm outlined by Florence Nightingale—the client, the nurse, health, and the environment—remains central even today. *Notes on Nursing—What It Is and What It Is Not* (Nightingale, 1859/1969) provided the foundation for modern nursing. Even today, nurses are looking to Nightingale for wisdom and guidance as they chart the future of the profession. Nurses work to put children and families in the best position to improve health. Our concern with the client's environment can be traced to Nightingale, who believed that modifying the environment was essential to improve health. As the demographics of the populations we care for change in this century, it will be imperative that nurses have a greater understanding of cultural and ethnic diversity and how this affects the delivery of care. As we work to modify the environment, we will need to have a greater understanding of how the heritage of families influences their health beliefs and practices. As we synthesize nursing knowledge about health, the client, and the environment, the nurse will become a powerful agent in promoting the health of children and families.

With all the changes facing health care in the future, the one constant in nursing is caring. Nursing pulls together the client, the family, and the health care system with the ultimate goal of improving health. This all occurs in an environment in which nurses advocate for the child and the family in providing needed services. Nurses are committed to providing compassionate, excellent care. Through such care, they make a difference in the lives of the children and families whose lives they touch.

The Nursing-Sensitive Outcomes Classification research reported in this book was assisted by grants from Sigma Theta Tau International and the National Center of Nursing Research (NIH 1R01NR03437-01) (M. Johnson and M. Mass, coprincipal investigators).

We thank a very special person who made this book possible: Linda Curran. Her administrative and editorial support was invaluable throughout the process of compiling and editing this book. Her abilities and positive attitude made the long process enjoyable. Furthermore, her response and the response of her family after losing their home to a tornado during the final stages of this book provided inspiration to her colleagues and to all families who face uncertainty due to a crisis. Linda, you were an inspiration to us all.

REFERENCES

Craft, M. J., & Denehy, J. A. (Eds.). (1990). *Nursing interventions for infants and children.* Philadelphia: W. B. Saunders.

Iowa Intervention Project. (2000). *Nursing interventions classification (NIC)* (J. C. McCloskey & G. M. Bulechek, Eds.; 2nd ed.) St. Louis, MO: Mosby-Year Book.

Iowa Outcomes Project. (2000). *Nursing outcomes classification (NOC)* (M. Johnson, M. Maas, & S. Moorhead, Eds.). St. Louis, MO: Mosby-Year Book.

Nightingale, F. (1969). *Notes on nursing—What it is and what it is not.* New York: Dover. (Original work published 1859)

PART I

Interventions for Infants and Childbearing Families

One of the biggest challenges nursing faces in the new millennium is making sure knowledge and the services available are accessible to all children and families. As child advocates, nurses need to ensure that every child has a healthy start, ideally beginning with preconception counseling, which will safeguard that future parents are as healthy as possible prior to childbearing. Such counseling not only identifies potential genetic risks but also provides parents information on lifestyle behaviors, such as nutrition, that affect their health status as well as having a potential impact on their future offspring. Once pregnancy occurs, nurses must ensure that all families have access to early and consistent prenatal care. This is particularly important for those mothers at high risk, the very young, the poor, and those with risk factors that may have a negative effect on pregnancy outcomes. Although the infant mortality rate has steadily declined in the United States, this country still ranks behind many other developed nations on this vital public health marker. In addition, many infants continue to be born prematurely, putting them at risk for developmental and health problems and costing the nation precious health care dollars.

For families who find conception a challenge, reproductive technology is making parenthood a reality. Nurses are often part of the multidisciplinary team that assists during this process and provides not only physical care but also emotional support and counseling throughout the often long and emotional fertility program. The holistic perspective of the nurse is valuable in understanding the many stresses experienced by the prospective family as they face medical testing and procedures as well as the financial strains and frequent disappointments in their quest for a family.

When an infant is stillborn or is born with genetic conditions, the nurse is often the first to support the family during these difficult moments. The nurse's wisdom and compassion are often manifested in his or her quiet presence, comforting words, and genuine concern. The chapters "Grief Work Facilitation: Perinatal Loss" and "Genetic Counseling" illustrate how sensitive, knowledgeable nurses have an impact on families who are experiencing a loss—the loss of a child through death or the loss of the dream of a perfect child. These chapters point out how nurses can use the strengths and resources of families in coping with their crisis by turning this difficult time into an opportunity for family growth.

For infants born preterm, nursing has provided leadership in implementing developmental care that will promote the growth and development of the infant. In addition to manipulating the environment in the neonatal intensive care unit, nurses are providing opportunities for parents to get to know their preterm infants through kangaroo care and early breast-feeding. These are both examples of autonomous nursing interventions that have changed practice during the past decade. Nursing research is beginning to show the benefits of these interventions not only to the infant but also on the development of the parent-infant relationship.

Other nursing interventions supportive of the childbearing family are Prenatal Care, Fathering Promotion, Lactation Counseling, and Early Intervention. These interventions are likely to support the development of family functioning and the health of the newborn. Parenting Promotion assists high-risk families in developing the parenting role and in identifying and using needed resources and support systems to become self-sufficient. The interventions in Part I are designed to give infant and family a healthy start, which is very important in today's society.

1

Preconception Counseling

Lynn Eidahl

Nurses should consider providing screening, information, and support to individuals prior to conception for several reasons. The earliest that females present for prenatal care is at 8 to 10 weeks gestation. By this time, options to optimize the pregnancy may be limited. The developing fetus may have already been detrimentally affected by poor maternal nutrition, environmental factors, a preexisting medical condition, genetic disease, or lifestyle behaviors such as alcohol or elicit drug use. The ideal time to intervene in any of these situations is before conception rather than during pregnancy. The value of prenatal care should not be diminished. Rather, preconception counseling and care should be a compliment and a precursor to prenatal care. Also, individuals need information prior to pregnancy so that they can make informed reproductive decisions. Both prospective parents need to be fully cognizant of the awesome responsibility that is part of choosing to conceive a child.

As more is learned about preconception health promotion strategies and preconception risks, it will become even clearer that nurses should take the initiative to provide preconception counseling to the target population—all individuals of childbearing age. Preconception counseling should include males in addition to females because of the increasing scientific evidence regarding male preconception risks. Also, a male's life-style can influence his partner's lifestyle and consequently affect the pregnancy outcome. *Healthy People 2000* (U.S. Department of Health and Human Services, 1991), which includes the national health promotion and disease prevention objectives for the Year 2000, supports preconception care and counseling. One stated objective is to "increase to at least 60% the proportion of primary care providers who provide age-appropriate preconception care and counseling" (p. 273).

LITERATURE REVIEW

Optimizing Changes for a Healthy Pregnancy

Individuals of childbearing age can optimize their chances for a healthy pregnancy by living healthy lifestyles and reducing preconception risks. Steps can be taken with regard to nutrition, weight status, exercise, medical conditions, medications, contraception, immunization, substance use, genetics and family history, and environmental exposure to reduce risks and promote health before a pregnancy.

Experts recommend that a female's nutritional status be evaluated before pregnancy. Iron deficiency is the most common nutritional deficiency. Vegetarianism, other special diets, and dieting to lose weight can lead to decreased nutritional status. In these situations, dietary changes or supplements can ensure that a female's body will be nutritionally sound at the time of conception (Hally, 1998; Maternal and Child Health Bureau, 1990).

Maternal folic acid consumption has been found to reduce the incidence of neural tube defects (NTDs), which occur in approximately 1 or 2 per 1,000 live births in the United States. The Centers for Disease Control and Prevention (CDC) recommends that females who have already had a child with a NTD should take 4 mg of folic acid daily starting 1 month before conception and continuing for 3 months into pregnancy, under the guidance of a physician. The CDC also recommends that all females of childbearing age consume 0.4 mg of folic acid daily, the recommended daily allowance for adults. This amount has been shown to decrease the first occurrence risk for NTDs by 50% to 70% (Locksmith & Duff, 1998).

A female's weight prior to conception and consequently during pregnancy can have an impact on pregnancy outcome. Underweight females (≤90% of the ideal weight for height) are at risk for amenorrhea and consequent infertility as well as problems during pregnancy and preterm delivery. Intrauterine growth retardation, lower Apgar scores, and low birth weight are also more common among infants of mothers who are underweight. Overweight females (≥ 35% of the ideal weight for height) are at increased risk for problems during pregnancy such as diabetes, and they are more likely to have a cesarean section delivery. Neonatal complications can include macrosomia, shoulder dystocia, difficulty regulating glucose levels, and mortality (Hally, 1998; Maternal and Child Health Bureau, 1990). Because of the increased risks associated with underweight and overweight status and the complicated physical and psychological issues regarding weight, the best time for a female to deal with her weight status is before a pregnancy occurs.

Exercise prior to pregnancy can promote ideal weight for height, increase a sense of well-being, and motivate a female to continue exercising during pregnancy. Experts generally agree that mild or moderate exercise during pregnancy, preferably at least three times per week, is safe and beneficial. It is best for a female to have an exercise regimen in place before pregnancy. Pregnancy is not the time to exercise to lose weight or begin a strenuous exercise program. Exercises or activities that pose any risk of abdominal injury may need to be replaced with safer activities. Hydration should be adequate, appropriate clothing should be worn, and the environment should be optimal for exercise in the first trimester to promote heat dissipation (Wang & Apgar, 1998). Exposure to heat, particularly hot tub or sauna use in early pregnancy, has been associated with an increased risk of NTDs (Milunsky et al., 1992).

There are numerous medical conditions, including diabetes and phenylketonuria (PKU), that can be treated prior to pregnancy to reduce the risk to a pregnancy and the developing fetus. Studies have concluded that education coupled with glycemic control in the preconception period and the early weeks of pregnancy can decrease maternal and fetal risks, particularly congenital anomalies (Herman, Janz, Becker, & Charron-Prochownik, 1999). PKU is a recessive disorder that causes profound mental retardation if untreated. Neonatal screening is currently the standard to detect affected infants, who are then put on a phenylalanine-restricted diet. Until the late 1970s, the dietary treatment was discontinued by the time a female reached her childbearing years. Females with PKU who are no longer on a phenylalanine-restricted diet and have high circulating phenylalanine levels (>20 mg/dl) are at risk to have a child with secondary effects, including mental retardation, microcephaly, congenital heart defects, and low birth weight. If these females are identified, however, dietary treatment can be reinstituted to lower phenylalanine levels at the time of conception and early pregnancy, which appears to decrease the risk of fetal malformations (Kirby, 1999).

Medications can also pose a risk to a developing fetus and should be discontinued or replaced with safer alternatives prior to conception when possible. For example, Isotretinoin (Accutane), which is used to treat cystic acne, can cause central nervous system, cardiac, and thymus abnormalities along with fetal demise. All the antiepileptic medications cross the placenta and are potentially teratogenic. To decrease the risks related to antiepileptic medication use, it is recommended that a single medication be used, if possible, at the lowest dose necessary. Discontinuing medication treatment should be considered if a female has been seizure free for at least 2 years (Shuster, 1994). The Food and Drug Administration categorizes medications according to their safety, but it is still not possible to guarantee the safety of any medication for use during pregnancy. Therefore, it is important to carefully evaluate the teratogenicity and necessity of any medication if pregnancy is a possibility (Thacker, 1999).

It is well-known that many infectious diseases, including sexually transmitted diseases (STDs), can have deleterious effects on fertility and fetal development. Screening for STDs such as chlamydia, herpes, gonorrhea, and syphilis through history taking and laboratory testing is important so that treatment or counseling can occur before pregnancy. The option of HIV testing, with appropriate consent and counseling, should be available to all females prior to conception, with particular emphasis on those who are considered high risk (American College of Obstetricians and Gynecologists [ACOG], 1995).

Immunization and screening are available to prevent the effects of several infectious diseases. It is recommended that "all females of childbearing age be immune to measles, rubella, mumps, tetanus, diphtheria, and poliomyelitis" (ACOG, 1993, p. 40). Experts also advocate for hepatitis B screening and immunization before pregnancy as well as screening for tuberculosis and cytomegalovirus among high-risk populations. Rubella deserves special attention because the rates of congenital rubella syndrome have been increasing since 1988, and 6% to 11% of females of childbearing age are seronegative. If rubella immunity is not known, antibody titers should be done, and those females who are not immune should be vaccinated. The rubella vaccine, as well as the mumps and measles vaccine, should be given at least 3 months prior to pregnancy because they are live vaccines (ACOG, 1993; Summers & Price, 1993).

Toxoplasmosis is an infectious disease that can result in mental retardation, chrorioretinitis, hearing loss, or fetal demise in a child whose mother was infected during pregnancy from contact with oocytes excreted in cat feces or found in raw meat. It is possible to test females prior to conception to identify those who are already immune. Those females who are not immune can be counseled about preventive measures when dealing with raw meat, cat litter, or soil that could contain the infecting oocytes (Beazley & Egerman, 1998).

Preventing Injury to the Fetus

The literature is full of reports on the devastating effects that can result if particular substances are used into pregnancy. The effects of the two substances most commonly used by females, alcohol and tobacco, are discussed here. Although fetal alcohol syndrome (FAS) is entirely preventable, it is recognized as the leading known cause of mental retardation. Characteristics include a distinctive facial appearance, prenatal and postnatal growth retardation, intellectual and behavioral difficulties, and other birth defects. Both heavy drinking (an average of two or three drinks per day) and moderate drinking (an average of one or two drinks per day) pose an increased risk for a child to be affected by FAS or fetal alcohol effects. Research has not definitively shown that the consumption of smaller amounts of alcohol is harmful. To be safe, however, abstinence is recommended for those who are pregnant or planning pregnancy (Bagheri, Burd, Martsolf, & Klug, 1998; Hanson, Streissguth, & Smith, 1978; Swan & Apgar, 1995).

Maternal cigarette use is the leading cause of low birth weight and is also associated with spontaneous abortion, stillbirth, and maternal pregnancy problems such as preeclampsia, abruptio placentae, and placenta previa. The incidence of sudden infant death syndrome and respiratory illnesses is also higher among children whose mothers smoked cigarettes during pregnancy. Females may smoke to relieve stress, control weight, combat depression, or because they are addicted to the habit and the nicotine. To prevent the negative effects of maternal smoking, it is desirable to address smoking cessation before pregnancy because quitting can be difficult and time-consuming (ACOG, 1995; Floyd, Rimer, Giovino, Mullen, & Sullivan, 1993). Certainly, the male's smoking habit may make it difficult for his female partner to abstain, and there is evidence that passive smoke can be detrimental to the fetus and children (Gergen, Fowler, Maurer, Davis, & Overpeck, 1998).

Individuals or couples may have multiple risks related to genetics or family history that are best addressed before the first prenatal visit. For example, carrier screening is available for specific diseases among individuals in high-risk populations. Those of Ashkenazi Jewish heritage can be tested for Tay-Sachs disease, African American individuals can be tested for sickle cell disease or trait, Mediterranean or Asian individuals can be screened for thalassemia, and those who have a relative with cystic fibrosis or who have a reproductive partner who is a carrier can be tested to determine their own carrier status. Another high-risk population is females ages 35 years or older, who are at increased risk to have a child with Down syndrome or other chromosome abnormalities. For example, at 25 years of age the risk of having a child with Down syndrome is 1 in 1,250, whereas the risk at 49 years of age is 1 in 11. Genetic counseling should be made available to help prospective parents sort out the risks, understand prenatal testing options, and make informed family planning decisions outside the emotional context of pregnancy (ACOG, 1995).

Evidence is gradually accumulating to implicate environmental exposure as a potential causative factor for fertility problems, spontaneous abortion, birth defects, and childhood cancer in offspring. For example, high exposure to lead and resultant toxic blood lead levels have been associated with reduced sperm counts, spontaneous abortion, low birth weight, and developmental problems in children. Research from animal and bacterial studies has shown that ionizing radiation can be teratogenic, although standard X rays that deliver less than 5 rads are not believed to be teratogenic. Even so, experts recommend that females who think they may be pregnant avoid X rays when possible (Fisher & Vessey, 1998; Kelcher, 1991). Certain parental occupations have been associated with adverse outcomes. For example, exposure to anesthetic drugs in the female's work setting has been associated with an increased risk of spontaneous abortion. Studies also link childhood leukemia and paternal exposure to solvents, paints, and employment in the automotive-related industry (Colt & Blair, 1998).

Preconception Counseling Strategies

A variety of different strategies have been used to provide preconception counseling (Table 1.1), including specific prepregnancy clinics, primary care and family planning initiatives, prepregnancy class outlines, and written preconception guides. There is even a company that will create a personalized preconception guide for a female considering pregnancy.

NURSING DIAGNOSES AND OUTCOMES DETERMINATION

Nursing diagnoses can be used to guide the nurse in providing preconception counseling. The diagnoses chosen will depend on the particular concerns identified by the nurse based on an assessment of each situation. Assessment can be done through verbal communication with individuals or couples, a review of records or family history, written questionnaires, or lab screening tests.

In almost every situation, Knowledge Deficit will be an appropriate diagnosis based on the fact that much of the information supporting preconception risk prevention and health promotion is quite new. Knowledge Deficit is also appropriate because many preconception decisions will depend, in part, on the information that individuals understand regarding specific issues. Informed decisions can be made only if individuals have a clear understanding regarding the potential impact of nutrition, folic acid supplementation, exercise, genetic factors, maternal disease, environmental exposure, lifestyle behaviors, and health insurance coverage.

Some individuals or couples may be genuinely anxious about preconception risk factors, such as a family history of genetic disease or exposure to chemicals in the workplace. Anxiety would be an appropriate diagnosis in these cases, for which the nurse can provide information, support, or referral to help them to alleviate or cope with the anxiety.

There may be situations in which individuals are aware of a specific preconception risk such as a 25% risk for a future child to have cystic fibrosis. They may experience Decisional Conflict regarding whether they want to attempt pregnancy while knowing the risk, try assisted reproductive technology, adopt a child, or make the decision not to have children at all.

Other more specific diagnoses may also fit the situation. For example, Altered Nutrition: More Than Body Requirements would be an appropriate diagnosis for a female who is identified to be morbidly overweight prior to conception. Potential for Infection would be an appropriate diagnosis for females who are not immune to rubella or who are at risk for toxoplasmosis infection during a pregnancy. Potential for Injury: Fetal could be used in the case of a female who is planning pregnancy and who is also taking Coumadin or another highly teratogenic medication. A couple who has a history of violent acts within their family, such as child abuse or spousal battery, could have the diagnosis of Potential for Violence applied to their situation. The situation could occur in which one partner does not want them to become pregnant while the other partner is set on their becoming pregnant. The diagnosis of Altered Family Processes could be used to guide counseling to help them work through their differences.

Couples who do not have any identifiable preconception risks may seek information regarding health-promotion activities that can be done before conception to promote a healthy pregnancy and baby. Health-Seeking Behaviors: Preconception would be an appropriate diagnosis for these couples. They may just need affirmation that they are doing everything possible to ensure the health of a future child (North American Nursing Diagnosis Association, 1999).

Any diagnosis should be accompanied by outcomes that can be measured by the nurse. Verbal or written statements made that indicate an understanding of information regarding preconception risks and preconception health-promotion activities are measurable outcomes. It is also possible to identify whether or not individuals take action to decrease

TABLE 1.1   Preconception Counseling Strategies

Reference	Strategy	Sample/Target Audience	Findings/ Implications
Chamberlain (1981)	First preconception clinic	130 females	Previous neonatal death (33%), previous pregnancy problems (20%), previous infant with a congenital anomaly (10%), and past multiple gestation (5%): The most common medical concerns were uterine fibroids and seizure disorders.
O'Conner (1988)	Preconception clinic run by a midwife	154 couples	Funding was a problem.
Cox, Whittle, Byrne, Kingdom, & Ryan (1992)	Preconception clinic	1,075 couples seen in the clinic; analyzed outcomes of 63 females	Previous pregnancy loss (45%), previous fetal anomaly (20%), and maternal disease (22%). A live birth rate of 81% was significantly higher after preconception counseling than the previous live birth rate of 42%.
Jackson & Bash (1994)	Preconception counseling in ambulatory clinic	Clients with uncomplicated diabetes	This was an effective means to provide information about insulin metabolism and the implications of high-circulating glucose for mother and fetus, and to recommended preconception and prenatal diabetes management.
Jack, Campanile, McQuade, & Kogan (1995)	Preconception counseling with negative pregnancy test	136 females	Psychosocial risk (93%), cigarette smoking (59%), nutrition risk (55%), reproductive or medical risk (52%), genetic risk (50%), HIV risk (29%), barriers to medical care (29%), hepatitis B risk (26%), recent use of elicit substance (26%): At least one risk was reported by 94% of the females, and 80% reported more than one preconception risk.
Barron, Ganong, & Brown (1987)	Preconception counseling in primary care setting by nurse practitioners	15 nurse practitioner interviews	Nurse practitioners' teaching responses to an audiotaped client interview indicated a lack of teaching regarding preconception issues.
Steinberg-Warren, Jones, & Huelsman (1993)	Preconception counseling in primary care	Survey responses from 55 professionals	58% did not address even two preconception issues per week. Barriers included low client receptivity and education levels, delayed presentation for health care, and lack of time.
Moos (1989)	Preconception counseling in family planning clinics	1,761 preconception health appraisals and comments by 344 females	There was an average of 6.8 preconception risks per female. Comments from 89% of the females indicated interest in the information and indicated that the information was new to them.

TABLE 1.1   *Continued*

Reference	Strategy	Sample/Target Audience	Findings/Implications
Lea, Gardiner, & Guttmacher (1992)	Preconception counseling to family planning clients through the Family Health Evaluation Program	529 family planning clients	Alcohol use (57%), potential for toxoplasmosis exposure (49%), smoking (35%), personal or family history of reproductive loss (12%), kidney problems (9%): The 10 minutes needed to address the screening questionnaires was reported to be worthwhile by family planning professionals and "improved the comprehensiveness of patient care."
Bushy (1992), Frede (1993), Summers & Price (1993), March of Dimes Birth Defects Foundation (1986-1993)	Prepregnancy class outlines	All individuals of childbearing age	These are available to help professionals educate about preconception risks and health-promoting activities.
Cefalo & Moos (1988), ACOG (1990), Swan and Apgar (1995)	Written guides	All individuals of childbearing age	These are available to educate individuals about preconception risks and health-promoting activities.
Perinatal Health, Inc. (1992)	Preconception risk assessment service	Females planning pregnancy	A personalized "Before Pregnancy Planning Guide" is created by this company after a self-administered inventory is completed by the female.

their preconception risk and promote preconception health. For example, the nurse can follow a female's preconception nutrition and exercise regimen to determine if progress is being made toward a healthy prepregnancy weight. The nurse can also measure whether folic acid intake was adequate during the periconceptual period; whether alcohol, cigarettes, or illicit drugs were discontinued; or whether the rubella vaccination was obtained as recommended. Whether or not a referral is accepted and there is follow-through by the client are good outcome indicators (e.g., genetic counseling, marriage counseling, or a rehabilitation program). It is also possible to determine whether an individual's or couple's anxiety is decreased after preconception counseling by simply asking them or by using specific tools to measure anxiety. Participation in prenatal care, as well as pregnancy outcome, can also indicate the effectiveness of preconception counseling. The only outcome may be that an individual or a couple decide not to become pregnant and state that they are happy with this decision, or a teenager may relate that he or she is going to take steps to prevent an unplanned pregnancy. Measurable outcomes described in the Iowa Outcomes Project (2000) include Decision Making, Risk Detection, Immune Status, Anxiety Control, Health-Seeking Behavior, Compliance Behavior, Risk Control: Drug Use, Tobacco Use, Alcohol Use, and Knowledge: Diet or Health Behavior.

INTERVENTION: PRECONCEPTION COUNSELING

Preconception Counseling can be defined as the use of an interactive helping process that involves providing screening, education, and support to promote health and reduce risks before pregnancy. The screening, education, and support provided by the nurse may involve many different activities.

Screening

Screening may involve obtaining a client history regarding substance use, diet, weight status, potential environmental exposures, medical conditions, prescription drug use, and family history. It may be important to explore with clients whether or not they are truly ready for pregnancy, birth, and parenting. Screening may also involve inquiring about physical abuse among partners or the abuse of children in a family. It may be important to obtain a thorough sexual history, including frequency and timing of intercourse, use of spermicidal lubricants, and postcoital habits such as douching, all of which can affect the likelihood of conception. The nurse can also identify real or perceived barriers to family planning services or prenatal care. The information obtained from a client history can be used to develop a preconception health risk profile that will guide the nurse through the process of preconception counseling.

Clinical and lab testing may be appropriate preconception screening measures in conjunction with the client history. Laboratory testing is appropriate to evaluate Rh status and hemoglobin and hematocrit levels, as well as to check for hepatitis and rubella immunity. A urine dipstick test may be done to check for protein and glucose in the urine. It is also possible to test for toxoplasmosis susceptibility. Carrier testing for Tay-Sachs, sickle cell disease, thalassemia, or cystic fibrosis is available for individuals at risk, and those at risk for tuberculosis or STDs such as AIDS can be offered testing. It is also important to determine the need for a Pap smear, dental examination, or a screening mammogram.

Education

Preconception counseling also involves educating individuals and couples. They should understand the relationships among fetal development and personal habits such as substance use, specific teratogens, self-care requisites, and folic acid supplementation in the periconceptual period. Individuals need to understand the reasons for other preconception recommendations. For example, a dental exam prior to conception is recommended to minimize exposure to X-ray examinations and anesthetics. Recommendations regarding self-care prior to pregnancy, including exercise and diet, can be provided to promote health prior to pregnancy and establish patterns that will continue through pregnancy. Information can also help them to understand the importance of avoiding pregnancy until appropriate treatments have been received, such as rubella vaccination or a course of antibiotics. In addition, individuals should be aware of the importance of early entry into prenatal care, including high-risk programs when appropriate.

Clients may need to learn about ways to avoid specific teratogens. For example, those who may be at risk for toxoplasmosis infection during pregnancy should be educated regarding the appropriate handling of cat litter and raw meat. There are a variety of resources that can assist a professional in providing information about other environmental risks before conception. Swan and Apgar (1995) provide a complete list of occupational reproductive hazard resources that includes the computer databases Medline, Toxline, Reprotox, and the On-Line Catalog of Teratogenic Agents. Material data sheets, which are required by law to be available to employees, may provide helpful information by describing the potential detrimental effects of any substance present in a workplace.

Preconception counseling may include providing information about contraception, fertility, and pregnancy, depending on the situation. It may be appropriate to discuss the cessation of specific birth control measures. For example, it is recommended that birth control pills be discontinued 3 months before trying to conceive for the body to regain a normal ovulatory cycle and to maximize dating of the pregnancy (ACOG, 1990). Methods for identifying fertility, such as mittelschmerz, spinnbarkeit, temperature elevation, and ovulation kits, can be discussed. It may also be important to ensure that individuals are aware of the early signs of pregnancy, such as missed menstrual period, breast tenderness or tingling, fatigue, frequent urination, and nausea. Information about available reproductive technology options or adoption may be appropriate for some individuals.

Support

Providing support to individuals or couples is also a part of preconception counseling. For those individuals who are not ready for pregnancy, the nurse can encourage contraceptive measures or abstinence until they are prepared for pregnancy. The nurse can also support individuals and couples in their decision making regarding the advisability of pregnancy based on their particular situation and identified risk factors. The nurse can discuss specific ways for individuals and couples to prepare for pregnancy relating to the social, financial, and psychological demands of childbearing and child rearing. Encouraging individuals to learn the details of their health insurance coverage with regard to prenatal care, delivery, pediatric care, waiting periods, and provider options is appropriate. Support may include encouraging attendance at prenatal and parenting classes. If barriers to family planning or prenatal services are identified, the nurse can assist individuals in discovering ways to overcome them. Providing and recommending follow-up are also a part of preconception counseling. A written plan of care should be provided to clients whenever possible.

Support may also include referrals. Any female with a chronic medical condition, such as diabetes, PKU, or epilepsy, should be referred to an appropriate specialist for prepregnancy management. Some couples may need to be referred to learn about prenatal diagnostic testing that is available with regard to specific genetic, medical, or obstetric risk factors. A referral to a genetic counseling center or a teratogen information service may be important for those individuals who need information about specific environmental exposures. Referrals to other community resources, such as a smoking cessation program or a weight loss program, may also be appropriate (Iowa Intervention Project, 1996).

INTERVENTION APPLICATION

Pamela, age 36, presented for her annual Pap smear at her family practice clinic where she is seen by the nurse practitioner (NP). Before the gynecological exam, the NP asked if Pam had any health concerns that she would like to discuss. Pam stated that she has been healthy and that she made the appointment to get her birth control prescription refilled. With further discussion, Pam related that she and her husband "plan to get pregnant within the next year because we are feeling the clock ticking."

The NP took this opportunity to discuss the concept of preconception counseling, and Pam agreed that she would like to learn if there is anything she and her husband can do to promote a healthy pregnancy and baby. The NP then proceeded with a client history and identified several preconception risk factors: rubella immunity status unknown, 5'6" tall at 175 lb, no regular exercise, and the husband's nephew has cystic fibrosis.

Several nursing diagnoses were appropriate in this situation to guide the NP's actions: Knowledge Deficit, Potential for Infection (rubella), and Altered Nutrition: More Than Body Requirements. Because Pam's rubella status was unknown, blood was drawn for a rubella titer, and the NP encouraged her to continue oral contraceptives because she might need the live vaccination if she was found to be seronegative. The NP talked with Pam about the increased risks related to overweight maternal status, and she related information regarding healthy exercise regimens and dietary changes that may help with weight loss. The NP also discussed Pam's age-related risk to have a child with Down syndrome—1 in 287. She provided Pam with information and written materials about the prenatal testing that she would be offered if she did become pregnant, including maternal α-fetoprotein and amniocentesis. She talked with Pam about the availability of carrier testing for cystic fibrosis and offered to make a referral to a genetic counseling center so that she and her husband could learn more about carrier testing and her age-related risks. Pam agreed to the referral. Because Pam was taking oral contraceptives, the NP recommended that she discontinue them for at least 3 months before trying to get pregnant to allow her body time to return to an ovulatory cycle and to maximize dating of a pregnancy. She also discussed the potential benefit of folic acid supplementation starting 1 month before pregnancy. The NP provided Pam with a list of her recommendations.

The nursing outcome Knowledge: Health Behaviors was used to evaluate the effectiveness of the nursing intervention Preconception Counseling (Iowa Outcomes Project, 2000). The Pap smear was normal, but Pam's rubella titer showed that she was not immune. The NP contacted her and scheduled her for a vaccination. At that time, Pam stated that she and her husband were going to see a genetic counselor. She had also started swimming at the local YMCA three times per week.

PRACTICE AND RESEARCH IMPLICATIONS

One of the most significant practice questions is how to ensure that individuals of childbearing age have access to preconception counseling. Those who could benefit most from preconception counseling and care are often disadvantaged and face many of the same barriers common to prenatal care. Also, clinics designed solely to provide preconception counseling and care are rare. To increase access, nurses in every setting should consider providing Preconception Counseling whenever appropriate. For example, the obstetric nurse should consider the first postpartum day also the first day of the preconception period. A postpartum clinic visit may also provide opportunities for Preconception Counseling. Routine gynecology visits are opportune times to inquire about childbearing plans and preconception risks. Occupational health centers and health-promotion programs are places in which nurses have contact with many individuals of childbearing age who may be receptive to preconception information. Community centers and churches or synagogues are other settings in which high-risk groups could be targeted for screening. Family planning clinics provide a setting for low-income clients and adolescents, and school-based clinics also provide an opportunity to reach adolescents. Family practice visits for routine health maintenance, school physicals, well child visits, or a negative pregnancy test in any setting are all times when preconception issues might be addressed.

Several research issues need to be addressed regarding preconception counseling. It still needs to be determined which risks are the most important to identify, and how best to intervene once risks are identified. Although a few tools have been developed, there is no standard for assessing preconception risks. Research is also needed to measure outcomes that show the value and effectiveness of preconception counseling in different settings. These are all areas that nurses can address through their own research or in collaboration with other professionals.

It is still hotly debated as to how the United States will deal with increasing health care costs and health care coverage for Americans. This country may adopt some form of national health care, or health maintenance organizations (HMOs) may continue to provide health care for increasingly more Americans. Either way, it will be important for researchers to show the benefits of preconception care and counseling in measurable terms. If preconception counseling and care can be shown to yield positive results that also save health care dollars, HMOs and other insurance companies will acknowledge the importance of this preventive strategy. They may then recognize its value through reimbursement and by encouraging providers and consumers to address preconception health issues. Nurses can play an essential role in providing the evidence to support preconception counseling through research endeavors and strong practice leadership.

REFERENCES

American College of Obstetricians and Gynecologists. (1990). *ACOG guide to preconception care*. Washington, DC: Author.

American College of Obstetricians and Gynecologists. (1993). Immunization during pregnancy. *International Journal of Gynecology and Obstetrics, 40,* 69-79.

American College of Obstetricians and Gynecologists. (1995). Preconceptional care. *International Journal of Gynecology and Obstetrics, 50*(2), 201-207.

Bagheri, M., Burd, L., Martsolf, J., & Klug, M. (1998). Fetal alcohol syndrome: Maternal and neonatal characteristics. *Journal of Perinatal Medicine, 26*(4), 263-269.

Barron, M., Ganong, L., & Brown, M. (1987). An examination of preconception health teaching by nurse practitioners. *Journal of Advanced Nursing, 12*(5), 605-610.

Beazley, D., & Egerman, R. (1998). Toxoplasmosis. *Seminars in Perinatology, 22*(4), 332-338.

Bushy, A. (1992). Preconception health promotion: Another approach to improve pregnancy outcomes. *Public Health Nursing, 9,* 10-14.

Cefalo, R., & Moos, M. (1988). *Preconception health promotion: Practical guide.* Rockville, MD: Aspen.

Chamberlain, G. (1981). The use of a pre-pregnancy clinic. *Maternal Child Health, 6,* 314-316.

Colt, J., & Blair, A. (1998). Parental occupational exposures and risk of childhood cancer. *Environmental Health Perspectives, 106*(Suppl. 3), 909-925.

Cox, M., Whittle, M., Byrne, A., Kingdom, J., & Ryan, G. (1992). Prepregnancy counseling: Experience from 1075 cases. *British Journal of Obstetrics and Gynaecology, 99*(11), 873-876.

Fisher, A., & Vessey, J. (1998). Preventing lead poisoning and its consequences. *Pediatric Nursing, 24*(4), 348-350.

Floyd, L., Rimer, B., Giovino, G., Mullen, P., & Sullivan, S. (1993). A review of smoking in pregnancy: Effects on pregnancy outcomes and cessation efforts. *Annual Review of Public Health, 14,* 379-341.

Frede, D. (1993). Preconceptional education. *AWHONN's Clinical Issues in Perinatal and Women's Health Nursing, 4,* 60-65.

Gergen, P., Fowler, J., Maurer, K., Davis, W., & Overpeck, M. (1998). The burden of environmental tobacco smoke exposure on the respiratory health of children 2 months through 5 years of age in the United States: Third National Health and Nutrition Examination Survey, 1988-1994. *Pediatrics, 101*(2), E8.

Hally, S. (1998). Nutrition in reproductive health. *Journal of Midwifery, 43*(6), 459-470.

Hanson, J., Streissguth, A., & Smith, D. (1978). The effects of moderate alcohol consumption during pregnancy on fetal growth and morphogenesis. *Journal of Pediatrics, 92*(3), 457-460.

Herman, W., Janz, N., Becker, M., & Charron-Prochownik, D. (1999). Diabetes and pregnancy. Preconception care, pregnancy outcomes, resource utilization, and costs. *Journal of Reproductive Medicine, 44,* 33-38.

Iowa Intervention Project. (2000). *Nursing interventions classification (NIC)* (J. C. McCloskey & G. M. Bulechek, Eds.; 3rd ed.). St. Louis, MO: Mosby-Year Book.

Iowa Outcomes Project. (2000). *Nursing outcomes classification (NOC)* (M. Johnson, M. Maas, & S. Moorhead, Eds.; 2nd ed.). St. Louis, MO: Mosby.

Jack, B., Campanile, C., McQuade, W., & Kogan, M. (1995). The negative pregnancy test: An opportunity for preconception care. *Archives of Family Medicine, 4*(4), 340-345.

Jackson, P., & Bash, D. (1994). Management of the uncomplicated pregnant diabetic client in the ambulatory setting. *Nurse Practitioner, 19*(12), 64, 66-73.

Kelcher, K. (1991). Occupational health: How environments can affect reproductive capacity and outcome. *Nurse Practitioner, 16,* 23-38.

Kirby, R. (1999). Maternal phenylketonuria: A new cause for concern. *Journal of Obstetric, Gynecologic, and Neonatal Nursing, 28*(3), 227-234.

Lea, D., Gardiner, G., & Guttmacher, A. (1992). Preconceptional family health evaluation: A regional education program for family planning clients and health professionals. *Journal of Genetic Counseling, 1*(3), 251-258.

Locksmith, G., & Duff, P. (1998). Preventing neural tube defects: The importance of periconceptual folic acid supplements. *Obstetrics and Gynecology, 91*(6), 1027-1034.

March of Dimes Birth Defects Foundation. (1986-1993). Series of seminar guides. 1275 Mamaroneck Avenue, White Plains, NY 10605.

Maternal and Child Health Bureau. (1990, December 6-8). *Call to action: Better nutrition for mothers, children, and families.* Washington, DC: National Center for Education in Maternal and Child Health.

Milunsky, A., Ulcickas, M., Rothman, K., Willett, W., Jick, S., & Jick, H. (1992). Maternal heat exposure and neural tube defects. *Journal of the American Medical Association, 268,* 882-885.

Moos, M. (1989). Preconceptional health promotion: A health education opportunity for all women. *Women and Health, 15*(3), 55-68.

North American Nursing Diagnosis Association. (1999). *Nursing diagnoses: Definitions & classification 1999-2000.* Philadelphia: Author.

O'Conner, S. (1988). Should pre-pregnancy advice be the norm. *Midwife-Health-Visit-Community Nurse, 24*(4), 112-113.

Perinatal Health, Inc. (1992). *Before pregnancy.* Citrus Heights, CA: Author.

Shuster, E. (1994). Seizures during pregnancy. *Emergency Medicine Clinics of North America, 12*(4), 1013-1023.

Steinberg-Warren, N., Jones, D., & Huelsman, K. (1993). Preconceptional health information: A survey of local primary health care providers. *Journal of Genetic Counseling, 2*(4), 328-329.

Summers, L., & Price, R. (1993). Preconception care: An opportunity to maximize health in pregnancy. *Journal of Nurse-Midwifery, 38*(4), 188-198.

Swan, L., & Apgar, B. (1995). Preconceptual obstetric risk assessment and health promotion. *American Family Physician, 51*(8), 1875-1885, 1888-1890.

Thacker, H. (1999). Medical aspects of pregnancy. *Journal of Women's Health, 8*(3), 335-346.

U.S. Department of Health and Human Services. (1991). *Healthy people 2000: National health promotion and disease prevention objectives* (DHHS Publication No. PHS 91-50312). Washington, DC: Government Printing Office.

Wang, T., & Apgar, B. (1998). Exercise during pregnancy. *American Family Physician, 57*(8), 1846-1852.

2

Reproductive Technology Management

Sandra Jane Hahn

Reproductive Technology Management is an intervention encompassing clusters of complex activities performed by nurses caring for patients seeking technological assistance in family building. Procreation has been described as a fundamental facet of being human. The current emphasis on "family values" reflects our society's expectation for married couples to become parents—a rite of passage into adulthood. The loss of a dream and sense of powerlessness that accompany infertility can have devastating results; human responses to the inability to conceive or to give birth include damaged self-esteem, depression, guilt, and anxiety (Applegarth, 1996). Thus, it is not surprising that when basic treatments have been exhausted many infertile couples choose assisted reproductive technologies (ARTs) despite their complexity and costliness. In 1996 in the United States and Canada, 300 ART programs reported 65,863 initiated cycles, 9,610 frozen embryo transfers, and 3,768 donor oocyte cycles with a total number of resulting deliveries of 14,702 (more than 21,000 offspring) (Society for Assisted Reproductive Technology, 1999). In addition, a 1987 Office of Technology Assessment (U.S. Congress, Office of Technology Assessment, 1988, as cited in English, 1996) survey revealed approximately 86,000 donor insemination cycles performed in 1987, resulting in 33,000 live births.

Candidates for reproductive technology management include couples and individuals who require technical assistance or nontraditional means to bring children into their families or both. In addition to infertile couples, candidates include couples who seek family-building alternatives to reduce the risk of transmitting a genetic disorder, people whose reproductive potential is threatened by cancer or its treatment, and single women and lesbian couples who desire children. Egg donors and gestational carriers (surrogates) are also targets for reproductive technology management.

Healthy People 2000 (U.S. Department of Health and Human Services [USDHHS], 1991) goals most central to this intervention are those for maternal and infant health, including reduction of infant mortality and low birth weight, severe complications of pregnancy, and cesarean delivery rate. The chief avenue toward these goals is prevention of multiple gestations through counseling (a) regarding the number of embryos to transfer that will minimize risk of multiple gestation and (b) regarding the option of multifetal reduction should a high-order multiple gestation occur. Other efforts toward maternal and infant health include assessing obstetric risks in older women, such as diabetes or cardiovascular disease, prior to treatment with ARTs.

Intervention activities related to preconception assessment and counseling also address *Health People 2000* (USDHHS, 1991) goals for physical activity and fitness, nutrition, tobacco use, alcohol use, use of other drugs, violent and abusive behavior, and HIV and STD risk assessment as well as goals for maternal and infant health. For example, ensuring maternal immunity to rubella prior to application of ARTs and advising all women of reproductive age to take folic acid supplements are activities that clearly prevent morbidity. The intervention furthers family planning goals related to reducing the prevalence of infertility through infertility preservation efforts. Mental health goals are addressed through counseling activities that strive to prevent mental disorders and adverse effects from stress.

THEORETICAL FRAMEWORK AND LITERATURE REVIEW

Human responses to infertility have both physical and psychosocial components that dynamically interact with the environment. Olshansky (1996a) asserts that infertility has meaning for the entire family and potential family, requiring care-provider sensitivity to larger family issues. Such issues include (a) stress on a marital or partner relationship, (b) stress on "potential grandparents," (c) confrontation with the meaning of genetic link, and (d) confrontation with the traditional definition of family (Olshansky, 1996a). Thus, a logical framework for Reproductive Technology Management is family systems theory, a unitary approach in which the family is viewed as an irreducible whole that is not understood by knowledge of individual family members alone (von Bertalanffy, 1968; Whall & Fawcett, 1991). As an open system, the family exchanges materials, energy, and information with its social, physical, and cultural environment; it is a dynamic entity ever changing and growing (Friedman, 1986; von Bertalanffy, 1968).

An early conceptualization of the intervention Reproductive Technology Management was that of Bernstein (1991), who described the origin of the infertility nursing role as follows:

> As patients with infertility "came out of the closet" in the late 1970s and early 1980s and sought medical care in unparalleled numbers, there was an intense demand for nursing intervention. Physicians were simply unable to provide for the varied needs of couples receiving high-tech medical care, and the team concept developed out of necessity. Today, nurses function as patient educators, as program coordinators, as physician extenders, as well as phlebotomists and ultrasound technicians. . . . They perform postcoital tests and intrauterine inseminations, and run artificial insemination programs. They are a major source of emotional support for couples, and often function as informal counselors. (p. 170)

In categorizing activities of the nurse's role in ARTs, James (1992) included the following: coordinator, educator, counselor, provider of hands-on care, researcher, and professional.

NURSING DIAGNOSIS AND OUTCOME DETERMINATION

The overarching diagnosis for which Reproductive Technology Management is an appropriate intervention is Altered Family Building, and the corresponding proposed outcome is Family Building. Both the diagnosis and the intervention were proposed by me. Closely related diagnoses, interventions, and outcomes are displayed in Table 2.1. Other related interventions are in the Health System Domain (Iowa Intervention Project, 2000), including Telephone Consultation, Multidisciplinary Care Confer-

TABLE 2.1   Diagnoses, Related Interventions, and Outcomes Applicable to
Reproductive Technology Management

Diagnoses[a]	Interventions[b]	Outcomes[c]
Altered Family Building[d]	Reproductive Technology Management[d]	Family Building[d]
Ineffective Individual Coping	Coping Enhancement, Emotional Support	Coping
Body Image Disturbance	Body Image Enhancement	Healthy Body Image
Self-Esteem Disturbance	Self-Esteem Enhancement[d]	Self-Esteem
Powerlessness	Empowerment	Health Belief: Perceived Control
Dysfunctional Grieving	Grief Work Facilitation	Grief Resolution
Anxiety	Anxiety Reduction	Anxiety Control
Decisional Conflict	Decision-Making Support	Decision Making
Knowledge Deficit: Infertility Prevention[d]	Teaching: Infertility Prevention[d]	Fertility Preservation
Knowledge Deficit: Preconception Issues	Preconception Counseling	Knowledge: Preconception Issues
Knowledge Deficit: Reproductive Technology	Teaching: Reproductive Technology	Knowledge: Reproductive Technology[d]
Knowledge Deficit: Parenteral Medication	Teaching: Parenteral Medication	Self-Care: Parenteral Medication
Pain	Pain Management	Comfort
Altered Tissue Perfusion	Shock Prevention; Shock Management Volume	Tissue Perfusion
Fluid Volume Excess; Fluid Volume Deficit	Fluid and Electrolyte Monitoring and Enhancement	Fluid Balance; Electrolyte and Acid-Base Balance

a. From the North American Nursing Diagnosis Association (1999).

b. From the Iowa Intervention Project (2000).

c. From the Iowa Outcomes Project (2000).

ence, Insurance Authorization, Laboratory Data Interpretation, Health
Policy Monitoring, and Research Data Collection.

Intervention: Reproductive Technology Management

Reproductive Technology Management (RTM) is defined as "assisting a patient through the steps of complex infertility treatment" (Iowa Intervention Project, 2000, p. 470). The following discussion highlights
RTM activities validated for the nursing interventions classification

(Iowa Intervention Project, 2000), including clusters of teaching, counseling, coordination, and technology-implementation activities.

Teaching Activities

Teaching activities are the essence of RTM. Validated activities related to teaching encompass preconception and prevention issues as well as teaching about the treatment process.

Preconception Teaching

Infertility care providers have a responsibility and unique opportunity to address preconception issues in educative processes. Not only do providers care for a population during the period preceding a hoped-for conception but also they diagnose pregnancies before or early in the period of organogenesis and cell differentiation. The challenge is to educate patients about the potential influence of lifestyle and health status on embryonic cells and the risks pregnancy may pose to the health of the woman.

Teaching Related to Genetics

Many genetic issues must be addressed preconceptionally in RTM teaching, including (a) genetic risks associated with advanced paternal or maternal age, (b) risks related to ethnic background (Ashkenazi Jewish, Tay-Sachs; African, sickle cell anemia; Asian or Middle Eastern, α-thalassemia), and (c) identifying family histories with a high incidence of ovarian or breast cancer (Jones, 1996). The absence of the vas deferens may represent the expression of an altered gene for cystic fibrosis; thus, genetic screening for cystic fibrosis should be offered to the couple prior to aspiration of sperm from the epididymis or testes for in vitro fertilization (IVF). Intracytoplasmic sperm injection (ICSI), injecting a single sperm into an egg to achieve fertilization, bypasses physiologic selection of sperm in fertilization. Although there has been no increase in birth defects in resulting offspring, ICSI is undergoing scrutiny for possible transmission of chromosome abnormalities or genetic mutations associated with male infertility, and such concerns should be shared with couples (Go, 1996). Couples at risk for a genetic disorder may desire biopsy of embryos for genetic diagnosis prior to transferring embryos to the uterus. Preimplantation diagnosis has been used for X-linked disorders, fragile X syndrome, cystic fibrosis, Tay-Sachs, and Marfan's disorder (Jones, 1996).

Teaching Fertility Preservation

Many opportunities for teaching fertility preservation arise in RTM. Examples are (a) imparting the need for cessation of smoking and (b) detection and treatment of chlamydia infections, because both smoking and chlamydia adversely affect fertility and gestational outcomes.

Provide Education About
Various Treatment Modalitites

Couples must understand the treatments available to them to make appropriate choices; they must master the steps of treatment to optimize their chances for pregnancy. Many couples request instruction in administration of parenteral medications, which are prescribed daily for weeks to months. They need preparation for possible emotional responses associated with assisted reproductive technology and for ethical dilemmas they will face. They may need assistance understanding cost implications and their insurance coverage for assisted reproductive technologies—IVF is covered by only 14% to 17% of insurance plans (Ginsburg, 1996).

Teaching About Risks,
Benefits, and Alternatives

Nurses collaborate with the ART team in assisting couples to make informed decisions. Every effort must be made to give patients a realistic estimate of their chances of conception and live birth for all of the alternatives open to them. Ensuring that patients understand the risks associated with ART is a priority teaching activity that must occur well before initiation of treatment and continue as each milestone is reached.

Risks Associated With Fertility Drugs

The prominent complication related to fertility drug use is severe ovarian hyperstimulation syndrome (OHSS), which occurs in 1% to 5% IVF cycles (American Society for Reproductive Medicine, 1996a). Although potentially life threatening without intervention, symptoms of severe OHSS (hypovolemia, hemoconcentration, and electrolyte imbalance) can be effectively managed by the ART team. Hospitalization and considerable discomfort are possibilities that should be acknowledged, and patients should be provided a written list of OHSS symptoms to report.

Studies have inconsistently reported an association between ovarian cancer and fertility drugs. It is important for infertile women and egg donors to be aware of this possible association. They should also recognize that pregnancy is protective against ovarian cancer.

Concerned patients can be advised that if fertility drugs do increase risk for ovarian cancer, it amounts to a two- or threefold increase over baseline risk, which translates to a lifetime risk for exposed U.S. women of 4% or 5% (compared to a lifetime risk for breast cancer of 12%) (Whittemore, 1993).

Risk for Multiple Gestation

Transferring multiple embryos in IVF enhances the probability of achieving pregnancy but also increases risk for multiple gestations. In the United States and Canada in 1995, 28.8% of IVF procedures resulted in 28.8% twins, 5% to 6% triplets, and 0.6% higher-order multiple deliveries (Society for Assisted Reproductive Technology, 1999). Couples need to be told the risks of multiple gestation, including pregnancy-induced hypertension, maternal hemorrhage, premature rupture of membranes, cesarean delivery, premature labor, premature delivery, and stillbirths (Olshansky, 1996b). They need to understand that premature birth places infants at risk for increased morbidity and mortality. To decide on the number of embryos to transfer, couples need ART program statistics to allow them to weigh pregnancy rates against multiple birth rates by number of embryos transferred. They need to know about the option for multifetal reduction and the associated risks. If a higher-order pregnancy persists to 10 weeks of gestation, couples may choose reduction to twins or triplets, accepting a risk of less than 10% that the entire uterine contents may be lost (Vauthier-Brouzes & Lefebvre, 1992).

Other Risks

Although risks of procedure-related hemorrhage, injury to pelvic structures, or infection are very small, patients must be informed of them. The risk of ectopic pregnancy is 5% following IVF (American Society for Reproductive Medicine, 1996b). Patients must be taught symptoms to report, and that after transfer of multiple embryos a tubal pregnancy can exist even when a gestational sac has been identified in the uterus. Recipients, donors, and surrogates must be informed about who will be responsible for costs associated with complications or injuries in an egg donor or gestational carrier. Donors and recipients and parties to surrogacy arrangements must acknowledge the legal uncertainty about whether intentions to exclude the donor or surrogate from all rearing rights and duties will be legally binding. Only five states clarify parental rights and responsibilities for egg donation. Thirty states address sperm donation (Robertson, 1996).

Counseling Activities

Many counseling activities have been validated for RTM, commensurate with the psychosocial impact of altered family building. The life crisis of infertility can immobilize immediate plans and desires, overtax existing resources, and threaten long-term life goals (Braverman & English, 1992). Emotional responses become more profound as the couple pursues more intense and aggressive forms of therapy, such as ARTs. Braverman and English (1992) discuss these unique concerns of subgroups: (a) older people may fear genetic defects and be concerned about their longevity or the stigmatization of older parents, (b) women with multiple births may feel ill equipped to manage the unique needs of each child, and (c) parents electing fetal reduction may have to live with a painful memory of terminating one or more fetuses without knowing if they were viable or healthy. Braverman (1994) stated that, for couples using donor eggs, the question of whether or not to disclose donor egg origins to the child "is considered in the midst of a crisis comprised of the woman's loss of her genetic contribution to the child and the couple's loss of the biological child they had planned to have together" (p. 145).

Olshansky (1996a) suggests that anticipatory guidance is a useful counseling activity because knowing that stresses are common can be therapeutic. Self-esteem and identity issues warrant counseling attention. Olshansky (1992) theorized that people who experience infertility take on an identity of themselves as infertile at the expense of more positive identities, such as spouse, friend, or career person. It is helpful to assist individuals and couples to focus on areas of their lives in which they view themselves as successful. Associated with identity as infertile is a view of self as a failure. Language such as "failed treatment" is often internalized and should be avoided. Olshansky recommends follow-up with patients who do not become pregnant, who may feel health care providers are not concerned about them after they "have failed" IVF. Couples may need help recognizing when to stop infertility treatment and go on to other options. When there is a pregnancy loss, the ART nurse needs skill in bereavement counseling. The chapters on grief work facilitation provide useful suggestions on what is helpful for and what not to say to grieving families.

Another counseling activity is to facilitate a couple's acceptance of their means of family building. Mahlstedt and Greenfeld (1989) asserted that couple acceptance of the means of conception is imperative for a positive adjustment of the child. To accept family-building alternatives, couples must take time (several months are recommended) to mourn losses and heal the wounds created by infertility (Mahlstedt & Greenfeld, 1989). The grief process can be facilitated by acknowledging that a loss has occurred and that grief is a normal and appropriate response and then providing support as the couple works through painful feelings. It is helpful to validate that successful parenting is dependent on accepting differences, love, and shared experiences rather than biological ties.

Decision-making support is an important activity in RTM, especially in light of the many ethical dilemmas faced by couples. Couples can be assisted to clarify values that will be crucial to decision making by asking questions to promote reflection, such as how do they view cryopreservation of embryos and how do they view multifetal reduction? Many couples need help identifying issues and systematically weighing pros and cons to make decisions. One way to facilitate thinking is to write each decision-making issue at the top of a piece of paper that is divided into two columns, for listing advantages and disadvantages of decision alternatives.

Couples may need referral to support groups or to mental health professionals. An important aspect of infertility counseling is helping families identify their own support systems, which may include family members, friends, spiritual advisers, and mental health professionals in their home communities. Counseling may be beyond the scope of the ART nurse in the face of the following: (a) symptoms of depression, (b) suicidal ideation, (c) increased use of alcohol and drugs, (d) marital discord, and (e) inability to make a treatment decision.

Coordination Activities (Indirect Intervention Activities)

Many ART nurses are called "IVF coordinators," reflective of central activities in RTM. Validated coordinating activities include (a) scheduling tests as needed, based on the menstrual cycle; (b) coordinating activities of the multidisciplinary team for treatment process; (c) collaborating with the IVF team in screening and selecting gamete donors; (d) coordinating synchronization of donor and recipient hormonal cycles; (e) participating in team conferences to correlate test results for evaluating oocyte maturity; (f) assisting with hormonal and ultrasound monitoring of early pregnancy; (g) scheduling follow-up medication, tests, and ultrasound exams; and (h) participating in reporting data about treatment outcomes to the national registry.

Particularly demanding is the coordination of third-party reproduction processes. Coordination and management of a donor-recipient cycle is estimated to require a fourfold increase in nursing time compared to that of a standard IVF cycle, thus requiring additional nursing support (English, 1996). First, egg and sperm donors, surrogates, and infertile couples must be screened for compliance with selection criteria, health problems, infertility factors, and sexually transmitted and blood-borne disease. Attempts are then made to match donors and recipients according to physical characteristics and medical histories. For egg donation and surrogacy, it is necessary to synchronize the donor's egg retrieval with the recipient's hormone replacement regimen to create an optimally receptive uterine lining at the time of embryo transfer. To meet this coordination challenge, detailed checklists and protocols are essential.

Technology Implementation Activities

RTM activities include hands-on technical procedures, often in an expanded role. Validated activities include (a) drawing specimens for endocrine determination; (b) performing ultrasound exams to ascertain follicular growth; (c) setting up equipment for oocyte retrieval; (d) assisting with freezing and preservation of embryos, as indicated; (e) assisting with fertilization procedures; (f) preparing the patient for embryo transfer; and (g) performing pregnancy tests.

RTM activities also encompass emergency and acute care of ART patients with ovarian hyperstimulation syndrome, ectopic pregnancy, ovarian torsion, miscarriage, and postoperative complications.

INTERVENTION APPLICATION

Meg and Tom Johnson were aware of their diagnosis of Altered Family Building (proposed by me) before they married because Meg had Turner's syndrome and ovarian dysgenesis. The option of using donated eggs appealed to them because Tom would be genetically related to the resulting children and Meg would undergo pregnancy, birth, and breast-feeding as well as parenting. They had not experienced infertility evaluation or treatment prior to entering an anonymous donor egg program; therefore, education activities were prominent in the use of the intervention RTM. At their initial visit, they met with multiple team members. With a counselor, they explored issues regarding family building with donor eggs. Because their families were aware of Meg's medical problems, they planned to share the origins of potential children with family members, but they had many worries about this issue. They viewed a videotaped presentation about the donor egg program and then spent time with Karen, an ART nurse, for preconception counseling and discussion of the treatment process, including risks, benefits, and alternatives. The ART physician recommended that Meg be evaluated for renal and uterine anomalies that can be problems for Turner's patients, and Karen coordinated the testing. Collecting a semen specimen for analysis and cryopreservation was very stressful for Tom. Karen explored with the couple ways to make this more comfortable for him on the day the donor's eggs would be retrieved. They signed a consent form stating their intentions to assume all rearing rights and responsibilities for offspring and to exclude the donor from the same. Meg was given written instructions for her hormone replacement regimen, and Karen explained how her cycle would be synchronized with the egg donor's ovarian stimulation. Karen also taught Tom how to give progesterone injections, which would be essential for maintenance of a pregnancy through the first trimester. They selected a donor who had physical features similar to Meg's and were provided with nonidentifying information about the donor's medical history and attributes. Twenty eggs were retrieved from the donor, 18 of which fertilized normally with Tom's sperm. Three embryos were transferred to Meg's uterus, and 15 embryos were cryopreserved. Against the odds, a triplet pregnancy resulted, and after counseling by specialists in high-risk obstetrics and neonatology, they made an agonizing decision to reduce the number of fetuses to two. The outcome, Family Building (proposed by me), meant in this case use of donated eggs to build a family of four. They sent photos of the twins to, and stayed in contact with, the ART team. Tom and Meg were encouraged to call as needed to further discuss disclosure to the children. They pondered what to do with their remaining frozen embryos—transfer, discard, or donate to another couple—and tentatively deciding to use their frozen embryos for one more pregnancy and to donate any that remained.

RESEARCH AND PRACTICE IMPLICATIONS

Research Implications

Because the duration of ART experience is less than 20 years, little is known about the impact of reproductive alternatives. Well-designed, multicenter longitudinal studies are needed to evaluate the outcomes for the parties involved. Several important questions need to be answered, including the following: (a) Will outcomes for families using anonymous donors be different from outcomes of families using identified donors? (b) Will outcomes be different for families that disclose birth origins to children and families that keep birth origins private? (c) How many offspring will search for their donors and other offspring of their donors? and (d) What will be the outcomes for all parties when searches occur? ART nurses who participate in the introduction of new technologies have a responsibility to participate in evaluating the impact of the technologies on individuals, families, and society.

Ethical Issues in Reproductive Technology Management

Reproductive technology raises many questions that challenge traditional assumptions about the beginning of life, family building, and defining parenthood. Although the government has avoided these politically sensitive issues, professional organizations have made efforts to examine ARTs for ethical repercussions and potential to cause harm. Two sources of ethical guidelines are the American Society for Reproductive Medicine (ASRM) and the National Advisory Board on Ethics in Reproduction. Another resource is the Nurses' Professional Group within the ASRM, which offers educational programs addressing ethical considerations in RTM. In addition to maintaining awareness of guidelines, it is advisable for ART programs to develop a structure that includes an ethics advisory committee that can consider ethical dilemmas and issues carefully in a framework of ethical principles. Facilitating such a committee is an appropriate activity for RTM by ART nurses.

Reproductive Technology Management is an intervention for the future. It needs to be tested for effectiveness. This intervention offers hope for family building integrating innovative technology. Nurses of the current and future generations need to have the skills necessary to carry out this intervention.

REFERENCES

American Society for Reproductive Medicine. (1996a). *Side effects of gonadotropins* [Fact sheet]. Birmingham, AL: Author.

American Society for Reproductive Medicine. (1996b). *Risks of in vitro fertilization (IVF)* [Fact sheet]. Birmingham, AL: Author.

Applegarth, L. D. (1996). Ethical issues in infertility nursing practice. *Infertility and Reproductive Medicine Clinics of North America, 7,* 611-621.

Bernstein, J. (1991). Development of the nursing role in reproductive endocrinology and infertility. In C. Garner (Ed.), *Principles of infertility nursing* (pp. 169-178). Boca Raton, FL: CRC Press.

Braverman, A. M. (1994). Oocyte donation: Psychological and counseling issues. *Clinical Consultations in Obstetrics and Gynecology, 6*(2), 143-149.

Braverman, A. M., & English, M. E. (1992). Creating brave new families with advanced reproductive technologies. *NAACOG's Clinical Issues in Perinatal and Women's Health Nursing, 3*(2), 353-362.

English, M. E. (1996). Third-party reproduction: Nursing issues. *Infertility and Reproductive Medicine Clinics of North America, 7,* 587-609.

Friedman, M. M. (1986). *Family nursing: Theory and assessment.* Norwalk, CT: Appleton-Century-Crofts.

Ginsburg, K. A. (1996). Infertility insurance: Status, myths, and strategies for change. *Infertility and Reproductive Medicine Clinics of North America, 7,* 553-564.

Go, K. J. (1996). An insider's look at the ART laboratory. In *Course XI reproductive and gynecologic health across the life-span: Nursing approaches,* 29th Annual Postgraduate Program (pp. 143-148). Boston: American Society for Reproductive Medicine.

Iowa Intervention Project. (2000). *Nursing interventions classification (NIC)* (J. C. McCloskey & G. M. Bulechek, Eds.; 3rd ed.). St. Louis, MO: Mosby-Year Book.

Iowa Outcomes Project. (2000). *Nursing outcomes classification (NOC)* (M. Johnson, M. Maas, & S. Moorhead, Eds.; 2nd ed.). St. Louis, MO: Mosby-Year Book.

James, C. A. (1992). The nursing role in assisted reproductive technologies. *NAACOG's Clinical Issues in Perinatal and Women's Health Nursing, 3,* 328-334.

Jones, S. L. (1996). Advances in human genetics: Implications for infertility nursing practice. *Infertility and Reproductive Medicine Clinics of North America, 7,* 577-585.

Mahlstedt, P. P., & Greenfeld, D. A. (1989). Assisted reproductive technology with donor gametes: The need for patient preparation. *Fertility and Sterility, 52,* 908-914.

North American Nursing Diagnosis Association. (1999). *Nursing diagnoses: Definitions and classification 1995-1996.* Philadelphia: Author.

Olshansky, E. (1992). Redefining the concepts of success and failure in infertility treatment. *NAACOG's Clinical Issues in Perinatal and Women's Health Nursing, 3*(2), 343-346.

Olshansky, E. (1996a). A family approach to infertility care. In *Course XI reproductive and gynecologic health across the life-span: Nursing approaches,* 29th Annual Postgraduate Program (pp. 79-84). Boston: American Society for Reproductive Medicine.

Olshansky, E. (1996b). Follow-up with children of assisted reproductive technology: Summary of the Mental Health Professional Group course from 1995. In *Course XI reproductive and gynecologic health across the life-span: Nursing approaches,* 29th Annual Postgraduate Program (pp. 185-190). Boston: American Society for Reproductive Medicine.

Robertson, J. A. (1996). Legal uncertainties in human egg donation. In C. Cohen (Ed.), *New ways of making babies* (pp. 175-187). Bloomington: Indiana University Press.

Society for Assisted Reproductive Technology and the American Society for Reproductive Medicine. (1999). Assisted reproductive technology in the United States and Canada: 1996 results generated from the American Society for Reproductive Medicine/Society for Assisted Reproductive Technology Registry. *Fertility and Sterility, 71,* 798-807.

U.S. Congress, Office of Technology Assessment. (1988). *Artificial insemination practice in the U.S.: Summary of the 1987 survey* (Publication No. 3-368). Washington, DC: Government Printing Office.

U.S. Department of Health and Human Services. (1991). *Healthy people 2000: National health promotion and disease prevention objectives* (DHHS Publication No. PHS 91-50312). Washington, DC: Government Printing Office.

Vauthier-Brouzes, D., & Lefebvre, G. (1992). Selective reduction in multifetal pregnancies: Technical and psychological aspects. *Fertility and Sterility, 57,* 1012-1015.

von Bertalanffy, L. (1968). *General systems theory: Foundation, development, application.* New York: George Braziller.

Whall, A. L., & Fawcett, J. (1991). The family as a focal phenomenon in nursing. In A. L. Whall & J. Fawcett (Eds.), *Family theory development in nursing* (pp. 7-29). Philadelphia: F. A. Davis.

Whittemore, A. S. (1993). Fertility drugs and risk of ovarian cancer. *Human Reproduction, 8,* 999-1000.

3

Reproductive Counseling

Disclosure About Birth Origins

Sandra Jane Hahn

Reproductive technology has enabled the separation of the genetic, gestational, and social components of parenting. In addition to adoption and foster parenting, alternative means of bringing a child into the family include donated sperm, eggs, or embryos; gestational carrier (or host uterus) arrangements, in which a woman carries the pregnancy for the intended and genetic parents; and traditional surrogacy, in which the intended father is the source of sperm, and the surrogate is the egg donor and carries the pregnancy. Parents who choose alternative means of bringing a child into a family are faced with the difficult decision of whether to disclose the means of conception or gestation or both to children with nontraditional origins. The nurse caring for families built through assisted reproductive technology (ART) must address many important psychosocial and emotional consequences, including potential adverse effects of disclosure or nondisclosure about birth origins. Reproductive

Counseling: Disclosure About Birth Origins consists of telling children conceived with donated gametes or gestated by a surrogate about genetic or gestational connections or both though an interactive helping process focusing on informational needs, problems, and feelings. The purpose of the intervention is to enhance or support coping, decision making, and interpersonal relationships.

THEORETICAL FRAMEWORK AND LITERATURE REVIEW

Theoretical Framework

Because the family is the unit of care, family systems theory with its hierarchy of systems, conceptualization of boundaries, and subsumed communication theory is the logical framework for this intervention focusing on communication of novel family relationships in the context of the family environment. Related theory of family secrets is also instructive for the intervention. Extending these theories is speculative literature about origins disclosure from the fields of mental health, law, ethics, and philosophy.

The family as an open system exchanges materials, energy, and information with its social, physical, and cultural environment; it is a dynamic entity, ever changing and growing (Friedman, 1986; von Bertalanffy, 1968). Family systems and subsystems have boundaries. The hierarchy of systems includes suprasystems, such as the community and larger society, and subsystems, such as parent-child, spousal, and sibling subsystems.

Although I favor the use of words such as "privacy" or "disclosure" to reduce a sense of bias, family secrecy theory is helpful in understanding the family phenomena regarding disclosure decisions. Family secrecy theory is also about family relationships structured by boundaries. According to Karpel (1980), "Secrets involve information that is either withheld or differentially shared between or among people" (p. 295). Internal family secrets, in which at least two people keep a secret from at least one other, strengthen subsystem boundaries in the family but result in estrangement between secret-holders and the unaware. Shared family secrets, when all members of the family know, strengthen boundaries separating the family from the outside world, impeding alliances between family members and persons outside the family. Consequences of family secrets result in deception, distortion, and mystification. At the emotional level, consequences include generation of anxiety for both secret-holders and unaware. The secret-holder fears disclosure and is uncomfortable with deceit. The unaware experiences anxiety relative to unexplainable tension that develops when areas relevant to the secret are discussed with secret-holders. Karpel (1980) stated, "Secrets contribute to a vague, but tenacious sense of shame or guilt in the unaware" (p. 300).

Birth origins disclosure has been discussed in the literature from the fields of mental health, law, ethics, and philosophy. From these discussions, three positions can be identified: (a) prodisclosure, (b) defense of privacy, and (c) best fit, maintaining that disclosure decisions are contextual. In each position, the benefits and risks must be weighed in light of the family's beliefs and values and of the sociocultural community in which children are likely to be raised.

Prodisclosure proponents assert that honesty will have the best outcomes in terms of mental health. They note the pathological effects of family secrets, the burden of secrecy for the family, and the cost of living a lie. They point to the effects of closed adoption; the overrepresentation of adoptees at mental health clinics, the self-identity and self-esteem problems of adoptees, and the compulsion of adoptees to search for their biological origins (Baran & Pannor, 1989; Demick & Wapner, 1988). They also note the experiences of children conceived with donor sperm—reports of sensing a family secret that had to do with them in a shameful way, and reports of the pain of having been lied to (Baran & Pannor, 1989). This group expresses concerns about the trauma of accidental disclosure, as can occur during a family argument. Prodisclosure advocates also object to the denial facilitated by secrecy, which obstructs resolution of infertility issues and impedes acceptance of the means of conception (Mahlstedt & Greenfeld, 1989). Furthermore, according to Gordon (1993), loss of genetic connectedness can be minimized by provision of information, explanations, and truthfulness.

Some authors in the mental health and ethical-legal literature defend privacy. The rationale for this includes the experience of families with children conceived with donor sperm in which parents are less likely to disclose donor origins. These families seem to have done well in terms of low rates of divorce and psychological morbidity (Braverman, 1993). Humphrey and Humphrey (1986) observed that where the quality of adoptive family relationships is sufficient to meet a child's emotional needs, ancestral knowledge is not requisite to mental health. Some fear that children may be psychologically harmed by knowledge of birth origins. For example, adoption reform advocate Allison Ward speaks of the anguish of donor sperm offspring on the discovery that their fathers sold the "essence of their lineage for forty dollars or so, without ever intending to love or take responsibility for them" (as quoted in Macklin, 1991, p. 11). There is concern that parent-child bonds may be threatened by knowledge of birth origins. Braverman and English (1992) allude to technology shock related to conception in a test tube with donated gametes. For these children, the thought of beginning life in a "test tube" or being gestated by a surrogate may result in their feeling isolated and unique.

The third position argues for a "best fit" contextually based decision about birth origins disclosure, consistent with Broderick's (1990) assertion that "a family's process is constrained by the nature of the larger suprasystem . . . of which it is a constituent element" (p. 196). Legal, religious, societal, health care, and cultural contexts constrain decisions regarding origin disclosure. Although 30 states have legislation related to sperm donation, only 5 have legislation addressing egg donation, embryo donation, and surrogacy (Mead, 1999), and there is little judicial precedent dealing with parental rights and responsibilities in reproductive alternatives. Families may view this lack of legal clarity regarding parental rights and responsibilities as either permissive or leaving them vulnerable to legal action by a donor or surrogate to claim parental rights with offspring. Furthermore, religious influences can be important. For example, Roman Catholicism and Orthodox Judaism oppose noncoital means of conception, generating discomfort and guilt for some parents. Disclosure decisions are also constrained by social context. People in the United States are generally uncomfortable with infertility and have a preference for biological ties (Mahlstedt & Greenfeld, 1989). There is stigma attached to family-building alternatives; for example, Demick and Wapner (1988) noted the suffering of adoptees in response to derogatory comments resulting in the child's feeling angry, embarrassed, or depressed. Often, the social attitudes of greatest concern are those of extended families. If supportive, families can enable confidence, conviction, and courage in dealing with donor conception; a history of parental rejection and criticism, however, may leave parents reluctant to disclose birth origins (Mahlstedt & Greenfeld, 1989). Parents fear that grandparents, aunts, and uncles aware of novel birth origins may reject the child or treat the child differently than other children in the family. The health care system also affects disclosure decisions. Advances in the field of genetics may lead to revelation of birth origins in the process of diagnostic genetic testing. Cultural elements, such as beliefs and values, are additional constraints in disclosure decisions. The belief that children have a right to know their birth origins, the valuing of honesty, or the valuing of a strong sense of family are variables in disclosure decisions (Hahn, 1996).

Empirical Literature About Birth Origins Disclosure

A review of 23 sperm donation studies worldwide (Brewaeys, 1996) revealed that 47% to 92% of parents did not intend to disclose donor origins to their children. These studies found well-adjusted parents with stable marriages and children showing rates of emotional disturbances similar to those of controls. Furthermore, the quality of the parent-child relationship was better in donor insemination groups than in fertile controls. A few studies polled attitudes toward disclosure of donor egg origins, and fewer than half of respondents favored disclosure to the child (Bolton, Golombok, Cook, Bish, & Rust, 1991; Oskarsson, Dimitry, Mills, Hunt, & Winston, 1991). Reasons for privacy about birth origins identified empirically include the following: (a) to avoid psychological harm to the child from confusion, stigmatization, or the inability to obtain information about the donor; (b) to avoid impairment of parent-child attachment; (c) to maintain privacy about infertility; and (d) to avoid uncertainty regarding when and how to disclose donor origins (Brewaeys, 1996; Leiblum & Hamkins, 1992; Pettee, 1993). Reasons for disclosure of donor origins identified empirically (Hahn, 1996; Leiblum & Hamkins, 1992) were as follows: (a) viewing secrets as inherently destructive, (b) believing the child has a right to know, (c) viewing disclosure as important for medical reasons, (d) acknowledging the potential for inadvertent disclosure, and (e) believing that "honesty is the best policy."

NURSING DIAGNOSIS AND OUTCOME DETERMINATION

The intervention discussed in this chapter is linked to some existing North American Nursing Diagnosis Association (NANDA, 1999) diagnoses and Nursing Outcomes Classification (Iowa Outcomes Project, 2000) outcomes. In addition, I propose others. The diagnosis that can be treated by this intervention is Altered Family Building (proposed by me). Potential outcomes include Disclosure of Birth Origins and Privacy About Birth Origins. Related diagnoses, interventions, and outcomes can be found in Table 3.1.

INTERVENTION: REPRODUCTIVE COUNSELING: DISCLOSURE ABOUT BIRTH ORIGINS

The language used to discuss disclosure issues may color parental thinking and influence choices (Braverman, 1994). Negative connotations of the term "secrecy" and positive connotations of the term "openness" may bias decision making. Braverman recommends presenting choices, such as between the more neutral terms "disclosure" and "privacy," to encourage objective exploration.

Although Bernstein (1994) recommends using the terms "genetic mother" for egg donors, "genetic father" for sperm donors, and "birth mother" for surrogates, Leon (1992) asserts that use of the terms "parent," "mother," or "father" to refer to third parties in reproduction is

TABLE 3.1   Diagnoses, Interventions, and Outcomes Related to Reproductive
Counseling: Disclosure About Birth Origins

Diagnosis	*Intervention*	*Outcome*
Altered Family Building[a]	Reproductive Counseling: Disclosure About Birth Origins[a]	Disclosure of Birth Origins; Privacy About Birth Origins[a]
Decisional Conflict[b]	Decision-Making Support[c]	Decision Making[d]
Knowledge Deficit: Birth Origins Disclosure[b]	Teaching: Birth Origins Disclosure[c]	Knowledge: Birth Origins Disclosure[d]
Anxiety[b]	Anxiety Reduction[c]	Anxiety Control[d]
Self-Esteem Disturbance[b]	Self-Esteem Enhancement[c]	Self-Esteem[d]
Family Coping: Potential for Growth[b]	Coping Enhancement[c]	Coping[d]
Dysfunctional Grieving[b]	Grief Work Facilitation[c]	Grief Resolution[d]

a. Proposed by the author.
b. From the North American Nursing Diagnoses Association (1999).
c. From the Iowa Intervention Project (2000).
d. From the Iowa Outcomes Project (2000).

confusing to children. The terms "ovum donor," "sperm donor," and
"gestational carrier" are clear and more neutral. Although children may
not be able to understand these terms until they develop concrete operational thinking at approximately age 7 years (Braff, 1977; Brodzinsky,
1984), children can learn the accurate labels as parents begin to tell the
child's story with simple facts. Probasco (1992) gave the following example: "The donor is a person who wanted to help us become your parents"
(p. 10).

Although some parents find disclosure issues to be important in their
decision about using donor eggs, others are primarily focused on achieving pregnancy and find early discussion of birth origins disclosure less relevant (Hahn, 1996). In the second case, it may be advisable to limit pre-
treatment discussions regarding disclosure to (a) the need to match blood
types and physical characteristics if the couple wants to keep open the option for privacy and (b) discouraging disclosure to persons other than the
child until a clear choice has been made to tell the child. For some parents,
the time for detailed discussion of the disclosure issue is after a healthy
pregnancy is established or as children approach an age when disclosure
might begin.

Anxiety can interfere with learning. Parents may have attention deficits because of preoccupation with other concerns and cognitive deficits
such as misinterpreting information or blocking of memory and recall
(Mesenhelder as cited in Suderman, 1995). Confronting and acknowledg-

ing the learner's anxiety frees the learner to discuss feelings and lessen anxiety. It is advisable to discuss disclosure issues repeatedly with anxious learners to facilitate recall.

This discussion is essential even when parents say they have already decided about disclosure. Parents frequently overlook important considerations, such as the fact that when many persons know of the child's birth origins, disclosure by a nonparent is highly probable. Written handouts for future reference are important because disclosure to the child may not begin for several years.

The ART nurse can improve the quality of disclosure decisions by teaching parents steps in systematic decision making and by assisting parents to identify and weigh alternatives in the context of their family environments. Parents may need help in determining what questions to ask: Do they believe the child has a right to know his or her genetic origins? How will the child's family and community react to the use of a donor? Can they live with a secret? Who else knows about the child's birth origins?

Not knowing how or when to tell children of their birth origins is a pervasive concern for parents contemplating disclosure. The appropriate age at which to tell a child has not been determined (Braverman & English, 1992). Furthermore, there are no proven scripts for disclosure. Probasco (1992) suggests that in early years efforts can be made to teach children about unconditional love with messages such as, "We wanted you, we are so glad to be your parents, you can depend on us" (p. 5). Children can be told of the many ways that families come together, and that for their family to get together mom and dad needed medical help. Explanation of simple facts of reproduction can also be given during early years. The following are signs that children may be ready for information about their beginnings: They begin to ask "baby-making" questions and recognize gender differences. Probasco (1992) advocates telling children how they came into the family before adolescence, when identity readjustment is occurring. Start with the simple, adding details later. Probasco suggests the following explanation:

> There are some people who are not able to make a baby, their sperm or egg does not work properly or the mother's body cannot carry a baby. Remember we told you we got help from a doctor and this is what happened for you to be born. (p. 10)

In later years, parents can explain their reasons for choosing their means of family building, sharing the pain and sadness of infertility and giving personalized descriptions of how the conception occurred and their reactions to the pregnancy. Donor offspring need information about why donors decide to help families, and medical and personal information about their donors. Probasco (1992) offered the following script: "We think your donor must have artistic and musical talents because you have these qualities. We have very positive feelings about the donor who assisted us in becoming your parents" (p. 10).

Considerations of timing disclosure include potential reactions. In a potentially disapproving family, parents may want to wait until the child understands the concept of protecting privacy (Resolve, 1995). In families with two or more children with donor origins, parents may want to tell the children at the same time because telling one child will raise questions in the other(s).

Parents who choose privacy about their child's birth origins need strategies for dealing with contingencies. Many questions require only a superficial or general answer, and details considered to be private can be concealed (Resolve, 1995). Parents can respond to many of a child's questions about beginnings by giving information about how life begins for us all—a sperm and egg get together and a baby grows in a woman's uterus. When the pediatrician asks about family history, what is known about the donor's medical history can be woven in. When the child is assigned a family tree project in school, the history of the rearing parents can be used honestly within a broad definition of family. Parents must accept, however, that to answer some of their children's questions they will have to lie, and this may be difficult. If the child eventually learns of his or her birth origins, parents need to be prepared to explain their choice of privacy. One suggestion to help explain the privacy choice is to keep a journal over time about reasons for choosing privacy.

How a child will react to disclosure of his or her birth origins is a pervasive concern for parents. Parents must recognize that feelings of confusion, sadness, and pain are appropriate responses; the child will have identity issues and questions because of the parents' choice. Children will need preparation to deal with cruel remarks, prejudice, and ignorance— "Some people might not understand our personal decision to become involved in donor conception" (Probasco, 1992, p. 10). Children will need guidance about whom they choose to tell and what details would be appropriate to share, but children need to feel positive about who they are and how they joined their families (Resolve, 1995). To discuss privacy without implying shame about their child's birth origins, parents might say, "This is your story and we feel proud of the way you came to our family. If it is your wish to be private regarding your beginnings, you have our support for that choice" (Probasco, 1992, p. 10).

Books for children such as Gordon and Clo's (1992) *Mommy, Did I Grow in Your Tummy?* and books for parents such as Bernstein's (1994) *Flight of the Stork* will help parents with the disclosure process. A current list of disclosure-related reading material should be provided. Resources can be identified by queries to Resolve (an infertility support organization) and by searching library databases and the World Wide Web. The adoption literature is a source of guidance if children choose to search for information about or contact with their donor.

Disagreement between partners about whether to disclose may block a couple's decision about birth origins disclosure and warrant referral to a counselor. Some donor egg recipients report painful feelings over loss of genetic connectedness to their children and may benefit from counseling. A mother of twins conceived with donor eggs expressed such loss as follows (Hahn, 1996):

> I wish it were me going into the future, genetically, and that will never happen. . . . Because of that I would rather not talk about it to anybody. The worry is that I will somehow convey that there is something not right about this because it kind of taps into an emotional sadness of mine. (p. 63)

For recipients of donated eggs, it may be helpful for nurses to emphasize the powerful biological connection afforded by pregnancy, giving birth, and breast-feeding while still acknowledging the significant loss of genetic continuity. Both parents and children may need counseling support during the process of disclosure.

Because there is so little guidance for parents using reproductive alternatives, they may need continued support from the ART team as they live with their disclosure decisions. The need for confidentiality mandates obtaining informed consent during the treatment process for future contact from team members. Long-term follow-up not only allows ongoing support but also facilitates research exploring effects of the disclosure and privacy decisions on families and children. Patients want to hear stories of other families and their disclosure decisions and how their decisions affected them. Nurses can collect these stories over time and share them with families in written or audiotaped form. Some patients are interested in confidential telephone networks or support groups, and nurses can help them get started.

INTERVENTION APPLICATION

John and Mary Green conceived their first child without assistance, but due to Mary's premature ovarian failure they decided to use donor eggs to have another child. In their second treatment cycle, pregnancy was achieved, and they had a daughter. In the course of their treatment process, nurses and counselors in the ART program discussed disclosure of donor egg origins with them. They assisted in examining and weighing the pros and cons of disclosure and privacy in light of the Greens' unique situation.

The nursing diagnosis was Decisional Conflict (NANDA, 1999). They had strong convictions about the child's right to know her genetic origins, and they believed there was a need for the child to know for medical reasons. They lived in a conservative and largely Catholic community, however, which gave them concerns about negative attitudes toward their means of conception. More important, there was a history of members of John's family treating an adopted niece differently from other children in the family—insensitive remarks were made at family gatherings. Through the use of the intervention Reproductive Counseling: Disclosure About Birth Origins, they arrived at a decision to tell their child and received guidance from their nurse about how and when to tell (Iowa Intervention Project, 2000). Thus, they were able to conduct Decision Making, the desired outcome (Iowa Outcomes Project, 2000). They decided to tell no one outside the family about using donor eggs and to delay full disclosure of her birth origins to their daughter until she could understand the need to be discriminating in sharing her story. When she started to ask baby-making questions, they began the disclosure process. This process included providing basic reproductive information and telling her they needed medical help to bring her into their family and how happy they were that she was their child. They talked to both children about the many ways families are formed, all equally good. They talked often to each other about their feelings about using donor eggs and about the telling process.

RESEARCH AND PRACTICE IMPLICATIONS

Little is known about effects of disclosure or privacy, the importance of knowledge of one's birth origins, or intervention with birth origins disclosure. The need for research in all these areas is urgent, and nurses have a responsibility to collaborate with team members and colleagues in other ART centers to do this work.

In this new frontier of reproduction, parents often do not know what questions to ask or the issues. Provision of educational materials about disclosure issues should be included in the initial packet of information provided candidates at entry into an ART program. Counseling about disclosure of birth origins begins with the initial visit and continues at nurse-patient encounters throughout treatment and early pregnancy. To ensure that disclosure discussions occur, it is helpful to schedule specific blocks of time dedicated to this purpose. Provision of privacy is important for discussion of this very personal issue. The anxiety experienced by candidates for ART procedures calls for repetition in educational efforts. Timing of counseling in response to the couple's readiness for learning will enhance the counseling process.

5

Ongoing follow-up allows the sharing of much needed information and resources as they become available, and it creates opportunities to refer families to counselors who can assist them in coping with disclosure choices. To clarify family boundaries and legitimize the roles of mother and father for the people who intend to raise and nurture the child, ART nurses have a responsibility to advocate for legislation specifying parental rights and responsibilities for parties to family-building alternatives.

REFERENCES

Baran, A., & Pannor, R. (1989). *Lethal secrets*. New York: Warner.

Bernstein, A. C. (1994). *Flight of the stork: What children think (and when) about sex and family building*. Indianapolis, IN: Perspectives Press.

Bolton, V., Golombok, S., Cook, R., Bish, A., & Rust, J. (1991). A comparative study of attitudes towards donor insemination and egg donation in recipients, potential donors and the public. *Journal of Psychosomatic Obstetrics and Gynecology, 12*, 217-228.

Braff, A. M. (1977, July/August). Telling children about their adoption: New alternatives for parents. *Maternal Child Nursing Journal*, 254-259.

Braverman, A. M. (1993). Psychological issues for recipients: Privacy versus secrecy. In *Proceedings of the sixth national conference for IVF nurse coordinators and support personnel* (pp. 7-10). Marco Island, FL: Serono Symposia.

Braverman, A. M. (1994). Oocyte donation: Psychological and counseling issues. *Clinical Consultations in Obstetrics and Gynecology, 6*(2), 143-149.

Braverman, A. M., & English, M. E. (1992). Creating brave new families with advanced reproductive technologies. *NAACOG's Clinical Issues in Perinatal and Women's Health Nursing, 3*(2), 353-362.

Brewaeys, A. (1996). Donor insemination, the impact on family and child development. *Journal of Psychosomatic Obstetrics and Gynecology, 17*, 1-13.

Broderick, C. B. (1990). Family process theory. In J. Sprey (Ed.), *Fashioning family theory: New approaches* (pp. 171-206). Newbury Park, CA: Sage.

Brodzinsky, D. M. (1984). New perspectives on adoption revelation. *Early Child Development and Care, 18*, 105-118.

Demick, J., & Wapner, S. (1988). Open and closed adoption: A developmental conceptualization. *Family Process, 27*, 229-249.

Friedman, M. M. (1986). *Family nursing: Theory and assessment*. Norwalk, CT: Appleton-Century-Crofts.

Gordon, E. (1993). Disclosure and secrecy in gamete donation: Disclosure. In *Proceedings of the twenty-sixth annual postgraduate course: Course XIII: Clinical assessment and counseling in third-party reproduction* (pp. 89-100). Montreal: American Fertility Society.

Gordon, E. R., & Clo, K. (1992). *Mommy, did I grow in your tummy? Where some babies come from*. Santa Monica, CA: Greenberg.

Hahn, S. J. (1996). *Parental decisions regarding disclosure of donor egg origins*. Unpublished master's thesis, University of Iowa, Iowa City.

Humphrey, M., & Humphrey, H. (1986). A fresh look at genealogical bewilderment. *British Journal of Medical Psychology, 59,* 133-140.

Iowa Intervention Project. (2000). *Nursing interventions classification (NIC)* (J. C. McCloskey & G. M. Bulechek, Eds.; 3rd ed.). St. Louis, MO: Mosby-Year Book.

Iowa Outcomes Project. (2000). *Nursing outcomes classification (NOC)* (M. Johnson, M. Maas, & S. Moorhead, Eds.; 2nd ed.). St. Louis, MO: Mosby-Year Book.

Karpel, M. A. (1980). Family secrets: Conceptual and ethical issues in the relational context. *Family Process, 19,* 295-306.

Leiblum, S. R., & Hamkins, S. E. (1992). To tell or not to tell: Attitudes of reproductive endocrinologists concerning disclosure to offspring of conception via assisted insemination by donor. *Journal of Psychosomatic Obstetrics and Gynecology, 1*(3), 267-275.

Leon, I. (1992). Will the real parents please stand up? *Resolve National Newsletter, 18,* 10.

Macklin, R. (1991, January/February). Artificial means of reproduction and our understanding of the family. *Hastings Center Report,* 5-11.

Mahlstedt, P. P., & Greenfeld, D. A. (1989). Assisted reproductive technology with donor gametes: The need for patient preparation. *Fertility and Sterility, 52,* 908-914.

Mead, R. (1999, August 9). Annals of reproduction: Eggs for sale. *The New Yorker,* 56-65.

North American Nursing Diagnosis Association. (1999). *Nursing diagnoses: Definitions and classification 1995-1996.* Philadelphia: Author.

Oskarsson, K. T., Dimitry, E. S., Mills, M. S., Hunt, J., & Winston, R. M. L. (1991). Attitudes towards gamete donation among couples undergoing in vitro fertilization. *British Journal of Obstetrics and Gynaecology, 98,* 3531-3536.

Pettee, D. (1993). Reflections on families formed through egg donation. *Resolve National Newsletter, 18,* 3.

Probasco, K. A. (1992, Summer). Discussion with children about their donor conception. *Insights Into Infertility: A Newsletter,* 5-10. (Available from Serono Symposia, USA, Norwell, MA)

Resolve. (1995). *Donor insemination: Facts and decision-making.* Somerville, MA: Author.

Suderman, E. (1995). Downsizing: Implications for nursing educators in a hospital setting. *Journal of Nursing Staff Development, 11,* 7-12.

von Bertalanffy, L. (1968). *General systems theory: Foundation, development, application.* New York: George Braziller.

4

Prenatal Care

Carol Loan

Low birth weight is the third leading cause of infant mortality in the United States. Women who do not receive prenatal care are three times more likely to have a low-birth-weight baby than those who do (Children's Defense Fund, 1995). Lack of prenatal care is associated with premature delivery of the neonate and increased maternal and infant mortality and morbidity (McClanahan, 1992; York, Grant, Gibeau, Beecham, & Kessler, 1996). Early prenatal care is so important to the nation's health that it has been included in the goals of *Healthy People 2000* (U.S. Department of Health and Human Services [USDHHS], 1991). It is critical to the health of mother and baby because it allows for early detection and treatment of existing conditions, provides the opportunity of encouraging healthy behaviors, and prevents disease by educating women about factors that might affect the pregnancy outcome (U.S. Public Health Service [PHS], 1989). To achieve the goal of 90% of women initiating prenatal care in the first trimester as set by *Healthy People 2000,* access to prenatal care needs to be in place for all American women. Improving access to prenatal care has the potential to influence the following objectives from *Healthy People 2000:* (a) reducing infant mortality; (b) reducing low birth weight; (c) reducing rates of fetal death, maternal mortality, and fetal alcohol syndrome; (d) increasing the number of women who gain adequate weight during pregnancy; (e) increasing the number of women who breast-feed their infants; (f) reducing severe complications of pregnancy and cesarean delivery rates; and (g) improving the management of high-risk cases (USDHHS, 1991).

The cost benefit of prenatal care has been clearly demonstrated. For every dollar spent on prenatal care, an estimated $2 to $11 are saved by reducing prenatal hospitalization, increasing infant birth weight, reducing the costs of neonatal intensive care, reducing the need for subsequent hospitalization, and preventing chronic conditions such as cerebral palsy, blindness, mental retardation, and learning disabilities (Fischler & Harvey, 1995; Haas, Berman, Goldberg, Lee, & Cook, 1996; Maloni, Cheng, Liebl, & Maier, 1996). Only 58.5% of pregnant women in the United States have private insurance that covers all or part of their care. Medicaid provides for approximately 34% of all deliveries (Abma, Chandra, Mosher, Peterson, & Piccinino, 1997). Other programs to assist poor pregnant women and their children include Maternal Child Health block grants that fund services for pregnant women and children (Alan Guttmacher Institute, 1989) and the Women, Infant, and Children (WIC) program, which provides supplemental foods, nutrition education, and health care to low-income women who are pregnant, breast-feeding, or new mothers as well as to infants and children up to the age of 5 years (Iowa Department of Public Health, 1996).

Prenatal care should be available to all pregnant women. In 1994, however, only 80% of all infants in the United States were born to mothers who initiated care in the first trimester of pregnancy (USDHHS, 1996). Poor women were less likely than those with higher incomes to obtain adequate prenatal care. Women who were young, unmarried, and those who have completed less than 12 years of education were less likely to obtain adequate prenatal care than those who were older, married, and better educated (Brown, 1989; USDHHS, 1996; Witwer, 1990). Battered women and women who abuse substances were also at risk for inadequate prenatal care (Taggart & Mattson, 1996; York et al., 1996), as were women who lived in rural areas (McClanahan, 1992).

Research indicates that African Americans, Hispanics, and Native Americans use prenatal services less frequently than Caucasians, with 87% of Caucasian mothers receiving care in the first trimester compared to 68% of African Americans, 69% of Hispanics, and 65% of Native Americans. Japanese and Cuban women obtain early prenatal care at high rates of 89% and 90%, respectively (USDHHS, 1996).

Although America's infant mortality rate is at an all-time low, a persistent difference in the number of deaths per race has been reported. Nationally, 7.2% of all newborns have been reported as weighing less than 2500 g and 11% born prematurely. Among African Americans, 13.3% have been reported as low birth weight and 18.5% reported as premature (USDHHS, 1995). Hispanics and Native Americans also have higher rates of low-birth-weight infants and prematurity than do Caucasians, whereas Asians have had the lowest rates (LaVeist, Keith, & Gutierrez, 1995). African American infants have been reported to be 4.5 times more likely to die as a result of low birth weight than Caucasian infants (Children's Defense Fund, 1995), but even normal-weight African American babies have had a greater risk of death. Mortality rates for some Native American tribes and Puerto Ricans were also reported to be higher than those for Caucasians. The maternal death rate for African American women has been shown to be three times higher than that of Caucasian women (USDHHS, 1991).

LITERATURE REVIEW

The Health Belief Model has been used to examine many health behaviors, including the use of prenatal care (Bluestein & Rutledge, 1993; Janz & Becker, 1984; Leatherman, Blackburn, & Davidhizar, 1990). This model proposes that an individual's behavior is dependent on perceptions of susceptibility to a particular illness or condition; the severity of the consequences of that condition; the likelihood of the health behavior preventing or reducing susceptibility or severity of the condition; and physical, psychological, financial, and other barriers related to the behavior. A cue or stimulus must occur to trigger the behavior, and modifying factors, such as demographic, social-psychological, and structural variables, serve to condition the individual's perception of the benefits of the behavior.

The first cue or stimulus that must occur to trigger entry into prenatal care is suspicion or recognition of pregnancy. Advice from peers and family to seek prenatal care and media campaigns regarding the importance of prenatal care can also provide stimulus for obtaining prenatal care. A woman's decision to seek prenatal care will be influenced by her perception of her susceptibility to pregnancy and by concern regarding a poor pregnancy outcome. Women may fail to recognize the signs of pregnancy and factors that make them at high risk. In one study, low-income women did not consider that their experience of giving birth to more than five children and their experience of giving birth to a low-birth-weight infant put them at high risk (York et al., 1996). A woman's perception of pregnancy-related health consequences, such as having a low-birth-weight or premature infant, will also influence her behavior. Her beliefs about the likelihood that prenatal care will prevent or reduce her susceptibility to a poor pregnancy outcome are an additional determinant. Not all women view prenatal care as important, however. Some women view pregnancy as a normal condition that does not require medical attention (Leatherman et al., 1990). Maloni et al. (1996) stated that the most influential barrier to prenatal care is a negative attitude about prenatal care and a limited understanding of its value.

Barriers to Prenatal Care

No single factor is responsible for inadequate use of prenatal care. Prenatal care should be available to any pregnant woman; the literature, however, documents that access to prenatal care is limited by many barriers (Groutz & Hagay, 1995; Maloni et al., 1996). Many studies have shown that insufficient money was the primary reason given for not obtaining adequate prenatal care (Leatherman et al., 1990; Maloni et al., 1996). Approximately 37 million Americans are without health insurance, and women of childbearing age are disproportionately represented among the uninsured (York et al., 1996). Although Medicaid provides funding for prenatal care, the system is frequently criticized for its cumbersome enrollment process. There are long waiting periods from entry into the system to enrollment in the program, and a woman may be well into her pregnancy before eligibility is established. In 1986, the Medicaid program was expanded with the aim of improving access to prenatal care. Findings from studies since that time, however, have documented that the expanded coverage did not increase the use of prenatal care during the first trimester (Dubay, Kenney, Norton, & Cohen, 1995; York et al., 1996). This lack of improvement suggests that significant barriers to prenatal care remained even when the financial barrier was reduced.

A variety of sites and practitioners are available for prenatal care. Settings include private offices, public health and county hospital clinics, and clients' homes. Practitioners include public health nurses, obstetrical nurses, nurse practitioners, nurse midwives, family practitioners, obstetricians, and perinatologists (Johnson, Walker, & Niebyl, 1996). Characteristics of the health care delivery system that may act as barriers to pregnant women include uncoordinated care, inconvenient locations and hours of service, inadequate reimbursement systems, inadequate outreach and follow-up, maldistribution of providers, inadequate support for and use of midwives and nurse practitioners, lack of transportation and child care, and multiple eligibility requirements for benefits (American Nurses' Association [ANA], 1987; Maloni et al., 1996).

Frequently, prenatal clinics are very busy, and this situation results in fragmented, uncoordinated care. Uncoordinated care can result from poor communication among health care providers, or it might result from the woman seeing a different health care provider at each visit. In addition, clinics are frequently unable to schedule appointments promptly. Women often have to wait 6 to 8 weeks before being seen for their first visit, which can result in a missed opportunity to change maternal behaviors that might affect fetal development (Maloni et al., 1996; York et al., 1996). Many women have to travel a great distance for care because many clinics are not in their communities but rather in large cities that are convenient for the provider. The women may also have to travel to multiple sites for testing, treatment, and social services (Maloni et al., 1996). Some women are limited in their choice of providers because many physicians do not accept Medicaid due to inadequate reimbursement, delayed payments, and extensive paperwork. Other physicians do not practice obstetrics because of the high cost of liability insurance (Maloni et al., 1996). Most clinics have daytime hours and no day care available, which make it difficult for working women or women with small children to use them. Long waiting periods before being seen by a health professional affect women's satisfaction negatively, and women frequently complain about long waits in the office followed by a short doctor visit (Handler, Raube, Kelley, & Giachello, 1996). Even in metropolitan areas, lack of transportation is a problem (Leatherman et al., 1990).

Personal barriers to care may include inadequate incentives to seek and remain in care, previous unsatisfactory experience with prenatal care, lack of knowledge regarding the importance of prenatal care, ambivalence about the pregnancy, fear of the system and providers, personal stress, drug abuse, and competing life demands (Brown, 1989). Many women delay prenatal care due to a fear of hospitals, health providers, medical procedures, others' reactions to pregnancy, or discovery of their illegal status in the country (York et al., 1996). Homeless women, those who abuse substances, and those who have eating disorders are often reluctant to seek care because of possible criticism or pressure to change their lifestyles (Brown 1989; Maloni et al., 1996). Adolescents may fear medical procedures, the pregnancy itself, or parental response to the pregnancy (Brown, 1989). Data have shown that women covered by Medicaid and those without health insurance are more likely to fear telling others of their pregnancy (York et al., 1996).

Stress also decreases the likelihood that a woman will seek prenatal care. Women who receive inadequate prenatal care are more likely to report being worried or upset about lack of money, problems with the baby's father, housing problems, lack of emotional support, and related burdens (Giblin, Poland, & Sachs, 1986). It may be that they view prenatal care as important, but it is difficult to place a priority on prenatal care because they are having difficulty meeting basic needs (Poland, Ager, & Olson, 1987). Depression and denial are also associated with inadequate prenatal care (York et al., 1996), with unplanned pregnancies occurring 60% of the time. Women with unplanned pregnancies are more likely to delay care (USDHHS, 1996) and engage in the use of tobacco, alcohol, and other drugs (Schor, 1997). The delay of care may also be related to failure to recognize the signs of pregnancy or to a decision on whether to continue the pregnancy (Brown, 1989). Denial of pregnancy is most often reported in pregnant teens (York et al., 1996).

COMPONENTS OF PRENATAL CARE

Three recommended components of prenatal care are early and continuing risk assessments, health promotion and education, and interventions with follow-up (PHS, 1989). Once pregnancy is suspected, contact with a prenatal provider is necessary to confirm the pregnancy and initiate interventions to avoid possible insult to the fetus during the critical period of fetal development (Maloni et al., 1996). An individualized risk assessment is the most meaningful indicator for the pattern, timing, and content of prenatal visits. Most morbidity and mortality will come from women with risk factors. The major risk are social and demographic characteristics. Other risk factors include (a) preexisting illness, (b) previous poor pregnancy outcomes, and (c) evidence of maternal malnutrition (Groutz & Hagay, 1995; Johnson et al., 1996).

The infant mortality rate is higher for teenagers, African Americans, unwed women, and mothers of low socioeconomic status (McClanahan, 1992). The pregnant teenager tends to delay entry into prenatal care until the second, and sometimes the third, trimester of her pregnancy for reasons such as attempts to conceal, unemployment, single parenthood, psychological stress, conflicts with the baby's father, and family crises (Lee & Grubbs, 1995). The pregnant teenager is at risk for delivering a low-birth-weight baby (USDHHS, 1991), whereas a woman older than age 35 has an increased risk of delivering a chromosomally abnormal child (Johnson et al., 1996). Cigarette smoking during pregnancy is a risk factor for low birth weight, prematurity, miscarriage, sudden infant death syndrome, and other maternal and infant health problems (USDHHS, 1991). Taggart and Mattson (1996) found that battered women sought prenatal care 6.5 weeks later than the nonabused sample. The battered woman's delay in seeking care may be due to threats, isolation, lack of transportation, or fear of exposing the obvious signs of abuse. Violence often begins or increases during pregnancy (Taggart & Mattson, 1996), and extreme violence in pregnancy may cause trauma or even death to the fetus (Schei, Samuelsen, & Bakketeig, 1991). In addition, the battering of women has been associated with a two to four times greater risk of delivering a low-birth-weight infant (Bullock & McFarlane, 1989). Children of unwanted pregnancies are at higher risk of prematurity, low birth weight, developmental problems, and mortality (Schor, 1997).

Preexisting illness and a history of poor pregnancy outcomes also place a woman at risk. Women with a history of diabetes, hypertension, tuberculosis, seizures, hematological disorders, multiple pregnancies, congenital anomalies, infectious disease, previous abdominal or pelvic operation, or cesarean section are at increased risk for poor pregnancy outcomes. Other indicators that place a woman at risk are previous miscarriage, preterm delivery, perinatal mortality, fetal growth retardation, malformations, placental accidents, maternal hemorrhage, incompetent cervix, uterine anomalies, and previous fetal macrosomia (Groutz & Hagay, 1995; Johnson et al., 1996).

NURSING DIAGNOSES AND OUTCOME DETERMINATION

Numerous nursing diagnoses are appropriate for women and their families during pregnancy. Those most appropriate for the woman who might delay or receive inadequate prenatal care include Knowledge Deficit, Caregiver Role Strain, Fear, Anxiety, and Ineffective Denial (North American Nursing Diagnosis Association [NANDA], 1999).

Outcomes to measure the effectiveness of improving access to prenatal care listed in *Health People 2000* (USDHHS, 1991) include (a) an increase in the percentage of pregnant women initiating care in the first trimester and (b) reductions in infant mortality, maternal mortality, and infants born with low birth weight. Associated outcomes with early prenatal care might be abstinence from substances, including alcohol and tobacco; a reduction of complications of pregnancy and cesarean deliveries; and an increase in the number of women breast-feeding. Outcomes from the Nursing Outcomes Classification (NOC) (Iowa Outcomes Project, 2000) that can be used in determining the effectiveness of interventions designed to improve access to prenatal care are Health Beliefs: Perceived Resources, Health Beliefs: Perceived Threat, Decision Making, and Risk Control. Indicators of these outcomes focus on awareness of the need for care, access to care, perception of risk and susceptibility, and ability to minimize risk behaviors and engage in health-promoting behaviors.

INTERVENTION: PRENATAL CARE

Prenatal Care is defined as "monitoring and managing of patient during pregnancy to prevent complications of pregnancy and promote a healthy outcome for both mother and infant" (Iowa Intervention Project, 2000,

p. 449). James (1994) defines a pregnancy as high risk when there is a likelihood of an adverse outcome to the woman or her baby that is greater than the incidence in the general population. *High-risk pregnancy care* is the "identification and management of a high-risk pregnancy to promote healthy outcomes for mother and baby" (Iowa Intervention Project, 1996, p. 318). Although all pregnant women should receive Prenatal Care, it is especially important for the woman at increased risk of poor birth outcomes. Access to and use of prenatal care for certain subgroups of the population continues to be a problem. Pregnant women are a diverse population; therefore, it is clear prenatal programs must be comprehensive and flexible to meet the differing needs of these women and their families. Prenatal care not only must be available but also must be affordable, accessible, and acceptable (Johnson et al., 1996).

Interest in solving access problems has led to the development and evaluation of numerous models of prenatal care. Primary approaches include (a) decreasing financial obstacles to care, (b) expanding the capacity of the prenatal care system, (c) improving institutional practices to make services more acceptable and accessible to clients, (d) continuing efforts to recruit women into prenatal care and keep them in care, and (e) providing social support to encourage continuation in prenatal care (York et al., 1996). Nurses can have an impact on improving access to and use of prenatal care in each of these areas.

One of the strongest motivators to prenatal care is the belief that it will make a difference (Handler et al., 1996). Therefore, increasing public awareness of the importance of prenatal care is important. Nurses should be involved in school-based health clinics that include pregnancy prevention, pregnancy recognition, and prenatal care at middle and high schools to improve teens' access to health information and preventive health care. Because pregnant adolescents who seek early prenatal care tend to have more family support and more knowledge about pregnancy than those who delay, nurses should provide information about pregnancy and the importance of prenatal care to preadolescent girls and their families (Lee & Grubbs, 1995).

The capacity of the prenatal care system can be expanded through the development of comprehensive programs located in the community that are population specific. The positive impact of comprehensive prenatal programs on access to prenatal care and birth outcomes has been documented. There are many benefits of comprehensive care, such as improved maternal and infant outcomes; a decrease in repeat pregnancy in adolescents; individualized care; reductions in premature rupture of membranes, premature deliveries, low-birth-weight infants, and neonatal intensive care unit admissions; and a decrease in hospital charges (Fischler & Harvey, 1995). Nurses should be instrumental in developing prenatal programs that are comprehensive, encompassing psychosocial and medical aspects of care. Services provided in the community would allow care to be designed to meet the specific needs of the population. A broad range of health services and other services needed in the community should be offered at one site. Miller, Margolis, Schwethelm, and Smith (1989) found that providing multiple services at one site promoted client enrollment and retainment. Comprehensive services for pregnant teenagers should be school based to keep adolescents in school and to provide care in a setting in which the teens do not require a car or have to rely on others for transportation to prenatal care.

Nurses should also become involved in planning educational media programs aimed at increasing the viewer's knowledge of pregnancy and the importance of early prenatal care. Some authors suggest disseminating information on prenatal care as early as the preschool years to promote the health of women at the time of conception (Leatherman et al., 1990). Byrne, Allensworth, and Price (1991) suggest that positive pregnancy reports be accompanied by information on prenatal care and that an insert on prenatal care information should be included in the packages of early pregnancy testing kits.

Increased participation in care is central to the access issue, and several activities can be attempted. Case finding improves participation in care. The number of women recruited, however, is often low and the cost per patient high. An exception is case finding using telephone hotlines, which appears to be successful and less expensive (York et al., 1996). Other activities include providing community outreach workers, providing incentives, advertising prenatal services more, locating the services near public transportation, subsidizing or providing transportation, and encouraging participants to recruit clients. Referral services include cross-agency referrals, services that make prenatal appointments and assist the caller in arranging services and those that foster referral ties between prenatal programs and other services, such as family planning clinics, schools, housing programs, WIC, welfare and unemployment offices, homeless shelters, and substance abuse and treatment centers (Brown, 1989).

Programs emphasizing social support enhance the use of prenatal care especially among populations at greatest risk for insufficient care (York et al., 1996). Linking a high-risk woman to a caseworker to help ensure that the client gets the services she needs through advocacy, follow-up, and tangible assistance, such as transportation or child care, is one possible activity (Brown, 1989). Paraprofessionals or peers also can offer social support through home visits. Personal and cultural barriers could be reduced by using lay community members for social support (Maloni et al., 1996). Evaluations of programs using home visits show a reduction in the preterm delivery rate, increased use of prenatal care, and a decrease in the number of low-birth-weight infants.

Activities to carry out the interventions of Prenatal Care and High-Risk Pregnancy care can be divided into the three basic components of prenatal care: risk identification, health promotion, and education. Risk identification ideally begins prior to pregnancy and continues throughout the pregnancy and labor. Identification of women "at risk" is made from their history and physical assessment, including social and behavioral factors. The risk identification provides a basis for planning individualized care with mutual goals for each prenatal visit (Maloni et al., 1996). Specific activities include identifying medical, obstetrical, and sociodemographic factors related to poor pregnancy outcome. Families should be asked about family history of Down syndrome, neural tube defects, hemophilia, hemoglobinopathies, mental retardation, and other birth defects. Tobacco and alcohol use, substance abuse, and occupational hazards should be determined (Johnson et al., 1996). A woman's physical status should be monitored throughout pregnancy. Nutritional status and weight gains are important parameters to monitor because weight gain is an important correlate of fetal weight gain (Johnson et al., 1996). Other physical parameters to monitor include blood pressure, urine glucose and protein levels, hemoglobin level, fundal height, and fetal heart rate. The woman should be observed for edema of ankles, hands, and face, and deep tendon reflexes should be checked regularly. She should also be questioned about the presence of other risk factors, such as nausea, vomiting, vaginal bleeding, symptoms of preterm labor, and anxiety (Witwer, 1990).

The woman's psychosocial status should also be monitored throughout the pregnancy. The practitioner should identify the patient's and family's social support system and monitor their adjustment to the pregnancy. In the case of an unplanned pregnancy, the practitioner should determine the patient's feelings and determine whether the family approves of the pregnancy. Also important is the identification of indicators of prenatal attachment by determining the image that the mother has of her unborn child and if the parents have names picked out for the baby (Iowa Intervention Project, 1996).

Health promotion during pregnancy includes instruction on the importance of regular prenatal care throughout the pregnancy, nutrition, smoking and alcohol avoidance, appropriate exercise and rest, desired weight gain, and danger signs that warrant immediate reporting. The father or significant other should be encouraged to participate in prenatal care. The family should be instructed on physiological and emotional changes in pregnancy, sexuality, fetal growth and development, self-help strategies for discomforts during pregnancy, and monitoring fetal activity. Breast-feeding should be promoted and attendance at childbirth classes encouraged. The family should receive information on preparing for labor and birth, information on family roles, and education on newborn care, parenting, and infant car seats (Iowa Intervention Project, 2000; Witwer, 1990).

Other educational activities based on the risk identification may include encouragement to stop smoking, to refrain from alcohol intake, and to decrease exposure to occupational hazards. In addition, nutritional counseling, counseling on safer sex practices, and preparation for diagnostic tests are all part of prenatal care (Johnson et al., 1996; Witwer 1990). For the woman and family determined to be at risk, additional educational activities may be appropriate. Educational materials specific to the risk factor and any anticipated tests and procedures can be provided. Instruction on prescribed medication and self-monitoring skills may also be appropriate (Iowa Intervention Project, 2000). For example, a woman who develops gestational onset diabetes needs instruction on the importance of diet and normalization of blood sugars. She may need to learn to monitor her own blood glucose level and receive instruction on administration of insulin.

Health teaching is appropriate in several areas. A woman with a previous preterm delivery should receive information on labor suppression, medication administration, and fetal risks associated with preterm birth at various gestational ages. Other high-risk women might benefit from information about what might occur during and following the birth process, such as fetal monitoring, labor induction, and cesarean section care. Information about common experiences during the postpartum period, such as exhaustion, depression, chronic stress, partner discord, and sexual dysfunction, also should be given as appropriate (Iowa Intervention Project, 2000). Other activities that might be indicated for a high-risk pregnancy include instruction about alternate methods of sexual intimacy gratification and written guidelines for signs and symptoms requiring immediate medical attention, teaching fetal movement counts, interpreting medical explanations for tests and procedure results, encouraging early enrollment in prenatal classes, or adapting educational materials for patients on bedrest (Iowa Intervention Project, 2000).

INTERVENTION APPLICATION

Julia is an 18-year-old single white female with a 16-month-old son, Ezra. Since Ezra's birth, Julia has been involved periodically with a support group for young single mothers through the United Action for Youth (UAY). Julia had lived with her divorced mother until Ezra was 1 year old, at which time she moved into an apartment with her current boyfriend, André. Julia appeared upset at one of the support group meetings and revealed she thought she might be pregnant again.

The nursing diagnoses of Fear, Anxiety, Caregiver Role Strain, and Knowledge Deficit were all appropriate for Julia and her family (NANDA, 1999). She expressed feelings of fear to the group, saying that she was afraid of André's reaction: "He doesn't always have a lot of patience with Ezra, let alone another one!" In addition, she was afraid to tell her mother: "I've finally gotten out on my own, but I'm not sure how I can handle another baby!" A caseworker encouraged her to make an appointment at the family planning clinic after Julia's initial concerns about being pregnant were expressed, and the UAY program helped her with transportation to her appointment and provided care for Ezra.

After the pregnancy was confirmed, Prenatal Care was initiated. Julia continued to attend the support meetings and share her feelings with the group. Initially, she considered terminating the pregnancy, but Andre was excited about the pregnancy and encouraged her to have the baby. Although Julia was relieved that André was excited about the pregnancy, she still worried about their ability to parent another child and frequently asked child-rearing questions about Ezra. Julia, André, and Ezra continued to use the services, which assisted them with transportation and child care so Julia could attend her prenatal appointments. They also were referred to the "Nest" program, a community-based incentive and educational program designed to increase the use of maternal and infant health care services. As participants, Julia and her family could earn points for keeping prenatal appointments and attending childbirth and parenting classes. They attended a series of classes with topics on nutrition, prenatal care, parenting, healthy lifestyle and stress management, and other issues such as self-esteem and consumer information. The points they earned were used to buy a car seat for the new baby, a safety gate, diapers, and baby clothes.

Julia delivered a healthy 8-pound baby girl, Chloe. Outcomes of care were evaluated by the NOC outcomes Knowledge: Health Resources and Risk Control (Iowa Outcomes Project, 2000). Indicators of awareness of the need for care, access to care, perception of risk and susceptibility, and ability to minimize risk behaviors and engage in health-promoting behaviors were apparent. The family continues to use the services of the UAY and is still earning points by keeping Chloe's well child and immunization appointments and continuing to attend parenting classes.

RESEARCH AND PRACTICE IMPLICATIONS

Barriers to prenatal care have been studied extensively. Improvements in the rate of early prenatal care occurred in the early 1990s, but wide disparities among populations of Americans remain. Additional research must focus on how to improve the use of prenatal care among the high-risk groups, including African Americans, Hispanics, Native Americans, and young, unmarried women with little formal education. It is also important to identify strategies that are effective in influencing women's perceptions that prenatal care is important, because women will not seek prenatal care, no matter how accessible, if they do not believe it is important. Investigators must examine what motivates women in each particular group to seek prenatal care in the first trimester. Research should focus on strategies designed to increase access to and use of prenatal care for high-risk groups and the effects of increased use on pregnancy outcomes.

Although many strategies have been suggested and seem to have potential, it is obvious that one strategy will not solve the problems of access to prenatal care. Studying different combinations of strategies specific to the community's population is likely to be more successful. Strategies that warrant further research include (a) comprehensive community-based programs that offer a range of services at one site, (b) the use of caseworkers (peers or paraprofessionals) to offer assistance and troubleshoot the need for tangible assistance such as transportation, and (c) home visitation and the use of interpreters when appropriate (Olds & Kitzman, 1993).

Expanding Medicaid eligibility has decreased financial obstacles to care, but there is more that can be done. Through their professional organizations, nurses can encourage and support legislation that provides more generous funding for state and local health departments and federal grant programs to provide free or reduced fees for prenatal care. Insurance coverage should be expanded to more completely cover prenatal care, and the process of applying for Medicaid must be shortened and simplified. Finally, the availability of Medicaid funds should be advertised to increase women's knowledge of its availability.

Increasing the use of nurse practitioners and certified nurse midwives can expand the capacity of the prenatal care system. There is no evidence that an obstetrician needs to be involved in every pregnancy. Nurse practitioners and midwives have a more holistic approach to prenatal care, have more time to spend on patient education and parenting preparation, are willing to work in underserved areas, and are less costly than obstetricians. Research indicates that midwives can manage normal pregnancies as well as can physicians (Fischler & Harvey, 1995). The use of nurse providers, however, is limited by barriers that prevent consumers from selecting them as their care providers. Nurse providers have difficulty obtaining direct reimbursement for services, and their prescriptive authority varies by state (Spatz, 1996). Nursing groups at the state and national levels need to promote legislation to support the role of advanced nursing practice by lobbying for changes in nurse practice acts and third-party reimbursement.

There is a well-established relationship between satisfaction and use of care: Women who are satisfied with their care are more likely to continue care (Handler et al., 1996). Nursing activities can include measures to ensure policies and procedures in institutions promote satisfaction with care, including technical competence of the practitioner, continuity of caregivers, and minimal waiting time in the clinic. Women also value being respected as individuals and having their personal experiences and cultural values understood. Interpreters should be available when appropriate, child care offered, and registration procedures expedited. Staff courtesy should be monitored, and clinic hours should be flexible and include evening and weekend hours (ANA, 1987; Brown, 1989; Handler et al., 1996).

Nurses in all settings must continue their efforts to recruit and keep pregnant women in prenatal care. Nurses in prenatal settings can be very innovative in finding ways to increase the capacity of the system and make services more accessible, affordable, and acceptable to women. They must be knowledgeable about the population they serve and generate creative ideas for providing social support to encourage continuation in prenatal care. Only through improving access to prenatal care will we achieve the goal set for the nation in *Health People 2000* (USDHHS, 1991) of 90% of women initiating prenatal care during their first trimester of pregnancy.

REFERENCES

Abma, J. C., Chandra, A., Mosher, W. D., Peterson, L., & Piccinino, L. (1997). Fertility, family planning and women's health: New data from the 1995 National Survey of Family Growth. National Center for Health Statistics [On-line]. *Vital Health Statistics, 23*(19). Available: http//www.cdc.gov/nchswww/datawh/statab/pubd/2319_69.htm

Alan Guttmacher Institute. (1989). *Prenatal care in the United States: A state and county inventory.* New York: Author.

American Nurses' Association. (1987). *Access to prenatal care: Key to preventing low birth weight,* Report of Consensus Conferences, Kansas City, MO, January/February, 1986. Kansas City, MO: Author.

Bluestein, D., & Rutledge, C. (1993). Psychosocial determinants of late prenatal care: The health belief model. *Family Medicine, 25*(4), 269-272.

Brown, S. S. (1989). Drawing women into prenatal care. *Family Planning Perspectives, 21*(2), 73-80.

Bullock, L., & McFarlane, J. (1989). The birthweight/battering connection. *American Journal of Nursing, 89,* 1153-1155.

Byrne, I., Allensworth, D., & Price, J. (1991). *Preparenting and prenatal care: First steps to high level wellness.* White Plains, NY: March of Dimes.

Children's Defense Fund. (1995). *The state of America's children*. Washington, DC: Author.

Dubay, L. C., Kenney, G. M., Norton, S. A., & Cohen, B. C. (1995). Local responses to expanded Medicaid coverage for pregnant women. *Milbank Quarterly, 73*(4), 535-563.

Fischler, N. R., & Harvey, S. M. (1995). Setting and provider of prenatal care: Association with pregnancy outcomes among low-income women. *Health Care for Women International, 16,* 309-321.

Giblin, P., Poland, M., & Sachs, B. (1986). Pregnant adolescents health information needs: Implications for health education and health seeking. *Journal of Adolescent Health Care, 7,* 168.

Groutz, A., & Hagay, Z. J. (1995). Prenatal care: An update and future trends. *Current Opinion in Obstetrics and Gynecology, 7,* 452-460.

Haas, J. S., Berman, S., Goldberg, A., Lee, L. W., & Cook, E. F. (1996). Prenatal hospitalization and compliance with guidelines for prenatal care. *American Journal of Public Health, 86*(6), 815-819.

Handler, A., Raube, K., Kelley, M. A., & Giachello, A. (1996). Women's satisfaction with prenatal care settings: A focus group study. *Birth, 23,* 31-37.

Iowa Department of Public Health. (1996). *WIC makes a difference*. Des Moines, IA: Women, Infant and Children program.

Iowa Intervention Project. (2000). *Nursing interventions classification (NIC)* (J. C. McCloskey & G. M. Bulechek, Eds.; 2nd ed.). St. Louis, MO: Mosby-Year Book.

Iowa Outcomes Project. (2000). *Nursing outcomes classification (NOC)* (M. Johnson, M. Maas, & S. Moorhead, Eds.; 3rd ed.). St. Louis, MO: Mosby-Year Book.

James, D. (1994). Organization of prenatal care and identification of risk. In D. K. James, D. T. Steer, C. P. Weiner, & K. B. Gohi (Eds.), *High risk pregnancy: Management options* (pp. 21-33). London: W. B. Saunders.

Janz, N. K., & Becker, M. H. (1984). The health belief model: A decade later. *Health Education Quarterly, 11,* 1-47.

Johnson, T. R., Walker, M. A., & Niebyl, J. R. (1996). Preconception and prenatal care. In S. Gabbe, J. Niebyl, & J. Simpson (Eds.), *Obstetrics: Normal and problem pregnancies* (pp. 161-184). New York: Churchill.

LaVeist, T. A., Keith, V. M., & Gutierrez, M. L. (1995). Black/white differences in prenatal care utilization: An assessment of predisposing and enabling factors. *Health Services Research, 30,* 43-58.

Leatherman, J., Blackburn, D., & Davidhizar, R. (1990). How postpartum women explain their lack of obtaining prenatal care. *Journal of Advanced Nursing, 15,* 256-267.

Lee, S. H., & Grubbs, L. M. (1995). Pregnant teenagers' reasons for seeking or delaying prenatal care. *Clinical Nursing Research, 4,* 38-49.

Maloni, J. A., Cheng, C., Liebl, C. P., & Maier, J. S. (1996). Transforming prenatal care: Reflections past and present with implications for the future. *Journal of Obstetric, Gynecologic, and Neonatal Nursing, 25,* 17-23.

McClanahan, P. (1992). Improving access to and use of prenatal care. *Journal of Obstetric, Gynecologic, and Neonatal Nursing, 21*(4), 280-284.

Miller, C. L., Margolis, L. H., Schwethelm, B., & Smith, S. (1989). Barriers to implementation of a prenatal care program for low income women. *American Journal of Public Health, 79,* 62-64.

North American Nursing Diagnosis Association. (1994). *Nursing diagnoses: Definitions and classification 1995-1996.* Philadelphia: Author.

Olds, D. L., & Kitzman, H. (1993). Review of research on home visiting for pregnant women and parents of young children. *Future of Children, 3*(3), 53-92.

Poland, M. L., Ager, J. W., & Olson, J. M. (1987). Barriers to receiving adequate prenatal care. *American Journal of Obstetrics & Gynecology, 157,* 297-303.

Schei, B., Samuelsen, S., & Bakketeig, L. (1991). Does spousal physical abuse affect the outcome of pregnancy? *Scandinavian Journal of Social Medicine, 19,* 26-31.

Schor, E. (1997, March). The pediatrician and unintended pregnancy. *American Academy of Pediatrics: News from the Iowa Chapter,* 2-3.

Spatz, D. (1996). Women's health: The role of the advanced practice nurse in the 21st century. *Nursing Clinics of North America, 31*(2), 269-277.

Taggart, L., & Mattson, S. (1996). Delay in prenatal care as a result of battering in pregnancy: Cross-cultural implications. *Health Care for Women International, 17,* 25-34.

U.S. Department of Health and Human Services. (1991). *Healthy people 2000: National health promotion and disease prevention objectives* (DHHS Publication No. PHS 91-50312). Washington, DC: Government Printing Office.

U.S. Department of Health and Human Services. (1995). *Monthly vital statistics report: Advance report of final natality statistics, 1993.* Washington, DC: Centers for Disease Control and Prevention.

U.S. Department of Health and Human Services. (1996). *Vital and health statistics: Prenatal care in the United States, 1980-94.* Washington, DC: Government Printing Office.

U.S. Public Health Service. (1989). *Caring for our future: The content of prenatal care: A report of the Public Health Service Panel on the Content of Prenatal Care.* Washington, DC: Government Printing Office.

Witwer, M. B. (1990). Prenatal care in the United States: Reports call for improvements in quality and accessibility. *Family Planning Perspectives, 22,* 31-35.

York, R., Grant, C., Gibeau, A., Beecham, J., & Kessler, J. (1996). A review of problems of universal access to prenatal care. *Nursing Clinics of North America, 31*(2), 279-292.

5

Lactation Counseling

Pamela D. Hill

The American Academy of Pediatrics (AAP) and the U.S. Department of Health and Human Services, Public Health Service (USDHHS-PHS) support human milk as the superior and ideal nutrition for infants (AAP, 1997; USDHHS, 1991). Ideally, mother's milk is the preferred source of feeding for almost all infants for at least the first year of life (AAP, 1997). Two objectives in *Healthy People 2000* (USDHHS, 1991) are to increase to at least 75% the proportion of mothers who breast-feed their infants in the early postpartum period and to increase to at least 50% the proportion who continue to breast-feed until their infants are 5 or 6 months of age. Nationwide survey data indicate that the incidence of in-hospital breast-feeding is 64% and continued breast-feeding decreases to 29% at 6 months (Ross Products Division of Abbott Laboratories, 1999). An increase in the establishment and maintenance of breast-feeding is needed to meet the *Healthy People 2000* objectives. Lactation Counseling is essential to assist in meeting this objective.

This chapter addresses lactation counseling as it applies to the mother who desires to breast-feed a normal, healthy, term infant and the role of family members in the breast-feeding process. For the mother who delivers a preterm infant, the establishment and maintenance of breast-feeding are different. Although this chapter will not address the special considerations of these mothers and infants, the health professional is referred to Meier and Brown (1996), who describe the benefits of breast-feeding for both mother and infant as well as research-based nursing interventions specific to this vulnerable population.

THEORETICAL FRAMEWORK AND LITERATURE REVIEW

Breast-feeding is an interactive process whereby mother and infant work together to produce a living biological substance that nourishes the infant, which benefits both mother and infant and establishes a warm and nurturing relationship between them (Baumslag & Michels, 1995). The nutritional, immunological, developmental, psychological, social, economic, and environmental benefits of human milk are well documented and unmatched by other feeding options (AAP, 1997). Human milk provides optimal nutrition for normal growth and development of the brain and central nervous system. Epidemiological studies suggest an association among breast-feeding and decreased rates of infant gastrointestinal illness, respiratory infection, otitis media, asthma (Dewey, Heinig, & Nommsen-Rivers, 1995), and atopic disease, including eczema, food allergy, and respiratory allergy (Saarinen & Kajosaari, 1995). For the mother, breast-feeding promotes the uterine contraction after childbirth and helps shed the extra pounds of the pregnancy. Women who have breast-fed have lower rates of breast, ovarian, and uterine cancers, urinary tract infections, and osteoporosis (Short, 1992). In addition to being more economical than formula feeding, breast-feeding offers psychological and physiological benefits to the mother (Baumslag & Michels, 1995).

Successful breast-feeding is a complex phenomenon that involves the mother, infant, family members, and health care providers. Family members, such as the father or significant other, and health care providers play an important role in successful breast-feeding through supporting and assisting the mother and providing the necessary knowledge about lactation management (McNatt & Freston, 1992). The mother's perception of the breast-feeding experience is a key element in determining breast-feeding success (Leff, Gagne, & Jefferis, 1994). Duration of breast-feeding is a commonly used criterion for success; duration alone, however, may not be an accurate reflection of the mother's feelings of satisfaction with the breast-feeding experience. For example, a mother who breast-feeds for only a few weeks may express a high level of satisfaction if her intent was to breast-feed for that length of time. If the infant is weaned or if breast-feeding is terminated earlier than planned, regardless of duration, the mother may feel unsuccessful or less than satisfied. Successful breast-feeding can be defined as adequate milk production and milk transfer to the infant for age-appropriate weight gain in addition to maternal and infant satisfaction with the breast-feeding process.

Several sociodemographic characteristics are associated with the profile of the successful breast-feeding mother. Such women tend to be married, Caucasian, have a college education, middle to upper class, in their twenties or thirties, and have a family income of more than $25,000. The successful breast-feeding mother also tends to be a nonsmoker (Hill & Aldag, 1996). Although more multiparas continue to breast-feed, duration is affected by maternal employment, with twice as many nonemployed mothers compared to employed mothers continuing to breast-feed at 6 months. The successful breast-feeding mother is one who receives support from her spouse, family, and friends as well as health care providers. Motivation, commitment, and positive beliefs about breast-feeding are essential ingredients for successful breast-feeding. Mothers committed to the belief that human milk is superior to artificial milks seem to have more perseverance when difficulties occur. Pain and emotions, such as anxiety or stress, may block the milk ejection reflex and lead to inadequate breast emptying, an unsatisfied infant, and nipple problems (Newton & Newton, 1967).

Numerous perinatal factors play a significant role in breast-feeding success. The first hour after delivery is usually one of quiet alertness for the newborn. With uninterrupted mother-baby contact during the first hour of life, the infant is likely to suck correctly (Righard & Alade, 1990). The imprinting of this early feeding on both mother and baby boosts maternal confidence and may be crucial to the continuance of breast-feeding. Early initiation and frequent, unrestricted suckling at each feeding stimulate a faster increase in milk production and the development of prolactin receptors in the mammary gland. Moreover, the effects of frequent feeding include increased infant weight gain, decreased incidence of neonatal hyperbilirubinemia, and decreased nipple and breast tenderness.

Several perinatal factors have a negative influence on breast-feeding success. The use of formula or artificial milks during the hospital stay is significantly related to early termination of breast-feeding. Routine supplementation with glucose and artificial milks following breast-feeding is common practice that is based on the belief that the infant needs extra fluids. In addition, a significantly greater number of mothers who supplement with artificial milks in the early postpartum period terminate breast-feeding earlier when compared to mothers who exclusively breast-feed (Hill, Humenick, Brennan, & Woolley, 1997). Other perinatal influences include factors related to the infant. Low-birth-weight infants have difficulty sustaining breast-feeding and have a unique set of problems compared to term infants (Hill, Hanson, & Mefford, 1994). Mother-infant separation related to the infant's health also has a negative effect on

lactation, continues during this phase of lactation. If the mother returns to work or school, she should be able to safely collect and store her milk. The family should express satisfaction with the breast-feeding experience and available support.

INTERVENTION: LACTATION COUNSELING

Lactation Counseling is defined as the "use of an interactive helping process to assist in maintenance of successful breast-feeding" (Iowa Intervention Project, 2000, p. 418). Lack of knowledge and support are the two biggest obstacles to successful breast-feeding. Therefore, the myriad of lactation counseling activities are grouped into two categories, support and education.

Education

Education is critical to successful breast-feeding. Particularly for the first-time breast-feeding mother, regardless of parity, the nurse has a responsibility to provide education about breast-feeding during the antepartum and postpartum period. This education should include information about maternal breast care and infant and maternal feeding activities. Breast-feeding is not instinctual but rather is a learned behavior. The decline in the number of mothers' breast-feeding has reduced the likelihood of modeling for a new mother. Thus, the need for knowledge and expert assistance with breast-feeding is necessary. Pregnancy is an appropriate time to support the mother's decision to breast-feed and provide her with educational materials. Such materials may be in the form of pamphlets, books, visual aids, audiovisual programs, group discussion, and one-to-one teaching (Bocar & Shrago, 1999). The numerous benefits of breast-feeding should be explained to prospective parents. In addition, nurses may recommend that mothers begin breast-feeding classes in the antenatal period and continue with breast-feeding support groups during the postpartum period.

Education About Breast Care

Nipple pain is a frequently encountered problem and is responsible for early termination of breast-feeding for some mothers. Confusion exists in the research literature regarding whether prenatal nipple preparation decreases or prevents subsequent nipple pain (Hill & Humenick, 1993). Should the mother have flat or inverted nipples, breast shells, unlike nipple shields, may be worn to make the nipples more protractile.

Postnatal care of the breasts involves adequate personal hygiene and careful monitoring of nipple skin integrity.

Some mothers experience engorgement and are at risk for a breast infection. The breasts become tender, swollen, and may feel hard, painful, and hot. Breast-feeding frequently (8 to 12 times in 24 hours) and the avoidance of supplements of water or artificial milks for the first 3 or 4 weeks unless medically indicated will help prevent engorgement. If feedings are missed, the mother should express her milk mechanically or by hand. Ice packs help relieve pain and swelling and can be applied after each feeding for approximately 20 minutes. Hand or pump expression of milk will help soften the nipple and areola for easier latch-on by the infant.

A breast-feeding mother needs to know the difference between a plugged milk duct and mastitis. Tenderness, heat, and possibly redness in one area of the breast or a palpable lump with well-defined margins without fever suggest a plugged duct. Also, a tiny white plug may be seen at the opening of the duct on the nipple. In contrast, the early signs and symptoms of mastitis include redness, fatigue, fever, and chills. The mother should be instructed to report to a health care provider if she experiences such symptoms. Fatigue, stress, plugged ducts, and a change in the number of feedings are factors associated with mastitis. Rest, fluids, continued frequent breast-feeding, and moist warm packs at the site and nipple are recommended. In addition, antibiotics are usually prescribed (Thomsen, Espersen, & Maigarrd, 1985).

Education Related to Infant Feeding Activities

For infant breast-feeding establishment, the mother needs to recognize infant feeding cues. Subtle cues include rapid eye movements during sleep, stretching, soft sounds or increased signs of restlessness indicating that the infant is moving into a lighter sleep level, and sucking movements of the mouth and tongue. Rooting is also a cue that the infant is interested in feeding.

The best measure for establishing and maintaining breast-feeding is proper attachment of the infant to the breast. Failure to position the infant correctly on the breast may lead to problems such as nipple soreness and inadequate milk transfer. The nurse must observe a breast-feeding session to monitor and teach, if necessary, the mother about proper infant alignment, areolar grasp, areolar compression, and audible swallowing. The infant should be in a flexed position with body and head at breast level. Regardless of position (cradle, football, side-lying, or other positions), the body is correctly aligned if an imaginary line can be drawn from the baby's ear to shoulder to iliac crest (Shrago & Bocar, 1989). The infant should be encouraged to open wide, with the tongue down and forward before being placed on the breast. The baby's chin should press into the breast with the head erect and tilted back slightly. The entire nipple and most of the areola should be drawn into the infant's mouth. After milk ejection, nutritive sucking can be observed, characterized by rhythmic slow mandibular motion (approximately one per second). If sucking is strong and regular with audible swallowing and the mother is pain free, positioning is correct (Renfrew, 1989). Some babies hold their tongue up in the roof of their mouths, biting and chafing the nipple. Should this occur, the nurse can demonstrate suck training, a procedure easily accomplished with a finger. Suck training involves insertion of the trainer's index finger, nail down, pad up. Gently begin rubbing the hard palate and progress to the soft palate to initiate sucking. As the infant sucks, gently press down and forward with the fingernail portion of the finger. Alternate rubbing the baby's hard palate with downward and forward pressure while giving praise and encouragement to the infant for proper motion (Marmet & Shell, 1984).

Length of feeding time will vary with the infant's particular nursing style. It is inappropriate to tell a mother exactly how long a feeding should last because milk transfer may occur at a fast or slow rate, and the infant will suckle a correspondingly shorter or longer amount of time. A typical routine is 5 to 10 minutes of swallowing at each breast each feeding every 2 or 3 hours, with 8 to 10 or more feedings a day in the early weeks. Frequent feedings are important for establishing and maintaining supply. The infant should be allowed to empty the first breast so that the rich, high-calorie hindmilk is received. If the infant is still hungry, offer the second breast (Righard, Flodmark, Lothe, & Jakobsson, 1993). The mother should be reassured that it is normal if her infant breast-feeds several times within a few hours for short intervals and repeats a cluster of feedings (M. Walker, personal communication, November 26, 1991).

Breast-feeding mothers should be instructed that frequent stools indicate adequate milk intake. During the first few days after birth, stools are dark and tarry. The breast-fed infant voids colorless urine eight or more times a day and passes soft, yellow, seedy stool after most feedings compared to less frequent, firmer, darker, odorous stool of formula-fed infants. After 1 or 2 months, the infant may pass stool less frequently. On the average, the infant should gain about 4 to 7 ounces a week or at least 1 pound per month. Some infants take 2 or 3 weeks to regain their birth weight.

Infants experience growth spurts at approximately 2 or 3 weeks, 6 weeks, 3 months, and 6 months of age (Mohrbacher & Stock, 1997). A mother who is uninformed about infant growth spurts may perceive that she does not have an adequate breast milk supply when her infant desires to nurse more often than usual. The nurse can explain that breast-feeding more frequently builds her milk supply to meet the infant's growth needs during these times; introducing artificial milks or solids or both is not necessary.

Education Related to Maternal Feeding Activities

The milk ejection reflex or letdown is key to maternal breast-feeding establishment and is more likely to occur when the mother is relaxed. The nurse should inform the mother about the signs of milk ejection: tingling sensation resembling pins and needles, sudden fullness or tightening in the breasts, leaking from the opposite breast while feeding, uterine cramping, and long, slow sucks with regular swallowing by the infant. A quiet environment away from distractions, a warm drink, relaxing music, breathing techniques, warm and moist compresses applied on the breasts, and breast massage may enable the mother to relax and "let down" her milk. The nurse can instruct the mother to gently massage her breast near the armpit without removing the infant from the nipple. Breast massage is used if the mother notices the infant is using shallow mouth movements or sleeping during most of the feeding. The infant will usually begin nutritive sucking to obtain the milk in the sinuses. Breast massage facilitates the milk ejection reflex and a more complete emptying of the breast (Bowles, Stutte, & Hensley, 1988).

For the first 2 to 4 weeks postpartum, the mother should be encouraged to avoid the use of supplemental artificial milks and solids, water, juice, and glucose water. Substances other than mother's milk interfere with the infant's desire to feed at the breast and may convey to the mother that her breast milk is not adequate (Chute, 1992). Pacifiers should be discouraged until lactation is well established (Barros et al., 1995). Many infants introduced to the bottle or artificial nipple may experience nipple confusion (Neifert, Lawrence, & Seacat, 1995). Regular pacifier use is more common among those with breast-feeding problems. When sucking on a pacifier, the infant opens his mouth very little and may find it difficult to switch to grasping the breast with a wide-open mouth (Righard & Alade, 1992). The breast-feeding mother should also be cautioned about the use of nipple shields that can interfere with positioning the baby properly at breast. Nipple shields reduce stimulation of the nipple and areola that interferes with release of prolactin and oxytocin (Walker & Auerbach, 1999). Moreover, nipple shields reduce milk transfer and lead to reduced milk volume (Auerbach, 1990). Breast shells, however, which are two-piece plastic devices worn over the nipple and areola prenatally to evert flat or retracted nipples, may be used in the postpartum period. Worn approximately 30 minutes prior to feeding, shells help relieve excess milk buildup in the lactiferous sinuses by inducing slow leaking (Walker & Auerbach, 1999).

The mother returning to work or school should be encouraged to continue lactation should she desire. Expression of breast milk, either manually or with a breast pump, is an important skill for the breast-feeding mother. A variety of hand-operated, battery-operated, and electric breast pumps are available. The nurse can assist the breast-feeding mother in choosing a pump appropriate for her needs (Walker & Auerbach, 1999). In addition, knowledge of proper collection, storage, and thawing techniques is essential. Occasionally, the mother may be unable to express enough breast milk and may need to introduce limited amounts of artificial milk at times when her milk supply is temporarily low. As a result, guilt and a sense of failure may be expressed by the mother. It is important that the health care provider be sensitive to these feelings and the ambivalence of the breast-feeding mother who returns to work or school.

For the mother who has ceased lactating and desires to relactate for reasons such as the infant being intolerant to most commercially prepared milks, premature birth, or maternal illness, the knowledgeable nurse or lactation consultant (LC) can assist the mother in resuming lactation. The mother's milk supply can be reestablished with regular, sufficient stimulation. It is important for the mother to have realistic expectations, however. To assist the mother with relactation, the health care professional needs to have an understanding of when lactation began and ceased, why lactation was terminated, age of the infant when lactation ceased, and how much time has passed since the last breast-feeding episode. Although the mother may have a strong desire to relactate, the infant may not be interested.

Support

A mother's decision to breast-feed is affected by societal values, acquired attitudes, and support from others (Baumslag & Michels, 1995). A mother, particularly inexperienced at breast-feeding, requires a supportive network to lactate successfully. Support may be in the form of reassurance, praise, encouragement, or an understanding attitude.

The mother who has a supportive person present is more likely to initiate breast-feeding and continue than a mother who does not have a supportive person present (Barron, Lane, Hannan, Struempler, & Williams, 1988; Perez-Escamilla, Segura-Millan, Pollitt, & Dewey, 1993). Support for breast-feeding may come from a variety of sources, such as a husband or significant other, the woman's mother, other family members, friends, and health care professionals. The role of social support from significant others cannot be overemphasized. Research suggests that persons viewed by the breast-feeding mother as influential in providing support for the initiation and continuation of lactation vary with the mother's ethnic and socioeconomic status. For low-income Anglo-American mothers, the male partner is the single most important source of support in promoting breast-feeding. Among African Americans, a best friend or peer is the most important source of support, and among Mexican Americans the woman's mother is the primary source of social support for lactation (Baranowski et al., 1983). Moreover, recent research indicates that low-income African American and Hispanic mothers without breast-feeding experience rely primarily on the babies' fathers and family members for social support (Humphreys, Thompson, & Miner, 1998). Thus, the mothers' social support network is influential in improving the breast-feeding rate among low-income mothers. Clearly, breast-feeding classes for educating these influential social contacts about the benefits of breast-feeding are warranted.

For maternal breast-feeding establishment, rest and naps when the infant is sleeping should be encouraged. In addition, the mother should set realistic priorities, simplify daily chores, and keep outside activities to a minimum. The male partner (Sears, 1992) and other family members and friends should be included in the teaching about their supportive role during breast-feeding. These individuals can demonstrate support by assisting with household responsibilities and child care and by encouraging the mother to rest and eat a well-balanced diet.

INTERVENTION APPLICATION

Julianna, a 30-year-old primigravida, delivered a baby girl, weighing 6 pounds 14 ounces, 38 weeks' gestational age, on a Thursday evening. A spontaneous vaginal delivery, vacuum extraction with no labor analgesia or anesthesia, occurred after 14 hours of labor. Approximately 7 hours after delivery, baby girl Chelsey attempted to nurse at the breast. She nursed for a few minutes and then "came off the breast." Julianna indicated that her baby did not seem interested in breast-feeding. Chelsey would "fight against" Julianna, moving her head toward the breast when trying to latch on. On Saturday, Julianna and her baby were discharged from the hospital. Chelsey had lost 10% of her birth weight. On Monday, Chelsey was seen by the pediatrician. Chelsey had lost 11% of her birth weight. The pediatrician referred the mother to the LC at the hospital. The lack of weight gain, feelings of frustration with the breast-feeding process, and lack of effective establishment of lactation indicated a nursing diagnosis of Ineffective Breast-Feeding. The intended outcome for the mother and infant was to establish breast-feeding.

The LC checked Chelsey's suck with her little finger, which indicated that Chelsey was not bringing her tongue forward. The LC worked with Chelsey by stroking the bottom lip and chin so that she would open her mouth wide to latch onto the breast. Chelsey latched on and nursed for 20 minutes. Two hours later, Julianna and Chelsey visited the LC as instructed. Chelsey's mouth was small, and she continued to have difficulty latching on. Also, Chelsey's head "bobbed a lot"; therefore, Julianna would have to control the baby's head when breast-feeding. The LC used water from a bottle to drop onto Chelsey's tongue and Julianna's nipple. The LC also had Julianna use a breast shield but explained the controversy regarding this intervention. By Tuesday, Chelsey had gained 1 ounce. Julianna continued breast-feeding Chelsey, using the nipple shield at times and using water on Chelsey's tongue and her nipples for the purpose of latch-on. During this time, Julianna's nipples had become sore and cracked. Julianna indicated that Chelsey would not open her mouth wide enough and would "pinch the nipple." On a few occasions, Julianna fed Chelsey pumped breast milk in a bottle to obtain relief from nursing. On Friday, a visit to the pediatrician was made, at which it was determined that Chelsey had lost 1 ounce. Julianna indicated that Chelsey was rooting more and seemed "to be getting the idea about nursing." The pediatrician said to return to his office on Monday for a weight check. Julianna was instructed to breast-feed every 2 hours around the clock. She continued to use the water to get Chelsey to latch on. At times, this would take as long as 30 minutes. By Monday, Chelsey had gained 4 ounces. During this difficult time, Julianna's husband supported her by doing household chores and told her "do not give up breast-feeding—hang in there." At 3 weeks of age, Chelsey regained her birth weight, and by 11 weeks of age she weighed 12 pounds. Julianna indicated that it took 2 weeks for Chelsey "to figure out what to do." The outcome of effective breast-feeding establishment was met as determined by proper alignment and latch-on and weight gain.

RESEARCH AND PRACTICE IMPLICATIONS

Barriers exist with respect to the initiation and continuance of breast-feeding. Bottle feeding rather than breast-feeding is portrayed by the media as the norm. One approach to change is a media campaign that stimulates public support for breast-feeding promotion and is geared toward the specific needs of the targeted population. One possible target populations is low-income mothers due to the lower breast-feeding incidence and the absence of support for this vulnerable group. Clearly, other barriers are the lack of knowledge, lack of appropriate clinical management, and attitude of health care providers (Freed et al., 1995). Improved support and consistent advice from knowledgeable health care providers are needed.

Hospitals can take the initiative to provide breast-feeding mothers with the information and skills needed to successfully initiate and continue breast-feeding their babies by becoming Baby-Friendly hospitals (World Health Organization/United Nations International Children's Emergency Fund, 1989). The Baby-Friendly initiative includes 10 steps, including a written policy for promoting and supporting breast-feeding, the training of health care staff on breast-feeding and lactation management, the absence of institutional promotion of infant foods or drinks other than mother's milk, and the practice of rooming-in. Prior to hospital discharge, the breast-feeding mother needs to know who to telephone for advice and support. With early hospital discharge, ideally a community health nurse should visit the mother during the first week postpartum to monitor the breast-feeding process, provide information and support, and refer the mother to lactation support groups in the community. Hospital-to-home programs for new mothers need to be evaluated for their effectiveness in meeting the needs of the breast-feeding mother. In addition, research suggests that most mothers cease lactation earlier than planned. Education and support on how to increase milk supply and how to accurately determine milk supply may be beneficial during lactation crisis periods. Intervention studies could be designed to evaluate if such support and education in the home do make a difference with respect to breast-feeding duration.

Another important barrier to breast-feeding is the lack of work policies and facilities that support the lactating mother. With an ever-increasing percentage of mothers of infants and young children working outside the home, efforts should focus on employers providing mothers with an environment in the workplace that is conducive to breast-feeding. Nurses can work with employers in setting up family-friendly environments that include private lactation rooms for breast-feeding or pumping. Breast pumps and refrigerators should be available, and mothers should be allowed flexible schedules that allow them to breast-feed during the day. Evaluation of these programs should focus on the ability of the mother to make a smooth transition back into the workplace after giving birth, the duration of breast-feeding, and maternal and employer satisfaction. Such programs provide opportunities for valued employees to return to work while meeting their goals for maintaining breast-feeding.

In conclusion, although there is much research to support the physiological and psychological benefits of breast-feeding for infants, most mothers do not choose this option; among those who do, few continue to breast-feed for 6 to 12 months. Nurses need to use the knowledge about the benefits of breast-feeding for both the infant and the mother so that families can make informed choices. In addition, nurses can assist parents in gaining the information needed and ensuring they have the family, community, and workplace support essential to successful breast-feeding.

Lactation Counseling can make a vital contribution to the health of mothers and infants and may help reestablish breast-feeding as the norm.

REFERENCES

American Academy of Pediatrics. (1997). Breast-feeding and the use of human milk. *Pediatrics, 100(6),* 1035-1039.

Auerbach, K. G. (1990). The effect of nipple shields on maternal milk volume. *Journal of Obstetric, Gynecologic, and Neonatal Nursing, 19,* 419-427.

Baranowski, T., Bee, D., Rassin, D., Richardson, J., Brown, J., Guenther, N., & Nader, P. (1983). Social support, social influence, ethnicity and the breast-feeding decision. *Social Science Medicine, 17*(20), 1599-1611.

Barron, S., Lane, H., Hannan, T., Struempler, B., & Williams, J. (1988). Factors influencing duration of breast-feeding among low-income women. *Journal of the American Dietetic Association, 88*(12), 1557-1561.

Barros, F. C., Victora, C. G., Semer, T. C., Filho, S. T., Tomasi, E., & Weiderpass, E. (1995). Use of pacifiers is associated with decreased breast-feeding duration. *Pediatrics, 95*(4), 497-499.

Baumslag, N., & Michels, D. L. (1995). *Milk, money, and madness.* Westport, CT: Bergin and Garvey.

Bocar, D., & Shrago, L. (1999). Breast-feeding education. In J. Riordan & K. G. Auerbach (Eds.), *Breast-feeding and human lactation* (pp. 241-277). Boston: Jones and Bartlett.

Bowles, B. C., Stutte, P. C., & Hensley, J. H. (1988). Alternate massage in breast-feeding. *Genesis, 9*(6), 5-9, 17.

Chute, G. E. (1992). Promoting breast-feeding success: An overview of basic management. *NAACOG's Clinical Issues in Perinatal and Women's Health Nursing, 3*(4), 570-582.

Dewey, K. G., Heinig, M. J., & Nommsen-Rivers, L. A. (1995). Differences in morbidity between breast-fed and formula-fed infants. *Journal of Pediatrics, 126,* 696-702.

Elander, G., & Lindberg, T. (1984). Short mother-infant separation during the first week of life influences the duration of breast-feeding. *Acta Paediatricia Scandinavica, 73,* 241-247.

Freed, G. L., Clark, S. J., Sorenson, J., Lohr, J. A., Cefalo, R., & Curtis, P. (1995). National assessment of physicians' breast-feeding knowledge, attitudes, training, and experience. *Journal of the American Medical Association, 273*(6), 472-476.

Hill, P. D. (1991). The enigma of insufficient milk supply. *MCN: American Journal of Maternal Child Nursing, 16,* 312-316.

Hill, P. D., & Aldag, J. C. (1996). Smoking and breast-feeding status. *Research in Nursing and Health, 19,* 125-132.

Hill, P. D., Hanson, K. S., & Mefford, A. L. (1994). Mothers of low birthweight infants: breast-feeding patterns and problems. *Journal of Human Lactation, 10*(3), 159-166.

Hill, P. D., & Humenick, S. S. (1993). Nipple pain during breast-feeding: The first two weeks and beyond. *Journal of Perinatal Education, 2*(2), 21-36.

Hill, P. D., & Humenick, S. S. (1994). The occurrence of breast engorgement. *Journal of Human Lactation, 10*(3), 79-86.

Hill, P. D., Humenick, S. S., Brennan, M., & Woolley, D. (1997). Does early supplementation affect long-term breast-feeding? *Clinical Pediatrics, 36*(6), 345-350.

Hill, P. D., Humenick, S. S., & West, B. (1994). Concerns of breast-feeding mothers: The first six weeks postpartum. *Journal of Perinatal Education, 3*(4), 47-58.

Humphreys, A., Thompson, N., & Miner, K. (1998). Intention to breastfeed in low-income pregnant women: The role of social support and previous experience. *Birth, 25*(3), 169-174.

Iowa Intervention Project. (2000). *Nursing interventions classification (NIC)* (J. C. McCloskey & G. M. Bulechek, Eds.; 2nd ed.). St. Louis, MO: Mosby-Year Book.

Iowa Outcomes Project. (2000). *Nursing outcomes classification (NOC)* (M. Johnson, M. Maas, & S. Moorhead, Eds.; 2nd ed.). St. Louis, MO: Mosby-Year Book.

Leff, E., Gagne, M., & Jefferis, S. (1994). Maternal perceptions of successful breast-feeding. *Journal of Human Lactation, 10*(2), 99-104.

Loughlin, H., Clapp-Channing, N., Gehlbach, S., Pollard, J., & McCutchen, T. (1985). Early termination of breast-feeding: Identifying those at risk. *Pediatrics, 75*, 508-513.

Marmet, C., & Shell, E. (1984). Training neonates to suck correctly. *MCN: American Journal of Maternal Child Nursing, 9*, 401-407.

McNatt, M. H., & Freston, M. S. (1992). Social support and lactation outcomes in postpartum women. *Journal of Human Lactation, 8*(2), 73-77.

Meier, P. P., & Brown, L. P. (1996). State of the science. Breast-feeding for mothers and low birth weight infants. *Nursing Clinics of North America, 31*(2), 351-365.

Mohrbacher, N., & Stock, J. (1997). *The breast-feeding answer book* (Rev. ed.). Schaumburg, IL: La Leche League International.

Neifert, M., Lawrence, R., & Seacat, J. (1995). Nipple confusion: Toward a formal definition. *Journal of Pediatrics, 126*, 5125-5129.

Newton, N., & Newton, M. (1967). Psychologic aspects of lactation. *New England Journal of Medicine, 277*, 1179-1188.

North American Nursing Diagnosis Association. (1999). *Nursing diagnoses: Definitions and classification 1995-1996*. Philadelphia: Author.

Perez-Escamilla, R., Segura-Millan, S., Pollitt, E., & Dewey, K. (1993). Determinants of lactation performance across time in an urban population from Mexico. *Social Science Medicine, 37*(8), 1069-1078.

Renfrew, M. J. (1989). Positioning the baby at the breast: More than a visual skill. *Journal of Human Lactation, 5*, 13-15.

Righard, L., & Alade, M. O. (1990). Effect of delivery room routines on success of first breast-feed. *Lancet, 336*, 1105-1107.

Righard, L., & Alade, M. O. (1992). Sucking technique and its effect on success of breast-feeding. *Birth, 19*(4), 185-189.

Righard, L., Flodmark, C., Lothe, L., & Jakobsson, I. (1993). Breast-feeding patterns: Comparing the effects on infant behavior and maternal satisfaction of using one or two breasts. *Birth, 20*(4), 182-185.

Ross Products Division of Abbott Laboratories. (1999). *Ross Laboratories mothers' survey updated breast-feeding trend through 1998.* Columbus, OH: Author.

Saarinen, U., & Kajosaari, M. (1995). Breast-feeding as prophylaxis against atopic disease: Prospective follow-up study until 17 years old. *Lancet, 346,* 1065-1069.

Sears, W. (1992). The father's role in breast-feeding. *NAACOG's Clinical Issues in Perinatal and Women's Health Nursing, 3*(4), 713-716.

Short, R. (1992). *Breast-feeding, fertility and population growth,* ACC/SCN Symposium Report, Nutrition Policy Discussion Paper No. 11, ACC/SCN 18th session symposium, February 1991 (pp. 33-46). New York: United Nations.

Shrago, L., & Bocar, D. (1989). The infant's contribution to breast-feeding. *Journal of Obstetric, Gynecologic, and Neonatal Nursing, 19*(3), 209-215.

Thomsen, A. C., Espersen, T., & Maigarrd, S. (1985). Course and treatment of milk stasis, noninfectious inflammation of the breast, and infectious mastitis in nursing women. *American Journal of Obstetrics and Gynecology, 149*(5), 492-495.

U.S. Department of Health and Human Services. (1991). *Healthy people 2000: National health promotion and disease prevention objectives* (DHHS Publication No. PHS 91-50312). Washington, DC: Government Printing Office.

Verronen, P. (1982). Breast feeding: Reasons for giving up and transient lactational crises. *Acta Paediatrica Scandinavica, 71,* 447-450.

Walker, M., & Auerbach, K. G. (1999). Breast pumps and other technologies. In J. Riordan & K. G. Auerbach (Eds.), *Breast-feeding and human lactation* (pp. 393-448). Boston: Jones and Bartlett.

World Health Organization/United Nations International Children's Emergency Fund. (1989). *Protecting, promoting and supporting breast-feeding: The special role of maternity services.* Geneva: World Health Organization.

6

Fathering Promotion

Arnette Marie Anderson

The role of fathers has not been studied to the extent that the role of mothers in parenting has been studied. Fathers appear to hold a lower position of influence and importance than mothers in the lives of children (Ehrensaft, 1995; Vanier Institute of the Family, 1994). The role of fathers has changed, however. It has evolved from that of the father as a moral teacher during the Puritan times to that of the father as a breadwinner during the industrial revolution. Following World War II, the father's role became that of a male role model, especially for sons (Lamb, 1986). Although Lamb suggested the roles of teaching values and morals and being the breadwinner are still important, fathers have become viewed as more nurturant and involved in the father-infant relationship since the mid-1970s. In recent studies, researchers reported that fathers are interested in their infants and express caring, sensitive feelings to their infants. Research has shown that sound father-child relationships positively influence the development of the child's sense of self, attitudes toward achievement, and the quality of the child's future relationships (Klaus & Kennell, 1982; Scull, 1992). Conflicting demands between breadwinning and individual success for men at the expense of nurturing children, however, are a concern in some cultures (Vanier Institute of the Family, 1994). These views are changing in many cultures, but the issues are still real for families.

As the health care system moves from an illness to a wellness focus, there is an increasing shift in the practice setting from the institution to community and an increased focus on health promotion and disease prevention strategies (Boyle & Letourneau, 1995). Nurses are in the business of health promotion, and their practice should reflect the practice of promoting healthy relationships within the family system. Unfortunately, there are very few existing programs in health care settings to assist fathers in developing their fathering role. Researchers suggest that fathers need parenting programs and assistance by health care professionals to promote a smoother transition to fatherhood (Battles, 1988; Tiller, 1995; Tomlinson, 1987a). This chapter will assist the reader to gain greater insight into an understanding of the father-infant relationship. Furthermore, it contains an intervention, Fathering Promotion, for nurses to use to anticipate and to meet the needs of fathers.

THEORETICAL FOUNDATION

Father-Infant Relationship in the Postbirth Period

The development of keen interest in and intense redundant preoccupation with newborns by fathers is a phenomenon that has been described and explicated into a model called engrossment (Greenberg & Morris, 1974). From their analysis of data collected during interviews of 30 first-time fathers, these researchers described the characteristics of engrossment as (a) visual awareness of the newborn in which the fathers perceive their infants as beautiful or attractive; (b) extremely pleasurable perception of touching, picking up, or playing with their newborns; (c) awareness of the distinct characteristics of their newborns to the point of stating they can distinguish their infants from others or can describe their infants in detail; (d) perception of their infants as perfect, even though infants are uncoordinated and awkward in their movements; (e) a strong attraction to their infants and an extreme elation regarding the birth of their infants; and (f) an increased awareness of a positive sense of self-esteem. In addition, Greenberg and Morris concluded that these feelings of love and engrossment were universal and innate in all fathers. Lewis (1986) criticized this study because he believed the birth of an infant does not occur in a vacuum. Although some fathers become totally engrossed in their infants, other fathers may be psychologically distant from their infants because of events surrounding the birth. Anderson (1996a) found that events such as an emergency cesarean section, concerns about their wives' health, or infant complications brought forth feelings of anxiety, anger, and helplessness in some fathers that initially overshadowed their positive feelings toward their infants. One father commented about the birth experience:

> I can't imagine how anyone could design anything that could create so much pain for one person and have the other person stand helplessly by and watch it. And the idea of watching my wife go through that again is just an absolutely disgusting thought for me. (Anderson, 1996a, p. 90)

In the past decade, researchers have reported data suggesting that birth attendance and extended father-infant contact during the postpartum period have positive effects on later father-infant interaction and father involvement. In one study, fathers who held infants within 1 hour of birth were found to exhibit more nonverbal communication when their infants were 1 month old compared to fathers who did not have early contact. The fathers' perceptions and attitudes toward their infants, however, did not differ significantly in these two groups of fathers (Jones, 1981). Palkovitz (1982) corroborated the previous findings to some extent. He found that fathers who spent more time with their newborns in the hospital demonstrated greater overall involvement and social play with their infants 5 months postpartum. Other studies, however, have not supported the hypothesis that fathers have increased interaction or display attachment behaviors toward their infants following early or extended contact during the birth or early postpartum period (Pannabecker, Emde, & Austin, 1982; Toney, 1983).

Researchers have not only examined the effect of extended father-infant contact on father-infant interaction but also explored how the infant contributes to this interaction. They also examined variables such as infant state, physical attractiveness, and temperament. Although Keller, Hildebrandt, and Richards (1985) found that infant characteristics did not affect the father-infant interaction, these researchers did find that the extended contact fathers engaged in greater amounts of interaction and infant care-taking responsibilities; they also had higher self-esteem scores as measured by the Tennessee Self-Concept Scale at 6 weeks postpartum. Analysis of covariance yielded significant effects for the total self-concept scale $F(1,24) = 5.36$, $p < .05$. Conversely, the research findings of Jones and Lenz (1986) supported the hypothesis that infant state is an important predictor of affection, touch, and comforting behaviors displayed by fathers during a videotaped interaction with their newborns. In addition, fathers who perceived themselves as competent were found to be more likely to stimulate their newborns by talking to and touching them than fathers with lower competence scores as measured by the paternal

Differences in Mother and Father Interactions

Data from studies have indicated that interactions between fathers and children center around play activities, whereas maternal interactions center around caretaking activities, such as feeding, bathing, and changing clothes and diapers (Clarke-Stewart, 1978; Kotelchuck, 1976; Lamb, 1995; Lewis, 1986; Rendina & Dickerscheid, 1976). In several studies, the fathers' play style was observed to be different than that of the mothers (Lamb, 1976). Fathers tended to play more physical rough-and-tumble games, whereas mothers played more conventional games such as peek-a-boo and patty cake. The mothers' play was observed to be less physical and arousing. Mothers tended to be more verbal and didactic, using play for educational purposes. Fathers held their babies more to play with them, and mothers primarily held infants for caretaking purposes (Clarke-Stewart, 1978; Lamb, 1976; Lewis, 1986). Anderson (1996a) described fathers holding their infants occasionally at a distance from their bodies or like a football. The rationale given for doing this is that they wanted to teach their infants independence and that babies exist separately from others. It is speculated that holding the baby away from the father's body may be a forerunner of the process of differentiation in which infants learn they exist without being attached to someone. Osherman (1992) suggested the father is the bridge to the outside world in which he reassuringly says to his child that "you can let go of mom, there's a whole world beyond mother that is exciting and interesting and ultimately manageable" (p. 210).

ASSESSMENT

Nurses are in a position to support an important dimension of an infant's nurturing environment—the father-infant relationship. A clear understanding of the ingredients of this relationship will assist nurses in selecting the appropriate assessment and intervention strategies. Although fathers want to provide a nurturing relationship, they do not feel as adept as mothers in establishing that relationship. Often, fathers lack role models, and they would like to have a closer relationship than they may have experienced with their own fathers (Anderson, 1996b; Daly, 1995).

Friedman (1992) suggests that "parenthood is the only major role for which little preparation is given, and difficulties in role transition adversely affect the quality of the marital and the parent-infant relationships" (p. 61). Some of the difficulties experienced in role transition include the father's lack of competence, confidence, and preparation for

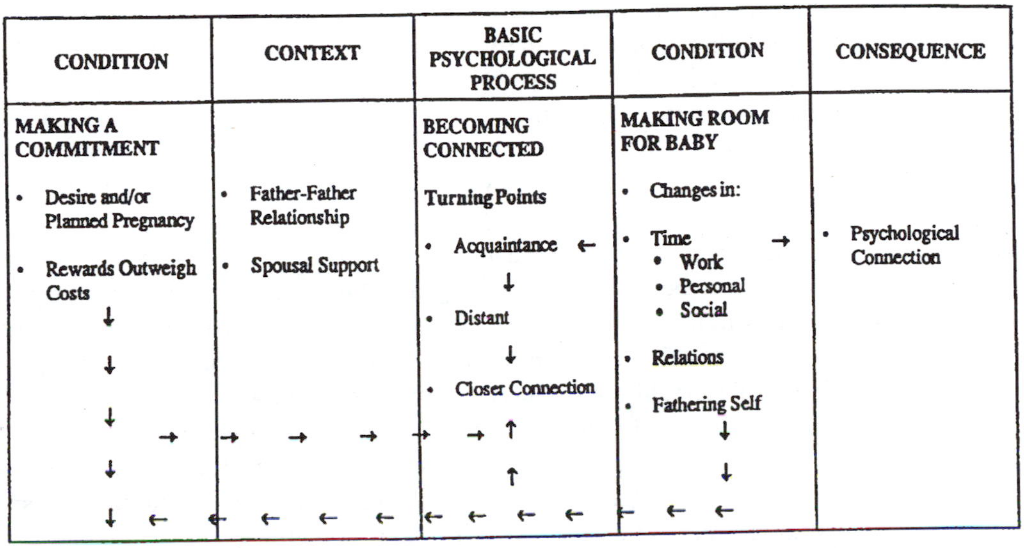

CONDITION	CONTEXT	BASIC PSYCHOLOGICAL PROCESS	CONDITION	CONSEQUENCE

MAKING A COMMITMENT
 	
• Desire and/or Planned Pregnancy
 	
• Rewards Outweigh Costs
 	
↓
 	
↓
 	
↓
 	
↓   →
 	
↓   ←
	• Father-Father Relationship
	
	• Spousal Support
	
	→ → →
	
	← ← ← ←
		BECOMING CONNECTED
		
		Turning Points
		
		• Acquaintance ←
		
		↓
		
		• Distant
		
		↓
		
		• Closer Connection
		
		→ → ↑
		
		↑
		
		← ← ← ←
			MAKING ROOM FOR BABY
			
			• Changes in:
			
			• Time →
			  • Work
			  • Personal
			  • Social
			
			• Relations
			
			• Fathering Self
			
			↓
			
			↓
			
			← ←
				• Psychological Connection

Figure 6.1. Conceptual Model of the Father-Infant Relationship

parenting; feelings of neglect and jealousy of the baby; lack of support; disruption and diminishment of social and sexual life; feelings of tiredness due to caring for the infant; and little time for other children and the marital relationship (Anderson, 1996b; Bronstein & Cowan, 1988; Friedman, 1992). McBride (1989) suggested that the lack of preparation in developing skills to become a nurturing parent results in undue stress in fathers and limits their ability to become involved with their children. A qualitative research project that I conducted provides a conceptual model from which to base assessment (Figure 6.1).

The grounded theory study described and provided a theoretical analysis of first-time fathers' experiences in developing a relationship with their infant (Anderson, 1996a, 1996b). The three major categories operative in the father-infant relationship were making a commitment, becoming connected, and making room for the infants (Figure 6.1).

Making a Commitment

Commitment was expressed by fathers as their willingness to invest in and take responsibility for nurturing the relationship with their infants despite parenting difficulties or other life pressures. According to Brickman (1987), commitment has two dimensions that occur simultaneously: "a sense of having to" and a "sense of wanting to." It is important to assess the nature of the relationship between the sense of having to and the sense of wanting to because the nature of this connection determines the nature of the commitment and, in turn, influences the relationship between the father and the infant. If the commitment is perceived by the fathers as primarily obligatory, the father-infant relationship will take on a character that is much different from that based on enjoyment and pleasure. Fathers in the study found that the rewards gained in the relationship with their infants far outweighed the costs or sacrifices. There were times, however, when fathers believed they had to care for their infants when they would rather have been doing something else, but these feelings were not predominant. It was evident that these fathers found it extremely pleasurable to interact with their infants. Emde (1980) suggests that health care professionals should take a "pleasure inventory" to assess how much pleasure parents are finding in their interactions with their infants.

For all fathers, the desire to have a baby and the feelings of readiness expressed by the fathers were a precursor to the commitment phase. Also, if fathers stated that they were involved in planning the pregnancy, this statement gave some indication that they were psychologically ready to raise children and to share their wives' attention with their infants. It would be important to assess the decision making regarding the planning of the pregnancy because Brickman (1987) suggests that if people perceive they have a range of choices and control over these choices, they will have a higher level of commitment than those who do not. Although some pregnancies are unplanned, fathers can be resilient and adapt positively to unexpected pregnancies if they view the situation as rewarding.

Becoming Connected

Becoming connected was the process that began with the father's intense, euphoric emotions at birth if there were no complications associated with the birth experience. Because of the close mother-infant bond and breast-feeding, fathers reported they were connected to their infants at a distance during the first 5 weeks. The turning point in the relationship occurred when fathers perceived their 2-month-old infants as more responsive, predictable, and familiar. These perceptions of their infants fueled the development of a closer connection. An impetus that encouraged fathers to participate more in the care of their infants was the increased responsiveness of the infant, especially the appearance of the infant's smile. Possibly, fathers then perceived their infants more as interactive human beings who were giving specific, positive feedback through their interactions rather than as objects who primarily slept and breast-fed during the first few weeks of life. Once the fathers could do more for their infants, their relationship deepened. Another way fathers connected with their infants was through identification. Fathers compared their infants' features and characteristics to those of someone in the family. Most of the infant's attributes were made using the mother and father's characteristics in a positive, complimentary fashion. Also, the predictability of the infants' behavior and routines gave fathers positive feedback about their parenting abilities that helped the relationships flourish.

Several questions arose in the initial stage of relationship building using the model: (a) To what extent are fathers encouraged to share their personal concerns and feelings during the birth process? (b) Do fathers feel excluded, jealous, or like outsiders during breast-feeding or during the infant's first few weeks of life? (c) How does the mother encourage and support the father in becoming involved when the father feels most vulnerable? (d) To what extent does the father become involved in the caretaking of the infant? (e) What does the father think and feel about the father-infant relationship? and (f) To what extent do fathers identify with their infants?

Making Room for Baby

Making room for baby consisted of fathers making changes or adjustments in their lives or both to make psychological and physical room for their infants. Fathers also made adjustments in their work and social and personal time and in relationships with their wives. Other factors that influenced the father-infant relationship were the relationship they had with their own fathers and the informational and emotional support they received from their wives.

The following are questions to use in the assessment phase: (a) How has being a parent affected your life? (b) What preparation have you had for parenting? (c) Who are your role models? (d) How have your parents influenced your parenting role and your relationships with your children? (e) What does your wife say or do that helps you develop a relationship with your baby? (f) What hinders you in getting to know your baby? and (g) What do you wish people would do or say to help you in your parenting role?

The primary concern for fathers today is not their roles but rather their relationships with their children. Fathers want a closer relationship than they experienced with their fathers (Anderson, 1996b). The nursing diagnosis that seems appropriate is Risk for Altered Parent-Infant Attachment (North American Nursing Diagnosis Association [NANDA], 1999). The Nursing Outcomes Classification (NOC) outcome is Parent-Infant Attachment, which includes the following indications: (a) fathers develop a close nurturing relationship with their infants and hold their infants close, (b) fathers develop a satisfactory coparenting relationship with their wives through feeding and caring for their infants, and (c) infants respond to parents' cues (Iowa Outcomes Project, 2000).

FATHERING PROMOTION

Fathering Promotion intervention activities directed toward support and education should include (a) providing support from spouses and health care professionals, (b) focusing on individual and parent family strengths, (c) facilitating the couple relationship, (d) enhancing father-infant communication, (e) teaching typical issues in infant development and caretaking skills, and (f) discussing common stresses that families encounter (Palm, 1997).

Nurses are in an ideal position to promote Family Integrity Promotion (Iowa Intervention Project, 2000), to integrate an infant into the family system through supportive and educative activities. Rogers (1990) states that "the purpose of nurses is to promote health and well-being for all persons wherever they are" (p. 6). The profession of nursing should emphasize ways of nurturing healthy relationships in the family and society. Human beings are actualized through relationships built on respect and caring. Specifically, the community health nurse is in a good position to work with families in an ongoing way, extending over many years as families face one transition after another in the developmental cycle. The community health nurse may not make home visits when families are in a stable condition but will enter when families face transitions, such as the birth of a baby. Schecket (1995) states that to provide supportive care for families, health care professionals must view fathers "not merely as support people for their wives, but as men in the midst of a powerful life transition, who have unique needs" (p. 143).

The importance of providing a supportive environment to fathers from their spouses, health care professionals, and institutions can play a critical role in enhancing the capacity of fathers to provide a nurturing environment for their children. There are many barriers that deter fathers from becoming full participants in their infants' lives.

Research has shown that fathers feel on the periphery or distanced from the relationship of their wives and infants, especially during the breast-feeding experience. Fathers believe that mothers have built-in mechanisms, such as the mother-fetus bond and breast-feeding, that facilitate the development of their relationship with the infant, whereas they as fathers have to work more intensely at developing the relationship. Fathers should be encouraged to discuss their feelings of exclusion so that these feelings can be dealt with in an open, direct manner. A mother can encourage a father's involvement by putting him in charge of supplemental feedings, giving him private time with the infant that seems to be a crucial factor in getting to know the infant. A father needs to spend time alone with his infant without feeling that someone is looking over his shoulder. One father remarked,

I felt that I was able to bond a little bit because I was in charge of the supplement. And that was my time with my baby rather than just playing, holding, and changing her. It was like her and me, and we were the only ones in the room at that time for the first month and half.

Women can be gatekeepers in that they, unwittingly, keep their children at a distance from fathers because they believe the nurturing of children lies within the woman's domain (Swigart, 1991). Women manage the infant's care, but they request help from their husbands, and in doing so they set the standards and prescribe what is to be done and how. Many women, however, will not give up the responsibility. The partners are seen as "supporting actors rather than costars" (Hawkins & Dollahite, 1997, p. 12). Nurses must encourage women to make space for their husbands and challenge parents to think differently about the way they approach their parenting roles. Jordan (1995) advocates that "in order to effect change in the degree of paternal involvement, attention must be given to altering the mind-sets of both mothers and fathers in order to change the dynamics and division of labor within the adult couple relationship" (p. 71). Support must be given to families as they negotiate new roles, problem solve, and make decisions about parenting issues during the transition to parenthood.

In my study, wives assisted their husbands in getting to know their infants through giving advice and guidance in the area of infant care and through sharing information about daily events and progress of the infant's development while fathers worked outside the home. In addition to informational support, husbands reported that their wives gave them emotional support by encouraging involvement with their infants, which in turn gave them confidence in their nurturing abilities and raised their self-esteem.

During clinic visits and home visits, fathers should be included. Nurses cannot assume, presume, or assign meanings to what and how fathers think and feel about parenting. Fathers should be authors of their own experiences rather than having mothers talk for them. For example, a father recounts his experience during a visit to an immunization clinic with his infant. The nurse asked him if his wife gave him the child's health care card before he left home and if she told him how much the child weighed. Although he was knowledgeable on both accounts, he did not say anything to the nurse. The nurse's condescending attitude sends a message that fathers are deficient and uninvolved and does not support the promotion of a competent and participating father. Hawkins and Dollahite (1997) issue a caveat:

An intervention strategy that consists mainly of holding up a mirror to men's faces so they can see their paternal warts more clearly is neither visionary nor empowering. The harsh glare of role deficiency may prompt men to retreat into the shadows of resentment rather than illuminate other paths of personal growth. (p. 12)

Nurses can make a difference in fathers' lives if they have an attitude that fathers play a significant role in their children's lives and if they fully support fathers' endeavors to become involved parents. Nurses may develop support groups that assist fathers to deal with other issues, including lifestyle changes, role overload, parental fatigue, and career demands. It is the nurse's responsibility to identify families who are lacking in support and develop plans to augment or compensate for the deficiencies by identifying and referring them to appropriate social support systems within the community.

Providing an Educative Environment

A nurse's responsibility to parents who are integrating an infant into their lives is to provide them with educational resources that ease this transition. It is a time of stress and change in their lives. In the past few decades, parent education programs mainly focused on mothers; educators, however, suggest there is a need to focus on developing programs for fathers. Palm (1997) advocates developing specific programs for fathers that recognize the gender differences, thus making programs sensitive to fathers' needs. Fathers have specific strengths and needs that should not be ignored. It may be advantageous to have male nurses involved in teaching parenting programs because fathers may feel more comfortable attending the programs. Men do not have extensive exposure to male parental role models; therefore, male nurses can provide this positive role model.

Family Strengths

Nurses can create an accepting and encouraging approach by working with the family's strengths and moving away from what the family cannot do. Nurses must reinforce positive parenting behaviors. Mothers and fathers need encouragement to honor their differences in parenting and balance their individual strengths to accommodate their active lives. Nurses can help them acknowledge what each one brings to caring for the infant. Fathers are aware that they offer different stimulation to their infants, and mothers acknowledge and accept this different style, which in turn encourages more involvement on the part of the father. The difference in infant stimulation compared to that provided by mothers was deemed to be necessary for fathers, and it provided a special place in the infant's life. One father told of how he offered a different type of stimulation:

> I know that I can provide a certain kind of stimulation for her. I can carry her with more strength in my arms; I can swing her in certain ways that my wife can't because she can't hold her that way. I'm sort of giving her that experience and saying well, "Here's something different. I know your mother probably doesn't do this with you."

Marital Relationship

Research suggests that a strong marital relationship influences the development of the father-infant relationship. It is important to work with the couple to explore what each contributes to the parenting role that works for them, what does not work, and what each family member can do to make it work (Dienhart & Dollahite, 1997). It may be necessary to assist young couples to listen to one another and respect each other's differences and needs in parenting, which will strengthen the family bond.

Father-Infant Communication

Brazelton (1969) and Barnard (1976) developed excellent videotapes that can be used to demonstrate newborn capabilities to parents, how to read infant cues, and unique ways in which infants interact with parents. Their research indicates that both the infant and the caregiver bring unique communication styles to this relationship, and that the communication heightens the parent awareness of infant competence and maturity. Teaching sessions that include unique behavioral capabilities of the infant enhance the communication and involvement of the father with the infant. It is essential that fathers recognize the social behaviors of infants because it gives pleasure and a strong incentive for fathers to be with the baby (Emde, 1980). One father remarked about his 2-month-old baby,

> I feel that I'm more engaged with her now because she is capable of more things than she was. She can focus now, and she can see my face and grin at me . . . and so I feel she recognizes me, and I'm pulled in and I want to play longer and do things longer.

Nurses should point out to fathers that they can develop a close relationship with their infants by rocking, playing, singing, or holding them. Generally, men feel better when they are actively doing something for people rather than freely expressing their emotions. Fathers should be encouraged to express their emotions to their children. In our society, women are encouraged and permitted to communicate on an emotional level, whereas men are encouraged not to display their emotions (Hendrick & Hendrick, 1992).

Teaching

Nurses are important role models when teaching fathers about caretaking skills, such as feeding, bathing, and diapering, and teaching about infant development. Content emphasizing anticipatory guidance and health promotion will increase the father's competence, confidence, and comfort while caring for the infant. To ensure the participation of fathers in classes, nurses should schedule the teaching sessions at various times. Nurses need to be careful not to reinforce stereotypical gender beliefs that promote "mother knows best." Nurses should examine their values about what they think are the correct roles in families to set aside these biases during teaching sessions. Also, the teaching sessions will provide an opportunity for parents to meet other parents with common concerns.

INTERVENTION APPLICATION

A community health nurse makes a postpartum visit to a young couple who had their first newborn, Julie, 1 week ago. Sally, a hairdresser, is not employed outside the home at the current time. Bob, a mechanic, has taken time off work to be present at the home visit because he has some concerns about caring for Julie.

During the assessment, Sally's primary concerns have to do with her husband's lack of involvement in caring for the baby. She openly berates her husband in front of the nurse about his inability to change a diaper or feed the baby correctly. The nurse has the impression that there is little communication between the couple, and Sally discourages Bob's involvement in Julie's care. Sally believes that a mother's intuition and nurturing abilities give her an advantage over her husband. She says, "I boss him around, and I know he resents it. I am so frustrated because he doesn't burp and change the diaper the way that I do."

When the nurse asks Bob about parenting, he suggests that because of the negative feedback he is receiving from his wife he realizes he is not involved as much as he should be. He elaborates that he does not know much about caring for these "fragile human beings." Bob acknowledges his frustration about his inability to read the baby's cues of hunger and discomfort, and he would like to learn more about infant growth and development. When asked if he had any role models that influenced his parenting role, he quickly remarked that his father was not a good role model, tossed him out of the home when he was 17 years old, and repeatedly told him he was going to be a failure at everything he did. Bob said, "I don't want my daughter to go through what I did. I am a little insecure that she is going to grow up and hate me." Although Bob had feelings of delight when talking about Julie, he had significant anxiety about his relationship. Sally and Bob do not have parents or relatives who live in close proximity and asked the nurse about the benefits of joining a neighborhood parent support group.

Following the infant's physical assessment and discussion of the infant's feeding, elimination, sleep, and activity patterns, the nurse determined that Julie is a healthy newborn. The anxiety expressed by Bob about his relationship with the baby led to the nurse diagnosing Risk for Altered Parent-Infant Attachment (NANDA, 1999), and the intervention Fathering Promotion was initiated.

Through careful listening, the nurse acknowledged the parents' positive parenting behaviors and comments on the father's interest and resourcefulness in his attempts to feed Julie during the visit. The nurse encouraged the parents to see their individual and collective strengths as parents and asks them to each give an example of what they appreciate most about the other's parenting skills. The nurse pointed out that each parent may have a different approach to parenting, but it is important to respect these differences. The nurse explored Sally's idea that mother knows best and how she might let go of some of these feelings. Sally was able to express her feelings about parenthood and her expectations of herself as a supermom. She also realized she needs to be less critical of Bob's skills as a father and to give him more support and positive reinforcement. The nurse reinforced their interest in joining a support group in the community. Bob was able to openly discuss his relationship with his father and discuss his hopes and goals about his new role as a father.

The nurse, in collaboration with the family, decided to discuss infant growth and development the next week. To facilitate the development of the father-infant relationship, the nurse encouraged the father to touch, play, and speak to their infant; to identify family characteristics he sees in their infant; and to use eye contact. Using a video presentation, she pointed out infant cues that showed the infant's responsiveness to the father. The nurse did a follow-up visit 3 months later and charted the following outcomes: (a) the father is maintaining a close nurturing relationship with the infant; (b) the parents are expressing their ideas about parenting in supportive, appropriate ways to one another; (c) the mother recognizes the strengths that the father brings to the socialization of their infant; (d) the father has a better understanding of the infant's growth and development; and (e) the father has developed a support system with other parents. Furthermore, the father is kissing and smiling at the infant, and the infant responds to the father's cues—indicators of the NOC outcome Parent-Infant Attachment (Iowa Outcomes Project, 2000).

RESEARCH AND PRACTICE IMPLICATIONS

To date, most researchers have focused on the competency and nurturing ability of fathers, the similarities and differences between mothers and fathers in their behavior toward their infants, and the degree to which mothers and fathers resemble each other in their parental activities. It is necessary to direct research to more fully understand the development of the father-child relationship. Furthermore, this may be one of the reasons why assessment of the parent-infant relationship focuses mainly on the mother in hospital and community health settings. Specific guidelines for assessing the mother-infant relationship are available, but a research-based assessment guide for fathers is not.

There has been little research on how fathers perceive their spouses' support in the development of the father-infant relationship. The emphasis has been on how the father could support the mother to maintain an effective relationship with the infant. Understanding the nature of this supportive or nonsupportive spousal environment may give researchers an understanding of factors that may influence the development of the father-infant relationship.

Another way to broaden the current understanding of the parent-infant relationship is to focus on the father because attachment theory is primarily based on studies of the mother-infant relationship. In addition, few studies have paid attention to how mothers or fathers perceive this relationship. It would be useful to focus on the joint influence of mothering and fathering and the way the marital relationship influences the development of the father-infant relationship. In addition, longitudinal studies would be useful to examine the changes that occur in the father-infant relationship over time.

For the most part, studies have been conducted on well-educated, middle-class, white fathers who are committed to and value their relationships with their infants. Investigation of the father-infant relationship in situations in which fathers feel obligated to have children or in which they are not involved in the planning of the pregnancy is needed. Furthermore, researchers should study diverse groups of fathers of different cultural, racial, socioeconomic, and age groups.

Researchers need not only study changes happening inside the family but also can examine how the workplace, economic trends, and government policies facilitate or inhibit families in raising their children. Longitudinal research to track the changes over time, taking into account the slow changes in the parenting roles, is also warranted (Tiedje & Darling-Fisher, 1996).

To develop father-friendly programs, researchers should examine the short- and long-term effects of existing programs. Future research should address questions such as the following: (a) Do programs have important impacts on father-child relationships? (b) What types of methods work best with different groups of fathers? (c) Are there certain program formats that are more effective? and (d) What are the goals that are most important to pursue as perceived by fathers (Palm, 1997, p. 181)?

Nurses should promote a better image of fathers by dispelling the myths that all men are uninterested in and uninvolved with their children and by sharing success stories of active fathering. Attitudes in society emphasize the father's role as a provider and someone who is valued for career achievements. The employment of the father does play a major role in shaping fathering behavior and his involvement in the child's life just as employment shapes mothering behavior. Fathers are sometimes judged harshly. Fathers have been given a negative identity by being called absent, clumsy, uninvolved, and uninterested. One father describes how he was critically examined:

> There are times that I felt I was stepping into a woman's domain, which was odd. I find that in the reception room at the doctor's office. Like the women are all watching me, waiting for me to do something typically male like drop him, or hammer him too hard. You feel very much under the microscope, especially if you step out of the role. It's funny they want us to play new roles as fathers, but they don't trust you to be able to do it.

Health care professionals should work toward changing negative societal attitudes to fathering. Nurses should be advocates for fathers by promoting a work environment that is more father and family friendly. Nurses can also lobby the government for policies such as flexible working arrangements, paternity leaves, on-site day care programs, options for working at home, and education on family topics. Fathers should to be given the opportunity to discuss their experiences and concerns while they attempt to develop a relationship with their infants. They need to be given direction, opportunities, and support to learn how to develop a relationship with their infants just as mothers need opportunities to learn how to be mothers. Fathers need support in their families, in the health care system, and in their communities that encourage and reward their involvement and relationships with their children. Fathers are important, and nurses need to help them become successful and experience enjoyment in their role.

REFERENCES

Anderson, A. M. (1996a). The father-infant relationship: Becoming connected. *Journal of the Society of Pediatric Nurses, 1*(2), 83-92.

Anderson, A. M. (1996b). Factors influencing the father-infant relationship. *Journal of Family Nursing, 2*(3), 306-324.

Barnard, K. E. (1976). *NCAST II learners resource manual.* Seattle: NCAST.

Battles, R. S. (1988). Factors influencing men's transition into parenthood. *Neonatal Network, 6*(5), 63-66.

Belsky, J., Gilstrap, B., & Rovine, M. (1984). The Pennsylvania infant and family development project: 1. Stability and change in mother-infant and father-infant interaction in a family setting at one, three and nine months. *Child Development, 55*(3), 692-705.

Boyle, B., & Letourneau, S. (1995). *Workforce adjustment competencies for community nursing practice.* Edmonton, Alberta, Canada: Capital Health Authority.

Brazelton, T. B. (1969). *Infants and mothers.* New York: Dell.

Brickman, P. (1987). *Commitment, conflict and caring.* Englewood Cliffs, NJ: Prentice Hall.

Bronstein, P., & Cowan, C. (Eds.). (1988). *Fatherhood today: Men's changing role in the family.* New York: John Wiley.

Clarke-Stewart, K. A. (1978). And daddy makes three: The father's impact on mother and young child. *Child Development, 49*(3), 466-478.

Daly, K. J. (1995). Reshaping fatherhood. In W. Marsiglio (Ed.), *Fatherhood: Contemporary theory, research, and social policy* (pp. 21-40). Thousand Oaks, CA: Sage.

Dienhart, A., & Dollahite, D. (1997). A generative narrative approach to clinical work with fathers. In A. Hawkins & D. Dollahite (Eds.), *Generative fathering* (pp. 183-199). Thousand Oaks, CA: Sage.

Dumas, M. A. (1991). *A phenomenological investigation of the meaning of "being jealous" as experienced in fathers following the birth of their first child.* Paper presented at the Qualitative Health Research Conference, Edmonton, Alberta.

Ehrensaft, D. (1995). Bringing in fathers: The reconstruction of mothering. In J. Shapiro, M. Diamond, & M. Greenberg (Eds.), *Becoming a father* (pp. 43-59). New York: Springer.

Emde, R. (1980). Emotional availability: A reciprocal reward system for infants and parents with implications for prevention of psychosocial disorders. In P. Taylor (Ed.), *Parent-infant relationships* (pp. 87-115). New York: Grune & Stratton.

Friedman, M. (1992). *Family nursing: Theory and assessment.* Englewood Cliffs, NJ: Prentice Hall.

Frodi, A., Lamb, M., Leavitt, L., & Donovan, W. (1978). Fathers' and mothers' responses to infant smiles and cries. *Infant Behavior and Development, 1*(2), 187-198.

Gamble, D., & Morse, J. (1993). Fathers of breast fed infants: Postponing and types of involvement. *Journal of Obstetric, Gynecologic and Neonatal Nursing,* 22(4), 358-365.

Graham, M. V. (1993). Parental sensitivity to infant cues: Similarities and differences between mothers and fathers. *Journal of Pediatric Nursing, 8*(6), 376-384.

Greenberg, M., & Morris, N. (1974). Engrossment: The newborn's impact upon the father. *American Journal of Orthopsychiatry, 44*(4), 520-530.

Hall, W. A. (1992). Comparison of the experience of women and men in dual-earner families following the birth of their first infant. *Image: The Journal of Nursing Scholarship, 24,* 33-38.

Hawkins, A., & Dollahite, D. (1997). Beyond the role-inadequacy perspective of fathering. In A. Hawkins & D. Dollahite (Eds.), *Generative fathering* (pp. 3-16). Thousand Oaks, CA: Sage.

Henderson, A. (1991). The experience of new fathers during the first 3 weeks of life. *Journal of Advanced Nursing, 16,* 293-298.

Hendrick, S., & Hendrick, C. (1992). *Liking, loving and relating* (2nd ed.). Pacific Grove, CA: Brooks/Cole.

Hyman-Partnow, J. (1995). Shifting patterns of fathering in the first year of life: On intimacy between fathers and their babies. In J. Shapiro, M. Diamond, & M. Greenberg (Eds.), *Becoming a father* (pp. 256-267). New York: Springer.

Iowa Interventions Project. (2000). *Nursing interventions classification (NIC)* (J. C. McCloskey & G. M. Bulecheck, Eds.; 3rd ed.). St. Louis, MO: Mosby-Year Book.

Iowa Outcomes Project. (2000). *Nursing outcomes classification (NOC)* (M. Johnson, M. Maas, & S. Moorhead, Eds.; 2nd ed.). St. Louis, MO: Mosby-Year Book.

Jones, C. (1981). Father to infant attachment: Effects of early contact and characteristics of the infant. *Research in Nursing and Health, 4,* 193-200.

Jones, C., & Lenz, E. (1986). Father-newborn interaction: Effects of social competence and infant state. *Nursing Research, 35*(3), 149-153.

Jordan, P. (1990). Laboring for relevance: Expectant and new fatherhood. *Nursing Research, 39,* 11-16.

Jordan, P. (1995). The mother's role in promoting fathering behavior. In J. Shapiro, M. Diamond, & M. Greenberg (Eds.), *Becoming a father* (pp. 61-71). New York: Springer.

Jordan, P., & Wall, V. (1990). Breastfeeding and fathers: Illuminating the darker side. *Birth, 17*(4), 210-213.

Keller, W., Hildebrandt, K., & Richards, M. (1985). Effects of extended father-infant contact during the newborn period. *Infant Behavior and Development, 8*(3), 337-350.

Klaus, M., & Kennell, J. (1982). *Parent-infant bonding* (2nd ed.). Toronto: C. V. Mosby.

Kotelchuck, M. (1976). The infant's relationship to the father: Experimental evidence. In M. Lamb (Ed.), *The role of the father in child development* (pp. 329-345). New York: John Wiley.

Lamb, M. (1976). Interactions between eight-month-old children and their fathers and mothers. In M. Lamb (Ed.), *The role of the father in child development* (pp. 307-327). New York: John Wiley.

Lamb, M. (1986). The changing roles of fathers. In M. Lamb (Ed.), *The father's role: Applied perspective* (pp. 3-27). New York: John Wiley.

Lamb, M. (1995). The changing roles of fathers. In J. Shapiro, M. Diamond, & M. Greenberg (Eds.), *Becoming a father* (pp. 18-35). New York: Springer.

Lewis, C. (1986). The father-child relationship. In C. Lewis (Ed.), *Becoming a father* (pp. 112-129). Bristol, PA: Open University Press.

McBride, B. (1989). Stress and fathers' parental competence: Implications for family life and parent educators. *Family Relations, 38*(4), 385-389.

North American Nursing Diagnosis Association. (1999). *Nursing diagnoses: Definitions and classification 1995-1996*. Philadelphia: Author.

Osherman, S. (1992). *Wrestling with love*. New York: Fawcett.

Palkovitz, R. (1982). Fathers' birth attendance, extended contact, and father-infant interaction at five months postpartum. *Birth, 9*(3), 173-177.

Palkovitz, R. (1997). Reconstructing "involvement": Expanding conceptualizations of men's caring in contemporary families. In A. Hawkins & D. Dollahite (Eds.), *Generative fathering* (pp. 200-216). Thousand Oaks, CA: Sage.

Palm, G. (1997). Promoting generative fathering through parent and family education. In A. Hawkins & D. Dollahite (Eds.), *Generative fathering* (pp. 167-182). Thousand Oaks, CA: Sage.

Pannabecker, B. J., Emde, R. N., & Austin, B. C. (1982). The effect of early extended contact on father-newborn interaction. *Journal of Genetic Psychology, 141*, 7-17.

Parke, R., & Tinsley, B. (1981). The father's role in infancy: Determinants in caregiving and play. In M. Lamb (Ed.), *The role of the father in child development* (2nd ed., pp. 429-457). New York: John Wiley.

Pruett, K. D. (1993). The paternal presence. *Families in Society: The Journal of Contemporary Human Services, 74*, 46-50.

Rendina, I., & Dickerscheid, J. (1976). Father involvement with firstborn infants. *Family Coordinator, 25*(4), 373-377.

Rogers, M. (1990). Nursing: Science of unitary, irreducible, human beings. Update 1990. In E. A. M. Barett (Ed.), *Visions of Roger's science-based nursing* (pp. 5-11). New York: National League for Nursing.

Rustia, J., & Abbott, D. (1993). Father involvement in infant care: Two longitudinal studies. *International Journal of Nursing Studies, 30*(6), 467-476.

Schecket, P. (1995). Support for fathers: A model for hospital-based parenting. In J. Shapiro, M. Diamond, & M. Greenberg (Eds.), *Becoming a father* (pp. 135-143). New York: Springer.

Scull, C. (1992). The evolving father: From absence to presence. In C. Scull (Ed.), *Fathers, sons and daughters* (pp. 3-9). Los Angeles: J. P. Tarcher.

Shapiro, J. (1987). The expectant father. *Psychology Today, 21*, 36-42.

Swigart, J. (1991). *The myth of the bad mother*. New York: Doubleday.

Tiedje, L. B., & Darling-Fisher, C. (1996). Fatherhood reconsidered: A critical review. *Research in Nursing and Health, 19*(6), 471-484.

Tiller, C. (1995). Fathers' parenting attitudes during a child's first year. *Journal of Obstetric, Gynecologic, and Neonatal Nursing, 24*(6), 508-514.

Tomlinson, P. S. (1987a). Spousal differences in marital satisfaction during transition to parenthood. *Nursing Research, 36*(4), 239-243.

Tomlinson, P. S. (1987b). Father involvement with first-born infants: Interpersonal and situational. *Pediatric Nursing, 13*(2), 101-105.

Toney, L. (1983). The effects of holding the newborn at delivery on paternal bonding. *Nursing Research, 32,* 16-19.

Vanier Institute of the Family. (1994). Dad is the trailer. *Transition, 2,* 17.

Worth, C. (1988). *The birth of a father.* New York: McGraw-Hill.

7

Parenting Promotion

Janice Denehy

Nurses who care for children and families have long been interested in parenting and have provided information to parents on many aspects of child rearing and child development. This information has typically been presented to parents in the form of anticipatory guidance during routine child health care in ambulatory settings (Denehy, 1990), but it also has occurred in the community, hospitals, and other settings in which nurses encounter children and families. Anticipatory guidance, for the most part, is delivered to parents on a one-to-one basis, making it very customized to the needs of the individual family and targeted to the developmental and individual temperament of the child. Nurses in ambulatory settings often implemented this intervention, knowing they would see the family again at a subsequent visit, thus enabling them to provide carefully paced and measurable doses of information during the critical phases of child rearing. Recently, parenting education has become a component of prenatal care with the realization that perspective parents not only need information about the physical and psychological aspects of childbearing but also must be prepared for the responsibilities of parenting an infant the day they leave the hospital.

Today, the reality is that many individuals are assuming the parental role with little support or information about how to succeed in this role.

of services designed to (a) prevent child abuse and neglect, (b) promote optimal child development, (c) promote positive parenting, (d) enhance parent-child interactions, and (e) ensure medical follow-up for well child care as well as screening and treatment for developmental delays (Fuddy, 1989). The family support home visitation program began in 1975, and the Healthy Start Model began in 1985 under demonstration grants. The focus was on prevention of child abuse and reduction of associated downstream costs for social and juvenile correction services. Because most child abuse morbidity and mortality occurs in the first 5 years of life, the program focused on visiting families during these crucial years.

At-risk families were identified during the postpartum period, and these families voluntarily signed up for participation in the program. The level of service, defined as frequency of visitation, was determined by the status of parent-child interaction, frequency of family crises, and the ability of the family to use community services. Visits were made by trained paraprofessionals, who each handled a caseload of 15 to 25 families. Cases were reviewed regularly by supervisors to determine the level and types of services needed and to document progress toward program outcome goals. Home visits were made weekly, biweekly, monthly, or quarterly for 5 years. Visits focused on attachment and parent-child interaction as well as the needs of children at different stages of development and parental coping skills needed at the various stages. Parents also met in groups for parenting classes or parent-child play mornings designed to not only provide information but also model parenting skills, reduce social isolation, and develop self-esteem. In addition, a toy lending library, short-term respite care, and support groups were available. A male home visitor was assigned to work with fathers to reduce high-risk characteristics and behaviors. Community resource referral and coordination was an important component of the program to meet other pressing needs identified in the high-risk participants, including referrals for housing; substance abuse treatment; spouse abuse treatment or shelter; food and clothing distribution; Women, Infants and Children's program (WIC); employment training; and day care. Coordination of referrals was necessary to avoid duplication or overlap and to ensure accessibility to this population of services available. Home visitors often provided transportation to medical appointments and other referrals to assist program participants in taking advantage of services.

Evaluation of the outcomes of the Hawaii Family Support Services programs showed a decrease in the expected reports of child abuse or neglect, estimated to be 20%, in this population. In 3 years, the program served 241 infants; among those who were older than 1 year (175), there were no reports of child abuse and only 4 cases of neglect (2%) reported among participants (Fuddy, 1989). No statistics were reported relating to the other four goals of the program.

The Parenting Enhancement Program is a holistic patient-centered nursing practice model based on a synthesis of practice, teaching, and research done by its creator, Luz Porter. The model, used with pregnant adolescents in Pennsylvania and West Virginia, focused on health promotion and preservation and was designed to promote self-care and develop decision-making skills among high-risk pregnant teens (Porter, 1984). The program sessions were divided into three phases: the prenatal phase (six sessions), the natal phase (one session), and the postnatal phase (four sessions). Each session, 2½ hours long, had five to eight participants. The sessions were a series of health teaching units ranging from concerns and information about pregnancy to parenting topics of feeding, safety, and minor illness management. The first session also focused on expressing concerns, identifying family strengths and problems, and activating self-care agency. From this pilot program, the author recommended that sessions be held at the same location and on the day of prenatal visits, hourly breaks with healthy snacks and movement, and limiting the time of the program to 2 to 2½ hours (the original program had sessions of 3 hours, which proved to be too lengthy for the participants). She also noted that many of the participants did not show enthusiasm or active involvement—in fact, some were outwardly hostile—until the fourth session. Gradually, these pregnant teens opened up and became active participants in the group, underscoring the importance of being patient and supportive during this phase of the program. Program outcomes were determined for Phase 1 only and showed that participants in the treatment group (n = 10) had higher scores in self-esteem, self-care agency, and pregnancy acceptance and did not miss any prenatal appointments. Teens in the control group (n = 12) also showed an increase in the three measures over time, but not as great an increase as that of those in the treatment group, and they missed seven prenatal appointments during the study (Porter, 1984). This pilot validated the feasibility of such a project, and there are plans to extend the study, adding a home visitation component and additional measurement of study outcomes of both the mother and the infant for a year after birth.

In response to a review of public health nursing services that showed a lack of convincing evidence of the effectiveness of these services, a team of researchers in Montreal, Canada, designed a randomized controlled trial to test a home intervention designed to bring about changes in the home environments of low-socioeconomic-status mothers (Infante-Rivard et al., 1989). Control group parents (*n* = 26) received two routine postnatal visits, whereas the experimental group (*n* = 21) received three prenatal and five postnatal visits. The visits focused on teaching and counseling based on items included in the Home Observation for Measurement of the Environment (HOME). The goal was for the mother to discover her own potential for interaction with her infant by providing her with tools to maximize this interaction. At 9 months of age, the HOME inventory was administered, and at 15 months the Bayley Mental and Motor Scales of Development were administered and questions were asked about the child's health and immunization status.

It was thought the lack of significant findings in prior studies may have been related to participant selection, and those who were at lesser risk were least likely to gain from parenting interventions. Mothers for this study were selected because they were below the poverty level or had less than 12 years of schooling or both, making them more likely to benefit from early intervention. Outcomes of this study showed that scores on the HOME and Bayley Scales for the experimental group were higher than those of the control group, although the results were not statistically significant. Children of control group mothers had a greater number of hospitalizations, incomplete immunizations, and fewer were breast-fed, although again the differences were not statistically significant (Infante-Rivard et al., 1989). Although the authors suggest the small sample size or the lack of sensitivity of the HOME contributed to the nonsignificance of findings in this study, they do not recommend abandoning home visitation to promote maternal-child development, but rather, identify the need for innovative strategies to achieve outcomes.

A study to determine the outcomes and cost-effectiveness of a family support and parenting education program in the homes of inner-city, high-risk African American mothers found that families in the home visitation group showed improved compliance with well child care, fewer illness visits, and dramatic reductions in child hospitalizations and abuse and neglect compared to the control group (Hardy & Streett, 1989). The researchers noted that children who grew up in homes with unfavorable conditions, such as substandard housing, lack of transportation, welfare dependency, high fertility, and intergenerational teenage childbearing, experienced numerous health conditions that compromised their potential for normal development. Hardy and Street proposed that these problems were preventable if parents had the skills, information, and basic resources needed for parenting. Ten home visits were scheduled 2 or 3 weeks before routine child health visits. A college-educated African American woman from the community was trained to present anticipatory guidance pertinent to the child's development, feeding, and safety and to the care of the well and sick child. Also emphasized was the importance of regular clinic visits and preventive health care. A calendar reminded parents of upcoming visits and developmental milestones, and a series of pamphlets written at the fourth-grade level provided information on developmental and child care issues. Hardy and Streett suggest that funds for home visits to improve parenting skills and preventive services for high-risk parents should be considered as a method of reducing the overall cost of pediatric health care for the poor. They note, however, that the educational program in isolation is not sufficient because many parents need more than parenting information. The home visitor in this study soon found that the parents she visited had many crisis and survival issues that required immediate attention, such as the need for food, diapers, and transportation to health care; the threat of eviction; or lack of heat or electricity, before they were able to attend to parenting and child health issues. The home visitor quickly became an important resource, family advocate, and friend. Such support and the use of community resources are an essential and cost-effective component in the care of high-risk families.

Clarke and Strauss (1992) described a nursing program of role supplementation for teen parents that recognized the complexity of the parenting role when added to other transitions occurring during adolescence. To enact such a role, the individual must have a clear idea of expected role behaviors, which include the ability to understand the physical, emotional, social, and cognitive needs of infants. The role supplementation interventions included role modeling, role rehearsal, and viewing other parents, in addition to parenting information, support, counseling, and monitoring. Data on a battery of assessment data were compared pre- and postintervention. The role supplementation interventions are prescriptive nursing treatments derived from theory and related research and currently are being tested in a longitudinal study to examine the outcomes during the first 2 years of the child's life.

Olds, Henderson, Tatelbaum, and Chamberlin (1988) studied the effects of a comprehensive pre- and postnatal nurse home visitation program on the outcomes of pregnancy, early childbearing, and life-course development of socially disadvantaged mothers. Eighty-five percent of the 354 participants were teenagers, unmarried, or low-socioeconomic-status, first-time mothers. This randomized clinical trial was based on the premise that nurse home visitors are in an optimal position to identify and change factors that influence maternal health habits, child rearing, maternal education and work, as well as family planning. This study was designed to promote educational and work achievements and reduce subsequent unintended pregnancies. Mothers were randomly assigned to four cumulative treatment conditions, beginning with no treatment and advancing to free transportation for prenatal and well child care, the addition of nurse home visitation during pregnancy, and, finally, continuing nurse visitation until the child reached 2 years of age. Children in all treatment groups were screened for developmental and perceptual problems at 2 years of age. Home visits typically lasted 1 hour and 15 minutes and were conducted by specially trained registered nurses hired for the study. Objectives for the home visits were to build on the mothers' strengths and desires and to encourage them to continue their education, seek employment, and use contraception for family planning. Families were referred to other health and social services as needed. The study was conducted in the semirural community of Elmira, New York, in which there was a high

rate of child abuse, poor economic conditions, and few employment opportunities.

Four years after giving birth, mothers in the nurse-visited group returned to school more rapidly, showed an 82% increase in the number of
months they were employed, had 43% fewer subsequent pregnancies, and
postponed the birth of their second child by 12 months (Olds et al., 1988).
The increase in months of employment may be due to the postponement of
further childbearing and job training. For unmarried teenagers, the impact on employment was not realized until after the program ended, when
the teens became old enough to apply for and hold jobs. Other results of the
program were mixed over time. Although such a program may not have
dramatic effects on mothers, the authors state that such a public health
strategy of using nurses to visit high-risk families may be an effective way
to make improvements in maternal and child functioning as well as result
in substantial savings related to increased maternal employment, reductions
in unintended pregnancies, and a decrease in other social service costs.

In a 15-year follow-up of their randomized trial, Olds and colleagues
(1997) were able to question 324 of their original subjects. They reported
that, in contrast to the comparison groups, mothers who received nurse
visitation during pregnancy and for 2 years after the birth of their children
had less reported child abuse and neglect, more time between subsequent
births, fewer subsequent births, shorter duration on the Aid to Families
With Dependent Children Program, fewer impairments related to drug or
alcohol abuse, and fewer arrests, convictions, and days in jail. All these
findings were statistically significant. For the group that received visitation during pregnancy only, positive results were between those of the
comparison group (no visitation) and those of the group that received visitation during pregnancy and 2 years after birth, suggesting a dose-
response relationship for the level of home visits. The positive results were
most profound for those mothers who were unmarried and from lower-
socioeconomic-status households. These results indicate that parenting
programs could lead to substantial government savings over time, and the
costs of the program would be recouped by the time the children reach 4
years of age.

Kitzman and Olds collaborated with others (1997) in replicating
their study with a different population of mothers in another geographic
region. Subjects for this randomized controlled trial were 1,139 predomi-
nately African American woman identified as high risk due to two of the
three following factors: unmarried, unemployed, or less than a 12th-
grade education. The study was done in Memphis, Tennessee. The four
treatment groups of the original study were replicated. Results of this
replication indicated that nurse visitation reduced pregnancy-induced hypertension, childhood injuries, and subsequent pregnancies. In addition, mothers in the visitation group were more likely to attempt breast-

feeding, provide more growth-producing home environments, express greater empathy, have more realistic expectations of their children, and were less likely to value physical punishment as a method of discipline. There were no program effects reported on infant birth weight; child immunization rates, mental development, or behavior problems; or maternal education and employment.

The literature reviewed represents only a small number of studies done on parenting programs for high-risk families and includes those designed or implemented by nurses. The results indicate the need for enrolling high-risk parents in programs as soon as possible, ideally prior to the birth of the infant, and supplementing the usual services of giving health care and child development information with a more comprehensive program that stresses the context of parenting. Such comprehensive programs include support, counseling, and referral to existing community resources to meet families' immediate needs as well as long-term needs for continued education and employment. Without such a vision, services delivered to children and families will be incomplete, fragmented, and poorly coordinated. They will also not be able to address the complex needs of many of today's high-risk young families—needs that must be met if the family unit is to thrive and the children in the family are to reach their optimum potential.

NURSING DIAGNOSES AND OUTCOME DETERMINATION

Parenting Promotion is an appropriate nursing intervention for individuals at risk for Altered Parenting due to risk factors that may be present in the parent or the child. Table 7.1 is a synthesis of risk factors related to Altered Parenting. Other nursing diagnoses that lend themselves to this intervention include Parental Role Conflict, Self-Esteem Disturbance, Social Isolation, Caregiver Role Strain, Altered Family Process, Impaired Social Interaction, and Altered Family Process (North American Nursing Diagnosis Association [NANDA], 1999). Each has related factors that, coupled with defining characteristics, indicate the need for preventive intervention. Parenting Promotion is a comprehensive nursing intervention designed to meet the complex needs exhibited by high-risk families.

The Nursing Outcomes Classification (NOC) outcome *Parenting,* defined as "provision of an environment that promotes optimum growth and development of dependent children" (Iowa Outcomes Project, 2000, p. 332), provides a framework to evaluate parent-child interaction and the environment created by the parent. Indicators include "provides for child's physical needs," "interacts positively with child," and "eliminates

TABLE 7.1   Risk Factors for Altered Parenting[a]

Risk factors (parent)

Social factors
Single parent
Poverty
Low socioeconomic status
Lack of resources
Lack of transportation
Lack of access to resources
History of abuse
Poor parental role model
Poor home environment
Low value on parenthood
Lack of social support network
Stress
Maladaptive coping strategies
Low self-esteem
Inability to put child's needs before own
Unplanned or unwanted pregnancy
Marital conflict
Inadequate child care arrangements
Marital problems, declining marital satisfaction

Knowledge factors
Unrealistic expectations
Lack of knowledge of child growth and
    development
Lack of or inappropriate child-rearing skills
Lack of cognitive readiness for parenthood
Low educational level or attainment
Poor communication skills
Inability to recognize and act on infant cues
Preference for physical punishment for discipline

Physiological factors
Lack of or late prenatal care
Young age, adolescent
High number of or closely spaced children
Multiple birth
Difficult labor or delivery or both
History of substance abuse
History of mental illness
Depression
Physical illness
Low energy level

Risk factors (child)

Separation from parent at birth
Premature birth
Physical illness
Handicapping condition
Developmental delay
Difficult temperament
Lack of goodness of fit (temperament) with
    parental expectations
Attention deficit hyperactivity disorder
Unplanned child
Not gender desired
Multiple birth
Altered perceptual abilities

a. Synthesis of literature from 1991 to 1997.

controllable environmental hazards." Other indicators relate to provision of routine health care, use of community resources, having realistic expectations, having a functional support system, and self-esteem. The indicators not only relate to specifics of child rearing and behavior management but also take a more holistic perspective, including support and community resources used by the parent in carrying out the parenting role.

Other related NOC outcomes that could be used to evaluate the effectiveness of specific components of a parenting promotion program include Knowledge: Child Safety, Knowledge: Health Resources, Parenting: Social Safety, Self-Esteem, Social Support, and Role Performance. All these outcomes have indicators that would assist in the measurement of the effectiveness of a parenting program and related parental and child behaviors.

INTERVENTION: PARENTING PROMOTION

The nursing intervention Parenting Promotion is a synthesis of the activities outlined in comprehensive community-based programs for parents. The intervention has been accepted for publication in the third edition of the *Nursing Interventions Classification* (NIC; 2000) (Table 7.2). It includes traditional aspects of anticipatory guidance and health teaching as well as toy-lending libraries, referrals for substance abuse treatment, and job training. This intervention takes into account the realization that education is necessary but not sufficient to make a difference in parenting skills and desired outcomes in children. It is essential to attend to the pressing social needs of high-risk families, such as money to pay the rent and purchase diapers or transportation to get to work, before they are in a condition to be receptive to information about parenting (Hardy & Streett, 1989).

Early identification of high-risk parents, during the prenatal or postpartum period, is the key to this intervention (Fuddy, 1989). The sooner the intervention begins, the more likely the parent is to have the needed support and success in the parenting role. Also critical to the success of the intervention is a person to consistently coordinate the activities of the intervention and provide the continuity needed to build a trusting relationship, especially because long-term home visitation is a vital component of the intervention (Hardy & Street, 1989; Infante-Rivard et al., 1989). Such a trusting relationship is needed if the home visitor is to be welcomed into the home of the family, and the information given and referrals made are to fall on receptive ears. In addition, the nurse needs to be nonjudgmental because parents often share their feelings, problems, and concerns. Direct observation during home visitation can provide the nurse with valuable data, obtainable by no other method, about the strengths and the needs of the families.

Assisting parents with acquisition of the parental role involves time and information as well as developing realistic expectations and the skills necessary to undertake this role (Clarke & Strauss, 1992). Information about parenting can be provided through anticipatory guidance at times when development transitions occur, such as safety information as an

TABLE 7.2   Parenting Promotion

Definition

Parenting Promotion consists of providing parenting information, support, and coordination of comprehensive services to high-risk families.

Activities

Identify and enroll high-risk families in follow-up program.

Encourage mothers to receive early and regular prenatal care.

Visit mothers in the hospital before discharge to begin establishing trusting relationship and schedule follow-up visit.

Make home visits as indicated by level of risk.

Assist parents to have realistic expectations appropriate to developmental and ability level of child.

Assist parents with role transition and expectations of parenthood.

Refer to male home visitors to work with fathers as appropriate.

Provide anticipatory guidance needed at different developmental levels.

Provide pamphlets, books, and other materials to develop parenting skills.

Discuss age-appropriate behavior-management strategies.

Assist parents to identify unique temperament of their infant.

Teach parents to respond to behavior cues exhibited by their infant.

Model and encourage parental interaction with children.

Refer to parent support groups as appropriate.

Assist parents in developing, maintaining, and using social support systems.

Listen to parents' problems and concerns nonjudgmentally.

Provide positive feedback and structured successes at parenting skills to foster parents' self-esteem.

Assist parents to develop social skills.

Teach and model coping skills.

Enhance problem-solving skills through role modeling, practice, and reinforcement.

Provide toys through toy-lending library.

Monitor child health status, well child checks, and immunization status.

Monitor parental health status and health maintenance activities.

Arrange transportation to well child visits or other services as necessary.

Refer to community resources as appropriate.

Coordinate community agencies working with family.

Provide linkage to job training or employment as needed.

Inform parents where to receive family planning services.

Monitor consistent and correct use of contraceptives as appropriate.

Assist in arranging day care as needed.

Refer for respite care as appropriate.

Refer to domestic violence center as needed.

Refer for substance abuse treatment as needed.

Collect and record data as indicated for follow-up and program evaluation.

infant becomes more mobile or preparation for toilet training. In addition to information about child development, information about creating an environment that is safe and fosters optimum development of the child is needed by families establishing new households. Written materials or videotapes supplement verbal teaching and are available when needed by the family. It is essential that written materials are easy to read, and acceptable to the target audience, and provide concrete examples of how the information can be applied in many common situations. Pictures and diagrams are a valuable supplement to textual information.

In addition to information, role modeling and rehearsing interaction and behavior management skills are an important component of Parenting Promotion. Such activities use information as the basis for the behavioral skills needed for role acquisition (Clarke & Strauss, 1992). Modeling communicating and playing with an infant shows parents how to perform these important parental behaviors and gives them the opportunity for feedback as their skills develop. A toy-lending library provides parents with a variety of developmentally appropriate toys and ideas on how to use them in creative play with their infants (Fuddy, 1989). With practice, young parents experience success in parenting that not only increases their effectiveness as parents but also assists them in meeting the needs of the infant, which leads to role satisfaction, improved self-esteem, and role competence.

Involving the father of the infant in the parenting program is important because the father is a significant member of the family unit and a central figure in the development of the infant. Encouraging the father to attend a parenting group for young fathers or to be visited by a male home visitor will promote role acquisition and the skills needed for parenting (Fuddy, 1989). These strategies are tailored to the needs of the father and often emphasize the importance of the male as a role model for the developing child and support person for the mother. Fathering classes not only focus on parenting skills but may also include job training and placement as well as family planning, money management, and budgeting.

Child health maintenance visits are essential to promoting the health of the infant and preventing illness through immunization, monitoring growth and development, and providing information on child development and parenting skills. Parents not only need transportation to health care visits but also need resources to pay for the care provided. For those unable to afford these services, referral to alternate resources for health care are appropriate. Monitoring attendance at clinic visits and follow-through on recommendations is an important function of the nurse (Fuddy, 1989; Infante-Rivard et al., 1989). Often, parents are overwhelmed with the amount of information given or other conflicting demands or crises; therefore, follow-up reinforces the importance of health maintenance visits and immunizations (Hardy & Streett, 1989). When an infant is ill, home visits monitor the infant's health status and compliance with medication or other treatment regimes. In addition to child health, monitoring parental health status is important because parents must have the energy needed to fulfill their parenting roles. Often, nurses focus so much attention on the health of the infant that they overlook the health of the parent. Important considerations are nutrition, rest, work responsibilities, support systems, substance use or abuse, the use of both prescription and over-the-counter medications, and the energy level and mental health of the parents. Other factors to consider are overall appearance and affect of the parents and the condition of the household. For the parents to successfully parent, they should be in optimal health.

Another important component of Parenting Promotion is the development of social and coping skills. Often, adolescents have not yet learned social skills necessary to negotiate the services they will need as parents. Problem-solving skills are valuable for new parents. They also may require assistance in developing adaptive coping skills due to the number of crises they may experience for which their are ill prepared. Coping strategies appropriate for adolescents may no longer be adequate or acceptable in the parental role. Adolescent parents need information about the stresses they will experience and practice resolving conflicts (Clarke & Strauss, 1992).

Identification of social supports available to the family is another important aspect of Parenting Promotion. The availability of support is essential for all families, but it is particularly important for high-risk families. Support systems often provide needed resources, reinforcement, and encouragement to young families. In addition, they may provide information, stability, and respite for the family. The provision of diversion and companionship is often welcomed by today's stressed and isolated families. Often, high-risk families do not have the resources for entertainment or child care services; therefore, family, friends, neighbors, church members, or other individuals can comprise a network of support for high-risk families. This network also validates the worth and importance of the developing family, and the availability of these people in times of crisis is invaluable to families as they encounter expected and unexpected transitions and life events.

Referral and coordination of services are important nursing functions (Fuddy, 1989; Hardy & Streett, 1989; Infante-Rivard et al., 1989). To promote parenting, numerous services may be needed by high-risk parents. Social services, financial assistance, Aid to Families With Dependent Children, WIC, subsidized housing, and medical services might be required by the family. For mothers abusing substances or being abused by their partners, quick referral to appropriate services and shelters is essential (Fuddy, 1989). Although they may not be receptive to such referrals, mothers need to understand that their safety and functioning as parents are of crucial importance to the optimal development of their infants. Providing extra support through these difficult times is essential for parents to change coping patterns and to develop the self-esteem needed to separate from an abusive relationship. Other important services are education, job training and placement, and the day care and transportation needed if parents are to take advantage of these opportunities.

Knowing what resources are available and how to link families to appropriate services is an important nursing role in community-based practice. Care coordination is also essential to prevent duplication of services or to prevent families from not receiving needed services. Assisting parents in negotiating services, completing paperwork, and providing transportation to needed service providers is essential if parents are to benefit from referrals. Follow-up on referrals is essential for optimum outcomes of community-based interventions. The nurse is the ideal person to provide a holistic perspective to care and management of the wide variety of services delivered to families designed to promote parenting.

INTERVENTION APPLICATION

Antonio, newborn son of Maria and José, arrived after a difficult delivery. Maria is a 17-year-old who received minimal prenatal care. She was moving around with her fiancé, José, as he worked seasonal farming jobs. She is currently living with an aunt in a trailer at a migrant camp. José recently got a job in a nearby packing plant for the winter months. They plan to marry as soon as he saves some money and they can afford a place to live together. The neonatal nurse practitioner put Maria in contact with the Project Parenting nurse who follows up on high-risk parents and coordinates services needed. She visited with Maria and José soon after delivery to explain the project and benefits of participation. After the initial contact, the nursing diagnoses At Risk for Altered Parenting and Social Isolation were made (NANDA, 1999). An appointment was made prior to discharge to institute a home visit within 2 days. At that time, a physical exam will be done on the infant, and infant feeding and sleeping will be the main topics of teaching and discussion. The nurse will also assess the mother's health, access to services, and the home environment. A schedule for subsequent visits to begin the Parenting Promotion intervention will be mutually determined by the mother and nurse based on the concerns of the mother and needs identified by the nurse.

At the first visit, the nurse found Maria tired and discouraged by the amount of time needed to care for her infant. She was exhausted from lack of sleep the previous night, during which Antonio cried off and on. She states he seems satisfied after feeding but does not seem comfortable sleeping on his back. The nurse talks about the importance of positioning and other ways to provide comfort and security through swaddling and soothing Antonio. She demonstrated many different strategies to calm

Antonio; then she encouraged Maria to try the strategies to gain confidence in her ability to care for her newborn. Antonio quickly calmed down, giving Maria a sense of satisfaction and confidence she could meet the needs of her infant.

On subsequent visits, Maria's confidence was increasing with regard to understanding her infant's unique signals and needs. She was, however, isolated from her family and friends, who lived in another state. She was interested in getting out of the house but hesitated to ask her aunt to baby-sit for Antonio and to drive her where she wanted to go. José worked long hours and overtime; therefore, he was not able to visit with the family regularly. She believed that he was not very responsive to the needs of their son, and when he did come to visit them, he often fell asleep as a result of long hours of work. The nurse encouraged Maria to attend the Young Parent's Network support group meetings in a nearby community at which she could meet with other young mothers to share concerns and have a day out. The nurse arranged transportation with another mother who attended the group. Child care was provided during the meetings, during which parents shared ideas and concerns and were given information about child rearing and services available in the community. The meetings ended in a play session in which interacting and playing with infants were modeled by project nurses. Each parent was assisted in selecting age-appropriate toys and books from a toy-lending program. Attendance at these sessions was rewarded by door prizes of diapers and other child-related products as well as by a meal served during the meeting. Each session also had a short section focusing on the mother's unique self-care needs and health.

Maria gained new skills and greater confidence in herself through participation in the Young Parent's Network during the next 6 months. Not only did she make new friends but also she began serving as a mentor to another young mother who was having difficulty getting to know her infant. She demonstrated many of the skills the nurse had modeled for her during earlier visits. She also recommended different services she believed were helpful in providing child health care and financial assistance. Maria was very compassionate in trying to help other mothers in the group by listening to their concerns and then offering her support if they needed someone with whom to talk. In the past month, José attended a meeting with Maria and was becoming more involved in parenting activities. He had made a point to be present at two of the past three home visits to receive progress reports on Antonio's development and information needed for upcoming developmental events. Although he did not communicate much during the visits, the nurse observed increasing interest and involvement in his son's development as "Little Tony" became more alert, communicative, and mobile. He took pride in the fact that his son looked "just like him" and was particularly responsive to his efforts to play with him.

José also worked with the nurse in understanding the services available in the community and deciding what would be acceptable to them. The couple became involved in a church group for new families that provided opportunities for regular social events at which child care was provided; they met a few couples with similar interests. The church group was eagerly helping plan their upcoming wedding and welcoming the new family into their congregation.

Appropriate outcomes to evaluate the effectiveness of Parenting Promotion for the family included Parenting, Social Involvement, and Knowledge: Health Resources. Over time, data gathered would document the growth of individuals in the family unit to effectively perform their role as parents and to use appropriate community resources and participate in community life (Iowa Outcomes Project, 2000).

The nurse followed the family for 2 years until they moved to another community in which José had a new job. Maria planned to enter a job training program so that she could work part-time to supplement the family income. She and José were eager to have another baby but believed that they needed more financial security before they could take on the responsibility of another child—and they were so busy enjoying their active toddler, Antonio, that they did not want to miss a moment of these exciting years. A year after they moved, the nurse received a Christmas card from the family announcing that a new family member would be added in the Spring.

IMPLICATIONS FOR NURSING PRACTICE AND RESEARCH

In this era of downsizing and program elimination designed to contain costs, child health professionals need to show positive outcomes for interventions designed to promote parenting. Such evidence has been shown in many comprehensive programs targeting high-risk families (Fuddy, 1989; Kitzman et al., 1997; Olds et al., 1988, 1997). Comprehensive parenting programs not only increase parental skills through education and modeling but also foster family growth through the use of targeted community resources and family planning, job training, and employment. Home visitation has been a hallmark of these programs and provides the continuity and coordination needed by families during the crucial early childbearing years. Positive parental and child health outcomes have the potential to reduce health care costs and create an optimal environment for positive educational outcomes for the child in school as well as positive employment outcomes for parents. The acquisition of parenting skills develops confidence and self-esteem in parents and has been shown to reduce the costs associated with child abuse and neglect as well as later costs related to social and juvenile justice services (Fuddy, 1989). The benefits of parenting promotion through long-term home visitation during the critical early years have been shown to be cost-effective in high-risk families (Olds et al., 1997).

Questions about the content and duration of comprehensive parenting programs need further study with subjects from different geographical regions representing numerous cultural and racial groups. The identification of critical components of Parenting Promotion needs to be determined. Also crucial to program success will be the determination of what level of professional needs to deliver the intervention: Is a registered nurse essential or would a paraprofessional with training and supervision provide equally beneficial services? Lastly, the cost-effectiveness of parenting programs needs to be quantified for policymakers to take seriously the fiscal contributions that long-term comprehensive parenting programs make to the health of children and families and subsequently to the health of the nation.

Nurses must integrate many if not all the activities included in the intervention, Parenting Promotion, in their care of high-risk childbearing and child-rearing families. We must move beyond demonstration grants to the establishment of public policy that provides funds for proven preventive interventions in light of the demonstrated benefits to children and families. Nurses need to lobby for such programs and advocate for those who are unable to speak for themselves—children, the poor, and the disinfranchised—the high-risk families they serve. Nurses in the new millennium will require a broader perspective and the ability to work with many disciplines in planning, implementing, and evaluating care. The next generation of nurses need education focusing on health promotion, disease prevention, and community-based practice. Multidisciplinary education will prepare them to work as team members and case managers in a more complex, cost-conscious health care environment. They also need skills in influencing and formulating health policies related to services that affect families.

The status of women's and children's health continues to rank poorly, despite the high level of knowledge and technology available in today's health care system. Parenting Promotion is a low-tech intervention that emphasizes identification of families at risk, knowledge and skills needed to succeed in the parenting role, and provision and coordination of services needed by families. Nurses must make it their goal to ensure that families most in need of services are informed of service availability, guaranteed access and transportation to services, and given follow-up and support throughout their early childbearing and child-rearing years so that they get a healthy start and are able to achieve their optimum potential.

REFERENCES

Campbell, J. M. (1992). Parenting classes: Focus on discipline. *Journal of Community Health Nursing, 9*(4), 197-208.

Clarke, B. A., & Strauss, S. S. (1992). Nursing role supplementation for adolescent parents: Prescriptive nursing practice. *Journal of Pediatric Nursing, 7*(5), 312-318.

Denehy, J. A. (1990). Anticipatory guidance. In M. J. Craft & J. A. Denehy (Eds.), *Nursing interventions for infants and children* (pp. 53-67). Philadelphia: W. B. Saunders.

Fuddy, L. J. (1989). *A statewide system of family support for the prevention of child abuse and neglect. Family support for high risk infants: Prevention of child abuse.* Honolulu: State of Hawaii, Department of Health, Family Health Services Division, Maternal and Child Health Branch.

Hardy, J. B., & Streett, R. (1989). Family support and parenting education in the home: An effective extension of clinic-based preventive health care services for poor children. *Journal of Pediatrics, 115*(6), 927-931.

Infante-Rivard, C., Filion, G., Baumgarten, M., Bourassa, M., Labelle, J., & Messier, M. (1989). A public health home intervention among families of low socioeconomic status. *Children's Health Care, 18*(2), 102-107.

Iowa Intervention Project (2000). *Nursing interventions classification (NIC).* (J. C. McCloskey & G. M. Bulecheck, Eds.; 3rd ed.) St. Louis, MO: Mosby-Year Book.

Iowa Outcomes Project. (2000). *Nursing outcomes classification (NOC)* (M. Johnson, M. Maas, & S. Moorhead, Eds.; 2nd ed.). St. Louis, MO: Mosby-Year Book.

Kitzman, H., Olds, D. L., Henderson, C. R., Hanks, C., Cole, R., Tatelbaum, R., McConnochie, K. M., Sidora, K., Luckey, D. W., Shaver, D., Engelhardt, K., James, D., & Barnard, K. (1997). Effect of prenatal and infancy home visitation by nurses on pregnancy outcomes, childhood injuries and repeated childbearing: A randomized controlled trial. *Journal of the American Medical Association, 278*(8), 644-652.

North American Nursing Diagnosis Association. (1999). *Nursing diagnoses: Definitions and classification 1995-1996.* Philadelphia: Author.

Olds, D. L., Eckenrode, J., Henderson, C. R., Kitzman, H., Powers, J., Cole, R., Sidora, K., Morris, P., Pettitt, L. M., & Luckey, D. (1997). Long-term effects of home visitation on maternal life course and child abuse and neglect: Fifteen-year follow-up of a randomized trial. *Journal of the American Medical Association, 278*(8), 637-643.

Olds, D. L., Henderson, C. R., Tatelbaum, R., & Chamberlin, R. (1988). Improving the life-course development of socially disadvantaged mothers: A randomized trial of nurse home visitation. *American Journal of Public Health, 78*(11), 1436-1445.

Olds, D. L., & Kitzman, H. (1993). Review of research on home visiting for pregnant women and parents of young children. *Future of Children, 3*(3), 53-92.

Porter, L. S. (1984). Parenting enhancement among high-risk adolescents: Testing a holistic patient-centered nursing practice model. *Nursing Clinics of North America, 19,* 89-102.

Roosa, M. W., Fitzgerald, H. E., & Carlson, N. A. (1982). Teenage parenting and child development: A literature review. *Infant Mental Health Journal, 3,* 4-18.

U.S. Department of Health and Human Services. (1991). *Healthy people 2000: National health promotion and disease prevention objectives* (DHHS Publication No. PHS 91-50312). Washington, DC: Government Printing Office.

8

Developmental Care

Preterm Infant

Lou Ann Montgomery

Advances in neonatal care during recent decades have been made at a phenomenal pace. Today, it is possible to have survival of even the most fragile infant born at 24 weeks gestation, but the risk for neurodevelopmental impairment is high. An infant's response to any environment is affected by heredity, gestational maturity, illness status, and stress level (Robertson et al., 1996). These factors are not readily manipulated. The actual environment in which the infant receives care, however, the neonatal intensive care unit (NICU), can be manipulated and modified by the caregiver (Als, Lester, Tronick, & Brazelton, 1982). It includes people, light, sounds, handling practices, positioning, thermoregulation, and other aspects of the extrauterine environment (Graven, 1992). The caregiver with the most influence over this environment is the nurse (Jorgensen, 1996).

Care that promotes development, or Developmental Care, has evolved in the past decade as a standard of care for preterm infants (Merenstein, 1994). It is a philosophy that recognizes the complex interaction of the preterm infant with the environment and caregivers. It is a planned, consistent approach of care to optimize the infant's extrauterine growth and

119

development (Als et al., 1982). The goal is to maintain stability and ultimately enhance movement toward a more organized state in the preterm infant (McGrath & Conliffe-Torres, 1996). Developmental Care has been shown to dramatically reduce length of stay for preterm infants and enhance positive developmental outcomes (Als et al., 1986). It also reinforces a family-centered philosophy that integrates parents as equal partners in care. Including parents in Developmental Care can have a stunning empowerment effect on them and enhances the parent-infant bond (McGrath & Conliffe-Torres, 1996).

Developmental Care is designed for preterm infants ranging from approximately 24 weeks gestation to 40 weeks (term) gestation (Jorgensen, 1996). Its philosophy is in alignment with the goals of *Healthy People 2000* (U.S. Department of Health and Human Services [USDHHS], 1991). An important goal is the prevention of death and disability due to prematurity. Efforts to minimize risk of developmental delay and long-term disabilities will enhance infant health and save health care dollars and other resources (Als, Lawhon, Duffy, Gibes-Grossman, & Blickman, 1994; Buehler, Als, Duffy, McAnulty, & Liederman, 1995; Fleisher et al., 1995).

LITERATURE REVIEW

Knowledge of intrauterine development helps the nurse and other caregivers appreciate the level of physiological, sensory, and behavioral organization present for any preterm infant at a particular gestational age. In addition, it serves as a baseline for comparison for what is demonstrated by the infant during interactions with the environment and caregivers.

Fetal Development

Fetal development is driven by a process of genetically influenced differentiation, organization, and development. Environmental influences, however, such as teratogenic exposure or substances, can interfere with the progression. Although critical periods occur in fetal development of animal species, it is unclear whether such periods exist for human beings (Graven, 1996). There is a sequential development of the sensory system in utero that continues into neonatal life. The somatosensory, vestibular, and chemosensory systems show a degree of function and organization that allows for recall recognition early in brain development. They operate at the brain stem and basal ganglion level. Tactile reception is necessary to allow for intake and processing of information to the sensory system (Jorgensen, 1996). The somatosensory system, present at 20 weeks gestation, includes touch, pressure sensitivity, and pain, with particular focus on the palms of the hand, soles of the feet, and mouth and nasal areas (Graven, 1996; Jorgensen, 1996).

The chemosensory systems, including the gustatory and olfactory senses, are present before 24 weeks gestation (Graven, 1996). Suck, swallow, and breathing-like actions are detectable in utero at 15 to 17 weeks gestation and perhaps are used as a calming measure by the fetus. Sucking pressure and effectiveness vary with weight, gestational age, and illness state. At 26 to 28 weeks gestation, there is withdrawal from bitter tastes. At 35 weeks gestation, there is identification of the taste of glucose. Synchronization of all sucking activities does not occur in an organized, purposeful fashion until nearly 33 weeks gestation, when responses are more stable and comparable to those of term infants (Jorgensen, 1996).

The development of the auditory system occurs in relation to and in sequence with other sensory modalities (Robertson et al., 1996). In utero, sounds are rhythmic and continuous at approximately 72 decibels. Hearing and habituation to sounds can occur in utero. By 24 weeks gestation, the auditory apparatus is structurally intact and functional. By 25 to 27 weeks gestation, the auditory system is able to receive vibrations and sense stimulation in a manner that can result in physiological changes detected in heart rate, blood pressure, and other parameters (Graven, 1996; Jorgensen, 1996; Robertson et al., 1996). There is the ability to hear moderately low frequencies. Extremely high or low frequencies are not heard until later in gestation (Robertson et al., 1996). Auditory stimulation can be perceived by 32 weeks gestation with a memory created on the cortex (Graven, 1996).

The vestibular system, which mediates balance, is functional by 21 weeks gestation (Jorgensen, 1996). Flotation in utero promotes stimulation of the inner ear in preparation for future balance (Bozynski et al., 1996). The fetus interprets that being in a position horizontal to the uterine floor suggests sleep and being in a position vertical to the uterine floor suggests interaction (Jorgensen, 1996).

The visual system is the last sensory system to be developed. There is probably little visual stimulation of the fetus in utero. The fetal brain, however, creates an endogenous, although immature, stimulation to the visual cortex by 22 or 23 weeks gestation during rapid eye movement (REM) sleep (Graven, 1996). At 24 to 26 weeks gestation, there is a visual path but no pupil reflex. Response to light is primitive. At 30 to 34 weeks gestation, the iris sphincter becomes functional (Blackburn et al., 1996; Jorgensen, 1996). Bright light results in eyelid closure. Spontaneous eye opening occurs. Primitive attention and fixation are possible (Blackburn et al., 1996; Graven, 1996). By 36 weeks gestation, the infant is less myopic. If born at this time, the infant will be able to see best from a distance of 8 to 10 inches while looking at black-and-white contrast, a face, or a simple pattern (Blackburn et al., 1996; Jorgensen, 1996).

There are other related physical features of the preterm infant that affect sensory and neurodevelopmental response. Autonomic nervous system maturity is necessary for homeostatic effect. Sympathetic nervous system function is seen only after 32 weeks gestation, but will gradually mature as the infant nears 36 to 40 weeks gestation. Parasympathetic nervous system function also should be functional at this time and is possibly more mature than sympathetic function (White-Traut, Nelson, Burns, & Cunningham, 1994).

There is sequential development of tone. In utero, the fetus floats and is eventually held tight predominantly in a flexed position with hands brought to midline and near the face, often with thumb in mouth. Once birth occurs, the uterus is no longer present to maintain this nesting position. The infant born prematurely at 28 weeks gestation displays complete hypotonia with poor flexion capabilities. Hips and knees begin to show some flexion at 32 weeks gestation, although the rest of the body will remain in extension. Flexor tone appears in the legs by 34 weeks of gestation. There is loose flexion of arms and legs and early grasp development seen at 36 weeks gestation. By 40 weeks gestation, flexion is mature and is the preferred position of the infant. Reflex activities and maturity in the central nervous system help the infant practice extension (Gardner, Garland, Merenstein, & Lubchenko, 1993). Without uterine containment, the preterm infant is prone to the effects of gravity and immature tone. Deformities of the cranium, neck muscles, shoulder muscles, scapula, extremities, and feet may occur (Bozynski et al., 1996) (see Chapter 11, this volume). Improper unsupported positioning can also affect sleep, cardiovascular response, gas exchange, and feeding tolerance.

The Influence of a Premature Birth

Because there is such rapid growth of the brain and nervous system between 25 and 40 weeks gestation, premature birth can disrupt emerging organization (Graven, 1992). Infants born prior to 35 weeks gestation are forced to maintain a higher level of arousal and neurological activity than was required in utero to support basic physiological and sensorial systems. The impact is probably best described as an inverse relationship: The earlier the gestational age at birth, the more difficulty the infant will have attaining an organized state because of immature development the and energy expenditure required. Illnesses, such as respiratory distress syndrome, and the stress of the neonatal environment deplete the infant's reserve even more. The NICU environment can be sensory depriving, sensory overstimulating, or lacking contingent timing in caregiving (Kitchin & Hutchinson, 1996; McGrath & Conliffe-Torres, 1996).

There are no established safe levels of sound and vibration exposure for preterm infants (Robertson et al., 1996). Regular nursery care activities occur in approximately the 50- to 70-decibel range and can be exacerbated during crisis events (DePaul & Chambers, 1994). Preterm infants, however, can experience physiological and state changes as a result of inappropriate sound levels. Their stress response is one of increased secretion of serum adrenaline, cortisol, and ACTH; decreased secretion of growth hormone; and suppressed function of lymphocytes and altered inflammatory response (McCarthy, Ouimet, & Daun, 1991). The increased frequency of hearing loss in the preterm infant may or may not be due to response to sound. There is no direct evidence that links isolated environmental sounds to poor developmental outcomes or that the addition of sounds to the environment enhances development (Robertson et al., 1996).

Continuous light, often found in NICUs, can be detrimental to the preterm infant who has immature visual function and autonomic and central nervous system-response (Blackburn et al., 1996). It can lead to sleep deprivation, endocrine changes, and variations in biological and circadian rhythms. Other maladaptive responses may include apnea, bradycardia, desaturation, hypoxemia, color changes, perfusion changes, change in tone, feeding intolerance, irritability, inability to habituate, aversion behavior, and risk for retinopathy of prematurity (Glass, 1994).

There has been much concern that infants in NICUs receive little time to sleep due to overstimulation from the environment and caregivers. Studies have documented that infants may be disturbed, especially by the nursing staff, numerous times each day for as long as 1 hour at a time, whereas they receive only a few minutes per hour of "true care." Although considered "routine care," these interruptions may cause cold stress, increased metabolic demands, hypoxemia, metabolic acidosis, decreased glucose stores, and decreased pH (Ariagno et al., 1996).

The Organized Infant

Organization is a process integrating parts into a systematic and related whole (D'Apolito, 1991). For the preterm infant, integration between the physiological and behavioral systems must occur. Regulation through homeostatic processes and increasing competence of the infant leads to the goal of organization.

Researchers have helped neonatal health care providers recognize the necessity of assessing and monitoring the abilities and responses of the preterm infant prior to any intervention to avoid disorganization and stress. Early work in the area of Developmental Care was done by T. Berry Brazelton. His assessment tool, the Neonatal Behavioral Assessment Scale (NBAS), used mostly with near-term and term infants, examines the infant's entire well-being and interaction process (Brazelton, 1984). The NBAS assesses the behavioral capabilities of newborns to assist parents and caregivers to become better acquainted with the infant, promote interaction, and improve family functioning. The examiner is responsible for eliciting optimal behavior from the infant through specific interactions. NBAS activities are used as graded sequences of increasingly demanding environmental input, starting with the infant in a sleep state and advancing to full alertness. By assessing the infant's approach or avoidance response, the examiner determines how much structure and facilitation the infant requires.

Heidelise Als, a colleague of Brazelton, developed the synactive theory of infant behavior, which postulates that there is a focus on a dynamic, continuous interaction and feedback among the various subsystems within the organism (Als, 1986). The organism is the preterm infant, and the subsystems involved are the autonomic nervous, motor, state organization, attention-interaction, and self-regulatory systems. While following a gestational development plan, the infant is also trying to adapt to each change and develop more competence at that level. Developmentally appropriate environmental interventions support this process. The Assessment of Preterm Infant Behavior (APIB) was developed by Als as a refinement and extension of the NBAS to assess well and at-risk infants up until 36 weeks gestation. APIB activities allow for scoring of responses that identify differentiation and modulation for each of the subsystems before, during, and after examiner facilitation (Als et al., 1982). An infant's behavior and reactions can also be assessed by observation only (Als, 1984, 1995). The Naturalistic Observation of Newborn Behavior (NONB) facilitates the recording of infant behavior and reactions observed during a 60- to 80-minute period of time prior to, during, and after care is given to the infant. Information obtained from the APIB or NONB serves as the basis for recommendations to adjust the environment and caregiving practices to meet the infant's needs and abilities. Outcomes of the effectiveness of interactions can be measured and further refined, stopped, or continued during future interaction times. This approach is known as the Newborn Individualized Developmental Care and Assessment Program (NIDCAP) (Als, 1995). The use of a NIDCAP-based developmental program has been found in single and replicated studies to improve infant outcomes, decrease length of stay and cost of care, and promote favorable parent responses to their infant (Als, 1994; Als et al., 1986, 1994; Buehler et al., 1995; Fleisher et al., 1995).

TABLE 8.1   Risk Factors for the Organized Infant

Prenatal	*Postnatal*	*Individual*	*Caregiver*	*Environmental*
Congenital/genetic disorders	Premature delivery	Gestational age	Cue misreading	Sensory deprivation
Teratogenic exposure	Malnutrition	Postconceptual age	Cue knowledge deficit	Sensory overstimulation
	Feeding intolerance	Immature neurological system	Environmental stimulation	Sensory inappropriateness
	Oral/motor problems	Illness		Physical environmental inappropriateness
	Pain			
	Invasive procedures			

SOURCES: Als et al. (1994), D'Apolito (1991), Lawhon and Melzer (1988), and the National Association of Neonatal Nurses (1993).

NURSING DIAGNOSIS AND OUTCOME DETERMINATION

The nursing diagnosis for Developmental Care is *Disorganized Infant Behavior* (North American Nursing Diagnosis Association [NANDA], 1994), defined as "alteration in integration and modulation of the physiological and behavioral systems of functioning (i.e., autonomic, motor, state, organization, self-regulatory, and attentional-interactional systems)" (p. 71). Variations of this diagnosis are Risk for Disorganized Infant Behavior and Potential for Enhanced Organized Infant Behavior.

To establish if the nursing diagnosis Disorganized Infant Behavior is appropriate, an assessment of the preterm infant must be done. First, risk factors present should be determined. There are five categories of risk factors: prenatal, postnatal, individual, caregiver, and environmental factors (Table 8.1).

Second, the caregiver must assess the infant's baseline response to stimuli in the environment. Once these features are identified, they can be compared to defining characteristics of the diagnosis to determine if the infant is organized or disorganized (Table 8.2).

The most commonly used instruments to perform the assessment are the NBAS and APIB (Als et al., 1982; Brazelton, 1984). For the preterm infant, the APIB is more specific and the preferred tool for measuring

TABLE 8.2   Signs and Symptoms of the Organized and Disorganized Infant Behavior System

Organized Infant	Disorganized Infant
Physiological/autonomic system (comparison to baseline)	
Heart rate: stable to baseline	Heart rate: bradycardia, tachycardia, and arrhythmia
Respiratory rate: stable to baseline	Respiratory rate: bradypnea, tachypnea, and apnea
Color: pink	Color: pale, cyanotic, mottled, and flushed
Oxygen saturation: 85%-95%	Oxygen saturation: below desired limits
Feedings: tolerated with minimal aspirate	Feedings: aspirates and emesis
Time-out signals: individualized	Time-out signals: gazes, grasps, hiccoughs, coughs, sneezes, yawns, sighs, slack jaw, open mouth, and tongue thrust
Motor system	
Tone: balanced	Tone: increased, decreased, or limp
Movement: smooth, synchronous, and spontaneous	Movement: tremor, startle, twitches, jitteriness, jerkiness, and uncoordinated movements
Posture: flexed with hands to mouth	Posture: hyperextension, finger splay, fisting, hand to face, and altered primitive reflexes
State-organization system	
Deep sleep: near still with occasional suck or twitch, smooth regular breathing, and ability to arouse to intense stimuli	Deep and light sleep and drowsy: diffuse and oscillating
Light sleep: some activity, with REM eye flutter, closed lids, brief smiles/cries/fussiness, irregular breathing, and some response to stimuli	

avoidance and aversion responses (Als et al., 1982). If an infant cannot tolerate direct hands-on assessment, however, the NONB is preferred (Als, 1984, 1995). Use of the NBAS and APIB requires that the examiner be certified in the use of the instrument to ensure reliability and interpretability.

The goal of Developmental Care is to provide adaptation to the extrauterine environment for the infant born prior to full term of 40 weeks (term) gestation. A Developmental Care outcome Preterm Infant Organization has been accepted for inclusion in the next edition of the *Nursing Outcomes Classification* (Iowa Outcomes Project, 1997). Infant status is evaluated on a 5-point continuum that includes extreme instability, substantial instability, moderate instability, mild instability, and the ultimate goal of stability. There are five categories of indicators, each with several subindicators, that compliment the signs and symptoms of the diagnosis: physiological status, motor status, state status, regulatory status, and attention-interaction status (Table 8.3).

TABLE 8.2 *Continued*

Organized Infant	Disorganized Infant
Drowsy state: variable activity with mild startles, occasional eye opening and closing, heavy eyelids, dull-glazed appearance, still face, irregular breathing pattern, and delayed or changing response to stimuli	
Quiet-alert state: minimal activity, bright and wide eyes, bright/shiny/sparkling face, regular breathing, and attention toward most stimuli	Quiet-alert state: stare-and-display gaze aversion
Active-alert state: fussy with increased activity, open but less bright eyes, some facial brightness, irregular breathing, and increased sensitivity to stimuli	Active-alert state: fussy with a worried gaze
Crying state: increased motor activity, color changes, closed or open eyes, facial grimace, more irregular breathing pattern, and increased response to unpleasant or intense external and internal stimuli	Crying state: irritable or panicky
Regulatory system	
Sucks on fingers, brings hands to face, displays extremity anchoring, pays attention to voices and faces, changes position as needed, and alert for intake of the surroundings	Irritable and unable to inhibit
Attention-interaction system	
Alert and available for interaction with environment	Difficult to soothe and unable to sustain alert state

SOURCES: Blackburn and VandenBerg (1993), D'Apolito (1991), and the National Association of Neonatal Nurses (1993).

INTERVENTION: DEVELOPMENTAL CARE

Developmental Care for the preterm infant is the process of structuring the environment and providing care in response to behavioral cues and states of the preterm infant (Blackburn & VandenBerg, 1993). Nurses have a responsibility to therapeutically manipulate the environment for the infant who cannot do so alone. I have developed the intervention, Developmental Care: Preterm Infant, from a synthesis of the literature in the area (Table 8.4). This intervention has been accepted for inclusion in the next edition of the *Nursing Interventions Classification* (Iowa Intervention Project, 2000).

Prior to implementation, the nurse selects an assessment tool, such as the APIB or NONB, to determine the infant's cue for readiness to participate in the intervention, realizing that there may be variation even within a gestational age.

TABLE 8.4   Developmental Care: Preterm Infant

Definition

Structuring the environment and providing care in response to the behavioral cues and states of the preterm infant

Activities

Create a therapeutic and supportive relationship with parents.

Provide space for parents on unit and at infant's bedside.

Provide parents with accurate, factual information regarding the infant's condition, treatment, and needs.

Inform parents about developmental concerns and issues of preterm infants.

Assist parents in becoming acquainted with their infant in a comfortable, nonhurried environment.

Teach parents to recognize infant cues and states.

Demonstrate infant capabilities to parents when administering the APIB scale or other neurobehavioral observation tools.

Demonstrate how to elicit infant's visual or auditory attention.

Assist parents in planning care in response to infant cues and states.

Point out infant's self-regulatory activities (e.g., hand to mouth, sucking, and use of visual or auditory stimulus).

Provide "time out" when infant exhibits signs of stress (e.g., finger splaying, poor color, lowered state, and fluctuation of heart and respiratory rate).

Teach parent how to console infant using behavioral quieting techniques (e.g., hand on infant, positioning, and swaddling).

Develop individualized developmental plan for each infant and update regularly.

Avoid overstimulation by stimulating one sense at a time (e.g., avoid talking while handling and avoid looking at while feeding).

Assist parents to have realistic expectations for infant's behavior and development.

Provide boundaries that maintain flexion of extremities while still allowing room for extension (e.g., nesting, swaddling, bunting, hammock, hat, and clothing).

Provide supports to maintain positioning and prevent deformities (e.g., back rolls, nesting, bunting, and head donuts).

Reposition infant frequently.

Provide water pillow and sheepskin as appropriate.

Use smallest diaper to prevent hip abduction.

Monitor stimuli (light, noise, handling, and procedures) in infant's environment and reduce as appropriate.

Decrease environmental ambient light.

therapeutic touch can be soothed to sleep and experience less motor distress (Harrison, Olivet, Cunningham, Bodin, & Hicks, 1996).

Vestibular

To promote vestibular function, water mattresses or pillows can be provided as tolerated (Hemingway & Oliver, 1991). The infant should be held horizontally for sleep and vertically for interaction or Kangaroo Care (Barb & Lemons, 1989; Luddington-Hoe et al., 1991). Overstimulation should be avoided so as not to create a perception of vertigo for the infant.

TABLE 8.4   *Continued*

Activities (continued)

  Shield eyes of infant when using light with high foot-candles.
  Alter environmental lighting to provide diurnal rhythmicity.
  Decrease environmental noise (e.g., turn down and respond quickly to monitor alarms
       and telephones and move conversation away from bedside).
  Position incubator away from source of noise (sinks, doors, telephone, high activity,
       radio, and traffic pattern).
  Time infant care and feeding around sleep-wake cycle.
  Gather and prepare equipment used (for care) away from bedside.
  Cluster care to promote the longest possible sleep interval and energy conservation.
  Provide comfortable chair in quiet area for feeding.
  Use slow, gentle movements when handing, feeding, or caring for infant.
  Feed infant without looking at or talking to the infant if these overstimulate infant.
  Position and support through feeding maintaining flexion and midline position
       (shoulder and truncal support, foot bracing, hand holding, use of bunting, and
       swaddling).
  Feed in upright position to promote tongue extension and swallowing.
  Promote parent participation in feeding.
  Support breast-feeding if mother desires.
  Use a pacifier for nonnutritive sucking in feeding via gavage and between feedings as
       appropriate.
  Provide quiet environment after feeding to avoid gagging, hiccoughs, spitting, and
       aspiration.
  Facilitate state transition and calming during painful and stressful but necessary
       procedures.
  Establish consistent and predictable routines to promote regular sleep-wake cycles.
  Provide stimulation using tape-recorded instrumental music, mobiles, massage,
       rocking, and touch as appropriate.

Gustatory and Olfactory

The preterm infant can be offered small tastes of breast milk to the lips (Jorgensen, 1996). Oral care can be provided with sweet-flavored swabs dipped in sterile water. Promotion of close proximity of the parent to the infant, especially in the first week of life when olfactory sensation is high, is desirable (Barb & Lemons, 1989). At this time, the infant can be positioned near the odor of breast milk on the breast of the mother, her breast pad, or cotton-tipped applicator dipped in breast milk.

Auditory

Ideally, the noise in the extrauterine environment should simulate that heard in utero. Music therapy is a growing area of interest as researchers find that, when used properly, music can have an immediate organization response in the preterm infant. Audiotapes of placental sounds (swishes), alone or blended with soothing instrumental lullabies, are often used in nurseries. Some nurseries also encourage parents and family members to audiotape their voices for the infant to hear (Barb & Lemons, 1989; Jorgensen, 1996). Preterm infants must learn to habituate much of the stimuli heard in the environment as a survival tactic. Much effort has gone into monitoring and decreasing noise levels in nurseries. Targeted areas include monitor alarms, human conversation, sinks, doors, telephones, high staff activity and procedure areas, traffic areas, and bedside equipment (DePaul & Chambers, 1994). If the infant's bed cannot be moved or shielded from such areas, nurseries have used earmuffs, quiet hour, acoustical furnishings, wall separators, plastic bins and cupboards, and bed padding to decrease or absorb noise (DePaul & Chambers, 1994; Staunch, Brandt, & Edwards-Beckett, 1993; Zahr & de Traversay, 1995).

Visual

It is essential to monitor light. Environmental ambient light should be decreased. Eyes of infants less than 30 to 34 weeks gestation should be shielded from light with high foot-candles because of their immature iris sphincter control (Blackburn et al., 1996; Jorgensen, 1996). Incubators and warmer beds may be covered with dark quilts or blankets in a manner that shields light but allows for safe visualization. Environmental light can be altered to provide diurnal rhythmicity (Treas, 1993). Mobiles and other visual effects placed 8 to 10 inches away with black and white contrasts, faces, or patterned figures are most appropriate (Graven, 1996).

Physiologically Directed

Respiratory and Circulatory States

A variety of activities should be used in unison to provide support (Jorgensen, 1996), including clustering care to promote the longest possible sleep intervals and conservation of energy; establishing consistent and predictable routines to promote regular sleep-wake cycles; providing "time out" when the infant exhibits signs of stress (e.g., finger splaying, poor color, and fluctuation in heart and respiratory rate); and facilitating state transition and calming during painful and stressful but necessary procedures.

Gastrointestinal

A quiet-awake state promotes the most successful feeding experience and uses the least energy for physiological maintenance (VandenBerg, 1999). Nonnutritive sucking and breast-feeding should be supported if desired (see Chapters 5 and 9, this volume). Comfortable chairs for both parents should be located in a quiet area for feeding. Quiet conditions minimize gagging, hiccoughs, spitting, and aspiration.

Dermatological

Preterm infants differ from term infants in development of the stratum corneum (Siegfried, 1996). In preterm infants, it is much thinner, does not prevent transepidermal water loss or absorption of topical agents, and is easily injured. Therefore, it must be treated cautiously. Karaya-based products and other skin barriers that are not readily absorbed by the skin should be used. Products should be removed carefully with water; rarely is it necessary to use chemical-based removers, which may be topically absorbed. Care is taken not to remove tissue layers by limiting baths to once or twice a week or as needed. Soap is used sparingly.

INTERVENTION APPLICATION

Amy M. was born at 28 weeks gestation to Mrs. M., a gravida one, now para one, African American married female. Mrs. M. received prenatal care starting at the 6th week of pregnancy. Her pregnancy history was significant for the onset of preeclampsia diagnosed during her routine prenatal visit at the 27th week of pregnancy. On diagnosis, she was admitted to the antenatal high-risk unit in a tertiary care center. That day, she and Mr. M. spoke at length to the attending neonatologist of the NICU regarding predicted outcomes for an infant born at this and older gestations. The NICU charge nurse toured them through the unit, showing them equipment used in the nurseries, introducing them to staff they might meet in the future, and discussing care in the NICU.

Mrs. M. required bedrest and a magnesium sulfate infusion on the second day of her admission. A lactation consultant offered her information about breast pumping, routine use of colostrum for early feedings of preterm infants, and reserving an electric breast pump. Mr. M. was pleased to learn from the developmental care specialist that he could participate in Kangaroo Care with his infant. A volunteer from the NICU parent support group offered his support and assistance, promised to visit every few days, and left his parent support pager number in case they wanted to talk with him. After these contacts, both parents felt reassured that, even though they did not have a medical background, they had a very important role to play in their infant's birth, delivery, and possible stay in the NICU.

Mrs. M. delivered a baby girl at 28 weeks gestation. She received β-methasone within a day of the delivery to enhance the baby's lung maturation. Baby Amy had Apgar scores of 5 and 7. She weighed 1000 grams and was a ruddy-tan color, long, thin, with thick black hair and lanugo and dark black eyes. She required nasal pharyngeal continuous positive airway pressure after delivery and was transferred by incubator to the NICU. The nursing diagnosis Risk for Disorganized Infant was made due to Amy's premature birth (NANDA, 1999). Mr. M. came to visit immediately and took instant photos and videotapes of Amy for his wife. He also assisted Amy's nurse in taking footprints and handprints and snipping a lock of her hair for her baby book. The nurse explained that Amy would need to have intravenous lines put in during the next hour and then would be provided clustered care.

The next day, when Mrs. M. was feeling better, she began to pump her breasts to collect milk for Amy. The lactation consultant and a parent volunteer mother were of great assistance in helping her use the equipment properly, feel relaxed while using the pump, and store the milk properly.

When Mrs. M. visited Amy for the first time with Mr. M., Amy's nurse gave them her progress update, explained about equipment in use, and encouraged them to participate in Amy's care. Mr. and Mrs. M. sat in comfortable chairs that allowed them close proximity to Amy. The developmental specialist repeated some of Amy's APIB assessment for them. She showed them how Amy opened her eyes if they cupped their hand above Amy's brow. Amy liked to be nested in a bunting. Mrs. M. helped tuck the bunting ties around Amy. The developmental specialist showed them how Amy settled into a quiet state when touched with palms of hands lightly on her head and thighs. The parents were excited to learn this and looked forward to identifying other cues from Amy that could guide their interaction with her. They noticed the lights were dimmed and brightened in the nursery to match night and day hours. During nursery quiet time, they tried to visit and kangaroo with Amy. They identified that, after Kangaroo Care, Amy liked to return to bed positioned in a head donut for 30 minutes, followed by the flexed prone position for sleep until her next feeding. Her feedings started out as 1 ml of colostrum every 8 hours but soon advanced to continuous drip, bolus, and then nonnutritive times at breast. At about 2 or 3 weeks of age, Amy's suck was strong enough to be able to suck on a pacifier during her tube feedings. The parents also helped the staff provide visual stimulation for Amy. Initially, they chose a black-and-white patterned bumper pad from the unit toy-lending library. Later, they selected a mobile in primary colors and a bright red jingle ball. Amy's skin remained intact during her stay. Karaya-based products were used starting at admission. Her first bath did not occur until several days after her birth. Water and a small amount of dermatologically recommended soap were used. Soon, her parents did her routine baths once or twice a week. Amy's progress was monitored by the outcome Premature Infant Organization, which includes indicators on physiological measures and infant state as well as observations on interaction with caregiver (Iowa Outcomes Project, 2000). Soon, Amy was transferred to the transitional nursery, where she began nutritive breast-feeding and began to grow stronger in preparation to be discharged.

RESEARCH AND PRACTICE IMPLICATIONS

Future studies should continue to focus on Developmental Care assessment tools and activity. More studies should focus on the use of the APIB or other instruments as assessment tools. More knowledge is needed about the outcomes of Developmental Care for different gestations and populations. The effects of Developmental Care on the long-term development of the child should be studied. In addition, studies focusing on its effects on parenting abilities and parent-infant attachment are needed. As length of stay decreases and more care is provided at home, there will be a need to know how family home life is affected and how nurses can provide home activities and ongoing support.

Developmental Care is applicable to the entire prenatal, perinatal, and postnatal experience. Today, pregnancies are diagnosed early and parents often seek prenatal instruction and anticipatory guidance about medical care that can be expected with the birth. Developmental Care activities can be introduced prenatally to give parents information that may help support and empower them during the NICU stay. Developmental Care concepts need to be integrated in other pediatric areas caring for preterm infants and neonates in inpatient, outpatient, and home care settings.

Developmental Care promotes parent and family involvement in their infant's care. Family-centered care and Developmental Care may in fact be inseparable. Developmental Care is cost-effective, and outcomes appear promising for promoting better preterm infant development. It will save health care dollars by lessening disabilities and improving parenting skills. Developmental Care also helps in attaining the goal of *Healthy People 2000* (USDHHS, 1991)—the prevention of early death and disability. Nurseries that do not practice this type of care will be accountable for explaining to consumers why they do not and challenged to do their own studies to disprove its efficacy (Merenstein, 1994).

ment program in perinaFoundation/March of Dimes.## REFERENCES

Als, H. (1984). *Manual for the naturalistic observation of newborn behavior (preterm and term infants)*. Boston: Children's Hospital.

Als, H. (1986). A synactive model of neonatal behavioral organization: Framework for the assessment of neurobehavior in the premature infant for support of infants and parents in the neonatal intensive care environment. *Physical and Occupational Therapy in Pediatrics, 6*, 3-53.

Als, H. (1994, October). *Medical, neurobehavioral and family outcome at 2 weeks post-term of a multisite NICU trial of developmental care* [Research abstract]. 5th Annual NIDCAP Trainer's Meeting, Boston.

Als, H. (1995). *NIDCAP guide—Revised*. Boston: Harvard Medical School.

Als, H., Lawhon, G., Brown, E., Gibes, R., Duffy, F. H., McAnulty, G. B., & Blickman, J. G. (1986). Individualized behavioral and environmental care for the very low birth weight preterm infant at high risk for BPD: NICU and developmental outcomes. *Pediatrics, 78*(6), 1123-1132.

Als, H., Lawhon, G., Duffy, F. H., Gibes-Grossman, R., & Blickman, J. G. (1994). Infant developmental care for the very low birth weight premature infant. *Journal of the American Medical Association, 272*(11), 853-858.

Als, H., Lester, B. M., Tronick, E. Z., & Brazelton, T. B. (1982). Manual for the assessment of preterm infant behavior APIB. *Theory and Research in Behavioral Pediatrics, 1*, 65-132.

Ariagno, R., Anders, T., Evans, J., Frank, M., Holditch-Davis, D., Schechtman, V., & Scher, M. (1996). Sleep/deprivation group: Study results. In *Proceedings of the physical and developmental environment of the high risk infant* (pp. 78-79). Tampa: University of South Florida.

Barb, S. A., & Lemons, P. K. (1989). The premature infant: Toward improving neurodevelopmental outcome. *Neonatal Network, 7*(6), 7-14.

Blackburn, S. T., (1978). State-related behaviors and individual differences. In K. E. Barnard (Ed.), *Early parent-infant relationships—Module 3. A staff development program in perinatal nursing* (pp. 22-32). Washington, DC: The National Foundation/March of Dimes.

Blackburn, S. T., Glass, P., Keenan, W., Lotas, M., Reynolds, J., Sliney, D., & Wyble, L. (1996). Light studies: Group findings. In *Proceedings of the physical and developmental environment of the high risk infant* (pp. 62-65). Tampa: University of South Florida.

Blackburn, S. T., & VandenBerg, K. A. (1993). Assessment and management of neonatal neurobehavioral development. In C. Kenner, A. Brueggenmeyer, & L. P. Gunderson (Eds.), *Comprehensive neonatal nursing: A physiological perspective* (pp. 1094-1123). Philadelphia: W. B. Saunders.

Bozynski, M. E., Brown, J. V., Carlo, W., Darnall, R., Derriggui, P., Dulock, H., & Fernbach, S. A. (1996). Position and motion studies: Group findings. In *Proceedings of the physical and developmental environment of the high risk infant* (pp. 75-77). Tampa: University of South Florida.

Brazelton, T. B. (1984). *The neonatal behavioral assessment scale* (2nd ed.). Philadelphia: J. B. Lippincott.

Buehler, D. M., Als, H., Duffy, F. H., McAnulty, G. B., & Liederman, J. (1995). Effectiveness of individualized developmental care for low-risk preterm infants: Behavioral and electrophysiologic evidence. *Pediatrics, 96,* 923-932.

D'Apolito, K. (1991). What is an organized infant? *Neonatal Network, 2,* 23-29.

DePaul, D., & Chambers, S. E. (1994). Environmental noise in the newborn intensive care unit: Implications for nursing practice. *Journal of Perinatal and Neonatal Nursing, 8*(4), 71-76.

Fleisher, B. E., VanderBerg, K., Constantinow, J., Heller, C., Benitz, W. E., Johnson, A., Rosenthal, A., & Stevenson, D. K. (1995). Individualized developmental care for very low birth weight infants. *Clinical Pediatrics, 34,* 523-529.

Gardner, S. L., Garland, K. R., Merenstein, S. L., & Lubchenko, L. O. (1993). The neonate and the environment: Impact on development. In G. B. Merenstein & S. L. Gardner (Eds.), *Handbook of neonatal intensive care* (3rd ed., pp. 564-608). St. Louis, MO: C. V. Mosby.

Glass, P. (1994). The vulnerable neonate and neonatal intensive care environment. In G. B. Avery, M. A. Fletcher, & M. G. McDonald (Eds.), *Neonatology: Pathophysiology and management of the newborn* (4th ed., pp. 77-94). Philadelphia: J. B. Lippincott.

Graven, S. N. (Ed.). (1992). The high risk infant environment, Part 2—The role of caregiving: The social environment. *Journal of Perinatology, 12*(3), 267-275.

Graven, S. N. (1996). Concepts of fetal sensory development. In *Proceedings of the physical and developmental environment of the high risk infant* (pp. 56-61). Tampa: University of South Florida.

Harrison, L., Olivet, L., Cunningham, K., Bodin, M. B., & Hicks, C. (1996). Effects of gentle human touch on preterm infants: Pilot study results. *Neonatal Network, 15*(2), 35-42.

Hemingway, M. M., & Oliver, S. K. (1991). Waterbed therapy and cranial molding of the sick preterm infant. *Neonatal Network, 20*(3), 53-56.

Iowa Intervention Project. (2000). *Nursing interventions classification (NIC)* (J. C. McCloskey & G. M. Bulechek, Eds.; 3rd ed.). St. Louis, MO: Mosby-Year Book.

Iowa Outcomes Project. (2000). *Nursing outcomes classification (NOC)* (M. Johnson, M. Maas, & S. Moorhead, Eds.). St. Louis, MO: Mosby-Year Book.

Jorgensen, K. M. (1996, September). Developmental care of the newborn following delivery. In *Proceedings of the Cooperative Caregiving Conference* (unpaginated). Des Moines, IA: Blank Children's Hospital.

Kitchin, L. W., & Hutchinson, S. (1996). Touch during preterm infant resuscitation. *Neonatal Network, 15*(7), 45-51.

Lawhon, G., & Melzer, A. (1988). Developmental care of the very low birthweight infant. *Journal of Pediatric and Neonatal Nursing, 2,* 55-65.

Lehman, K. (1984, June). The toybrary concept: Expansion into the neonatal intensive care unit. *Neonatal Network,* 31-35.

Luddington-Hoe, S. M., Hadeed, G. C., & Anderson, G. C. (1991). Physiologic responses to skin-to-skin contact in hospitalized premature infants. *Neonatal Network, 11,* 19-24.

Lutes, L. (1996). Bedding twins/multiples together. *Neonatal Network, 15*(7), 61-62.

McCarthy, D. O., Ouimet, M. E., & Daun, J. M. (1991). Shades of Florence Nightingale: Potential impact of noise stress on wound healing. *Holistic Nursing Practice, 5*(4), 39-48.

McGrath, J. M., & Conliffe-Torres, S. (1996). Integrating family centered developmental assessment and interventions into routine care in the neonatal intensive care unit. *Nursing Clinics of North America, 31*(2), 367-385.

Merenstein, G. (1994). Commentary. *Journal of the American Medical Association, 272*(11), 890-891.

National Association of Neonatal Nurses. (1993). *Infant developmental care guidelines.* Petaluma, CA: Author.

North American Nursing Diagnosis Association. (1999). *Nursing diagnoses: Definitions and classification 1995-1996.* Philadelphia: Author.

Robertson, A., Bose, C., Engle, W. A., Hal, J., Karp, W., Martin, P., Philbin, M. K., Stockard, J., & Thomas, K. (1996). Sound studies: Group report. In *Proceedings of the physical and developmental environment of the high risk infant* (pp. 40-45). Tampa: University of South Florida.

Siegfried, E. C. (1996). Skin care and the high risk infant. In *Proceedings of the physical and developmental environment of the high risk infant* (pp. 108-129). Tampa: University of South Florida.

Staunch, C., Brandt, S., & Edwards-Beckett, J. (1993). Implementation of quiet hour: Effects on noise levels and infant sleep states. *Neonatal Network, 12*(2), 31-35.

Treas, L. S. (1993). Incubator covers: Health or hazard? *Neonatal Network, 12*(8), 50-51.

U.S. Department of Health and Human Services. (1991). *Healthy people 2000: National health promotion and disease prevention objectives* (DHHS Publication No. PHS 91-50312). Washington, DC: Government Printing Office.

VandenBerg, K. A. (1999). What to tell parents about the developmental needs of their baby at discharge. *Neonatal Network, 18,* 57-59.

White-Traut, R. C., Nelson, M. N., Burns, K., & Cunningham, W. (1994). Environmental influences on the development of the preterm infant: Theoretical issues and applications to practice. *Journal of Obstetric, Gynecologic and Neonatal Nursing, 23*(5), 393-401.

Zahr, L. K., & deTraversay, J. (1995). Premature infant responses to noise reduction by earmuffs: Effects on behavioral and physiologic measures. *Journal of Perinatology, 15*(5), 448-455.

9

Nonnutritive Sucking

Rita H. Pickler

Nonnutritive Sucking (NNS) is a nursing intervention that may assist the preterm infant in achieving physiologic homeostasis and behavior state modulation. It involves the ability to achieve and maintain healthy behavior states and to make smoother transitions between states. Its benefits include improved physical growth, shorter transition from gavage to bottle feeding, and improved feeding performance outcomes (shorter time for feeding and greater formula intake) in preterm infants. It also promotes behavioral organization abilities, including a reduction of behavioral manifestations of stress, in preterm and term infants (Anderson, Burroughs, & Measel, 1983; Bernbaum, Pereira, Watkins, & Peckham, 1983; Campos, 1994; Field & Goldson, 1984; Pickler, Higgins, & Crummette, 1993). Nonnutritive Sucking is an inexpensive, simple-to-use intervention.

Nonnutritive Sucking, a nurse-initiated direct care intervention, is defined as the "provision of sucking opportunities for [the] infant who is gavage fed or who can receive nothing by mouth" (Iowa Intervention Project, 2000, p. 472). Nonnutritive sucking has been studied extensively as a mechanism for calming preterm and term infants as well as promoting the transition from gavage to oral feeding (Anderson et al., 1983; Campos, 1994). Thus, NNS may be more broadly defined as the provision of sucking opportunities for infants that may or may not be associated with food intake.

Although the research clearly supports the use of NNS as an intervention for hospitalized preterm infants both as a calming technique and as a mechanism to enhance feeding transitions, NNS can be viewed as an intervention for all infants. The research supports NNS as an intervention appropriate for term infants during episodes of stress, such as circumcisions or immunizations. Recent research suggests that there is an innate motivational drive for newborn mammals to suck nonnutritively (Rushen & DePassille, 1995). The act of sucking appears to increase the secretion of hormones, which have both digestive and behavior-calming effects.

THEORETICAL FRAMEWORK

The use of NNS as an intervention should be considered within the framework of the synactive theory of development (Als, 1979). Als's hierarchical model includes four interrelated subsystems: autonomic, motoric, behavior state, and attentional (interactive). As a fetus matures to birth and continues to develop during the early newborn period, these integrated subsystems, which are reflective of the integrity of the child's neurobehavioral development, become more differentiated and controlled.

The autonomic subsystem matures first, at approximately 28 weeks postconceptional age (PCA), and is seen in the infant's increased ability to maintain steady heart and respiratory rates and to better tolerate enteric feedings. At approximately 36 weeks PCA, motoric differentiation occurs. The infant is now able to maintain muscle tone and posture for longer periods and balance body movements between extension and flexion. The behavior state subsystem is the next to develop mature differentiation. At approximately 44 weeks PCA, a full range of robust behavior states, from deep sleep to full arousal, is exhibited. Moreover, clear transitions between states are noted. At approximately 3 months of age, the infant is ready to engage fully in regulating social interaction, now providing clear cues for engagement or aversion.

Preterm infants have immature functioning in these subsystems. Moreover, they are unable to balance behaviors among subsystems (Als, 1979). Thus, when stressed, fatigued, or handled for extended periods of time, the infant may become disorganized in all subsystems. This also may be true of term infants, although theoretically their threshold for disorganization is much higher. Nonnutritive sucking has demonstrated effectiveness at improving the autonomic functioning and motor and behavior organization in both preterm and term infants (DiPietro, Cusson, Caughy, & Fox, 1994).

LITERATURE REVIEW

The research on NNS has focused on physiologic (autonomic) and behavioral (activity and state) outcomes. These outcomes have been examined in preterm and term infants under both stressful and nonstressful conditions. In addition, the research has studied the use of NNS as an intervention to modulate the feeding experience of preterm infants.

Data show that NNS increases transcutaneous oxygen levels in preterm infants at rest (Burroughs, Asonye, Anderson, & Vidyasagar, 1978; Paludetto, Robertson, Hack, Shivpuri, & Martin, 1984) and during gavage feedings (Bernbaum, Pereira, & Peckham, 1982; Nading & Landes, 1984). These effects have also been demonstrated in term and preterm infants who experienced invasive procedures such as heelstick blood drawing (Campos, 1994; Treloar, 1994).

Nonnutritive sucking has also been shown to decrease heart rate in term and preterm infants (Campos, 1994; Woodson & Hamilton, 1986), thereby decreasing energy expenditure. In part, the decrease in heart rate associated with NNS is related to the effect of sucking on behavior state. Nonnutritive sucking also results in a reduction in crying in both preterm and term infants (Campos, 1994; Field & Goldson, 1984). In fact, NNS has been shown to result in reduced crying and decreased heart rate in intubated preterm infants who were undergoing intravenous catheter insertion (Miller & Anderson, 1993). Although behavioral stress and some autonomic responsiveness may be mediated by the use of NNS, cortisol levels (indicating adrenocortical response to stress) do not appear to be affected (Gunnar, Connors, Isensee, & Wall, 1988).

In addition to general effects on autonomic outcomes, NNS has been shown to decrease restlessness in term (Kessen & Leutzendorff, 1963) and preterm infants (Anderson et al., 1983). The behavior modulating effects of the intervention have long been known. Crying infants calm when given a pacifier by ceasing to cry and by decreasing body movements. This knowledge has led to many investigations about the modulating effect of NNS on the feeding experience of preterm infants. The earliest studies in this area documented the use of NNS with gavage feedings in preterm infants resulted in more rapid weight gain and earlier transition to bottle feeding (Bernbaum et al., 1983; Field et al., 1982; Measel & Anderson, 1979). Recently, researchers have documented that the provision of NNS during gavage feedings results in more modulated behavioral state activity (DiPietro et al., 1994).

Several researchers have found that the use of NNS prior to bottle feedings resulted in optimal, or quiet awake, behavior states being achieved before, during, and after the feedings (Gill, Behnke, Conlon, McNeely, & Anderson, 1988; McCain, 1995; Pickler et al., 1993; Pickler,

Frankel, Walsh, & Thompson, 1996). In addition, research has documented that the use of NNS prior to bottle feedings in preterm infants resulted in improved feeding performance with a greater percentage of the prescribed formula being taken during a shorter period of time (Pickler et al., 1993) and a more rapid onset of the first nutritive suck (Pickler et al., 1996).

The mechanisms by which NNS affects the neurobehavioral subsystems of the infant are unclear. Although the literature has suggested relationships between NNS and the release of gastric hormones and increased gastric motility, there is insufficient evidence to support the existence of such relationships. The literature has also failed to support claims that the effectiveness of NNS is related to direct improvement of cardiac or respiratory mechanisms. Rather, the evidence increasingly supports the hypothesis that NNS is effective because it assists the infant in achieving a modulated behavior state (McCain, 1995; Pickler et al., 1996). Thus, by helping the infant to quiet behaviorally, there is less reactivity in the interrelated autonomic and motoric subsystems. The infant is calmer and is therefore less likely to experience tachycardia or apnea. Theoretically, providing more opportunities for improved neurobehavioral organization results in more rapid growth and better modulated organic functioning such as feeding.

NURSING DIAGNOSIS AND OUTCOMES DETERMINATION

Direct-care, nurse-initiated interventions such as NNS should be used with appropriate nursing diagnoses. Moreover, expected outcomes should be measurable and patient focused.

Nursing Diagnoses

Several nursing diagnoses may be treated by the nursing intervention Nonnutritive Sucking. In particular, the diagnosis of Altered Growth and Development (North American Nursing Diagnosis Association [NANDA], 1999) may be appropriate for the preterm infant whose early birth precludes the expected pattern of infant development. As research has demonstrated, use of NNS may enhance the growth and the neurobehavioral development of peterm infants.

The diagnoses of Disorganized Infant Behavior, Risk for Disorganized Infant Behavior, and Potential for Enhanced Organized Infant Behavior may also be made for both preterm and term infants. Each of these diagnoses suggests a need for interventions designed to promote modulation of neurobehavioral functioning. As noted previously, NNS hypothetically makes its most important contribution to infant well-being in this area. Numerous health conditions, environmental stimulation, or caregiving activity can result in disorganization of the preterm or sick term infant's vulnerable neurobehavioral function. Use of NNS has demonstrated effectiveness in promoting a return to more organized behavior and in avoiding disorganized behavioral patterns (Field & Goldson, 1984; Treloar, 1994).

Many preterm infants may be diagnosed with Ineffective Infant Feeding Patterns. Again, the research increasingly supports the effectiveness of NNS in promoting more effective feeding patterns. This effectiveness is supported by data demonstrating more rapid weight gain and transition to bottle feedings in preterm infants provided NNS during gavage feedings. The intervention has also been shown to effectively promote optimal behavioral organization in preparation for and during bottle feedings.

Other diagnoses for which NNS might be an appropriate intervention include Sensory/Perceptual Alterations (gustatory) and Impaired Swallowing (NANDA, 1999). These diagnoses are made when an infant is unable to receive fluid through normal channels, either gavage or nipple. Problems with fluid and food intake also occur in the very sick infant who has cardiac, respiratory, or gastrointestinal impairment. In some cases—for example, when the infant must have portions of the bowel removed due to necrotizing enterocolitis—enteral feedings are withheld for extended periods. Infants with severe respiratory conditions, such as bronchopulmonary dysplasia, lack the energy required for nipple feeding. In these cases, the infant may receive no oral feedings. At first, these conditions present as alterations in sensory input; over time, however, the actual ability to swallow may become impaired. Although research does not support the use of NNS as an effective cure for these problems, research clearly supports the need of an infant to suck nonnutritively for developmental purposes.

Nurse-Sensitive Outcomes

Several nurse-sensitive outcomes may be used when NNS is employed. Management of pain level is an expected outcome when use is made of the pacifying effects of NNS. Although psychological comfort might be difficult to measure in infants, physical comfort can be demonstrated by reduction in heart rate, increased oxygenation, and more restful behavior states. Preterm Infant Organization Adaptation, a newly developed outcome described in Chapter 8, may also be useful when examining outcomes of NNS. Autonomic and behavioral stability are well-documented effects of the intervention.

Growth may also be an outcome associated with NNS (Iowa Outcomes Project, 1997). The most recent research suggests this outcome can be anticipated only if the intervention is used consistently over an extended period of time (DiPietro et al., 1994). Sleep is another expected outcome of NNS. Although NNS is useful in bringing preterm infants to alert wakefulness prior to bottle feeding, it is most often used to promote sleep in infants following caregiving activities. The effectiveness of the intervention when used in this way is well established (DiPietro et al., 1994; Pickler et al., 1993; Woodson, Drinkwin, & Hamilton, 1985).

INTERVENTION: NONNUTRITIVE SUCKING

Providing NNS to an infant involves the following activities: pacifier selection, positioning of infant, positioning the pacifier and monitoring its use, determination of timing and duration, and parental involvement.

Selection of an appropriate pacifier is essential. The pacifier needs to be long enough to stimulate a vagal response (Anderson et al., 1983). Moreover, the nurse should consider using a pacifier with a shape similar to the nipple used for bottle feedings. Although there is no literature documenting the actual occurrence of "nipple confusion," it is possible that an immature feeder, such as a preterm infant, may have difficulty adjusting to differing nipple shapes, even though the mechanisms of nutritive sucking are completely different from those of NNS.

Infants can be held or positioned in incubators during NNS. Preterm infants and infants with compromised respiratory status are best positioned in prone or side-lying positions. The right side-lying position has been cited as particularly beneficial during gavage feedings because this position promotes the flow of fluid by gravity through the gastrointestinal tract. Following stressful procedures, the addition of swaddling may enhance the calming benefits of NNS; holding the infant while offering NNS may also be useful to help the infant associate holding with comfort or feeding. Most infants need little encouragement to suck nonnutritively. Activities to promote sucking should be gentle and as noninvasive as possible. Pacifiers should never be taped in place or positioned in such a way that the infant cannot disengage with ease.

My research supports the timing of offering NNS before, during, and after gavage feedings. Moreover, most research findings suggest that infants should be allowed to suck nonnutritively until satiated—that is, until they disengage from the pacifier on their own. In addition, as the research demonstrates, NNS should be offered to preterm infants prior to bottle feedings to promote a more alert behavioral state in readiness for feeding. These infants also benefit from postfeeding NNS because the intervention is effective in helping the infant return more rapidly to a restful state. Infants offered NNS during routine or invasive caregiving procedures consistently demonstrate more modulated behavioral organization. The intervention is also appropriately offered to infants undergoing painful procedures, such as heelsticks, circumcisions, or immunizations. Although NNS does not replace appropriate pharmacologic pain management, the behavioral benefits of the intervention may augment the effectiveness of other pain management strategies.

Parents need clear explanations about the benefits of NNS. They need assistance in interpreting their infant's cues indicating a need for NNS. They also may be concerned about potential negative effects of pacifier use. Parents can be reassured that pacifier use in young infants poses little risk for dental caries or permanent tooth malalignment. Mothers who wish to breast-feed their infant may raise concerns about pacifier use. Currently, there is no research to support never offering a pacifier to an infant. Recent research findings, however, have implicated the use of pacifiers in earlier breast-feeding termination for full-term infants (Righard & Alade, 1997). An individualized approach involving assessment of the infant's ability to adapt to differing nipples provided for different purposes may be best in these situations. In addition, nurses should also document effectiveness using research-supported effects of NNS: decrease in heart rate, improved oxygenation, decreased motor activity, and more organized behavior state.

Nonnutritive Sucking may be used in conjunction with other interventions, such as Nutrition Therapy, Enteral Tube Feeding, Sleep Enhancement, and Environmental Management: Comfort (Iowa Intervention Project, 2000).

INTERVENTION APPLICATION

Baby boy Sam was born at 25 weeks of gestation and at a weight of 650 g to a 25-year-old married primipara who received prenatal care throughout her pregnancy. Early delivery was the result of severe preeclampsia. Sam had no spontaneous respiration at delivery; he was intubated and given surfactant. On admission to the neonatal intensive care unit, he was placed on a ventilator and cardiorespiratory monitors.

Sam's progress was slow but steady. By the third day of life, he had been extubated and placed under an oxygen hood. He was also started on enteral feedings by gavage tube. Although Sam was neurologically capable of sucking, he was too young to master coordinated sucking, swallowing, and breathing. Thus, many weeks of gavage feeding were to follow before he would be ready to begin oral or nipple feedings. The diagnosis of Altered Growth and Development was made.

As part of Sam's plan of care, the intervention of Nonnutritive Sucking was used. Every 2 hours with each tube feeding, he was offered a pacifier. The nurses usually offered this source of NNS just before beginning the flow of formula. Sam sucked vigorously on the pacifier and often continued sucking for some time after the feeding had been completed. The nurses allowed Sam to keep his pacifier for as long as he seemed to desire it, observing that the pacifier promoted a more restful state.

The nurses and Sam's parents also found that a pacifier calmed him when he had to have invasive procedures, such as heelsticks for routine blood work. A pacifier in conjunction with swaddling or gentle containment helped Sam to maintain his heart, respiratory, and oxygen saturation rates within normal ranges. He also was offered a pacifier when he became fussy or had difficulty falling to sleep following routine caregiving activities, such as bathing or vital signs.

At approximately 35 weeks PCA, Sam was offered his first feeding by nipple. Prior to the feeding, his mother gave him a pacifier at the suggestion of the nurses, who had found that this strategy often helped preterm infants come to an awake behavior state in readiness for a feeding. This did help, and Sam was able to take approximately half of his prescribed formula by nipple; the remainder was given by gavage, again with NNS offered as an adjunct to the feeding. For the next 2 weeks, Sam was alternately fed by nipple and gavage, with NNS opportunities offered as appropriate for each type of feeding. By 37 weeks PCA, Sam was feeding fully by nipple and was ready for discharge. The outcome indicators for Growth and Child Development had been attained (Iowa Outcomes Project, 2000).

RESEARCH AND PRACTICE IMPLICATIONS

Nonnutritive Sucking has been clearly demonstrated to be a beneficial nursing intervention. It is a simple, inexpensive intervention with well-documented behavior-modulating effects in preterm and term infants. Nonnutritive sucking promotes restful behavior states in agitated infants, decreases heart rate, and increases oxygenation in a variety of circumstances, and it modulates behavior during invasive and painful procedures. It appears to have both short- and long-term effects on feeding progression, promoting more rapid weight gain and transition to nipple feeding when offered consistently with gavage feedings. Furthermore, NNS promotes optimal behavioral performance when offered before nipple feedings.

As with most studies involving preterm infants, almost all research on NNS has involved very small samples. Moreover, many studies are flawed by the short-term nature of the investigational use of NNS. In addition, integration of research findings is made difficult by the inconsistent application of the intervention, particularly the number and length of NNS opportunities.

Perhaps the most pressing need for research in this area is in discovering the mechanisms by which NNS results in effectiveness. Although findings of improved gastric transit (Widstrom et al., 1988), increased gastric secretion of hormones and enzymes (Marchini, Lagercrantz, Feuerberg, Winberg, & Uvnas-Moberg, 1987), and stimulation of vagal response (Widstrom et al., 1988) have been posited as explanations for how NNS works, these findings have not been replicated. The most consistent research findings to date suggest that NNS works by promoting behavioral organization, thus allowing the infant's other systems to function more effectively. Additional research aimed at testing this hypothesis is needed.

In today's health care climate, interventions that are likely to decrease hospital stay, are inexpensive, and are easily delivered are in great demand. Nonnutritive Sucking is one such intervention. The demonstrated effectiveness of this intervention in preterm and term infants adds to its attractiveness. As research continues to uncover benefits and mechanisms for those benefits, the use of NNS may become a standard of care to promote optimal neurobehavioral outcomes.

REFERENCES

Als, H. (1979). Social interaction: Dynamic matrix for developing behavioral organization. In I. Uzgiris (Ed.), *New directions for child development* (pp. 21-41). San Francisco: Jossey-Bass.

Anderson, G. C., Burroughs, A. K., & Measel, C. P. (1983). Nonnutritive sucking opportunities: A safe and effective treatment for preterm neonates. In T. Field & A. Sostek (Eds.), *Infants born at risk: Physiological, perceptual, and cognitive processes* (pp. 129-146). New York: Grune & Stratton.

Bernbaum, J., Pereira, G. R., & Peckham, G. J. (1982). Increased oxygenation with non-nutritive sucking during gavage feedings in premature infants. *Pediatrics Research, 16*, 278A. [Abstract No. 1199]

Bernbaum, J., Pereira, G. R., Watkins, J. B., & Peckham, G. J. (1983). Nonnutritive sucking during gavage feeding enhances growth and maturation in preterm infants. *Pediatrics, 71*, 41-55.

Burroughs, A. K., Asonye, U. D., Anderson, G. C., & Vidyasagar, D. (1978). The effect of nonnutritive sucking on transcutaneous oxygen tension in noncrying, preterm neonates. *Research in Nursing and Health, 1*, 69-75.

Campos, R. G. (1994). Rocking and pacifiers: Two comforting interventions for heelstick pain. *Research in Nursing and Health, 17*, 321-331.

DiPietro, J. A., Cusson, R. M., Caughy, M. O., & Fox, N. A. (1994). Behavioral and physiologic effects of nonnutritive sucking during gavage feeding in preterm infants. *Pediatric Research, 36,* 207-214.

Field, T., & Goldson, E. (1984). Pacifying effects of nonnutritive sucking on term and preterm neonates during heelstick procedures. *Pediatrics, 74,* 1012-1015.

Field, T., Ignatoff, M. S., Stringer, S., Brennan, J., Greenberg, R., Widmayer, S., & Anderson, G. C. (1982). Nonnutritive sucking during tube feedings: Effects on preterm neonates in an intensive care unit. *Pediatrics, 70,* 381-384.

Gill, N. E., Behnke, M., Conlon, M., McNeely, J. G., & Anderson, G. C. (1988). Effect of nonnutritive sucking on behavioral state in preterm infants before feeding. *Nursing Research, 37,* 347-350.

Gunnar, M. R., Connors, J., Isensee, J., & Wall, L. (1988). Adrenocortical activity and behavioral distress in human newborns. *Developmental Psychobiology, 21,* 297-310.

Iowa Intervention Project. (2000). *Nursing interventions classification (NIC)* (J. C. McCloskey & G. M. Bulechek, Eds.; 3rd ed.). St. Louis, MO: Mosby-Year Book.

Iowa Outcomes Project. (2000). *Nursing outcomes classification (NOC)* (M. Johnson, M. Maas, & S, Moorhead, Eds.; 2nd ed.). St. Louis, MO: Mosby-Year Book.

Kessen, W., & Leutzendorff, A. M. (1963). The effect of nonnutritive sucking on movement in the human newborn. *Journal of Comparative and Physiological Psychology, 56,* 69-72.

Marchini, G., Lagercrantz, H., Feuerberg, Y., Winberg, J., & Uvnas-Moberg, K. (1987). The effect of non-nutritive sucking on plasma insulin, gastrin, and somatostatin levels in infants. *Acta Paediatrica Scandinavica, 76,* 573-578.

McCain, G. C. (1995). Promotion of preterm infant nipple feeding with nonnutritive sucking. *Journal of Pediatric Nursing, 10,* 3-8.

Measel, C., & Anderson, G. C. (1979). Nonnutritive sucking during tube feeding: Effect on clinical course in preterm infants. *Journal of Obstetric, Gynecologic, and Neonatal Nursing, 8,* 199-200.

Miller, H. D., & Anderson, G. C. (1993). Nonnutritive sucking: Effects on crying and heart rate in intubated infants requiring assisted mechanical ventilation. *Nursing Research, 42,* 305-307.

Nading, J. H., & Landes, R. D. (1984). Oxygen tension changes due to nonnutritive sucking during orogastric tube feeding. *Pediatric Research, 18,* 206A. [Abstract No. 663]

North American Nursing Diagnosis Association. (1999). *Nursing diagnoses: Definitions and classification 1995-1996.* Philadelphia: Author.

Paludetto, R., Robertson, S. S., Hack, M., Shivpuri, C. R., & Martin, R. J. (1984). Transcutaneous oxygen tension during nonnutritive sucking in preterm infants. *Pediatrics, 74,* 539-542.

Pickler, R. H., Frankel, H. B., Walsh, K. M., & Thompson, N. M. (1996). Effects of nonnutritive sucking on behavioral organization and feeding performance in preterm infants. *Nursing Research, 45,* 132-135.

Pickler, R. H., Higgins, K. E., & Crummette, B. D. (1993). The effect of nonnutritive sucking on bottle-feeding stress in preterm infants. *Journal of Obstetric, Gynecologic, and Neonatal Nursing, 22,* 230-234.

Righard, L., & Alade, M. O. (1997). Breastfeeding and the use of pacifiers. *Birth, 24,* 116-120.

Rushen, J., & DePassille, A. M. (1995). The motivation of non-nutritive sucking in calves, *Bos taurus. Animal Behavior, 49,* 1503-1510.

Treloar, D. M. (1994). The effect of nonnutritive sucking on oxygenation in healthy, crying full-term infants. *Applied Nursing Research, 7*(2), 52-58.

Widstrom, A. M., Marchini, G., Matthiesen, A. S., Werner, S., Winberg, J., & Uvnas-Moberg, K. (1988). Nonnutritive sucking in tube-fed preterm infants: Effects on gastric motility and gastric contents of somatostatin. *Journal of Pediatric Gastroenterology and Nutrition, 7*(4), 517-523.

Woodson, R., Drinkwin, J., & Hamilton, C. (1985). Effects of nonnutritive sucking on state and activity: Term-preterm comparisons. *Infant Behavior and Development, 8,* 435-441.

Woodson, R., & Hamilton, C. (1986). Heart rate estimates of motor activity in preterm infants. *Infant Behavior and Development, 9,* 283-290.

10

Kangaroo Care

Kathryn Moore Breitbach

Kangaroo Care originated in Bogotá, Colombia, to counter the high rate of infant mortality and incidence of infant abandonment of preterm infants (Whitelaw, Heisterkamp, Sleath, Acolet, & Richards, 1988). This intervention encouraged mothers of preterm infants to nurse and bond with their infants. Before 1979, the mortality r.ate of preterm infants born in Bogatá was high. After Dr. Edgar Rey Sanabria and Dr. Hector Martinez introduced Kangaroo Care, the mortality rate was dramatically reduced and the incidence of abandonment became almost nonexistent (Anderson, Marks, & Wahlberg, 1986; Anderson, 1989b).

Kangaroo Care is an intervention that involves holding a preterm infant between the mother's breasts or on the father's chest. It involves skin-to-skin contact and simulates the intrauterine environment by providing warmth and the soothing rhythmic sound of a heartbeat. In addition, Kangaroo Care is a means of providing tactile stimulation to preterm infants in a natural way.

Prematurity continues to be the major cause of perinatal mortality in the United States. The high cost of care and the potential for developmental delays for preterm infants who survive are issues related to prematurity. Kangaroo Care is a positive, proactive, and preventive nursing intervention that may address these issues. The implications for decreasing preterm infant mortality, promotion of breast-feeding and attachment, promotion of family-centered care, decreasing the cost of care, and shortening the length of preterm infants' hospitalization are tremendous. There is a need to study this intervention to explore its feasibility, safety, and benefits to the preterm infant and the family unit.

Today, preterm infants may stay in a neonatal intensive care unit (NICU) or intermediate care nursery from a few weeks to several months. Visitation by parents is often limited by the distance from home to the hospital and by other responsibilities such as work or the need to care for siblings. There is considerable emphasis on getting parents involved in the care of their preterm infants, however, and most NICUs have unlimited visiting hours. Although care by parent is encouraged, technological equipment continues to place a barrier between parent and infant that could last for weeks or months. Health care professionals are concerned about the psychological consequences of prolonged separation and high-technological equipment, such as ventilators and monitors, on preterm infants and their parents. Therefore, interventions are needed to ameliorate this separation.

One of the three major initiatives set forth by *Healthy People 2000* (U.S. Department of Health and Human Services, 1991) to improve maternal and infant health is to reduce infant mortality to no more than 7 deaths per 1,000 births. Kangaroo Care can have an impact on this initiative by promoting growth and development of preterm infants, promoting healthy parent-infant attachment, and encouraging breast-feeding. Kangaroo Care not only promotes the health of preterm infants but also has the potential to reduce the length of hospitalization, thereby reducing health care costs.

REVIEW OF THE LITERATURE

To provide Kangaroo Care, a mother or father holds the diaper-clad infant in an upright prone position between the breasts. The skin-to-skin contact provided by Kangaroo Care is a means of affective touch, and therefore the concept of affective touch needs to be explained to clarify the potential benefits of Kangaroo Care for preterm infants. Ingham (1989) noted that "expressive (affective) touch is one kind of nonverbal communication that is essential for development of self-awareness and a concept of self interacting with other human beings" (p. 69). One's perception of touch is greatly influenced by past experiences with touch and the cultural environment.

Properties of Touch

Touch has the potential to play a major role in the development of a healthy state of mind and body. It is generally a positive behavior that produces a satisfying effect on the individual and is among the basic needs for healthy emotional and physical development (Clement, 1987). Weiss (1988) described classifications that included the following properties: the qualities of touch and the meaning of touch. There are two types of touch—direct and indirect. Direct touch is demonstrated when mothers touch their fingertips, face, or palms to the infant. Indirect touch is seen when mothers touch their infant's face with a diaper or bottle. The qualities of touch are based on location, duration, intensity, and sensation (Weiss, 1988). The meaning of touch has been studied from the perspectives of patients and nurses. Love, sympathy, hope, understanding, reassurance, caring, and the presence of another person as well as negativity all can be conveyed through touch.

Physiological Perspectives of Affective Touch

The earliest sense to develop in the fetus is the sense of touch (Hynd & Willis, 1988). The head is the first area to become sensitive to touch, and during a 7-week period sensitivity to touch descends down the body of the fetus until it reaches the toes. This is evidenced by reflexive activity of the embryo in response to touch beginning at the lips and ending with the legs and feet (Molsberry & Shogan, 1990). The myelinization process begins at 12 weeks of gestation (Hynd & Willis, 1988). Rapid brain development occurs during the third trimester of fetal life. According to Catlett and Holditch-Davis (1990), "the major events of this period include orientation and layering of cortical neurons, elaboration of dendritic and axonal processes, establishment of synaptic contacts, and proliferation and differentiation of glia" (p. 20). Barb and Lemons (1989) state that "the myelin sheath is a series of cell membranes surrounding the axon that enhances the conduction of nervous impulses. Myelination within the central nervous system, particularly the forebrain, generally develops after birth" (p. 8). At birth, the pathway mediating tactile sensation is myelinated in the spinal cord and brain stem to the level of the thalamus (Hynd & Willis, 1988).

Preterm infants have an immature nervous system, and the degree of immaturity is related to their gestational age. They are hypersensitive to touch; therefore, it is important not to overstimulate them. Physical decompensation, indicated by changes in respiratory rate, heart rate, color, and oxygen requirements, can be seen as a result of overstimulation (Catlett & Holditch-Davis, 1990; Molsberry & Shogan, 1990). The repetitious use of different types of touch can result in the compensation of preterm infant's tactile behaviors. The type of touch along with the qualities and meaning of touch all contribute to a preterm infant's response. Preterm infants need help in gradually integrating stimuli to respond appropriately (see Chapter 8, this volume). Hypersensitivity decreases as preterm infants approach their corrected gestational age due to the maturation of their nervous system.

Infant Development and Affective Touch

Development is influenced by affective touch. Amniotic fluid surrounds and bathes the human fetus in utero. Tactile stimulation necessary for the activation of an infant's vital organs comes with the onset of labor and uterine contractions. The infant is delivered into the hands of the health care provider and then is quickly placed into the mother's open arms. When an infant is born prior to 40 weeks gestation, the neuronal processes tend to reorganize or form alternative connections. The more preterm an infant is, the more exaggerated this response will be, especially the Moro reflex (Catlett & Holditch-Davis, 1990). Due to negative flexor tone and minimal opposition to range of motion, infants born at less than 37 weeks gestation will stay in any position in which they are placed (Volpe, 1987). This inability to reposition themselves causes discomfort and an inability to cope, resulting in responses that are dysfunctional (Catlett & Holditch-Davis, 1990).

Kangaroo Care

The literature on Kangaroo Care is based on the behavior of the kangaroo in the care of its young. The kangaroo is a large marsupial that carries its young in a pouch on the abdomen. A baby kangaroo, called a joey, is undeveloped and tiny at birth. The baby kangaroo is approximately 2 or 3 inches long and weighs only a few ounces at birth. Gradually, the joey finds its way into the mother's pouch and remains there for several weeks to 6 months until it can care for itself. While in the pouch, the baby kangaroo nurses, is kept warm, and grows rapidly (*World Book Encyclopedia*, 1995).

Kangaroo Care began with human infants when pediatricians at San Juan de Diós Hospital in Bogotá, Colombia, started sending preterm infants home with their mothers due to the shortage of equipment, the frequency of infection in the hospital, and the high incidence of abandonment (Whitelaw & Sleath, 1985). The infants were carried between the mother's breasts in a vertical position and fed only mother's milk. Whitelaw and colleagues (1988) carried out a randomized trial of Kangaroo Care at Hammersmith Hospital in London. Premature infants who received Kangaroo Care breast-fed 4 weeks sooner and cried less at 6 months of age than the infants who did not receive Kangaroo Care. Anderson (1989a) visited 11 countries in Europe to learn more about the studies being conducted and how Kangaroo Care was being practiced. She observed that infants participating in Kangaroo Care had adequate oxygenation, maintained stable temperatures, had a decrease in the incidence of periodic breathing and apnea, cried less at 6 months of age, were discharged home sooner, spent more time in deep sleep, and were more inclined to breast-feed. There was no indication that Kangaroo Care causes overstimulation or increased risk of infection in the preterm infant population.

Bosque, Brady, Affonso, and Wahlberg (1995) performed a study in which they continuously monitored the physiological status of infants receiving Kangaroo Care versus infants receiving incubator care in a tertiary-level nursery. The results showed that heart rate, respiratory rate, incidence of apnea, and oxygen saturation were similar during Kangaroo Care and while in the incubator. After providing Kangaroo Care, mothers stated that they believed they had emotionally completed their pregnancies and could better care for their infants. The researchers concluded that Kangaroo Care was safe and beneficial for selected infants and mothers in a NICU.

Ludington-Hoe (1990) studied the effects of Kangaroo Care on three indexes of energy expenditure: heart rate, behavioral state, and activity level. She hypothesized that Kangaroo Care would reduce heart rate, increase sleep, and lower activity level due to its soothing effects. The findings suggested that Kangaroo Care was a simple, cost-effective intervention that stabilizes the heart rate and reduces activity and state-related energy expenditure.

Affonso, Bosque, Wahlberg, and Brady (1993) studied the effects that Kangaroo Care had on mothers' emotional reactions in a tertiary-level intensive care nursery. Reconciliation and healing occurred when mothers provided Kangaroo Care to their preterm infants. Mothers stated that they were able to start adjusting to the fact that they had a preterm infant, and they began to work through the emotions associated with having a preterm infant, indicating Kangaroo Care helped initiate the process of healing. Kangaroo Care had the potential to facilitate mothers' awareness and expressions of their emotional reactions associated with having a high-risk infant.

The Nursing Intervention Classification (NIC) (Iowa Intervention Project, 2000) intervention Kangaroo Care was developed and validated by Breitbach (1994). Current literature continues to support the activities of this intervention and outcomes associated with Kangaroo Care. Bauer, Sontheimer, Fischer, and Linderkamp (1996) compared the effects of maternal and paternal Kangaroo Care on oxygen consumption, carbon

tion Project, 2000, p. 412). Kangaroo Care is a nursing intervention that emphasizes touch between parents and their high-risk infant. It promotes attachment behaviors, lactation, and comfort through touch. It is a unique nursing intervention that focuses on parents and their preterm infant.

Kangaroo Care is relatively easy to initiate in the hospital setting. Parents should be informed about the opportunity to provide Kangaroo Care to their infant on admission, but emphasis should be made on the need for the infant to be physiologically stable. Contradictions to Kangaroo Care include infants that cold stress easily and those who experience a decrease in heart rate or oxygen saturation or both with minimal stimulation and handling. It is important for parents to wear open-front clothing, for them to take care of their basic needs before starting, and that they are provided a comfortable chair and as relaxed an environment as is possible in the intensive care setting. Infants will receive the most benefit if they are provided Kangaroo Care for at least 20 minutes or longer. Parents should be instructed on how to transfer the infant from incubator, warmer bed, or bassinet and how to manage equipment and tubing; then the following steps should be taken. First, position the diaper-clad infant in a prone upright position on the parent's chest, and then wrap the parent's clothing around or place a blanket over the infant to maintain the infant's position and temperature. Next, encourage the parent(s) to focus on the infant rather than the high-technological setting and equipment. The parent may gently stroke, rock, or provide auditory stimulation and eye contact as appropriate once the infant's behavioral cues and state have been assessed. Privacy and comfort are a must. Postpartum mothers should be encouraged to change position and get up every 90 minutes to prevent thrombolytic disease. Both parents should be encouraged to provide Kangaroo Care because the feel of each of their chests is unique to an infant and provides the infant with different tactile sensations.

Another important aspect is to ensure that all health care workers in the NICU are educated about how and when to initiate Kangaroo Care and are knowledgeable about benefits of Kangaroo Care to both parents and preterm infant. Since the development and validation of Kangaroo Care as a nursing intervention, the guidelines have become less restrictive in NICUs. Because the comfort level of health care providers with Kangaroo Care has increased in recent years, infants on high-frequency ventilators and other high-tech equipment are now being allowed to kangaroo with their parents. Health care workers need to continue to monitor the parent's emotional reaction to Kangaroo Care and to monitor the infant's physiological status during Kangaroo Care. Should an infant show signs of overstimulation, distress, or avoidance, the parent should be instructed to decrease activity. Breast-feeding may also be encouraged during Kangaroo Care if the infant is developmentally ready (Iowa Intervention Project, 2000).

INTERVENTION APPLICATION

Baby H. was a 1,410-gram product of a 29-week-gestation pregnancy born by normal spontaneous vaginal delivery to a 19-year-old married white female. The pregnancy was complicated by premature labor and premature rupture of membranes 3 days prior to delivery. The infant's Apgar scores were 5 at 1 minute and 7 at 5 minutes. Mrs. H. received β-methasone 3 days prior to delivery. The infant was taken to the NICU and placed on nasopharyrgeal continuous positive airway pressure. Baby H. received a 7-day course of antibiotics. Because of the separation of the infant from her parents and the high-tech equipment used to sustain the infant during the first days of life, the nursing diagnosis At Risk for Altered Parents/Infant Attachment was made.

On the fourth day of life, Baby H. was stable enough to start Kangaroo Care at a weight of 1,360 grams. Baby H.'s mother would kangaroo with her infant for 30 to 50 minutes after the morning feeding. She implemented Kangaroo Care on a consistent basis. The following results show that there was no physiological compromise during Kangaroo Care:

Number of days participated in Kangaroo Care: 15

Average daily weight gain: 35 grams

Average heart rate: before, 143 beats per minute (bpm); during, 138 bpm; after, 139 bpm

Average axillary temperature: before, 36.7°C; after, 36.8°C

Average oxygen saturation: before, 98%; during, 99%; after, 99%

Oxygen supplement: room air

Statements by the parents indicated progress in achieving the outcome Parent-Infant Attachment. Mrs. H. believed that Baby H. was less irritable and slept better on the days that she implemented Kangaroo Care. She loved the closeness to her infant and believed that she was more relaxed after the experience. Mr. H. was very excited about how Kangaroo Care made him feel like he was truly a part of the baby's life. Nurses reported that the parents became very comfortable handling their infant, they were much more interested in their infant, and they were able to better assess their infant's behavioral cues and state changes after instituting Kangaroo Care.

RESEARCH AND PRACTICE IMPLICATIONS

Kangaroo Care is a nursing intervention used to enhance the growth and development of the preterm infant and to promote interaction between parent and infant. Continued research and education is needed for Kangaroo Care to become a widely accepted intervention in NICUs for preterm infants. Nurses must also continue to study the effects of touch on preterm infants and determine ways to decrease the negative outcomes of over-stimulation. The following are other research questions to be explored: (a) Does Kangaroo Care improve a preterm infant's long-term developmental outcome? (b) Does the postconceptual age of the infant make any difference in the level of benefit? (c) Does the preterm infant's behavioral state at the time of Kangaroo Care affect how it is tolerated? (d) Does Kangaroo Care benefit the "micropremie"? (e) Is Kangaroo Care cost-effective? (f) Will Kangaroo Care enhance patient and family satisfaction? (g) Will Kangaroo Care provide satisfaction to health care providers? (h) Is Kangaroo Care as effective for the term infant? (i) Should Kangaroo Care be discussed with parents prenatally? and (j) When does Kangaroo Care have the potential to decrease the length of stay in the hospital for preterm infants?

Implications for practice are in the areas of bereavement and surrogate Kangaroo Care. Several hospitals in the United States have used Kangaroo Care as a means to facilitate grief after fetal death. No research to date has been done in this area, and it would be interesting to learn more about parents' emotional responses and whether Kangaroo Care could facilitate the grieving process. Surrogate Kangaroo Care might focus on grandparents and siblings of high-risk infants. Do grandparents' or siblings' bodies have similar physiological reactions as those of parents? Do the infants have similar physiological reactions when they kangaroo with their grandparents or siblings? Could unrelated individuals provide surrogate Kangaroo Care?

Staff adjustment is another area to investigate. Staff resistance to Kangaroo Care stems from the fear that problems may occur and they will be blamed (Drosten-Brooks, 1993). It is difficult for some health care providers to comprehend that an infant's condition may improve in a parent's arms or that teaching should be initiated in an intensive care unit. According to Drosten-Brooks, nurses' attitudes tend to change as they observe the positive benefits of Kangaroo Care on their patients and families.

To provide the opportunity for Kangaroo Care, the design of most NICUs needs to be rethought. Families need an area that is both spacious and provides privacy when visiting their high-risk infant. Rocking chairs, recliners, pillows, decreased lighting, decreased noise, footstools, and screens need to be included in the nursery design. Also, NICUs need to redesign how they provide care to high-risk infants. Do we need to disturb the infant as often as we do? How can we enhance development through positioning, decreased handling, changing the environment, and enabling parents to hold and kangaroo with their infant?

Finally, research on the effectiveness of Kangaroo Care on infants and their parents needs to continue. With all the publicity Kangaroo Care is receiving in the media, the opportunity to explore some of these research avenues will occur as parents request the opportunity to participate in Kangaroo Care with their infants.

REFERENCES

Affonso, D., Bosque, E., Wahlberg, V., & Brady, J. (1993). Reconciliation and healing for mothers through skin-to-skin contact provided in an American tertiary level intensive care nursery. *Neonatal Network, 12*(3), 25-32.

Anderson, G. C., Marks, E., & Wahlberg, V. (1986). Kangaroo care for premature infants. *American Journal of Nursing, 86*(7), 807-809.

Anderson, G. C. (1989a). Skin to skin: Kangaroo care in western Europe. *American Journal of Nursing, 86*(5), 662-666.

Anderson, G. C. (1989b). Kangaroo care and breast feeding for preterm infants. *Breast Feeding Abstracts, 9*, 7-8.

Barb, S. A., & Lemons, P. K. (1989). The premature infant: Toward improving neurodevelopmental outcome. *Neonatal Network, 7*(6), 7-15.

Bauer, J., Sontheimer, D., Fischer, C., & Linderkamp, O. (1996). Metabolic rate and energy balance in very low birth weight infants during kangaroo holding by their mothers and fathers. *Journal of Pediatrics, 129*(4), 608-610.

Blaymore, J., Ferguson, A., Morales, Y., Liebling, J., Archer, D., Oh, W., & Vohr, B. (1996, December). Comparison of skin-to-skin contact with standard contact in low-birth-weight infants who are breast-fed. *Archives of Pediatric Adolescent Medicine, 150*, 1265-1269.

Bosque, E., Brady, J., Affonso, D., & Wahlberg, V. (1995). Physiologic measures of kangaroo versus incubator care in a tertiary-level nursery. *Journal of Obstetric, Gynecologic, and Neonatal Nursing, 24*(3), 219-226.

Breitbach, K. (1994). *Validation and development of the nursing intervention "kangaroo care."* Unpublished thesis, The University of Iowa, Iowa City.

Catlett, A. T., & Holditch-Davis, D. (1990). Environmental stimulation of the acutely ill premature infant: Physiological effects and nursing implications. *Neonatal Network, 8*(6), 19-26.

Clement, J. (1987). Touch: Research findings and use in preoperative care. *AORN Journal, 45*(6), 1429-1439.

Denehy, J. A., & Grafft, C. Q. (1999). Analysis of the nursing diagnosis Altered Growth and Development. In M. J. Rantz, & P. LeMone (Eds.), *Classification of nursing diagnoses: Proceedings of the thirteenth conference: North American Nursing Diagnosis Association.* Glendale, CA: CINAHL.

Drosten-Brooks, F. (1993, September/October). Kangaroo care: Skin-to-skin contact in the NICU. MCN: *American Journal of Maternal Child Nursing, 18,* 250-253.

Hynd, C. W., & Willis, W. G. (1988). *Pediatric neurophysiology.* Orlando, FL: Grune & Stratton.

Ingham, A. (1989). A review of the literature relating to touch and its use in intensive care. *Intensive Care Nursing, 5*(2), 65-75.

Iowa Intervention Project. (2000). *Nursing interventions classification (NIC)* (J. C. McCloskey & G. M. Bulechek, Eds.; 3rd ed.). St. Louis, MO: Mosby-Year Book.

Iowa Outcomes Project. (2000). *Nursing outcomes classification (NOC)* (M. Johnson, M. Maas, & S.Moorhead, Eds.; 2nd ed.). St. Louis, MO: Mosby-Year Book.

Ludington-Hoe, S. (1990). Energy conservation during skin-to-skin contact between premature infants and their mothers. *Heart & Lung, 19*(5), 445-451.

Molsberry, D., & Shogan, M. G. (1990). Communicating through touch. In M. J. Craft & J. A. Denehy (Eds.), *Nursing interventions for infants and children* (pp. 127-150). Philadelphia: W. B. Saunders.

U.S. Department of Health and Human Services. (1991). *Healthy people 2000: National health promotion and disease prevention objectives* (DHHS Publication No. PHS 91-50312). Washington, DC: Government Printing Office.

Volpe, J. J. (1987). *Neurology of the newborn* (2nd ed.). Philadelphia: W. B. Saunders.

Weiss, S. J. (1988). Touch. In *Annual review of nursing research* (Vol. 6, pp. 3-27). New York: Springer.

Whitelaw, A., Heisterkamp, G., Sleath, K., Acolet, D., & Richards, M. (1988). Skin to skin contact for very low birthweight infants and their mothers. *Archives of Disease in Childhood, 63*(11), 1377-1381.

Whitelaw, A., & Sleath, K. (1985). Myth of the marsupial mother: Home care of very low birth weight babies in Bogotá, Colombia. *Lancet, 1*(8439), 1206-1208.

The World Book Encyclopedia (Vol. 11). (1995). Chicago: Field Enterprises Educational Corporation.

11

Supportive Positioning

Christine L. Doyle

Cynthia S. Hockman

Infants have been spending more time on their backs since a task force for the American Academy of Pediatrics (AAP) recommended that healthy infants be positioned on their side or back for sleep. The recommendation was based on studies that suggested an increased risk of sudden infant death syndrome (SIDS) with the prone sleep position (Kattwinkel, Brooks, & Myerberg, 1992). A revised recommendation of supine position only for sleep was issued in 1996 because the side-lying position put the infant at a slightly greater risk for SIDS due to the potential for the infant to roll from side to abdomen (Kattwinkel, Brooks, Keenan, & Malloy, 1996). There is evidence that this recommendation may decrease the incidence of SIDS. The recommendation for supine positioning for sleep, however, also has a potentially negative impact on the neuromotor and musculoskeletal development of term infants and especially preterm infants.

Parents and primary caregivers of infants need education about neonatal positioning in the prone, side-lying, and supine positions. Education is especially important for parents of term infants younger than 3 months old and parents of preterm infants who are older because preterm infants are most susceptible to postural abnormalities from being positioned exclusively in one position.

According to *Healthy People 2000 Midcourse Review* (U.S. Department of Health and Human Services [USDHHS], 1995), infant mortality is 8.5 per 1,000 live births. This review further states that in 1992 low-birth-weight infants (<2,500 grams) represented 7.1% of infants born, whereas very low-birth-weight infants (<1,500 grams) represented 1.3% (USDHHS, 1995). Advancements in medical intervention have improved these infants' chances of survival. These data indicate that more infants are susceptible to influences of positioning on their neuromotor and musculoskeletal development. These findings and the recommendation for supine sleep to reduce the incidence of SIDS make neonatal positioning essential to the promotion of healthy growth and development of infants.

REVIEW OF EMPIRICAL LITERATURE

Infant growth and development will serve as the conceptual framework for this chapter. Studies of growth and development of premature infants and the impact that positioning had on that development will be reviewed. Finally, studies regarding SIDS and the potential role that sleep position may play in this syndrome will be discussed.

Growth is generally defined as an increase in size or change in structure. *Development* refers to the patterned, orderly maturation or increasing complexity of function. Vaughn and Litt (1990) note, however, that "no single description of growth and development . . . is adequate to the complexity of processes involved" (p. 1). Therefore, for the purposes of this chapter, only physiologic and neuromotor growth and development will be included.

Physiologic growth and development are the physical changes of structure and function (Vaughn & Litt, 1990). Weight, length, and head circumference are some of the measures of physiologic growth and development. The fetus nearly triples in weight and increases in length by approximately 50% during the last trimester of pregnancy (Vaughn & Litt, 1990). It is in this trimester that the fetus assumes "physiologic flexion" or the fetal position. The head is bent down slightly, the arms are brought forward and up near the face, and the hips and knees are flexed against the abdomen due to the mass of the fetus and limited elasticity and growth of the uterus (Fay, 1988; Updike, Schmidt, Macke, Cahoon, & Miller, 1986). The posture of the term newborn reflects this physiologic flexion. In the supine position, the infant generally has flexed knees and abducted hips, and the arms are flexed close to the trunk with hands fisted (Tappero, 1993).

Body proportions illustrate the cephalocaudal or head-to-toe progress of physiologic growth and development. At birth, an infant's head comprises one fourth of total body length compared to one eighth of adult height (Vaughn & Litt, 1990). Therefore, the head comprises a relatively large portion of total body weight of the newborn and young infant.

The second model of growth and development to be considered is neuromotor. This model considers the maturation or increasing complexity of neurobiological function that evolves with age (Vaughn & Litt, 1990). Gross and fine motor, social, and language growth and development are measures of this model. For the purposes of this chapter, both gross and fine motor development will be reviewed.

Gross motor development involves the maturation of muscle necessary for skills such as lifting the head in the prone position, sitting, standing, and walking. Fine motor development includes the evolution of skills such as tracking a visual stimulus, grasping, bringing hands together, and reaching. These skills evolve in a step-like, sequential progression. There is overlap in mastery in the evolution of these motor skills. An understanding of how an infant is affected by various positions (i.e., prone, supine, and side lying) is relevant to facilitating the neuromotor and musculoskeletal development of the infant. These effects illustrate the need for neonatal positioning interventions.

Premature infants have been deprived of last-trimester development in utero. The consequence of premature delivery is that physiologic flexion does not develop because the infant's body mass is not large enough to necessitate a posture of flexion and no longer has the containment of the uterus or the support of the amniotic fluid (Oehler, Strickland, & Nordland, 1991). Placing the infant in different positions with supports can help promote flexion, facilitate symmetrical postures, and enhance midline orientation.

The prone position is considered best for promoting flexion, symmetry, and midline orientation. It encourages flexion of the lower extremities and brings the shoulders forward and hands close to the body (Fay, 1988). Infants in the prone position lift their heads more frequently and therefore are able to change head position from side to side, diminishing the predominance of one-sided preference for head turning seen in infants maintained in a supine position (Konishi, Kuriyama, Mikawa, & Suzuki, 1987). Molding of the head, such as occipital bone or asymmetrical parietal bone flattening, is less likely to occur. The prone position, however, does have limitations. When infants younger than 33 weeks gestation are placed in the prone position, they abduct their hips into a frog-like position due to their physiologic hypotonia (Downs, Edwards, McCormick,

Roth, & Stewart, 1991). Therefore, while in this position the infant needs to have supports to maintain proper body alignment.

The side-lying position offers many of the same benefits as the prone position. Side lying eliminates the potential for hip abduction (Downs et al., 1991). This position also keeps the head in the midline, decreasing the potential for asymmetrical head-turning preference and facilitating the infant in bringing the hands to the midline (Perez-Woods, Malloy, & Tse, 1992). This midline activity enhances the infant's ability to self-quiet by finger or hand sucking. It is important, however, to alternate side-lying positions, using both right and left positions to minimize asymmetry of head shape. Konishi et al. (1987) found that premature infants maintained in a side-lying position were somewhat slower than prone-positioned infants in developing head control. This finding was not statistically significant and was probably due to the muscle strength required to lift the head when in the side-lying position.

Premature infants maintained in a supine position for prolonged periods of time are susceptible to the effects of gravity and weak muscle tone, and they can develop abnormal postures associated with flattening against the supporting surface. Specifically, these postures are generalized extension with hyperextension of the neck, flattening of the occiput, and retraction of the shoulders. Georgieff and Bernbaum (1986) noted that shoulder girdle abnormalities inhibit crawling, sitting, and object manipulation, which are important developmental tasks in the first year of life. Muscle tone abnormalities, such as shoulder girdle hypertonicity and lower extremity extension, may persist for the first 2 years of life (Gennaro & Bakewell-Sachs, 1991; Georgieff & Bernbaum, 1986). Normally, by 3 months of age infants in the prone position can raise their head and chest from a firm surface with their arms extended in front of them (Vaughn & Litt, 1990).

Recently, a study noted a significant increase in referral for plagiocephaly (asymmetric flattening of the occiput) without synostosis (Kane, Mitchell, Craven, & Marsh, 1996). This increase coincided approximately with the time that the supine position for sleep recommendation was made by the AAP. Hunt and Puczynski (1996) challenged this study's findings because they questioned the isolated occurrence of this increase. They did recommend, however, that parents should alternate infant head position between midline and partial turning to the left and right. They also recommended that supervised prone-position infant play be encouraged.

A study by Konishi et al. (1987) examined the effect of body position on postural and functional lateralities and found that infants maintained in a supine position demonstrated a head-turning preference twice as often as infants maintained in the prone position. Furthermore, of those infants who were in the supine position, more than one fourth continued to show a head-turning preference at 9 months of age. Typically, by 3 or 4 months of age, term infants demonstrate a posture with the head maintained in a midline position and hands often brought together in midline or at the mouth (Vaughn & Litt, 1990).

Supine is the least preferred position for facilitating flexion. Infants placed in this position, however, can be placed in nests made of soft foam or rolled blankets to facilitate flexion. These nests contain the infant's extremities to promote flexion and to maintain proper body alignment and midline head position (Fay, 1988; Grunwald & Becker, 1991; Oehler et al., 1991).

Research has been carried out to evaluate the use of supports to minimize the effects of gravity on premature infants' posture in a given position. Downs et al. (1991) found that the use of postural supports in the prone, side-lying, and supine positions reduced flattened posture and excessive hip flexion seen in the control group. Infants who received supportive positioning as a component of developmental care have demonstrated fewer disorganized movements and better flexed postures than infants who were not part of developmental care studies (Als et al., 1986; Becker, Grunwald, Moorman, & Stuhr, 1991) (see Chapter 8, this volume).

In the past several decades, a tremendous amount of effort has gone into trying to find possible causes for SIDS. Positioning appears to be a risk factor that must be considered and therefore is important to include in this review. SIDS is the leading cause of death in infants younger than the age of 1 year, with the peak incidence occurring between 2 and 4 months of age (Willinger, 1995). The cause of SIDS is unknown; several factors related to the risk of SIDS have been identified, however. One factor that has received much attention is the sleep position of the infant.

A task force from the AAP evaluated data from studies concerning positioning and SIDS (Kattwinkel et al., 1992). The data supported the possible relationship between prone sleep and SIDS. From this report came the recommendation for supine or side-lying positions for sleep. In 1996, the AAP revised this recommendation to the supine position only for sleep of infants (Kattwinkel et al., 1996). The change in recommendation was due to the risk that infants placed on their sides could potentially roll to their abdomens during sleep.

Two studies published in 1995 yielded different results on the impact of supine sleep position on the reduction of the incidence of SIDS. Data from a study in Tasmania revealed that after public health activities and verbal instruction to educate parents about supine sleep, the incidence of SIDS decreased from 7.6 to 4.1 deaths per 1,000 live births in the cohort studied (Dwyer, Ponsonby, Blizzard, Newman, & Cochrane, 1995). Klonoff-Cohen and Edelstein (1995), however, did not find an association between prone sleep and an increased risk of SIDS. They found that of the infants who died of SIDS, 80% were in a prone position when found. These and earlier studies reviewed by the AAP show multiple factors that could increase the risk of SIDS. Because a possible relationship between prone position for sleep and an increased risk for SIDS exists, however, supine is the recommended position for sleep for infants. It is important to remember that this recommendation for supine position is for sleep only, and the supine position is not exclusively the position of choice for infants at times other than sleeping.

The review of the literature revealed that no single position used exclusively is best. The goals of positioning are to promote flexion, facilitate symmetrical postures, and enhance midline orientation. These goals are best met by changing the infant's position regularly and using supports such as rolled blankets to maintain proper body alignment in all positions. Premature infants need assistance in maintaining proper posture because they lack the muscle tone to overcome the flattening effects of gravity.

NURSING DIAGNOSIS AND OUTCOME DETERMINATION

As part of the nursing process, appropriate nursing diagnoses must be identified. Two diagnoses are useful for infants susceptible to the effects of positioning. The first nursing diagnosis to be considered is *Altered Growth and Development* (North American Nursing Diagnosis Association [NANDA], 1999). This nursing diagnosis is defined as "the state in which an individual demonstrates deviations in norms from his or her age group" (p. 105). One of the major defining characteristics of this diagnosis is "delay or difficulty in performing skills typical of age group" (p. 105-106). The area of greatest concern is the potential impediment of the infant's gross and fine motor development. One of the tenets of growth and development is that the human organism develops in medial-distal and cephalocaudal directions. Therefore, infants need opportunities for midline play—that is, hands together to foster medial orientation. Likewise, the prone position allows natural opportunities for lifting the head and pushing up with the hands and forearms to lift the chest and to eventually get up on all four extremities.

From the physical growth perspective, infants will turn their heads to interact with their caregivers. If this is most often in the same direction, the infant will display a head-turning preference that can result in asymmetrical growth of the neck muscles and asymmetrical flattening of the occiput. The head-turning preference may present to the practitioner as a prolonged tonic neck reflex that typically disappears at 3 or 4 months of age. Similarly, infants 4 or 5 months of age should be able to visually track 180 degrees. If an infant has a head-turning preference, the child will track easily to the preferred side but may not turn much past midline to the other side.

A second nursing diagnosis that may be appropriate is *Impaired Physical Mobility*, which is defined as "a state in which the individual experiences a limitation of ability for independent physical movement" (NANDA, 1999, p. 84). Certainly, the young infant is largely dependent on the caregiver for a change of position. Defining characteristics of this diagnosis, however, include limited range of motion and decreased muscle strength, control, mass, or all three. This diagnosis would be considered for the infant with decreased range of motion of the neck due to muscle shortening of the preferred side. Also, the infant who demonstrated shoulder retraction due to prolonged supine position is unable to bring the hands forward to midline and often finds the prone position uncomfortable.

From these nursing diagnoses, certain nursing outcome measures would be appropriate. The outcome measures to be considered are Child Development: 2 Months and Child Development: 4 Months (Iowa Outcomes Project, 2000). *Child Development* is defined as milestones of physical, cognitive, and psychological progression by a specific age. These child development outcomes are determined by indicators that are measured on a 5-point Likert scale ranging from 1 ("extreme delay from expected range") to 5 ("no delay from expected age") (pp. 58-60).

Three indicators in the outcome classification for Child Development: 2 Months are appropriate for neonatal positioning. The first indicator is "lifts head, neck, and upper chest with support on forearms while in prone position" (Iowa Outcomes Project, 2000, p. 155). This indicator reveals the amount of opportunity the infant has had in prone position. The second indicator in this outcome is "some head control in upright position" (p. 155). Again, time in the prone position will play a part. Also, if the infant has a head-turning preference, this may be evident if the head tilts toward the preferred side when the infant is held upright. The third indicator, "shows interest in visual stimuli" (p. 155), is appropriate when evaluating the degree of visual tracking by the infant. Head-turning preference will become evident when the infant readily tracks the stimulus to one side but not the other.

The outcome measure of Child Development: 4 Months has four indicators that are appropriate: "in prone positions holds head erect and raises body on hands; controls head well; rolls from prone to supine; and holds own hands" (Iowa Outcomes Project, 2000, p. 156). The first two indicators are further development of activities that were emerging at 2 months. The infant needs opportunities to practice raising up on the arms, which also helps the infant strengthen neck muscles. The third indicator,

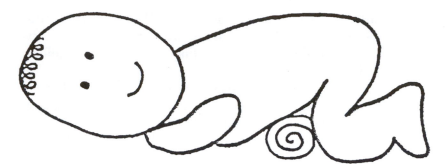

Figure 11.1. Prone Infant With Roll Under Hips

"rolls from prone to supine" (p. 156), requires that the infant has an opportunity to be prone. The fourth indicator addresses midline orientation. The infant is able to bring hands to the middle of the body and is able to grasp them together.

INTERVENTION: SUPPORTIVE POSITIONING

The nursing intervention *Supportive Positioning* is defined as aligning an infant's trunk and extremities with supports to promote flexion, facilitate symmetrical posture, and enhance midline orientation. These supports are tucked around the infant to assume and maintain a position. The supports can be soft, cotton terry cloth hand towels or small bath towels, depending on the size of the infant and the size and thickness of the towels. Cotton flannel receiving blankets are also a good choice for making a support. The support is created by starting at one edge of the blanket or towel and rolling it jelly-roll style into a tight roll. The site at which the support is to be used will determine how large and long the support should be and will also determine what size blanket or towel is best. Receiving blankets and towels are readily available to parents and other caregivers. The variety of sizes, ease of washing when soiled, and the fact that they can be reused make towel or blanket supports convenient to use.

Supportive Positioning includes activities that describe techniques for positioning infants in prone, side-lying, supine, and sitting positions. Prone position is to be used only when the infant is awake. For the very young infant, such as a newborn or preterm infant, a small rolled blanket or towel positioned under the hips helps keep the hips and knees flexed (Figure 11.1). Adjustment of the roll may be required to prevent external rotation of the hips causing the "frog-leg" appearance of the lower extremities.

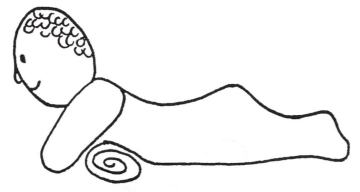

Figure 11.2. Prone Infant With Roll Under Chest

Placing a small roll under the infant's chest facilitates the infant's ability to change head positions from side to side (Figure 11.2). If the infant has difficulty with head raising or arms flailing out to the sides, use a roll large enough to curl around the infant to keep the arms midline (Figure 11.3).

The thickness of the roll is determined by the size of the infant. The roll under the hips needs to be thick enough to allow the infant to get good hip and knee flexion without putting pressure on the abdomen. The roll under the chest is smaller and should be approximately at the nipple line. Frequent monitoring and readjusting will be necessary as the infant moves or because the roll can become positioned under the abdomen or under the neck. Prone position helps the infant develop head control and upper-body strength. A toy or other colorful object in front of the infant can serve as a stimulus for the infant to attempt head lifting. As the neck muscles get stronger and head control improves, the infant will enjoy the

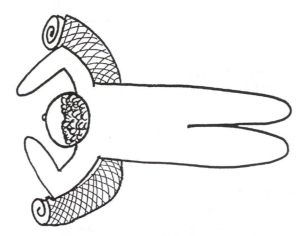

Figure 11.3. Prone Infant With Chest Roll Curled Forward

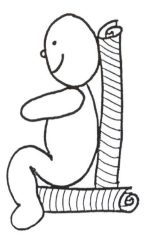

Figure 11.4. Side-Lying Infant With Back and Foot Rolls

ability to look around. This position is also important in the developmental milestones of rolling over and getting up on all fours for creeping and crawling.

The second position is side lying. This is no longer an acceptable position for sleep for infants because they could roll onto their abdomens, but it is suitable for awake or drowsy states. A long, large roll is placed firmly against the infant's back to prevent arching (Figure 11.4). The back roll, if long enough, or a second small roll can be placed under the infant's feet to maintain hip and knee flexion. Alternate positioning of the infant on the right and left side is needed to facilitate symmetrical development and for the prevention of head molding in the premature and the term infant. The side-lying position allows the infant to bring hands into midline, which facilitates passing an object from hand to hand. It also allows hand-to-mouth activities to enhance oral motor behaviors. The infant is able to observe the surroundings while keeping the head in a neutral position.

For the first 3 months of life, an infant spends an average of approximately 15 hours per day sleeping (Vaughn & Litt, 1990). Consequently, the infant should be in the supine position for these hours of sleep. Therefore, it is even more important that an infant is placed in other positions for the short amounts of awake time that occur. In the event the infant falls asleep in a prone position, the infant should be gently repositioned onto the back.

As was previously stated, supine is the recommended position for sleep. Small rolls should be placed under the shoulders to prevent hyperextension of the shoulders. The rolls need to be only thick enough to bring the arms slightly forward. Another roll should be placed just below the hips to facilitate flexion of the hips and knees (Figure 11.5). If the in-

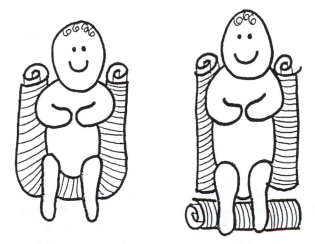

Figure 11.5. Supine Infant With Shoulder and Leg Rolls

fant tends to externally rotate the hips, the shoulder rolls can be made long enough to extend along the hips, or the roll under the hips can be curled up along the sides to keep the legs midline.

Just as it is important to place the infant on the right side and the left side for symmetrical development in the side-lying position, it is equally important to alternate head position when the infant is supine. Parents and primary caregivers tend to hold the infant so that the infant's head is predominantly cradled in the same arm, and therefore they lay the infant in the same place in the crib from this position. This pattern establishes the "head" and "foot" of the crib. Infants need to be placed so that their head is alternated between the head and foot of the crib because infants tend to turn toward the direction of the caregiver. This change of position helps the infant spend equal amounts of time with the head turned to the right, turned to the left, and in the neutral or midline position.

Rolls can also be used to maintain proper position when the infant is in a car or infant seat. Rolls placed behind the shoulders are similar to those used in the supine position. A small roll can also be placed around the infant's head to help maintain midline position. Rolls along the hips may or may not be necessary.

All positions require regular monitoring for signs of impaired circulation of arms and legs from rolls that are too big, improperly placed, or have become displaced. Likewise, the infant's respiratory effort should be monitored. After instruction, nurses need to demonstrate to parents how to place the infant in various positions. Parents need reinforcement of the use of supportive positioning through demonstration and offering rationale for each position and how it helps the infant. The case study discussed in the following section illustrates postural abnormalities from exclusive supine positioning of a preterm infant, the developmental delays that were identified, and how the use of supportive positioning by the parents helped the infant achieve developmental milestones.

INTERVENTION APPLICATION

Katie, a 1,240-gram female, was delivered at 29 weeks gestational age by emergency cesarian section for fetal distress with Apgars of 2 and 7 at 1 and 5 minutes, respectively. She was hospitalized in the neonatal intensive care unit (NICU) for 2 months, 3 days prior to her discharge to her parents' home. As per the protocol of the NICU, she was enrolled in a NICU developmental follow-up program. A nursing diagnosis of At Risk for Altered Growth and Development related to her premature birth was made. She was initially seen at 4 months, 1 week chronological age; development was within normal limits for her adjusted age of 1 month, 2 weeks. She demonstrated a right-side head-lying preference and mildly flattened right occipital area. No facial asymmetry was observed. She was able to right her head to midline with object stimulus and would visually track past the midline, but she was unable to turn her head independently to the left. She also demonstrated mild hyperextension of the shoulder girdle. The infant was bottle fed. She had minimal prone play activity while awake. The parents related that Katie disliked prone positioning, and they were unaware of head-turning preference. When the examiner revealed this preference, however, the parents stated that Katie did demonstrate a right-sided head-turning preference at home. The activities in the Supportive Positioning intervention were discussed and demonstrated to the parents. The parents were interested in the activities and demonstrated understanding of supportive positioning. This information was also provided in the form of a pamphlet, with simple illustrations of positions, that was given to the parents to refer to at home. The pamphlet was designed to be a reminder for the parents of how to use the supports for each position and to reinforce the benefits of each position. The Nursing Outcomes Classification outcome Child Development appropriate for age (Iowa Outcomes Project, 2000) was used along with other developmental tools to monitor Katie's development.

At 7 months, the infant's development was questionable for her adjusted age of 4 months, 1 week per the standard of the Denver II Developmental Screening Test. One delay was observed in the gross motor sector because the infant was unable to maintain her head in an upright steady position. She would tilt her head mildly to the right. Other significant findings on physical examination consisted of mild facial asymmetry as forehead protrusion noted on the same side of the occipital flattening and forehead flattening on the opposite side with subtle asymmetry noted in the fullness of cheeks. The parents related that Katie disliked prone positioning, and they had not followed through with alternate positioning. The parents stated that it was not comfortable to alternate holding the infant in the right and left arms for bottle feeding. They were also reluctant to place Katie in the prone position because it made her cry. The intervention activities for supportive positioning were reemphasized. In addition, the parents were instructed to passively exercise Katie's head from side to side four or five times at each diaper change to facilitate full range of motion. The examiner demonstrated how the passive exercises were to be done. Once the parents were aware of the subtle asymmetry and limited neck range of motion, they were again motivated to use the supportive positioning activities.

At 9 months chronological age (6 months, 1 week adjusted age), Katie's developmental behaviors were within normal limits for adjusted age. Katie was able to sit briefly without support and maintain her head in an upright position. The parents related that they had been quite dedicated to using supportive positioning and passive range-of-motion exercises for Katie during the first few weeks after the 7-month visit but had not been as diligent the past 2 or 3 weeks.

RESEARCH AND PRACTICE IMPLICATIONS

Additional research about supine positioning of term infants and the influence of position on neuromotor and musculoskeletal development needs to be undertaken. Similarly, additional research on the effect of the use of supports in positioning infants will determine whether supportive positioning facilitates symmetrical development or whether merely alternating positions can be as effective. Finally, additional evaluation of the pamphlet that was used in the case study is needed to understand its effectiveness as a tool for parent education.

Infants of younger gestational ages are surviving and going home as a result of advances in neonatology and perinatology. These infants are most susceptible to exclusive positioning and could benefit most from alternating positions. Nurses can serve as role models for parents. Nurses in NICUs are providing supported positions and alternate infant position, but parents also need to realize the importance of position change postdischarge.

Education about supportive positioning also needs to be provided for parents of healthy term infants. Discharge teaching for parents of newborn or premature infants should include supportive positioning and the demonstration of positioning with their infants after teaching. Tools such as a brochure with illustrations or a videotape could be used as a supplement to teaching and serve as a guide for parents after they take their infants home. We have a responsibility as health professionals to educate parents about positioning so that they can use the activities to foster their infant's growth and development and avoid potential problems associated with exclusive supine positioning.

REFERENCES

Als, H., Lawhon, G., Brown, E., Gibes, R., Duffy, F. H., McAnulty, G., & Blickman, J. G. (1986). Individualized behavioral and environmental care for the very low birth weight preterm infant at high risk for bronchopulmonary dysplasia: Neonatal intensive care unit and developmental outcome. *Pediatrics, 78*(6), 1123-1132.

Becker, P. T., Grunwald, P. C., Moorman, J., & Stuhr, S. (1991). Outcomes of developmentally supportive nursing care for very low birth weight infants. *Nursing Research, 40*(11), 150-155.

Downs, J. A., Edwards, A. D., McCormick, D. C., Roth, S. C., & Stewart, A. L. (1991). Effect of intervention on development of hip posture in very preterm babies. *Archives of Disease in Childhood, 66*(7), 797-801.

Dwyer, T., Ponsonby, A. L., Blizzard, L., Newman, N. M., & Cochrane, J. A. (1995). The contribution of changes in the prevalence of prone sleeping position to the decline in sudden infant death syndrome in Tasmania. *Journal of the American Medical Association, 273*(10), 783-789.

Fay, M. J. (1988). The positive effects of positioning. *Neonatal Network, 12*(3), 23-28.

Gennaro, S., & Bakewell-Sachs, S. (1991). Discharge planning and home care for low-birth-weight infants. *NAACOG's Clinical Issues, 3,* 129-145.

Georgieff, M. K., & Bernbaum, J. C. (1986). Abnormal shoulder girdle muscle tone in premature infants during their first 18 months of life. *Pediatrics, 77*(5), 664-669.

Grunwald, P. C., & Becker, P. T. (1991). Developmental enhancement: Implementing a program for the NICU. *Neonatal Network, 9*(6), 29-45.

Hunt, C. E., & Puczynski, M. S. (1996). Does supine sleeping cause asymmetric heads? *Pediatrics, 98,* 127-129.

Iowa Outcomes Project. (2000). *Nursing outcomes classification (NOC)* (M. Johnson, M. Maas, & S. Moorhead, Eds.; 2nd ed.). St. Louis, MO: Mosby-Year Book.

Kane, A. A., Mitchell, L. E., Craven, K. P., & Marsh, J. L. (1996). Observations on a recent increase in plagiocephaly without synostosis. *Pediatrics, 97*(6), 877-885.

Kattwinkel, J., Brooks, J., Keenan, M. E., & Malloy, M. (1996). Positioning and sudden infant death syndrome (SIDS): Update. American Academy of Pediatrics Task Force on Infant Positioning and SIDS. *Pediatrics, 98* (6, Pt. 1), 1216-1218.

Kattwinkel, J., Brooks, J., & Myerberg, D. (1992). Positioning and SIDS. *Pediatrics, 89*(6), 1120-1126.

Klonoff-Cohen, H. S., & Edelstein, S. L. (1995). A case-control study of routine and death scene sleep position and sudden infant death syndrome in southern California. *Journal of the American Medical Association, 273*(10), 790-794.

Konishi, Y., Kuriyama, M., Mikawa, H., & Suzuki, J. (1987). Effect of body position on later postural and functional lateralities of preterm infants. *Developmental Medicine and Child Neurology, 29*(6), 751-757.

North American Nursing Diagnosis Association. (1999). *Nursing diagnoses: Definitions and classification 1999-2000.* Philadelphia: Author.

Oehler, J. M., Strickland, M., & Nordlund, C. (1991). Beyond technology: Meeting developmental need of infants in NICUs. *MCN: American Journal of Maternal Child Nursing, 16*(3), 148-151.

Perez-Woods, R., Malloy, M. B., & Tse, A. M. (1992). Positioning and skin care of the low-birth-weight neonate. *NAACOG's Clinical Issues, 3,* 97-113.

Tappero, E. P. (1993). Musculoskeletal system assessment. In E. P. Tappero & M. E. Honeyfield (Eds.), *Physical assessment of the newborn: A comprehensive approach to the art of physical examination* (pp. 101-119). Petaluma, CA: NICU.

Updike, C., Schmidt, R. E., Macke, C., Cahoon, J., & Miller, M. (1986). Positional support for premature infants. *American Journal of Occupational Therapy, 40*(10), 712-715.

U.S. Department of Health and Human Services. (1995). *Healthy people 2000 midcourse review and 1995 revisions.* Washington, DC: Government Printing Office.

Vaughn, V. C., & Litt, I. (1990). The first year. In V. C. Vaughn & I. Litt (Eds.), *Child and adolescent development: Clinical implications* (pp. 163-178). Philadelphia: W. B. Saunders.

Willinger, M. (1995). Sleep position and sudden infant death syndrome. *Journal of the American Medical Association, 273,* 818-819.

12

Early Intervention

Marie L. Lobo

Early intervention consists of community-based services with a goal of minimizing the "impact of a child's disability or the impact of prevailing risk factors to strengthen families and to establish the foundation for subsequent development" (Guralnick, 1997a, p. xv). Programs that have emerged are complex and rely on numerous disciplines to implement the necessary interventions. With increased knowledge about the important influence of early environment on development, programs have incorporated more complex interventions that are delivered to the child and family as early as possible. In 1989, Savage and Culbert discussed the unique role that nurses can play in early intervention. They used the term *early intervention* to mean "educational and therapeutic services provided for infants and toddlers between birth and 3 years of age who have been identified as biologically or environmentally at risk for developmental delay" (p. 239). Families must work with nurses and other health professionals in the planning of the child's program of early intervention if it is to succeed (Crutcher, 1991; Roberts, Wasik, Casto, & Ramey, 1991; Rousch, Harrison, & Palsha, 1991). Interagency collaboration, nurses, and the family are all a part of the team approach that is critical if early intervention is to be successful (Bazyk, 1989; Reiss, Cameron, Matthews, & Shenkman, 1996).

Although many nurses are involved in implementing early intervention and in conducting research on early intervention, many of the reports are from interdisciplinary teams and are published in interdisciplinary journals. This strength of early intervention makes the determination of the unique nursing contribution difficult because nursing contributions are embedded within these interdisciplinary reports. This intricate interdisciplinary care, however, provides many resources for the child and family.

LITERATURE REVIEW

Early intervention consists of services provided to an infant and the family to promote optimal infant and child growth and development. These services are offered with the goal of enhancing social, cognitive, emotional, or physical growth and development or all these. The most successful programs occur over a period of time. They include the family and professionals who customize and implement the interventions. Successful programs include both home and institutional components. Some programs provide additional social services to parents that enhance the child's environment, such as job training or literacy classes. Characteristics of programs should include long-term contact with the families and many services to the families (Gallagher, 1991).

Minimum components for statewide comprehensive systems should include (a) definitions of developmental delay; (b) a timetable for services to all in need in the state; (c) comprehensive multidisciplinary assessment of needs of children and families; (d) individualized family service plans, child find, and referral systems; and (e) central directories of resources, experts, and services. In addition, policies and procedures need to be in place for implementation of the programs, personnel standards, and systems for compiling data. A public awareness campaign must also be developed (Sass-Lehrer & Bodner-Johnson, 1989). Each state can implement statewide comprehensive systems in its own manner, however. Agencies vary from education to health, social services, developmental disabilities, and interagency coordinating councils. It is not clear how individuals are referred for services to all these different agencies.

The diversity between states makes a comparison of the programs and their outcomes almost impossible. In a meta-analysis of early intervention programs, Bryant and Maxwell (1997) drew different conclusions than Innocenti and White (1993) when analyzing the same early intervention studies. There are different definitions of significant terms used in describing early intervention studies. "Intensity" and "duration" of the intervention are terms included in most studies. Some define intensity as the number of hours a child is seen in a program (Innocenti & White, 1993), whereas others examine the amount of resources available to the constituents being served (Wasik & Karweit, 1994). "High-intensity" programs are those with greater amounts of time and more services provided to both parents and child for a longer duration, whereas "low-intensity" programs usually last for a shorter period of time, focus on only the child or the parents, and have fewer components. As Bryant and Maxwell (1997) note, timing and duration are often intertwined. That is, the closer the child is to school-age at entry, the shorter the duration of the program. For most of the studies reported in the literature, the longer the child and family are in the program and the more comprehensive the program, the more positive and enduring are the outcomes (Barnett, 1995; Olds & Kitzman, 1993; Ramey & Ramey, 1992; Yoshikawa, 1995). The many program variabilities may also be affecting or influencing the outcomes in a way that is not measured. For example, if parents are receiving job training or receiving some other support services that might indirectly affect the outcome of the early intervention program, those services must be incorporated into the model.

Some programs enroll children by physical risk (i.e., prematurity or other physical handicapping conditions), whereas others identify social risks (i.e., maternal education, intelligence quotient, or family poverty) (Bryant & Maxwell, 1997; Powell, 1993; Yoshikawa, 1995). Some programs enroll mothers prenatally and follow the child after birth for some period of time, whereas others enroll children at various ages, up to and including kindergarten (Olds & Kitzman, 1993). This great variability makes comparisons difficult. Identifying the nurse's role in these diverse programs is a challenge because nurses are involved to very different degrees in the varied interventions and evaluations.

CHILDREN IN NEED OF EARLY INTERVENTION

Early intervention has been developed for children who are socially and physically at risk. The socially at-risk child may live in a single-parent home, with a family in poverty, with drug-using parents, with a mentally retarded parent, or in a community with environmental risks such as high lead levels (Bryant & Maxwell, 1997; Feldman, 1997). Physically at-risk infants may be born prematurely or have a genetic problem or other structural problem, such as prenatal exposure to human immunodeficiency virus; all these make them vulnerable to developmental delay (Cohen,

Grosz, Ayoob, & Schoen, 1997). Some may have technological dependencies in addition to prematurity (Als, 1997).

According to *Kids Count Data Book: 1997* (Casey, 1997), 21% of all children in the United States live in poverty, with 9% of all children living in extreme poverty—that is, in a family with income lower than 50% of the poverty level. The teen birth rate for 15- to 17-year-olds is 38 per 1,000 (Casey, 1997). Although the infant mortality rate in the United States has decreased to 8 per 1,000 live births, the percentage of low-birth-weight infants has increased to 7.3% (Casey, 1997). African American infants are twice as likely as white infants to be born low birth weight or die before their first birthday (Children's Defense Fund, 1997).

It has long been recognized that there are many challenges in identifying at-risk infants and their families (Ramey & Brownlee, 1981). Children born into families with the previously mentioned characteristics are at risk for developmental delays from physical, social, and environmental factors. These infants can have a better future with early intervention (Guralnick, 1997a).

Much of the research in nursing has focused on the premature infant or infant in the neonatal intensive care unit (NICU), although more children are at risk from social and environmental deprivation (Als et al., 1986; Barnard et al., 1987; Kang et al., 1995). Programs for premature or NICU residents often focus on enhancing parenting or stimulating optimum growth and development of the infant while they are in the NICU or both. Some programs continue for a defined period after discharge, but these vary greatly. Although targeted short-term programs help, they are not as effective as long-term early intervention.

Entry into early intervention programs may be dictated by the program rather than by the child's needs. For example, children born in Jones County School District are eligible to participate in a program such as Parents as Teachers (Carnegie Corporation of New York, 1994) offered to all new parents in the community. Children may enter from birth to 4 years of age, depending on the structure of the program. Most findings support the idea that the earlier the child begins the program, and the more intense and comprehensive the services, the stronger the long-term outcomes in terms of health (Barnett, 1995; Guralnick, 1997a).

The manner of implementation in these programs varies. The range of comprehensive services varies from a single lay visitor, providing the parent and infant with specific information, to multiple professionals providing very specialized information and strategies. Nurses have been identified as optimal early intervenors because of the broad base of physical, social, developmental, and health information that they can provide to the mother (Olds & Kitzman, 1993). A visit by a nurse can be flexible and meet the immediate needs of the child and parents.

LEGAL MANDATE FOR SERVICES

Beginning with the establishment of the Children's Bureau in 1912, there was a recognition by the federal government that it had a responsibility for the well-being of the children of the United States (Guralnick, 1997b). Many programs were initiated throughout the years for both socially and physically at-risk children. The most influential move to provide early intervention to infants and young children in the United States occurred in 1986 with the passage of Public Law (PL) 99-457, the Education of the Handicapped Act Amendment, which mandated that states provide early intervention programs for handicapped infants and toddlers (Downey, 1990a, 1990b; Meisels, 1989; Sass-Lehrer & Bodner-Johnson, 1989). These programs were to be comprehensive, multidisciplinary, and family focused. Part H of this federal law specifically targets the prevention or minimization of developmental delays in children. The goals include reduction in special education costs and assistance to families in meeting the needs of their handicapped child. Although identifying physically or mentally handicapped infants may be relatively easy, identifying the child at environmental risk is more challenging. Each state has developed its own early intervention program, which means that entry criteria and services available vary in each of the 50 states.

The passage of PL 99-457 brought two major changes in services for both the handicapped and other at-risk infants. First, this law required Individual Family Service Plans (IFSP) to be developed by the team of professionals in conjunction with the family (Downey, 1990b). The IFSP coordination is often handled by the professional with the most responsibility in the child's care. The inclusion of the family in planning was a primary difference from earlier programs for young children (Beckman & Bristol, 1991; Campbell, Strickland, & La Forme, 1992; Krauss, 1990). A second significant difference in this legislation was the inclusion of children from birth to 3 years of age. Earlier legislation had mandated services beginning at 3 years of age. In the early 1980s, it was recognized that valuable time in a child's development was lost when intervention did not begin at birth, influencing the development of legislation that mandated services from birth.

Public Law 99-457 was updated in 1990 with the passage of PL 101-476 (Individuals With Disabilities Education Act [IDEA]), which mandated additional services for disabled children (Pakala & Palmer, 1997). Pakala and Palmer noted, "This law provided financial incentives to states to establish comprehensive early intervention services, including screening, identification, referral, and treatment for infants and toddlers with or at risk for developmental disabilities" (p. 99). In addition,

family resources is essential to developing IFSP to meet the needs of the infant and family.

The infant's physical risk factors, such as low birth weight, prenatal exposure to drugs or alcohol, and known genetic factors, should be assessed before treatment is planned. Physical problems resulting from events in the perinatal period, such as intraventricular hemorrhage, might be central to care. Any physical or genetic problems that will affect cognitive development must also be identified and integrated into the treatment plan.

The home environment and other environments, such as day care or a grandparent's home where the child spends a significant portion of time, are also included in the assessment. The quality and quantity of toys and books should be assessed as well as the cleanliness and safety of the environment. A safe bed and access to adequate nutrition are also important. The infant should be in the least restrictive but safe environment possible, with the interventions integrated into the environment.

NURSING DIAGNOSIS AND OUTCOMES DETERMINATION

Diagnosis

The nursing diagnosis will flow from the assessment data. There are many diagnoses related to family functioning and family process, parenting, growth, and development that often fit infants and families needing early intervention. Examples of common nursing diagnoses used in early intervention include (a) potential for Altered Growth and Development of the infant related to Knowledge Deficit: Parental; (b) Altered Growth and Development of the infant related to prematurity; (c) alterations or potential alterations in family development related to an infant with a neurological deficit (or other identified health problem); (d) Altered Parenting related to single parent, unwanted child, child illness, or social isolation; and (e) Altered Family Processes related to birth of premature infant, drug abuse in a family member, and poverty (North American Nursing Diagnosis Association, 2000).

Outcomes

Evaluation of the outcomes of early intervention programs varies greatly. Because there are multiple tools and methods used in evaluating early intervention programs, comparing the outcomes of various programs is challenging ("The Future of Children," 1995). The frequency of post–early intervention evaluation also varies. Some programs are evaluated in the short term, 6 weeks or 3 months after completion, whereas other programs evaluate their participants for years, up to and including adulthood. Other early intervention programs have control groups that receive no treatment. There is great variability in the controls to program participants and the ability to recontact them after years have passed for additional outcome evaluation. Some believe it is imperative that investigators examine the long-term outcomes of early intervention programs to justify continued funding (Gomby, Larner, Stevenson, Lewit, & Behrman, 1995). It is difficult to compare programs that vary so greatly in their outcome indicators; therefore, standardized measures are needed to facilitate comparison.

Other standardized instruments used for outcomes include the Bayley Scales of Infant Development for physical and cognitive development, and the standard tests of intelligence, such as Cattel IQ, Stanford-Binet, or McCarthy, can be used (Aylward, 1995). Tools to measure the quality of parent-infant interaction include the Nursing Child Assessment Teaching and Feeding Scales (Sumner & Spietz, 1994a, 1994b). Qualities of the home environment are evaluated using the Home Observation for Measurement of the Environment (Caldwell & Bradley, 1978), and evaluation of language development is done with the Early Language Milestone Scale (Coplan, 1989).

According to the Iowa Outcomes Project (2000), the definition of *parenting* is "the provision of an environment that promotes optimum growth and development of dependent children" (p. 332). The following are examples of key indicators that reflect the outcomes of the parenting interventions: (a) provides for child's basic needs, (b) eliminates controllable environmental hazards, (c) provides regular preventative and episodic health care, (d) stimulates cognitive development, (e) stimulates social development, and (f) stimulates emotional development (Iowa Outcomes Project, 2000). This list is by no means inclusive of all the indicators one would like to see as a result of early intervention, but these outcomes do reflect some of the areas covered in program evaluation.

Outcomes related to *growth,* defined as "a normal increase in body size and weight" (Iowa Outcomes Project, 2000, p. 225), may also be included in the evaluation of early intervention programs. Selected indicators include (a) weight percentile for age, (b) weight percentile for height, (c) length and height percentile for age, (d) head circumference percentile for age, (e) rate of weight gain, and (f) rate of height gain (Iowa Outcomes Project, 1997). The goal is to have no deviations from the expected normal ranges for age and gender.

Child development outcomes are always changing. During the first year of life, a healthy infant acquires multiple new skills, from as simple as following an object with his or her eyes to reaching, grabbing, and manipulating the object; from being dependent on responsible caregivers to change his or her position to rolling over and walking; and from coos and babbling to saying words. One definition of *child development* is the attainment of milestones of physical, cognitive, and psychosocial progression appropriate for age (Iowa Outcomes Project, 2000). Child development indicators for a 12-month-old child are used here as an example. Some of the key indicators of accomplishment of expected tasks include (a) attempts to take steps alone, (b) precise pincher grasp, (c) bangs blocks together, (d) drinks from a cup, (e) feeds self with spoon, and (f) uses vocabulary of one to three words in addition to "mama" and "dada" (Iowa Outcomes Project, 2000). It should be noted that many of these indicators are included as items in the various tests and scales used to measure the effect of early intervention. Specific developmental outcomes would be expected based on the age of the child.

INTERVENTION: EARLY INTERVENTION

Early intervention is not a well-defined construct. Therefore, it is not surprising that implementation of early intervention varies extensively. Some programs are center based (i.e., implemented in an institution, day care, or child development center), some are home based, and some programs include both home- and center-based services (Carnegie Corporation of New York, 1994; Weiss, 1993). Although the physical environment may differ, the target of the intervention may also differ, with some aimed at parents, some at the child, and some including the parents, the child, and any other members of the household (Carnegie Corporation of New York, 1994; Weiss, 1993). It is important to note that early intervention is a family-centered activity. The child in need of intervention spends the majority of his or her time within the family unit. It is critical for the early intervention team to include the family in all aspects of their planning, acknowledging the complex nature of the impact of the child's disability or potential disability on the family (Trout & Foley, 1989). Many parents are angry and guilty about their loss of the expected "ideal" infant. These factors can interfere with the family dynamics, creating even more stress within the family system. Parents need (a) information about the amount of time it will take for them to work with their child and how outcomes will be assessed, (b) an opportunity to set goals with the early intervention team, (c) respect for their skills as parents, and (d) support for their commitment to their child if the early intervention team is to be successful (Musick, 1998).

Nursing activities for early intervention with children include the following assessment, intervention, and evaluation strategies:

1. Monitor the child by collecting information, tracking events, making nursing diagnosis, and identifying the problems and concerns of the family.

2. Provide information in verbal or written form to the client and provide role modeling information using a variety of media, including books, pamphlets, computer programs, and videotapes.

3. Provide support by validating behaviors, reinforcing care activities, and praising and encouraging the parents in caring for their infants. Support also includes listening and assisting in accessing supplies and other resources.

4. Provide therapy or services or both for a specific problem, such as feeding difficulties.

5. Develop a plan of action to achieve the goals set by the nurse with the interdisciplinary team.

6. Provide and seek consultation from other professionals involved in the case.

7. Serve as a referral source, directing families to other institutions within the community (Kang, Barnard, & Oshio, 1994).

These nursing activities have been demonstrated by Barnard and colleagues in many studies with the goal of improving outcomes for infants at risk. When reading the integrated review by Olds and Kitzman (1993), some or all of these intervention activities are noted in the successful programs.

Kang et al.'s (1994) early intervention activities for the nurse are comparable to those found in the National Standards of Nursing Practice for Early Intervention Services. The roles of the nurse as defined in the National Standards include (a) diagnosing and treating health problems with infants and families at risk for or with existing health or developmental needs; (b) screening and assessing the psychological, physiological, and developmental qualities of the child and family for early identification, referral, and intervention; (c) planning and coordinating with the family and interdisciplinary team; (d) providing interventions to improve the child and family health and developmental status; and (e) evaluating the effectiveness of nursing care provided to the child and family (Consensus Committee-Maternal Child Nursing, 1993, as cited in Collin, 1995, p. 530).

Parents are the key to early intervention implementation. Ramey and Ramey (1992) support the need for continuous educational intervention activities during the first 5 years of the child's life. They identified six essential types of experiences that optimize a child's growth and development: (a) encouragement of exploration; (b) mentoring in basic skills; (c) celebration of developmental advances; (d) guided rehearsal and extension of new skills; (e) protection from inappropriate disapproval, teasing, or punishment; and (f) provision of a rich and responsive language environment (Ramey & Ramey, 1992). Nurses can be key in encouraging these experiences through anticipatory guidance during routine well child care, immunization visits, and home visits (Green, 1994). By providing these experiences, the child will be better able to attain the desired outcomes of early intervention.

A major intervention activity developed and implemented by nurses in early intervention is the enhancement of parent-infant interaction. According to Barnard's (1997) analysis of multiple studies, there is a relationship between the quality of parent-infant interaction and later cognitive and language development in the child. Many of the intervention activities developed by nurses are short term, in the hospital, or based on limited home visits after discharge. Activities include reinforcing positive parenting behaviors and teaching parents about their infant's capabilities.

Activities for early intervention used successfully by nurses include educational and supportive activities with the caregiver of preterm or physically or socially at-risk infants. Some nurses have used videotapes as a method to teach parents about their child (Koniak-Griffen, Verzemnieks, & Cahill, 1992; Rich, 1990). The parents and child are videotaped together during a feeding or teaching activity, and the tape is then played back with commentary from the nurse. With the availability of portable video cameras and video cassette recorders in most homes and clinics, videotaped interventions can be used easily. Parents who observe their behavior, and who receive coaching by the nurse, can be encouraged to interact with their infant in a positive and stimulating manner.

Other educational activities include teaching the parents how to talk to their child. The importance of mothers talking to their infants is becoming more apparent every day. Demonstrating to the mother the infant's response to her voice is one strategy of enhancing parent-infant interaction. Lawhon (as cited in Barnard, 1997, p. 259) established a "therapeutic alliance" with the parents, focusing her interventions on the parents' interests. She demonstrated increased parental and infant competence with this strategy, and infants were discharged earlier than those not in the intervention program.

The following are activities that have been identified in the Nursing Interventions Classification (Iowa Intervention Project, 2000) for developmental enhancement: (a) build a trusting relationship with the child and family; (b) demonstrate activities that promote development to caregivers; (c) encourage child to interact with others by role-modeling interaction skills; (d) create a safe, well-defined space for the child to explore and learn; and (e) sing and talk to the child. Activities to improve parenting include the following: (a) teach normal physiological, emotional, and behavioral characteristics of child; (b) identify appropriate developmental tasks or goals for the child; (c) review nutritional requirements for the specific age; and (d) review developmentally appropriate safety issues (Iowa Intervention Project, 1996). The nurse going into the home or meeting with a family in the clinic has many opportunities to help parents gain the knowledge required to nurture their infant. Parents overwhelmed with the effects of poverty, drug use, or lack of education may not be sensitive to the needs of a child until these are reviewed with them. These activities help parents recognize and meet the appropriate needs of their child.

It should be noted that, to be effective, the activities suggested previously must be done together. None of these approaches will be as effective in isolation as multiple approaches to infants and families in need of early intervention. For example, telling the parents what they should expect in infant behavior at the next stage of development must be accompanied by suggestions of how the parents can help the child attain the next stage. Parents must be included as partners in their child's care if the interventions are to be successful.

INTERVENTION APPLICATION

Isaac is the preterm newborn son of Laurie Smith, a 26-year-old African American mother who teaches English to junior high school students, and her husband, Michael Smith, a 27-year-old African American engineer. Both parents and children are covered by health insurance from their jobs. The Smiths live in a suburban, single-family dwelling, which they are purchasing. They have one other child, Jacob, who is 3 years old, up-to-date on well child care, and healthy. Jacob is in day care while Laurie and Michael work. Isaac was the product of a planned pregnancy, and Laurie had routine prenatal care. She developed toxemia of pregnancy, however, and delivered Isaac at 29 weeks. After 6 weeks in the NICU, the Smiths brought Isaac home from the hospital. Isaac came home with tube feedings and an apnea monitor. Although Isaac received developmentally appropriate and state-related care, he experienced a Grade 2 intraventricular bleed in the hospital; thus, both his pediatrician and the Smiths knew he had the potential for developmental delays.

The initial nursing diagnoses were Potential for Alterations in Development Related to Preterm Birth and Potential for Alterations in Family Process Related to Stress of Birth of Preterm Child With Potential Developmental Disabilities. The Smiths were referred to Babynet, the state early intervention provider. After evaluation by a developmental pediatrician, in which physical delays and potential cognitive developmental delays were identified, Isaac was referred for multiple services. He received visits from a nurse, occupational therapist, physical therapist, speech therapist, education specialist, and an early interventionist. An early interventionist in many states is an individual who has graduated from college and has had additional training in developmental stimulation. This individual works as a member of the early intervention team. He or she assists in the provision of resources and services to the child and family. In some situations, this individual may be the coordinator of care.

Isaac's early intervention team was coordinated by the nurse case manager. She facilitated the planning meeting with all the members of his early intervention team, which included the parents. An IFSP was developed to incorporate Isaac's parents into the planning and implementation of his care. In the IFSP, goals were stated in a clear, measurable manner, and standardized tools such as the Bayley were identified that would be used to determine Isaac's developmental progress. Laurie quit her position as a teacher to care for Isaac, which caused the family income to decrease by approximately one third. Financial assistance was made available through the state because financial support for early intervention was not covered by their private insurance. (This coverage is guaranteed by the state under Part H of the Individuals With Disabilities Education Act, PL 99-457). Jacob also began staying home from his day care, which saved some money for the family. The family's patterns of interaction both within the family and with their friends and community were altered because of the amount of time required for Isaac's care.

Occupational therapists visited the home, focusing on fine motor and feeding issues. They visited twice a week and instructed Laurie in additional exercises to perform during the rest of the week. The physical therapist also visited twice a week and instructed Laurie in large motor exercises to implement with Isaac during the rest of the week. The speech therapist visited once a week, again asking Laurie to practice with Isaac certain exercises every day. The early interventionist worked with Isaac on integrating these skills and stimulating cognitive development. Although the educator attended the team meetings, she did not visit weekly because of the stimulation Laurie was already providing.

Home visits by the nurse case manager focused on coordination of all of Isaac's care, assessing and intervening with the family stresses occurring with decreased income, changes in child care for Jacob, and implementing the multiple strategies being used to enhance Isaac's development. The nurse also began focusing on enhancing the quality of parent-infant interaction and infant stimulation. Because of his neurological deficits, it was difficult at times to read Isaac's cues. His cries were high pitched, and it was not always possible to determine what he wanted. A decision was also made to schedule some of the visits from the providers late in the day or early evening so that Michael could participate in the intervention process.

The providers going into the home worked at building a trusting relationship with the child and family. The needs of the child and family had been identified in the hospital and transmitted to the home-based program staff. The intervention Developmental Enhancement activities were structured for the family that facilitated Isaac's cognitive, psychosocial, and physical development (Iowa Intervention Project, 2000). Materials useful for helping the Smiths learn to read Isaac's cues were provided from the program *Keys to Caregiving* (Barnard, 1997).

The intervention activities for Family Involvement focused on the parents and family and included identification of the strengths of the family to care for Isaac. The nurse monitored the family structure and roles to assist the family in sharing the challenges of implementing all the activities needed for Isaac to attain maximum functioning. She also worked with the family to ensure that they understood Isaac's medical condition and his potential for maximum growth and development. She also helped them identify and access resources within their network to assist them in the care of a special needs child (Iowa Intervention Project, 2000).

Indicators of adequate child development at 12 months include large motor capabilities, such as pulls to a stand, cruises around furniture, and attempts to take steps alone. Fine motor indicators of success include precise pincer grasp, points with fingers, and bangs blocks together. Oral motor indicators include the ability to ingest enough food to meet caloric needs. Combined oral and fine motor skills include feeding self finger food and feeding self with a spoon. Cognitive development can be indicated by a vocabulary that includes one to three words in addition to "mama" and "dada," imitating vocalization, and playing social games (Iowa Outcomes Project, 2000, p. 158).

Outcomes for parenting include the following: provides for the child's physical needs and provides regular and preventive health care. The Smiths demonstrated their abilities to use community resources and provide cognitive social-emotional and physical developmental stimulation. They expressed satisfaction with their roles as parents because they saw the growth Isaac had made in his first year of life (Iowa Outcomes Project, 1997, p. 229). In addition, by 1 year Isaac had all of his immunizations for age and had all of his well child visits. Also, Isaac had no emergency department visits or injuries during his first year. On the basis of the Bayley Scales of Infant Development, Isaac was at an appropriate developmental age, adjusted for prematurity, at the end of 1 year of early intervention. He was able to take all food orally and was making strides in meeting his gross and fine motor activities for age. He was also beginning to verbalize more frequently. His early intervention team would continue to work with Isaac and his family, adjusting the plans according to his achievement of developmental milestones. Plans were made to follow

Isaac in the follow-up developmental clinic through entry into elementary school.

PRACTICE AND RESEARCH IMPLICATIONS

Early intervention activities address complex issues related to cognitive, emotional, and biobehavioral dimensions. They can be summarized as (a) problem identification; (b) assisted referral; (c) care coordination in the hospital, community, or home or all three; (d) developmental intervention activities; and (e) parent education about health and developmental implications of the child's diagnosis (Robinson, 1997).

Early intervention programs are evolving as interdisciplinary programs. Nurses are the ideal professionals to intervene with young children because of the breadth of knowledge they bring to the situation (Olds & Kitzman, 1993). Nurses are accustomed to working with families in their homes and in the hospital. Nurses are also the professionals who spend the most time with high-risk infants in NICUs and other institutions. Nurses have the knowledge to assist these children to achieve a better quality of life.

Much more information is needed about optimal timing, intensity, and duration of interventions. Each provider, nurse, occupational therapist, physical therapist, and educator working with the parents must identify the specific areas on which to focus. Early intervention is often evaluated in the short term, such as 3 or 6 months after treatment is completed. To understand the true efficacy of early intervention, long-term studies with large numbers of infants and families must be conducted.

There is a great need for systematic evaluation of the effectiveness of early intervention programs. Many different intervention programs have been attempted, as have many evaluation strategies. There are several findings that need to be incorporated in future programs. Early intervention needs to begin as soon after birth as possible; for prematures, this may mean in the NICU. Early intervention needs to be intensive and ideally contain both a home- and center-based component, particularly for infants who are at risk because of poverty and inadequate home environments. Early intervention needs to occur over a sufficient length of time so that the intervention "takes," allowing the infant to benefit from the intervention for the longest period of time.

In reviewing the literature, there was no identified theoretical perspective used consistently between and among the programs. Furthermore, the operational definition for early intervention varies. For example, literature review inconsistencies were found with regard to the frequency and duration of visits. Differences in definition, combined with varying levels of providers, makes it difficult to compare and contrast various programs. In future studies, it is imperative for these issues to be addressed and for a standard definition of early intervention to be adopted.

This intervention is timely and significant for improving the quality and decreasing the cost of health care. The testing of the intervention for efficacy and effectiveness across settings will make a significant contribution to nursing sciences and policy decisions.

REFERENCES

Als, H. (1997). Earliest intervention for preterm infants in the newborn intensive care unit. In M. J. Guralnick (Ed.), *The effectiveness of early intervention* (pp. 47-76). Baltimore, MD: Brookes.

Als, H., Lawhon, G., Brown, E., Gibes, R., Duffy, F., McAnulty, G., & Blickman, J. (1986). Individualized behavioral and environmental care for the very low birth weight preterm infant at high-risk for bronchopulmonary dysplasia: Neonatal intensive care unit and developmental outcome. *Pediatrics, 78,* 1123-1132.

Aylward, G. P. (1995). *Bayley infant neurodevelopmental screener.* San Antonio, TX: Harcourt Brace.

Barnard, K. E. (1997). Influencing parent-child interactions for children at risk. In M. J. Guralnick (Ed.), *The effectiveness of early intervention* (pp. 249-268). Baltimore, MD: Brookes.

Barnard, K. E., Hammond, M. A., Sumner, G. A., Kang, R., Johnson-Crowley, N., Snyder, C., Spietz, A., Blackburn, S., Brandt, P., & Magyary, D. (1987). Helping parents with preterm infants: Field test of a protocol. *Early Child Development and Care, 27,* 256-290.

Barnett, W. S. (1995). Long-term effects of early childhood programs on cognitive and school outcomes. *Future of Children, 5*(3), 25-50.

Bazyk, S. (1989). Changes in attitudes and beliefs regarding parent participation and home programs: An update. *American Journal of Occupational Therapy, 43,* 723-728.

Beckman, P. J., & Bristol, M. M. (1991). Issues in developing the IFSP: A framework for establishing family outcomes. *Topics in Early Childhood Special Education, 11,* 19-31.

Blair, C., Ramey, C. T., & Hardin, J. M. (1995). Early intervention for low birthweight, premature infants; Participation and intellectual growth and development. *American Journal of Mental Retardation, 99,* 542-554.

Bradley, R. H., Whiteside, L., Mundfrom, D. J., Casey, P. H., Kelleher, K. J., & Pope, S. K. (1994). Early indications of resilience and their relation to experiences in the home environments of low birthweight, premature children living in poverty. *Child Development, 65,* 346-360.

Brooks-Gunn, J., McCarton, C. M., Casey, P. H., McCormick, M. C., Bauer, C. R., Bernbaum, J. C., Tyson, J., Swanson, M., Bennett, F. C., Scott, D. T., Tonascia, J., & Meinert, C. L. (1994). Early intervention in low-birth-weight premature infants. *Journal of the American Medical Association, 272,* 1257-1262.

Pakala, A. L., & Palmer, F. B. (1997). Early intervention for children at risk for neuromotor problems. In M. J. Guralnick (Ed.), *The effectiveness of early intervention* (pp. 99-108). Baltimore, MD: Brookes.

Powell, D. R. (1993). Inside home visiting programs. *Future of Children, 3,* 23-38.

Ramey, C. T., & Brownlee, J. R. (1981). Improving the identification of high-risk infants. *American Journal of Mental Deficiency, 85,* 504-511.

Ramey, C. T., Bryant, D. M., Wasik, B. H., Sparling, J. J., Fendt, K. H., & LaVange, L. M. (1992). Infant health and development program for low birth weight, premature infants: Program elements, family participation, and child intelligence. *Pediatrics, 89,* 454-465.

Ramey, C. T., & Campbell, F. A. (1984). Preventive education for high-risk children: Cognitive consequences of the Carolina Abecedarian Project. *American Journal of Mental Deficiency, 88,* 515-523.

Ramey, C. T., & Ramey, S. L. (1992). Effective early intervention. *Mental Retardation, 30,* 337-345.

Ramey, C. T., & Ramey, S. L. (1994). Which children benefit the most from early intervention? *Pediatrics, 94,* 1064-1066.

Reiss, J., Cameron, R., Matthews, D., & Shenkman, E. (1996). Enhancing the role public health nurses play in serving children with special health needs: An interactive videoconference on Public Law 99-457 Part H. *Public Health Nursing, 13,* 345-352.

Rich, O. J. (1990). Maternal-infant bonding in homeless adolescents and their infants. *MCN: American Journal of Maternal Child Nursing, 19,* 195-210.

Roberts, R. N., Wasik, B. H., Casto, G., & Ramey, C. T. (1991). Family support in the home: Programs, policy, and social change. *American Psychologist, 46,* 131-137.

Robinson, C. (1997). Early intervention services. *Journal for the Society of Pediatric Nursing, 2*(4), 191-192.

Rousch, J., Harrison, M., & Palsha, S. (1991). Family-centered early intervention: The perception of professionals. *AAD: American Annals of the Deaf, 136,* 360-366.

Sass-Lehrer, M., & Bodner-Johnson, B. (1989). Public Law 99-457: A new challenge to early intervention. *AAD: American Annals of the Deaf, 134,* 71-77.

Savage, T. A., & Culbert, C. (1989). Early intervention: The unique role of nursing. *Journal of Pediatric Nursing, 4,* 339-345.

Sumner, G., & Spietz, A. (1994a). *Nursing Child Assessment Feeding Scale (NCAFS).* Seattle: NCAST, University of Washington.

Sumner, G., & Spietz, A. (1994b). *Nursing Child Assessment Teaching Scale (NCATS).* Seattle: NCAST, University of Washington.

Trout, M., & Foley, G. (1989). Working with families of handicapped infants and toddlers. *Topics in Language Disorders, 10,* 57-67.

Wasik, B. H., & Karweit, N. L. (1994). Off to a good start: Effects of birth to three interventions on early school success. In R. E. Slavin, N. L. Karweit, & B. A. Wasik (Eds.), *Preventing school failure* (pp. 13-57). Needham, MA: Allyn & Bacon.

Wasik, B. H., Ramey, C. T., Bryant, D. M., & Sparling, J. J. (1990). A longitudinal study of two early intervention strategies: Project Care. *Child Development, 61,* 1682-1696.

Watson, J. E., Kirby, R. S., Kelleher, K. J., & Bradley, R. H. (1996). Effects of poverty on home environment: An analysis of three year outcome data for low birth weight premature infants. *Journal of Pediatric Psychology, 21,* 419-431.

Weiss, H. B. (1993). Home visits: Necessary but not sufficient. *Future of Children, 3*(3), 113-128.

Yoshikawa, H. (1995). Long-term effects of early childhood programs on social outcomes and delinquency. *Future of Children, 5*(3), 51-75.

13

Genetic Counseling

Janet K. Williams

An understanding of genetic aspects of health and disease is important for nurses who care for children and their families. Although clients with genetic concerns have traditionally consulted with professionals with advanced training in medical genetics, health professionals in all settings care for clients faced with genetic concerns, and nursing is a major resource for these families. When nurses have clients with inherited conditions or who are at risk for these conditions, genetic counseling may be indicated. This intervention encompasses not only identification of risks for inherited conditions but also health teaching, emotional support, decision-making support, maintenance and insurance of confidentiality, and referral for specific services. Because all individuals are believed to have several deleterious genes, genetic counseling may be indicated for any child or family. In this chapter, however, the discussion of genetic counseling as a nursing intervention will focus on situations in which the nurse recognizes the presence or the risk for a genetic or inherited disorder. Monitoring children and families for health risks is a basic component of *Healthy People 2000* (U.S. Department of Health and Human Services, 1991). This monitoring is focused on reducing mortality rates in infants through prenatal care and reducing exposure to environmental risks, recognizing and managing health problems in children, and minimizing additional health complications in children with disabilities.

THEORETICAL FRAMEWORK
AND LITERATURE REVIEW

Genetics

Recognition of risk for an inherited disorder is a basic element of genetic counseling, and an understanding of genetic principles is an important foundation. Principles of inheritance were initially identified by Mendel in his experiments with garden peas. Although the term "gene" was not coined until the early 1900s, Mendel's principles state that units of heredity are passed from parent to child; these units exist in pairs, but only one member of the pair is passed on to the next generation; and inherited characteristics are passed on independently of each other (Thompson, McInnes, & Willard, 1991). These laws explain inheritance of many genetic traits and are the bases of estimates of the likelihood that the gene for a specific condition will be inherited.

One Mendelian pattern of inheritance is autosomal dominant (AD). When the term *autosomal* is used, it refers to genes located on the non-sex chromosomes. An example of an AD condition is Marfan syndrome. A person with this disorder has a 50% chance of passing the gene for this condition on to each offspring. One characteristic of AD conditions is that the features of the disorder may vary in people who have the gene for the condition. For example, in Marfan syndrome, some individuals may have problems in one organ system such as the eyes, whereas others may have cardiac or skeletal problems.

A second Mendelian pattern of inheritance is autosomal recessive (AR). In AR inheritance, both members of a gene pair, also called alleles, contain a mutation leading to a disorder. Cystic fibrosis (CF) is inherited in an AR manner. Each parent is an obligate carrier, meaning that the parent has one normal and one abnormal CF gene. When these parents have a child, there is a 25% chance that the child will inherit both altered genes and have CF. The child could also be a carrier like the parents (a 50% chance) or inherit neither altered gene (a 25% chance).

Disease mutations can be present on the X chromosome. When females have a gene for an X-linked recessive disorder on one X chromosome, they are carriers. Carriers have a 50% chance of passing that gene on to a son, who will have the disease, or a daughter, who will be a carrier. Hemophilia A is an X-linked recessive disorder. When a male with an X-linked recessive disorder has children, all of his daughters will be carriers because he passes his X chromosome to female children. None of his sons can inherit the gene for this condition because they only inherit the Y chromosome, which does not contain the altered gene. Genes for a few diseases can also be inherited as X-linked dominant disorders. In these cases, both females and males would have signs of the conditions. An example of an X-linked dominant disorder is hypophosphatemic rickets.

Risk identification is also based on an understanding that genes are arranged on chromosomes. An alteration in the number or structure of chromosomes can cause serious disorders. Problems typically associated with an autosomal chromosome abnormality include alterations in growth, mental retardation, and multiple malformations (Thompson et al., 1991). An example of excess chromosome material is trisomy 21, also called Down syndrome, a condition in which an additional number 21 chromosome is present in each cell. When parents have a child with trisomy 21, the chances that they may have another child with this disorder are slightly increased. In some cases, another type of chromosome abnormality, a translocation, is present in the family. When this occurs, the recurrence risk can be markedly increased. Because it is not possible to determine the type of chromosome abnormality from a child's physical appearance, it is important that a chromosome analysis, or karyotype, be done to accurately determine the chance of recurrence for the child's parents.

As new information emerges about the identity and location of genes, it is becoming clear that multiple genes, often in combination with environmental factors, can lead to common disorders that appear in more than one family member. Most congenital malformations and many adult-onset diseases have genetic components but are not usually caused by single genes or chromosome abnormalities. This is termed *multi-factorial inheritance,* indicating that they are caused by numerous genetic factors with some influence from the environment. Examples of multi-factorial disorders include cleft lip and palate, neural tube defects, and diabetes mellitus (Thompson et al., 1991).

Much of this new information derives from research supported by the Human Genome Project. The identification and mapping of the estimated 50,000 to 100,000 genes and the determination of the sequence of 3 billion base pairs of nucleotides that make up human deoxyribonucleic acid (DNA) are two of the original goals of the Human Genome Project (Collins et al., 1998). Discovery of genes will allow for more accurate diagnosis of inherited conditions at the time or even before the onset of symptoms of the disorder. Identification of gene mutations and their functions may lead to new therapies to replace, correct, or supplement malfunctioning genes. An understanding of basic and newly identified genetic principles by nurses is an essential component of the Genetic Counseling nursing intervention. Knowledge of teaching and counseling also underlies this intervention.

Teaching and Counseling

Genetic counseling is defined by the American Society of Human Genetics as a communication process that deals with the human problems associated with the occurrence or the risk of occurrence of a genetic disorder in a family (Ad Hoc Committee on Genetic Counseling, 1975). In genetic counseling, information about a diagnosis, its cause, recurrence risk, and reproductive options and management alternatives are discussed by a team of health professionals with the individual or family. The genetic counseling process is based on a nondirective approach, especially when reproductive options are discussed. When people are at risk to have a child with a genetic disorder, genetic counseling may include information about a range of options, such as carrier testing, prenatal diagnosis, artificial insemination by donor, or a choice not to use these measures. Counselors endeavor to support individual client decisions about reproduction and to facilitate discussions about reproductive decision making. Support of family decisions is consistent with the central axiom of respect for persons that guides the practice of professional nursing as defined in the *Code for Nurses With Interpretive Statements* (American Nurses' Association, 1985).

Genetic counseling also helps the family cope with the presence of a genetic condition or the risk of its occurrence. When counseling is provided, the meaning of a genetic disorder for each person may be unique to that person's background and family values. For example, the belief that a person who resembles a family member with CF is a carrier is a common myth. Parental guilt and blame are additional deterrents to seeking carrier testing by healthy siblings (Fanos & Johnson, 1995). In a study of individuals with a family history of Huntington disease, however, family was frequently the primary source of information about new genetic testing services (Holloway et al., 1994).

When health teaching is provided, a more directive manner is generally followed. An example is the presentation of information regarding the prevention of neural tube defects (NTDs). Results of clinical studies showed that women with children with NTDs who received folic acid supplements prior to and following conception were less likely to give birth to other children with this disorder (Smithells et al., 1983). These findings led to recommendations from the U.S. Public Health Service that stated that all women of childbearing age should consume folic acid in their diets or in multivitamins supplements. When providing health teaching, nurses have found that supportive counseling is also needed. Learning about folic acid has been noted to trigger grief and past emotions in some women who already have children with NTDs (Romanczuk & Brown, 1994).

Nursing

Genetic counseling has appeared in the nursing literature since the early 1960s, when psychosocial support and case-finding responsibilities of nurses were emphasized (Forbes, 1966; Hillsman, 1966). Nurses concerned with genetic health care were generally found in public health or developmental disability settings. These nurses identified individuals who could benefit from genetic counseling and helped families understand management of their children's disorders. Recognition of nurses as members of genetic counseling teams is reflected in discussions during the 1970s and 1980s (Fibison, 1983; Sahin, 1976). Some nurses provided genetic counseling as advanced practice nurses, whereas others incorporated genetic counseling into their professional practice in the primary, acute, or community setting. During the 1980s, the need for educational preparation in genetic counseling for all nurses involved in pediatric nursing and other advanced nursing practice areas was identified (Monsen, 1984; Williams, 1983). This preparation is important so that nurses can recognize and intervene with children with genetic disorders. Genetic counseling became a part of nursing standardized language when it was included in the Nursing Interventions Classification (Iowa Intervention Project, 2000).

NURSING DIAGNOSIS AND OUTCOME DETERMINATION

Children with genetic conditions and their families are at risk for many nursing diagnoses for which nurses can apply components of genetic counseling. Although application of genetic information to patient care is not new in nursing, the language to reflect this activity is evolving. Thus, not all situations are reflected in the current nursing diagnosis literature, and some diagnoses are still in the development stages. This situation is even more evident when outcomes of this nursing intervention are considered. Conceptualization of the outcome process for genetic counseling is in its infancy, and researchers from a variety of professional disciplines are contributing to the development of this new body of knowledge. Understanding of recurrence risks and reproductive behavior have traditionally been used as outcome measures of genetic counseling effectiveness. Recent studies suggest that client satisfaction and the extent to which counseling meets client expectations may also be important factors in determining client outcomes (Michie, Axworthy, Weinman, & Marteau, 1996). An understanding of diagnoses and outcomes is essential, however, to assist nurses in becoming prepared to use genetic counseling as a nursing intervention.

Outcomes

Outcomes for individuals who receive genetic counseling are classified into several broad categories. Although knowledge is an outcome
that is desired in almost any nursing encounter, for some clients it is the
primary reason for requesting genetic counseling. In a study of individuals
who requested genetic carrier testing for CF and other inherited disorders,
satisfaction of curiosity regarding their risk status was an important reason for requesting the test information (Williams & Schutte, 1997).

A second outcome traditionally associated with genetic counseling is
Decision Making. This outcome, identified in the Nursing Outcomes
Classification (Iowa Outcomes Project, 2000), includes identifying relevant information and acknowledging the social context of the situation.
Decision Making has most commonly been associated with reproductive
decisions. Choices regarding presymptomatic and susceptibility testing,
however, will likely become important indicators of genetic counseling effectiveness as more genes are discovered that cause adult-onset diseases
(Bernhardt, 1997). Informed consent is part of making choices, and ensuring informed consent is an integral part of the responsibilities shared
by nurses when providing nursing care to people seeking genetic information (Scanlon & Fibison, 1995).

Relief of anxiety and concern about the issues that bring people to
health providers to receive genetic counseling is also identified as an outcome of the genetic counseling process (Michie, Bron, Bobrow, & Marteau,
1997). In one study, the most frequently mentioned benefit of learning
one's carrier status for specific inherited diseases was peace of mind and a
relief from fears regarding being a carrier (Williams & Schutte, 1997).
Those who learned that they were carriers felt relief to know their status
but expressed sadness regarding implications for their offspring. A related
outcome reflected in the nursing literature is Enhanced Coping as it relates to expressing one's feelings, feeling more able to care for a family
member with a genetic disorder, and being able to adjust to changes in
one's social relationships (Daack-Hirsch, 1995). Client Satisfaction and
the meeting of clients' expectations are also outcomes of genetic counseling (Daack-Hirsch, 1995; Michie et al., 1997).

Nursing Diagnoses

People who may benefit from genetic counseling may be At Risk for
Inherited Disorders. Factors that place an individual at risk to have a genetic disorder include a person's family health history and his or her ethnic background. A person who has a relative with a condition that has AD
inheritance might have that condition. If the person has a relative with an
AR condition, the person may not have the disorder but could pass the

gene on to offspring who might have the condition. When the relative has an X-linked recessive condition, males can be at risk to have the condition and females can be at risk to be carriers.

A person's ethnic background may also place him or her at an increased risk to carry a gene for a serious AR genetic disorder. Ethnic groups have evolved with their own characteristic sets of gene frequencies. Examples include an increased frequency of the gene for Tay-Sachs disease in people of Ashkenazi Jewish background, sickle cell disease in people of African background, and CF in people of European Caucasian background (Thompson et al., 1991). Knowing an individual's ethnic background is important in identifying if he or she may need information regarding the chances that they could be a carrier of a specific inherited disease.

Knowledge Deficit (North American Nursing Diagnosis Association [NANDA], 1999) is present in most individuals with or at risk to have a genetic disorder. A survey of the general public in Belgium noted that there is a widening gap between what is known by a relatively small group of genetics specialists and that of the general public, with misunderstandings regarding the inheritance of genetic disorders being particularly prominent (Decruyenaere, Evers-Kiebooms, & Van den Berghe, 1992). Geller (1995) reported that a major misconception among families is that one must have a family history of an AR disease, such as CF, to be at risk. As knowledge about genetics increases rapidly, it is likely that this knowledge gap will become even greater. Knowledge Deficit in family members is also a concern of nurses who manage health problems in clients who have an inherited disorder. For example, guidelines for teaching parents who have children diagnosed with sickle cell disease include teaching parents to recognize the early signs and symptoms of specific complications, a discussion of the genetics of the disorder, and explaining the need for administration of prophylactic penicillin to reduce the incidence of pneumococcal infections (Selekman, 1993).

A risk for alteration in one's peer relationships leading to Social Isolation (NANDA, 1999) is a consequence that is associated with many genetic disorders, especially those that result in alterations of appearance such as neurofibromatosis or cleft lip. Feelings of isolation may also result from being or having someone in the family who is different. In a study of children with hemophilia, some children were concerned about coping with being different and not being able to take part in some of the activities that were part of the lives of other children (Spitzer, 1992). Although individuals with specific genetic conditions are at risk for Social Isolation, this is not experienced by all who have these disorders. Individuals with CF report that they control the timing, the audience, and the nature of information they share about their disorder, lessening the need for concealing their condition (Admi, 1995). Another group that is at risk for Social

Isolation is those who learn through a genetic testing or screening process that they are carriers of genes for inherited conditions. Although these people are clinically healthy, consequences of this knowledge may lead to personal feelings of stigmatization or in some cases have been associated with social discrimination (Markel, 1992).

When a condition is genetic, it is a family concern, and Altered Family Process (NANDA, 1999) may occur. Experiences of guilt, marital stress, and difficulties in communicating with spouse, children, and extended family all may be present in families with a child who has a genetic disorder. Mothers of children with Turner's syndrome report that they and their spouses have difficulty in establishing expectations for home responsibilities and issues regarding discipline (Williams, 1995). Altered Family Process also occurs when communication regarding inheritance issues is raised within families. Results of one study note that parents and sisters are the most important source of information about the inheritance of hemophilia. Twenty percent of women who had a relative with hemophilia, however, reported that in their parental home the hereditary nature of this condition was never discussed (Varekamp, Suurmeijer, Brocker-Vriends, & Rosendaal, 1992).

The discovery of genes for inherited diseases makes it possible for people of all ages to have genetic testing to determine if they have one of these genes. This opportunity may lead to Decisional Conflict (NANDA, 1999). Decisions about having testing performed are especially controversial when the person who may need testing is a child. Because of potential risks for stigmatization, misunderstanding of test results, altered identity, and impact on parental expectations, a recent Institute of Medicine Committee recommended that "children should generally be tested only for genetic disorders for which there exists an effective curative or preventive treatment that must be instituted early in life to achieve maximum benefits" (Andrews, Fullarton, Holtzman, & Motulsky, 1994, p. 10). Despite general guidelines that discourage genetic testing of children, some parents have difficulty in considering decisions about the testing of their children. An additional factor that makes decisions difficult is the potential that a person undergoing genetic testing may experience insurance or employer discrimination based on his or her genetic makeup. This situation may be eased through legislation to protect individuals from genetic discrimination.

Many genetic conditions are associated with Altered Growth and Development (NANDA, 1999). For example, children with neurofibromatosis type 1 are more likely to have short stature; therefore, their adult height may not be consistent with parental expectations. Phenylketonuria (PKU) has well-documented negative effects on intelligence and behavior. These can partially or totally be eliminated by strict adherence to dietary treatments throughout childhood (Bowe, 1995). Children with inherited disorders should be carefully monitored to detect such alterations.

INTERVENTION: GENETIC COUNSELING

Genetic Counseling is defined as "use of an interactive helping process focusing on assisting an individual, family, or group, manifesting or at risk for developing for transmitting at birth defect or genetic condition, to cope," (Iowa Intervention Project, 2000, p. 357). This nursing intervention consists of activities to provide risk identification, health teaching, emotional support, decision-making support, confidentiality, and referrals for specific services. Many aspects of genetic counseling are interrelated, and one activity, such as health teaching, may also be a part of others, such as risk identification or promoting coping. Reviewing lifestyle behaviors and obtaining a genetic family history start this process.

Risk Identification

Obtaining a family history and recording the family pedigree offer the nurse the opportunity to observe family interactions and to determine the level of understanding they have about a disorder. This process takes time, and it is often necessary for a nurse to speak several times with a family because information may not be remembered at the first interview. Individuals may need to consult extended family members to obtain more detailed family history information. The health status of children, parents, and extended family members as well as the ethnic backgrounds of family members should be recorded. A standardized format for recording a genetic pedigree should be used when family history information is included in a client's health record (Bennett et al., 1995) (Figure 13.1).

Good interviewing skills are needed because risk identification requires a nonjudgmental approach. Risk identification begins with the nurse providing privacy and ensuring confidentiality. Genetic information is personal in nature; therefore, some individuals may be reluctant to reveal sensitive aspects of their family's background. The nurse may start the interview by saying, "I'd like to know about the health of each member of your family. Starting with your child, does he or she have any current or past health problems?" Health problems and causes of death of the parents, siblings, grandparents, and offspring should be recorded. The presence of mental illness, a child born outside of the current relationship, spontaneous or elective abortion, mental retardation, or nonpaternity should be documented. An example of how to elicit information about

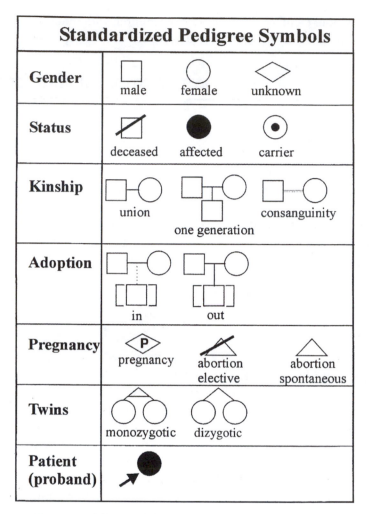

Figure 13.1. Standardized Pedigree Symbols (Reproduced from Bennett et al., 1995, *American Journal of Human Genetics,* by permission of the University of Chicago Press)

mental retardation is to say, "Does your child, or does anyone in your family, have a learning problem, or did they require any special help in school?" (Williams, 1996). The nurse should review the family history and consult with genetic specialists when a disorder appears to have a Mendelian pattern of inheritance or a condition is present in several family members.

The ethnic background of the child's ancestors should also be identified and recorded. This information may be useful in determining if family members have an increased chance of having inherited conditions that are more commonly found in people who share a specific heritage. Risk identification allows the nurse to determine with the family what other interventions they need. A component that is frequently needed is health teaching.

HEALTH TEACHING

Determining the individual's purpose, goals, and agenda for seeking genetic information is essential prior to providing health teaching. Information about many aspects of genetic conditions will be desired by parents and children. One topic of discussion desired by parents and children is how to manage the child's disorder. For example, teaching for children with metabolic disorders such as PKU begins at birth and continues throughout childhood and adolescence. At the time of the newborn screening test, nurses need to explain the purpose of the test. One study found that this required between 1 and 5 minutes of the nurse's time, and mothers were more knowledgeable about the procedure after this teaching (Faden, Chwalow, Holtzman, & Horn, 1982). Subsequent teaching includes how to manage a low-phenylalanine diet at home and at school. Issues such as how to handle overnight visits or what to do when there are special treats at school can be difficult for some children; therefore, health teaching is important in preparing the child for these situations. Adolescent and young adult females need information on relationships between diet and prevention of congenital anomalies associated with maternal PKU in their offspring (Wright, Brown, & Davidson-Mundt, 1992). Teaching by nurses about metabolic disorders in children takes place not only in specialty clinics but also in the home, in which it is combined with developmental assessment and psychosocial support (Phoenix, 1986).

Health teaching often begins at the time of a diagnosis of a genetic condition in a child and continues as new issues and concerns occur. For example, parents of children with Down syndrome must absorb a large amount of information as they begin to understand their children's unique features and problems. They will receive much of this information from specialists, such as medical geneticists, neonatalogists, developmental disability team members, and cardiologists. Health teaching by the nurse after these visits is important to help clarify and focus the parents' concerns and evaluate their level of understanding. The nurse draws on an understanding of human genetics to clarify basic facts about Down syndrome. For example, a nurse may clarify that trisomy 21 is a chromosomal disorder that was present in the egg or sperm prior to conception, and it is not known that anything either parent did caused this condition in their fetus. The presence of the extra number 21 chromosome affects numerous organs and body systems leading to a wide variety of alterations in the growth and development of the fetus. Although many parents ask for a

Parents may be asked to participate in genetic testing for the purposes of research, and the results may have no immediate clinical benefit to themselves or their child. When genetic testing is part of research, nurses must participate with others on the health team to ensure that parents give informed consent. When the purpose of the test is for genetic research, additional information is necessary. People should be given information regarding how the confidentiality and privacy of the specimen will be maintained, who has ownership of the specimen, and their future access to information that may emerge from ongoing studies (Weir & Horton, 1995).

Parents and children will also participate in decisions about the child's treatment options. Genetic researchers will continue to search for new and more effective treatment options for genetic disorders. With an increasing number of options, parents and children will need some assistance making decisions regarding these new treatments. Documenting the values and beliefs of children regarding their own care is one part of this process (Geller, 1995).

Ensuring Confidentiality

Genetic information is different from other health-related data in that it not only has implications for the individual for whom the information is gathered but also has implications for the health of other biological family members. Information regarding a genetic condition or carrier state for an inherited condition is part of an individual's health record, and nurses have a critical role in maintaining the confidentiality of this information (Scanlon & Fibison, 1995). This can be an especially difficult situation when other people requesting information are extended family members. For example, a relative may ask about genetic evaluations of other family members. The nurse is ethically obligated not to disclose information without the individual's permission. Family members can benefit, however, from nurses' efforts to help them plan how to discuss genetic information with others in their family.

Referrals for Specific Services

Providing referrals to genetic health care specialists and to community resources such as support groups is a component of Genetic Counseling (Iowa Intervention Project, 2000). Many families will need the services provided by a specialty genetic counseling evaluation and management team. The detection of unexplained alterations in growth or intellectual development is one indication for a genetic consultation referral. A referral is also important when a family has a child with a genetic disorder but who do not fully understand genetic aspects of the condition. Referral may be necessary at the time of diagnosis and also when there are changes in the family structure or new questions occur. It also will be important for those who received counseling several years ago because there could be new information that has emerged from ongoing research. Individuals often need help in understanding the relationship between new scientific discoveries and the time and effort involved in developing hoped-for treatments or cures.

In addition to initiating a referral, nurses help children and their parents understand the purposes of a genetic counseling consultation and can help them identify what questions to ask. For example, parents may want to know if their child's condition could occur in that child's offspring or in his or her siblings, if the condition could be detected prenatally, the features of this condition and its prognosis, and what treatment options are available. Nurses also help parents identify sources of family health information that is useful in their genetic consultation, such as family photographs and birth, death, or medical records (Williams, 1993). Nurses are also sources of information on community resources. These include not only diagnostic and management services but also services that help families with financial, educational, or emotional support needs. For example, nurses refer families to disease-specific organizations in which they learn more about the condition and others who have the disorder. The Alliance of Genetic Support Groups is an organization that provides information about a specific condition or more general support organizations for families (Mackta & Weiss, 1994).

INTERVENTION APPLICATION

At the beginning of the school year, the school nurse notes that Jenny, a new student, is much shorter than others in her 3rd-grade class. Jenny's mother, Kim, tells the nurse that she and Jenny's father are concerned that Jenny is not keeping up with other children her age. The school nurse obtains a family history and learns that Jenny is one of three girls, and all other family members are of average height. On the basis of the data gathered during the family history and Jenny's placement at below the 3rd percentile on the growth chart, a nursing diagnoses of Altered Growth and Development was made. She asks Jenny's mother if they would like help in identifying a specialist who could evaluate Jenny's growth. With Kim's consent, the nurse refers Jenny to a genetic clinic at which Jenny is diagnosed with Turner syndrome (TS). The nurse is aware that children with TS are at risk for learning disabilities and social isolation.

Components of the Genetic Counseling intervention for Jenny and her parents include risk identification, teaching, emotional support, and referral. She also talks with Jenny's mother about the need for a school psychology evaluation to help identify an educational plan for Jenny. In addition, she asks Kim if Jenny has had any difficulty in making friends. Kim states that she is very worried about this because Jenny did not have any friends in her old school, and she is hoping that things will be better at the new school. The nurse talks with Kim about helping Jenny become involved in structured peer activities, such as Brownies or church groups. She discovers that Jenny's parents have not agreed on what responsibilities Jenny is expected to have at home, and that their discipline efforts have been inconsistent. She helps Kim identify expectations that are appropriate for Jenny's age and develop a plan for rewards when Jenny completes her tasks at home. The nurse also talks with Jenny about what she understands about TS and about Jenny's attempts to make new friends in the school. She gives Jenny and Kim information about how to contact the Turner Syndrome Society of America.

Several months after school began, Kim states that she and Jenny's dad are much less anxious about Jenny's size, and they understand TS caused her slower growth. She is also appreciative of the counseling the nurse provided them regarding their expectations of Jenny at home; they are also pleased that Jenny is in a school program aimed at meeting her learning and social development needs. These statements indicate that the parents have gained substantial knowledge of the disease process—or outcome goal for the nursing intervention Genetic Counseling. As the school year progresses, the nurse will use the outcome Social Involvement to monitor Jenny's involvement with peers and school activities.

RESEARCH AND PRACTICE IMPLICATIONS

Activities of the nursing intervention Genetic Counseling are implemented by advanced practice nurses whose primary responsibilities are in genetic counseling programs and also by nurses who care for children in a variety of settings. The intervention is based on activities within the scope of practice of the professional nurse. Factors that influence the effectiveness of this intervention, however, are not known. Studies are needed to evaluate ways to provide genetic information that will make it meaningful and useful to families and children. The importance of variables such as prior knowledge, previously held attitudes about the cause of disease, the timing of the information, and its manner of delivery need to be clarified through scientific study. One promising area of research is identifying the kinds of information that children with genetic conditions need to enable them to better understand and cope with the effects of their disorders.

Factors that are associated with adaptive and maladaptive coping are not well understood. Factors such as family support, expectations for one's child, and burden of the disorder on the parents need additional investigation. Research is also needed to evaluate interventions to promote healthy coping among those who are unable to do this on their own. Characteristics of the decision-making process and its application to genetic situations need to be identified. Research is also needed to identify specific outcomes and means to measure these in recipients of the nursing intervention Genetic Counseling.

The integration of Genetic Counseling in nursing education at all levels is essential for nurses to more fully participate in this important area of professional nursing practice (Anderson, 1996). Although nurses can provide many aspects of genetic counseling, their use of this intervention will be limited if their educational backgrounds do not provide a foundation in genetics that includes its incorporation into nursing practice. This foundation is particularly limited when nurses do not have a good understanding of genetics principles. A lack of educational preparation in genetics and genetic counseling will result in inappropriate or lack of referrals by nurses for families in need of additional genetic counseling services. Genetics is a rapidly changing area, and nurses will need to update their education as new developments in genetic research and applications of these discoveries to nursing practice occur.

Opportunities to implement this nursing intervention are present in any institution or community-based setting in which nurses encounter children and their families. It is estimated that approximately one fourth to one third of pediatric admissions are for children with genetic diseases (Jorde, Carey, & White, 1995). Nurses who provide care to children in acute care units will continue to have the opportunity to provide components of genetic counseling to these children and their families. Nurses who provide care to children with chronic conditions, such as hemophilia, CF, or spina bifida, also need a strong foundation in genetics and genetic counseling to enable them to apply this knowledge to their practice. Nurses also provide genetic counseling to adolescents and their parents in family planning settings. School nurses can use this intervention with children who have genetic conditions and in their health teaching regarding genetic aspects of health and disease.

As the health care system continues to change, the primary care setting will increasingly be the site for provision of genetic information, especially related to risk identification and decision-making regarding genetic testing. Nurses are recognized as an important resource to help meet the demand for these genetic services (Andrews et al., 1994). As knowledge of the genetic aspects of health and disease continues to expand, so will the need for nurses to learn and apply this important nursing intervention.

REFERENCES

Ad Hoc Committee on Genetic Counseling of the American Society of Human Genetics. (1975). Genetic counseling. *American Journal of Human Genetics, 27,* 240-242.

Admi, H. (1995). "Nothing to hide and nothing to advertise": Managing disease-related information. *Western Journal of Nursing Research, 17*(5), 484-501.

American Nurses' Association. (1985). *Code for nurses with interpretive statements.* Kansas City, MO: Author.

Anderson, G. (1996). The evolution and status of genetics education in nursing in the United States 1983-1995. *Image, 28*(2), 101-106.

Andrews, L., Fullarton, J., Holtzman, N., & Motulsky, A. (1994). *Assessing genetic risks: Implications of health and social policy.* Washington DC: National Academy Press.

Bennett, R., Steinhaus, K., Ulrich, S., Sullivan, C., Resta, R., Lochner-Doyle, D., Markel, D., Vincent, V., & Hamanish, J. (1995). Recommendations for standardized human pedigree nomenclature. *American Journal of Human Genetics, 56,* 745-752.

Bernhardt, B. (1997). Empirical evidence that genetic counseling is directive: Where do we go from here? *American Journal of Human Genetics, 60,* 17-20.

Bowe, K. (1995). Phenylketonuria: An update for pediatric community health nurses. *Pediatric Nursing, 21*(2), 191-194.

Collins, F., Patrinos, A., Jordan, E., Chakravarti, A., Gesteland, R., Walters, L., & the Members of the DOE and NIH Planning Groups. (1998). New goals for the U.S. Human Genome Project: 1998-2003. *Science, 282,* 682-689.

Daack-Hirsch, S. (1995). *Nursing sensitive outcomes related to the nursing intervention genetic counseling.* Unpublished manuscript, The University of Iowa, Iowa City.

Decruyenaere, M., Evers-Kiebooms, G., & Van den Berghe, H. (1992). Community knowledge about human genetics. *Birth Defects: Original Article Series, 28,* 167-184.

Faden, R., Chwalow, J., Holtzman, N., & Horn, S. (1982). A survey to evaluate parental consent as public policy for neonatal screening. *American Journal of Public Health, 72,* 1347-1352.

Fanos, J. H., & Johnson, J. P. (1995). Barriers to carrier testing for CF siblings: The importance of not knowing. *American Journal of Human Genetics 59,* 85-91.

Fibison, W. (1983). The nursing role in the delivery of genetic services. *Issues in Health Care of Women, 4,* 1-15.

Forbes, N. (1966). The nurse and genetic counseling. *Nursing Clinics of North America, 1,* 679-688.

Geller, G. (1995). Cystic fibrosis and the pediatric caregiver: Benefits and burdens of genetic technology. *Pediatric Nursing, 21,* 57-61.

Hillsman, G. (1966). Genetics and the nurse. *Nursing Outlook, 14,* 34-39.

Holloway, S., Mennie, M., Crosbie, A., Smith, G., Raeburn, S., Dinwoodie, D., Wright, A., May, H., Calder, K., Barron, L., & Brock, D. (1994). Predictive testing for Huntington disease: Social characteristics and knowledge of applicants, attitudes to the test procedure and decisions made after testing. *Clinical Genetics, 46,* 175-180.

Iowa Intervention Project. (2000). *Nursing intervention classification (NIC)* (J. C. McCloskey & G. M. Bulechek, Eds.; 3rd ed.). St. Louis, MO: Mosby-Year Book.

Iowa Outcomes Project. (2000). *Nursing outcomes classification (NOC)* (M. Johnson, M. Maas, & S. Moorhead, Eds.; 2nd ed.). St. Louis, MO: Mosby-Year Book.

Jorde, L., Carey, J., & White, R. (1995). *Medical genetics.* St. Louis, MO: C. V. Mosby.

Mackta, J., & Weiss, J. (1994). The role of genetic support groups. *Journal of Obstetric, Gynecologic and Neonatal Nursing, 23*(6), 519-523.

Markel, H. (1992). The stigma of disease: Implications of genetic screening. *American Journal of Medicine, 93,* 209-215.

Michie, S., Axworthy, D., Weinman, J., & Marteau, T. (1996). Genetic counseling: Predicting patient outcomes. *Psychology and Health, 11,* 797-809.

Michie, S., Bron, F., Bobrow, M., & Marteau, T. (1997). Nondirectiveness in genetic counseling: An empirical study. *American Journal of Human Genetics, 60,* 40-47.

Monsen, R. (1984). Genetics in basic nursing program curricula: A national survey. *Maternal-Child Nursing Journal, 13,* 177-185.

North American Nursing Diagnosis Association. (1999). *Nursing diagnoses: Definitions & classification 1999-2000.* Philadelphia: Author.

Phoenix, B. (1986). The nursing role in metabolic management. In G. Felton (Ed.), *Proceedings of the national conference on nursing practice in clinical genetics: Prospects for the 21st century* (pp. 145-153). Iowa City: The University of Iowa.

Romanczuk, A., & Brown, J. (1994). Folic acid will reduce risk of neural tube defects. *MCN: American Journal of Maternal Child Nursing, 19,* 331-334.

Sahin, S. (1976). The multifaceted role of the nurse as genetic counselor. *Maternal Child Nursing Journal, 1,* 211-216.

Scanlon, C., & Fibison, W. (1995). *Managing genetic information: Implications for nursing practice.* Washington, DC: American Nurses' Association.

Selekman, J. (1993). Update: New guidelines for the treatment of infants with sickle cell disease. *Pediatric Nursing, 19*(6), 600-605.

Smithells, R. W., Nevin, N. C., Seller, M. J., Sheppard, S., Harris, R., Read, A. P., Fielding, D. W., Walker, S., Schorah, C. J., & Wild, J. (1983). Further experience of vitamin supplementation for the prevention of neural tube defect recurrences. *Lancet, 1*(8332), 1027-1031.

Spitzer, A. (1992). Coping processes of school-age children with hemophilia. *Western Journal of Nursing Research, 14*(2), 157-169.

Thompson, M., McInnes, R., & Willard, H. (1991). *Genetics in medicine* (5th ed.). Philadelphia: W. B. Saunders.

U.S. Department of Health and Human Services. (1991). *Health people 2000: National health promotion and disease prevention objectives* (DHHS Publication No. PHS 91-50312). Washington, DC: Government Printing Office.

Varekamp, I., Suurmeijer, T., Brocker-Vriends, A., & Rosendaal, F. (1992). Hemophilia and the use of genetic counseling and carrier testing within family networks. *Birth Defects: Original Article Series, 28,* 139-148.

Weir, R., & Horton, J. (1995). DNA banking and informed consent—Part 1. *IRB: A Review of Human Subjects Research, 17*(4), 1-4.

Williams, J. K. (1983). Pediatric nurse practitioners' knowledge of genetic disease. *Pediatric Nursing, 9,* 119-121.

Williams, J. K. (1993). New genetic discoveries increase counseling opportunities. *MCN: American Journal of Maternal Child Nursing, 18*(4), 218-222.

Williams, J. K. (1995). Parenting a daughter with precocious puberty or Turner syndrome. *Journal of Pediatric Health Care, 5,* 109-114.

Williams, J. K. (1996). *Genetic issues for perinatal nurses.* White Plains, NY: March of Dimes Birth Defects Foundation.

Williams, J. K., & Schutte, D. L. (1997). Benefits and burdens of genetic carrier identification. *Western Journal of Nursing Research, 19,* 71-81.

Wright, L., Brown, A., & Davidson-Mundt, A. (1992). Newborn screening: The miracle and the challenge. *Journal of Pediatric Nursing, 7,* 26-42.

14

Perinatal Substance Abuse Treatment

Michele J. Eliason

According to the *Healthy People 2000* report (U.S. Department of Health and Human Services, 1991), more than one half of infant deaths can be attributed to low birth weight, congenital anomalies, sudden infant death syndrome, and respiratory distress syndrome. Perinatal substance abuse is a significant risk factor underlying all these causes of infant mortality. Between 10% and 20% of children in the United States are exposed to alcohol or drugs or both during prenatal life (National Council on Alcoholism and Drug Dependence [NCADD], 1993; National Institute of Alcohol Abuse and Alcoholism [NIAAA], 1987), and many more are exposed after birth to the social and physical environment that a substance-abusing parent provides (Levy & Rutter, 1992; Steinglass, 1987). This chapter focuses on interventions for substance-abusng mothers and their newborns.

Alcohol is a widely accepted legal substance, and society not only encourages social use but also sometimes condones excessive use of alcohol, as at New Year's Eve and tailgate parties. Alcohol-related deaths are the third most common cause of death in adults, and alcohol is implicated in

50% of motor vehicle accidents, 60% of murders, and 66% of child sexual molestation cases (Goode, 1993). Despite these statistics, there is a tendency to view substance abuse in one of three ways (Sullivan, 1995): (a) to ignore, avoid, or deny the fact that alcohol is a problem; (b) to view alcohol abuse as a moral defect requiring punishment or censure or both; and/or (c) to view alcohol abuse as an illness requiring professional help. The public outcry about fetal alcohol syndrome and prenatal drug exposure leading to the jailing of pregnant substance abusers and the entire "Just Say No" campaign point to the prevalence of the second view. The view of nurses as represented in nursing education integrates a combination of the first and third views. Although the nursing curriculum often presents substance abuse as a disease, the time devoted to addictions in the typical curriculum is small. When 25% to 50% of patients in medical-surgical hospital beds are alcoholic and 50% to 60% of clients with mental disorders have coexisting alcohol disorders (Jack, 1993), denial must be responsible for lack of attention to the matter.

The majority of women drink at least some alcohol, although there are racial and ethnic differences in the prevalence of problem drinking. Contrary to stereotypes that alcohol abuse is higher in women of color, the rates of problem drinking are lowest among Asian American, African American, and Latino women and highest in Native American and European American women (Wilsnack & Wilsnack, 1993). The consequences of heavy drinking in women of color, however, are often greater because of lack of access to treatment due to the expense, lack of insurance coverage, lack of treatment facilities in their neighborhoods, and lack of culturally competent treatment.

One study (NIAAA, 1987) suggested that one in six mothers exposes her fetus to potentially dangerous levels of alcohol, whereas the NCADD (1993) found that one in nine women tested positive for drugs or alcohol at delivery. Slutsker, Smith, Higginson, and Fleming (1993) found that 5% of women giving birth in one state tested positive for illegal drugs, and 15% to 25% of adult and 40% of adolescent pregnant women smoke cigarettes (Davis, Tollestrup, & Milham, 1990; Hawkins & Catalano, 1992). In a nationally representative study of more than 2,600 pregnant women, racial and ethnic differences in alcohol and drug use patterns were identified. Rates of smoking (20% overall) were highest in white women (24%), followed by African Americans (20%) and Latinos (6%). Alcohol use (19% overall) was also highest in white women (23%), followed by Latinos (9%) and African Americans (6%). Crack cocaine use (1% overall) was highest in African Americans (4.5%), followed by Latinos (0.7%) and whites (0.4%) (National Institute on Drug Abuse [NIDA], 1994).

In the following sections, the potential perinatal effects of alcohol, tobacco, marijuana, cocaine, and heroin are discussed. Some substances are teratogens and have the potential for causing physical birth defects in the fetus (alcohol and probably nicotine, barbiturates, cocaine, benzodiazepines, volatile solvents and inhalants, caffeine, and dexedrine), whereas other substances can produce neonatal withdrawal syndrome (the opiates—heroin, methadone, codeine, Demerol, morphine, talwin, and barbiturates). All these substances, when used to excess, can impair parenting ability.

Alcohol

Alcohol has well-documented negative effects for mother and fetus. In the mother, chronic alcohol use can result in general health deterioration, nutritional deficiencies, and emotional problems (Coletti & Donaldson, 1996). Women who become alcoholics were often depressed and victims of sexual and physical abuse prior to the onset of alcohol abuse—factors that may also affect their ability to effectively parent (Eliason & Skinstad, 1995; Hurley, 1991). One study found that adolescent mothers who had been sexually and physically abused as children were seven times more likely to be substance abusers than adolescent mothers without childhood abuse (Berenson, San Miguel, & Wilkinson, 1992).

Alcohol freely crosses the placenta and causes a continuum of damage, called fetal alcohol effects (FAEs). At one end of the continuum is fetal death due to miscarriage or stillbirth, followed by severe birth defects (fetal alcohol syndrome), whereas at the other end are milder learning and behavioral problems. Fetal alcohol effects are the leading known cause of mental retardation, attention deficits, and learning disabilities (Eliason & Williams, 1990). Fetal alcohol syndrome (FAS) results in altered facial appearance, such as epicanthic folds, flattened or absent philtrum, thin upper lip, short nose; intrauterine-onset growth retardation that persists throughout life; physical birth defects, such as cardiac, renal, skeletal, and eye anomalies; and central nervous system abnormalities, such as mental retardation, learning impairments, fine motor dysfunction, and attention deficits (Center for Substance Abuse Treatment, 1993).

The incidence of FAS varies from 1 in 8 births in certain Native American groups to approximately 1 in 3,000 in the general U.S. population (Little & Wendt, 1993; Pagliaro & Pagliaro, 1996). Fetal alcohol effect is thought to be at least three times as common. The incidence data probably represent underestimates, however, because FAE is difficult to measure and some of the symptoms are not apparent until later in life. Fetal alcohol syndrome is six times more common in African American newborns than in white newborns, which could be related to economic class variables because several studies have found higher rates in poor women (Streissguth & LaDue, 1985).

Many health care providers are reluctant to make the diagnosis of FAE or FAS because they believe that the damage has already been done and they may alienate the mother. Another reason for misdiagnosis may be the denial or lack of awareness of alcohol problems by health care providers. Little, Snell, Rosenfeld, Gilstrap, and Grant (1990) found a 100% failure rate to identify FAS in infants whose mothers had informed their physicians that they drank alcohol during pregnancy.

In the first trimester, heavy drinking is most likely to cause physical birth defects, whereas in the second trimester spontaneous abortion, growth retardation, and central nervous system anomalies are the most common consequences. Even third-trimester drinking can inhibit growth, especially of the central nervous system. Longitudinal studies have revealed lower intelligence, impaired attention and memory, and behavioral problems in the absence of physical birth defects in children of mothers who drank at moderate levels (approximately two drinks per day), suggesting that prenatal alcohol exposure, even at relatively low doses, causes permanent damage (Streissguth, Barr, Sampson, Darby, & Martin, 1989; Streissguth, Darby, Barr, Smith, & Martin, 1984). Alcohol can continue to have effects after birth because it readily passes into breast milk. There is a myth that alcohol stimulates the letdown reflexes and produces a greater, richer milk supply. The fact is that alcohol has no positive influence on lactation and has potentially dangerous effects because the infant's nervous system continues to develop rapidly in the months after birth.

Tobacco

One in six deaths in the United States is linked to smoking, but tobacco remains legal and readily available. Most studies have focused on the effects of nicotine, a highly addictive substance. Cigarettes contain more than 200 different chemicals, however. The chemicals most linked to potential problems for the fetus include nicotine, nitrosamine, carbon monoxide, and cyanide. Tobacco effects on the mother include higher frequency of early menopause, osteoporosis, reduced fertility, cancer, and an interaction with birth control pills that increases the risk for stroke. Obstetric complications associated with tobacco include spontaneous abortion, vaginal bleeding, abruptio placentae, placenta previa, and premature aging of the placenta that decreases fetal nutrition and affects growth (DiFranza & Lew, 1995).

A fetal tobacco syndrome has been identified with growth retardation as its main effect. Tobacco is responsible for 14% of the cases of low birth weight (LBW) in the United States, and smokers have babies that weigh, on average, 200 grams less than the babies of nonsmokers (Pagliaro & Pagliaro, 1996). After birth, the infant is at higher risk for sudden infant death syndrome, upper respiratory infections, and otitis media (DiFranza & Lew, 1995). These problems could be the result of the prenatal exposure or passive smoke exposure after birth. Most of the chemicals in tobacco products also readily pass into breast milk. Nicotine causes reductions in prolactin and insufficient milk supply; thus, smoking mothers are unable to breast-feed for as long as nonsmokers, and more than one half of smoking mothers wean within 4 weeks (Hill & Aldag, 1993; Schulte-Hobein, Schwartz-Bickenbach, Abst, Plum, & Nau, 1992). Tobacco is also thought to potentiate the effects of alcohol in pregnant women. Recently, some studies have linked smoking during pregnancy with childhood neurodevelopmental impairments such as hyperactivity (Olds, Henderson, & Tatelbaum, 1994).

Marijuana

Marijuana, the most widely used illicit drug in the United States, is smoked by 27% to 31% of pregnant women (Hingson et al., 1986; Zuckerman et al., 1989). Chronic, heavy marijuana use in women is associated with anovulation, shortened luteal phase, and precipitate or prolonged labor. Marijuana readily crosses the placenta, and because of its long half-life it remains in the fetal system up to 30 days after an exposure. Marijuana smoke has five times the amount of carbon monoxide as tobacco, which reduces oxygen intake to the fetus (Hetteberg et al., 1995). Studies have not clearly identified marijuana as a teratogen, although some researchers have reported symptoms similar to FAS (Zuckerman et al., 1989). There are reports of increased frequency of meconium passage, tremors, startles, and altered visual responsiveness in the neonatal period, which resolve later (Gal & Sharpless, 1984). Dahl (1990) found sleep disturbances in the newborn that persisted for 3 or more years. Marijuana also passes into breast milk and decreases prolactin levels, making breast-feeding more difficult (Asch & Smith, 1983). The study of marijuana effects is complicated by the fact that women in the United States who are heavy marijuana users generally use other substances as well, making it difficult to identify which substance has what effect on the fetus (Hetteberg et al., 1995), and it is not clear whether marijuana use alone is harmful to the fetus (Dreher, 1997).

Cocaine

There is considerable controversy regarding the effects of cocaine on fetal development. In the mid-1980s, there was a general alarm about the cocaine epidemic, and dire predictions were made that babies exposed to cocaine would be born addicted and with severe physical and mental birth defects. These predictions have proved to be gross exaggerations (Kandall, 1997). Cocaine has many negative consequences, but most of the effects on the fetus are probably related to lifestyle factors of the addicted mother rather than direct effects of cocaine (Hetteberg et al., 1995). Like marijuana users, cocaine users invariably use other substances in combination with cocaine, complicating the study of its effects.

Heavy cocaine use in any form, crack or powder, smoked, inhaled, or injected, is associated with poor nutrition, higher rates of infections (especially sexually transmitted diseases and AIDS), poor general health, and putting oneself into potentially dangerous situations. The obstetric complications of spontaneous abortion, premature labor, abruptio placentae, preterm delivery, and LBW or small for gestational age (SGA) newborns are related to a combination of direct effects of cocaine, such as stimulation of smooth muscles, and lifestyle factors, such as poor nutrition and lack of prenatal care (Snodgrass, 1994).

Cocaine readily crosses the placenta, and some researchers have suggested that birth defects such as prune belly syndrome, ileal atresia, and urogenital anomalies are more common in cocaine-exposed infants (Brouhard, 1994; Good, Ferriero, Golabi, & Kobori, 1992; Udell, 1989). Cocaine is not nearly as potent a teratogen as alcohol, however, and few infants exposed to cocaine prenatally have any physical birth defects. The more common effects of cocaine on the infant are the direct stimulatory effects on the central nervous system: irritability, hypertonicity, hyper-responsiveness to stimuli, gaze aversion, poor state control (Chasnoff, Griffith, MacGregor, Dirkes, & Burns, 1989), and depressed habituation (Mayes, Granger, Frank, Schottenfeld, & Bornstein, 1993). These effects last for 8 to 10 weeks in most infants (Hetteberg et al., 1995). The major long-term risks appear to be related to the mother-infant attachment process and to the home environment. The hyperirritability of the mother and infant, compounded by separation if the infant requires close monitoring after birth or the mother enters inpatient treatment, can interfere with the normal bonding process. There is a relatively high rate of abandonment of these babies, and once home the infant is at higher risk for sudden infant death syndrome, neglect, and abuse. Cocaine exposure can continue after birth via breast milk and passive smoke, and there have been reports of accidental ingestion of crack "rocks" by infants and toddlers (Udell, 1989). Azuma and Chasnoff (1993) found that declines in IQ at age 3 in children who were exposed prenatally to cocaine were mediated by the home environment and child behavioral characteristics.

Heroin

Heroin can have significant effects on fertility, pregnancy, and the fetus and newborn. Chronic heroin users are more likely to suffer pregnancy-related hypertension, abruptio placenta, premature delivery, and postpartum hemorrhage (Hetteberg et al., 1995). Heroin causes vasoconstriction, which may reduce uteroplacental exchange and thus the amount of essential nutrients the fetus receives. These effects can result in stillborn, SGA, or LBW babies. Babies exposed to heroin rapidly become addicted. Signs of in utero withdrawal include irritability, agitation, and increased movement, which increase the energy requirements of the fetus at the same time as the mother's withdrawal causes uterine cramping and vasoconstriction. The result can be fetal hypoxia. Because the dangers of withdrawal are generally higher than the dangers of the heroin exposure, detoxification of the mother is not recommended until the fetus is viable (Hetteberg et al., 1995). Withdrawal symptoms in the neonate generally begin within 48 hours of birth. Some mothers are placed on methadone maintenance prenatally; methadone, however, produces even more severe withdrawal symptoms in the newborn than heroin and is associated with high risk for spontaneous abortion (Pagliaro & Pagliaro, 1996). If mothers are to be maintained on methadone, the lowest possible dose to decrease drug craving and avoid withdrawal symptoms is recommended (Bashore, Ketchum, Staisch, Barrett, & Zimmerman, 1981).

Other Substances

There are many other substances linked to pregnancy complications and fetal and infant problems, including other illegal drugs, such as methamphetamine, inhalants, and the hallucinogens; prescription drugs, such as Dilantin and Valium; and over-the-counter preparations, such as vitamins with megadoses of vitamin A. Even caffeine, which is widely accepted as a "safe" drug, may cause a higher risk for limb defects, fetal loss, LBW, and child hyperactivity at doses equivalent to about three cups of coffee or approximately 375 mg per day (Pagliaro & Pagliaro, 1996).

Alcohol and Drug Addiction and Parenting

Very little research has focused on mothers who are substance abusers, and even fewer studies have examined parenting per se because of the prevailing stereotype that the substance-abusing woman cannot be a good parent (Taylor, 1993). There has not been such close scrutiny of the parenting abilities of alcohol- or drug-addicted fathers. Substance-abusing women might not be adequate parents because (a) the majority come from homes in which they were abused or one or both parents were substance abusers and were not good parenting role models; (b) they are more likely to be single and the sole care provider for their children; (c) they are more likely to be in a relationship with a substance-abusing man who might be abusive; (d) they are more likely to be depressed, which interferes with nurturing their children; and (e) they experience high levels of shame and guilt that serve as a barrier to getting treatment and can lead to neglect or abuse of their children (Eliason & Skinstad, 1995). It is clear, however, that some substance-abusing women are, or can be taught to be, loving and responsible parents (Lief, 1985).

NURSING DIAGNOSIS AND OUTCOME DETERMINATION

Savage (1996) described many screening tests for alcohol and other drug use. One of these instruments should be part of the intake interview in every nursing setting. For example, the Alcohol Use Disorder Identification Test (Babor & Grant, 1989) was developed in a multinational study and contains 10 questions that can be administered face-to-face or on paper. For those with even more limited time, the CAGE has only 4 questions ("Have you ever felt the need to Cut down on your drinking?" "Do you feel Annoyed by people complaining about your drinking?" "Do you ever feel Guilty about your drinking?" and "Do you ever need an Eye-opener in the morning to relieve the shakes?"). These instruments have been well tested and have good sensitivity. Drug screening tests are just beginning to be tested empirically.

Once substance abuse has been identified, nurses should be alert to the common problems associated with substance abuse. Possible nursing diagnoses for substance-abusing mothers include Risk for Noncompliance, Altered Nutrition, Knowledge Deficits (parenting, social skills, vocational skills, and health maintenance), Self-Esteem Disturbance, Altered Parenting, Risk for Violence, Ineffective Denial, Ineffective Individual Coping, and Impaired Adjustment (North American Nursing Diagnosis Association [NANDA], 1999). Important outcomes for the substance-abusing mother might include Knowledge: Substance Use Control, Parent-Infant Attachment, and Parenting (Iowa Outcomes Project, 2000).

There are also checklists for identifying symptoms of FAS (Clarren & Aldrich, 1993) and fetal drug effects (Brazelton Neonatal Assessment Scale; Brazelton, 1991) in newborns. Infants born exposed to alcohol and drugs are at higher risk for feeding problems, altered growth and development, and altered parent-infant attachment. Some also have physical birth defects. Desirable outcomes for the prenatally exposed infant could include optimal child development, as indicated by norms for the child's chronological age, and consistent parent-infant attachment. The indicators of attachment in the infant with neurobehavioral irritability may be altered because three of the four indicators for infants are likely to be impaired in drug-exposed infants (infant looks at parent[s], infant responds to parent's cues, and infant seeks proximity with parent) (Iowa Outcomes Project, 2000). These indicators may not develop for several months, until the child can better handle environmental stimuli.

INTERVENTION:
PERINATAL SUBSTANCE ABUSE TREATMENT

The following sections highlight a cluster of nursing interventions for substance-abusing mothers and their infants. These interventions and specific activities are drawn from the Iowa Intervention Project (2000). It should be noted, however, that all substance-abusing women and their children are unique, and there is no specific intervention plan for all substance abusers or their children. Rather, interventions are based on the diagnoses and nurse-sensitive outcomes.

Interventions for the Mother

Prenatal Care

Prenatal care should be provided as early as possible, although this is more difficult in the case of the substance-abusing mother because drug use often impairs early detection of pregnancy, the mother may fear losing custody of her children if her substance abuse is detected, and she may lack financial resources for health care. Prenatal programs need to provide nonjudgmental care or substance-abusing women will avoid them. The following are some specific activities:

- Instruct patient on the importance of regular prenatal care throughout the entire pregnancy.
- Instruct patient on nutrition needed during pregnancy.
- Monitor nutritional status.
- Instruct patient on harmful effects of smoking on fetus and the harmful effects of alcohol and other drugs, legal and illegal.

Substance Abuse Treatment

Pregnancy may provide the needed motivation for substance-abusing women to reduce or stop their use (Starn, Patterson, Bemis, Castro, & Bemis, 1993). Nurses should consider that all clients could potentially be substance abusers and include the following activities in their intake procedures:

- Establish a therapeutic relationship with the client.
- Determine history of drug or alcohol use.
- Determine substance(s) used.

There are a few guidelines for interviewing about substance use. The first guideline is to be aware that clients are very sensitive to nurses' attitudes and will detect if nurses are judgmental. Second, there is a need to be very specific when interviewing about substances. For example, instead of asking "Do you drink?," ask "How much beer do you drink in a typical week (or month)?" Continue by asking separately about wine, wine coolers, hard liquor, cough syrups with alcohol or codeine, prescription medications, illegal drugs, over-the-counter medications, and tobacco. Be very specific about the amounts because one beer might mean a can of beer to one woman but a 36-ounce glass to another. In addition, ask about her significant other's substance use because this will be an important factor in discharge planning. The risk for relapse is much higher if the woman returns to live with a substance-abusing partner. Once a substance abuse problem has been identified, other appropriate activities might include the following:

- Assist the patient or family to identify the use of denial as a substitute for confronting the problem. Do this carefully because substance-abusing mothers may already feel overwhelming shame and guilt, and a confrontational approach may scare them away from treatment.
- Discuss with the patient the impact of substance use on medical condition or general health. Also mention the impact on the pregnancy and developing fetus, stressing that reduction or cessation of substance use at any point in the pregnancy will improve the outcome.
- Assist the client to identify the negative effects of substance abuse on health, family, and daily functioning.

There are few substance abuse treatment facilities that will accept pregnant women and many obstetricians who will not accept substance abusers; thus, many women must wait until after the birth of the baby to begin treatment. Child care while in treatment is also a major concern for most women because most treatment facilities do not provide it. Some states consider the woman's entry into treatment as child abandonment and remove her children from her custody. As of 1994, 200 women in the United States had been prosecuted for delivering a controlled substance to a minor (through the umbilical cord), and countless others had their children removed from their custody for actual or perceived child abuse and neglect (Kandall, 1997). These facts decrease the likelihood that women with children will voluntarily seek treatment for addictions (Kandall & Chavkin, 1992).

Nurses need to keep in mind that substance abuse in women is generally a symptom of some other underlying pathology (Tiedje & Starn, 1996), and treatment needs to address these underlying problems or relapse is inevitable. A recent volume of the *NIDA Research Monograph Series* (Rahdert, 1996) addresses some of the problems encountered by pregnant or parenting women in treatment, such as negative attitudes of health care providers, housing concerns, transportation, child care, involvement with the legal system, and the need of many women for vocational training. In summary, the problems of substance-abusing women are complex and require individual assessment, treatment planning, and aftercare services to be successful (Lanehart, Clark, Kratochvil, Rollings, & Fidora, 1994; Marr & Wenner, 1996).

Substance Use Treatment:
Alcohol or Drug Withdrawal or Both

Depending on the amount, frequency, and combinations of substances used, a pregnant woman should be hospitalized for detoxification so that the effects of withdrawal on the fetus can be closely monitored. All of the activities listed for Substance Abuse Treatment should be considered for the pregnant woman (Iowa Intervention Project, 2000, p. 616). Finding a treatment program for the pregnant addict may prove difficult. Of the "war on drugs" federal money, less than 1% is earmarked for treatment, and only a minuscule portion of that for programs targeting pregnant women (Kandall, 1997). If the woman is placed in a typical substance abuse treatment program, she will also need obstetric care from a specialist familiar with the problems of substance abuse.

Postpartal Care

Most of the usual activities for postpartal care are appropriate for the substance-abusing woman with a few exceptions. For example, if a woman continues to drink alcohol, smoke, or use drugs, breast-feeding should be discouraged. In addition, use of analgesics should be evaluated carefully, and the woman should be monitored for withdrawal or signs that she is continuing drug or alcohol use in the hospital. If possible, the substance-abusing mother and her infant should be kept in the hospital longer than usual to monitor for signs of withdrawal in mother and baby.

Attachment Promotion

A major risk for the often emotionally impaired substance-abusing mother is bonding with her possibly irritable, difficult to console, possibly unwanted baby (Taylor, 1993). Hanna, Faden, and Dufour (1994) found that pregnant women who were depressed and did not want the pregnancy were likely to maintain high levels of drinking and drug use during pregnancy, whereas those who were not depressed and had a positive attitude about the pregnancy reduced their use during pregnancy. Thus, interventions for depression and initiating attachment should begin as early as possible. Attachment Promotion activities include

- Discuss parents' reaction to pregnancy.
- Provide opportunities for the parents to see, hold, and examine the newborn immediately after birth.
- Reinforce caregiver role behaviors, or teach them to women who are not familiar with them.
- Assist parents in planning for early discharge (if necessary).
- Phone the patient to determine how she is coping with the transition to home, or engage a home health visitor to monitor her progress.

Alcohol- and drug-exposed newborns may give more confusing or ambiguous cues about their needs. Their mothers may need help and practice identifying their infants' cues.

Interventions for the Newborn

Substance Abuse Treatment: Drug Withdrawal

If the mother used barbiturates or opiates during the pregnancy, monitor the newborn for neonatal abstinence syndrome (withdrawal). The onset of symptoms varies from immediately after birth to approximately 6 days postpartum, and these include bradycardia, apnea spells, projectile vomiting, diarrhea, hyperirritability, shrill cry, poor suck, difficulty feeding, frequent yawning and sneezing, stuffy nose, and, rarely, seizures. Finnegan (1988) developed a scale to measure the severity of withdrawal symptoms that nurses might find helpful in identifying and monitoring the progress of drug-exposed infants. Interventions for neonatal withdrawal may include pharmacological, such as administration of paregoric, tincture of opium, or phenobarbital, depending on the drug being withdrawn; infection control and monitoring because of the mother's risk for sexually transmitted diseases, HIV, and other infectious diseases; maintaining fluid and electrolyte balance through intravenous or enteral feedings; and respiratory care. The activities listed under the intervention Substance Abuse Treatment: Drug Withdrawal pertain to adults and are not applicable to neonates. Substance Abuse Treatment: Alcohol Withdrawal is also unlikely to apply to the neonate, who rarely shows withdrawal from alcohol because it takes months or even years to develop alcohol dependence. Separate interventions are needed for substance abuse withdrawal in newborns and for perinatal drug exposure. Some appropriate activities for the drug- or alcohol-exposed infant might include the following:

- Decrease the amount of stimulation in the environment (e.g., light, noise, temperature changes, and hanging toys).
- Soothe the agitated infant with swaddling, by vertical rocking (hold away from the body and gently rock up and down), or by holding the infant with its back to the caregivers chest.
- Approach slowly and gradually increase the amount of stimulation.
- Monitor developmental progress carefully.

Whether the infant shows signs of withdrawal or not, comprehensive developmental assessment needs to be conducted at birth and periodically thereafter at least until the child is in school and longer if problems are identified.

INTERVENTION APPLICATION

Allison was just over 3 years of age when she was brought to the hospital emergency room (ER) after a sheriff in a nearby small town found her staggering down the street with alcohol on her breath. She was at the 10th percentile for height, weight, and head circumference, and she had epicanthic folds, small, rotated ears, and a flat philtrum. She had an innocent heart murmur and a mild clubfoot. Although difficult to assess in the ER in her frightened and intoxicated state, it soon became apparent that she had delayed expressive language skills and communicated by gesture. The sheriff located her 18-year-old mother (Jackie) and brought her to the ER. Jackie was approximately 5 ft 2 in. tall and weighed 95 pounds. She, too, had the facial features of FAS and seemed to be mildly retarded. She told the nurse that she was having a rum and coke at home when she remembered she was supposed to pick up her boyfriend at work. She left the house suddenly, leaving Allison alone with an open bottle of rum. Allison had consumed about 10 ounces of rum and wandered out of the house. Jackie acknowledged that she often gave alcohol to Allison to quiet her when she cried. Jackie learned this trick from her own mother, who was also an alcoholic. Later, Jackie revealed she was pregnant.

Nursing diagnoses appropriate for Allison were Risk for Injury due to lack of supervision and Altered Growth and Development related to her growth and delayed developmental milestones (NANDA, 1999). She was kept in the hospital for 5 days for extensive physical and psychological assessment. She was found to have no serious physical birth defects, and a brace was made for her clubfoot. Contact was made with local special education services, and she was placed in a preschool program for at-risk children for language stimulation and additional monitoring of cognitive development. The nursing outcomes Safety Behavior: Home Environment and Child Development: 3 Years were used to monitor Allison's home situation and development during the next year (Iowa Outcomes Project, 2000).

A nursing diagnosis of Altered Parenting was made for Jackie related to her alcohol use, lack of consistent supervision, and inability to provide an environment conducive to a developing child and fetus (NANDA, 1999). Jackie was referred for prenatal care and outpatient substance abuse treatment. The incentive for continuing treatment was continuation of custody of Allison and the unborn baby. A social worker was assigned to the case to monitor the family's progress. At the 1-year follow-up visit, Allison was talking and was at near-normal developmental levels for cognitive and behavioral growth as monitored by the nursing outcome Child Development: 3 Years (Iowa Outcomes Project, 2000). Jackie had given birth to a son, who appeared to be physically normal but was being closely monitored. Jackie had not stopped drinking entirely, but she was attending parenting classes and a vocational training program and seemed more motivated to stop drinking. Her care of her two children was considered adequate as monitored by the Nursing Outcomes Classification outcomes Parenting and Risk Control: Alcohol Use (Iowa Outcomes Project, 2000).

RESEARCH AND PRACTICE IMPLICATIONS

The direct effects of specific substances on fetal growth and development have been difficult to determine, making some researchers cautious in declaring substances as teratogens. This cautious approach, however, misses the point that no drug, legal or illegal, is healthy for the growing fetus. Nurses could study the general short- and long-term effects of drugs and alcohol on children and families, whether the drug is a teratogen or not. Nurses also need to identify and test interventions to reduce or eliminate drug use in pregnancy. For example, research on the effectiveness of prenatal interventions is needed. Also needed are studies on recruiting and retaining pregnant substance abusers into prenatal care, and data derived from these studies could be used to develop substance abuse treatment programs that could provide effective care for pregnant women.

Nurses can also take a central role in developing interventions aimed at healthy pregnancy and child rearing. First, however, nurses need better education about the hazards of substance abuse, and they need to overcome the heavy denial in our society and in our profession in which nurses have a high rate of addiction (Haack & Hughes, 1989). They also must face the reality that the most deadly drugs for mother and fetus are alcohol and tobacco rather than illegal drugs. As a society and as a profession, it is time to rethink our attitudes about the acceptability of mood-altering substances of all types, including tobacco and caffeine. Nurses are considered as role models for health. Therefore, they must be encouraged to reduce or eliminate unhealthy substances from their own lives and model healthy lifestyles for the children and families they serve.

REFERENCES

Asch, R., & Smith, C. (1983). Effects of marijuana on reproduction. *Contemporary OB-GYN, 28,* 217-225.

Azuma, S., & Chasnoff, I. (1993). Outcome of children prenatally exposed to cocaine and other drugs: A path analysis of three-year data. *Pediatrics, 92*(3), 396-402.

Babor, T., & Grant, M. (1989). From clinical research to secondary prevention: International collaboration in the development of the Alcohol Use Disorders Identification Test (AUDIT). *Alcohol Health and Research World, 13*(4), 371-374.

Bashore, R., Ketchum, J., Staisch, K., Barrett, C., & Zimmerman, E. (1981). Heroin addiction and pregnancy—Interdepartmental clinical conference. *Western Journal of Medicine, 134*(6), 506-514.

Berenson, A. B., San Miguel, V. V., & Wilkinson, G. S. (1992). Violence and its relationship to substance abuse in adolescent pregnancy. *Journal of Adolescent Health, 13*(6), 470-474.

Brazelton, T. B. (1991). What we can learn about the status of the newborn. In M. Kilbey & K. Asghar (Eds.), *Methodological issues in controlled studies on effects of prenatal exposure to drug abuse* [Research monograph] (p. 114). Rockville, MD: National Institute on Drug Abuse.

Brouhard, B. H. (1994). Cocaine ingestion and abnormalities of the urinary tract. *Clinical Pediatrics, 33*(3), 157-158.

Center for Substance Abuse Treatment. (1993). *Pregnant, substance-using women: Treatment improvement protocol* (DHHS Publication No. SMA-1993). Rockville, MD: U.S. Department of Health and Human Services.

Chasnoff, I., Griffith, D., MacGregor, S., Dirkes, K., & Burns, K. (1989). Temporal patterns of cocaine use in pregnancy: Perinatal outcome. *Journal of the American Medical Association, 261*(12), 1741-1744.

Clarren, S. K., & Aldrich, R. A. (1993). *A concise manual for fetal alcohol screening: Fetal Alcohol Checklist.* Seattle, WA: U.S. Department of Health and Human Services, Public Health Service, and Washington State Department of Health.

Coletti, S. D., & Donaldson, P. L. (1996). Maternal-child nursing. In K. Allen (Ed.), *Nursing care of the addicted client* (pp. 53-70). Philadelphia: J. B. Lippincott.

Dahl, R. E. (1990). Prenatal marijuana exposure remains evident in early childhood. *American Family Physician, 41*(2), 596.

Davis, R. L., Tollestrup, K., & Milham, S., Jr. (1990). Trends in teenage smoking during pregnancy. Washington State: 1984 through 1988. *American Journal of the Diseases of Children, 144*(12), 1297-1301.

DiFranza, J. R., & Lew, R. A. (1995). Effect of maternal cigarette smoking on pregnancy complications and sudden infant death syndrome. *Journal of Family Practice, 40*(4), 385-394.

Dreher, M. C. (1997). Cannabis and pregnancy. In M. L. Mathre (Ed.), *Cannabis in medical practice: A legal, historical and pharmacological overview of the therapeutic use of marijuana* (pp. 159-170). Jefferson, NC: McFarland.

Eliason, M. J., & Skinstad, A. H. (1995). Drug/alcohol addictions and mothering. *Alcoholism Treatment Quarterly, 12,* 83-96.

Eliason, M. J., & Williams, J. (1990). Fetal alcohol effects and the neonate. *Journal of Perinatal and Neonatal Nursing, 3*(4), 64-72.

Finnegan, L. (1988). The dilemma of cocaine exposure in the perinatal period. *National Institute of Drug Abuse Research: Monograph Series, 81,* 379.

Gal, P., & Sharpless, M. K. (1984). Fetal drug exposure—Behavioral teratogenesis. *Drug Intelligence and Clinical Pharmacy, 18*(3), 186-201.

Good, W., Ferriero, D., Golabi, M., & Kobori, J. (1992). Abnormalities of the visual system in infants exposed to cocaine. *Opthalmology, 99*(3), 341-346.

Goode, E. (1993). *Drugs in American society.* New York: McGraw-Hill.

Haack, M. R., & Hughes, T. L. (1989). *Addiction in the nursing profession.* New York: Springer.

Hanna, E., Faden, V., & Dufour, M. (1994). The motivational correlates of drinking, smoking, and illicit drug use during pregnancy. *Journal of Substance Abuse, 6*(2), 155-169.

Hawkins, J. D., & Catalano, R. F. (1992). *Communities that care: Action for drug abuse prevention.* San Francisco: Jossey-Bass.

Hetteberg, C., Bragg, E., Feblinger, D., Flandermeyer, A., Kenner, C., & Jamerson, P. (1995). Substance abuse in perinatal care. In E. J. Sullivan (Ed.), *Nursing care of clients with substance abuse* (pp. 191-233). St. Louis, MO: C. V. Mosby.

Hill, P., & Aldag, J. (1993). Insufficient milk supply among black and white breast-feeding mothers. *Research in Nursing and Health, 16*(3), 203-211.

Hingson, R., Zuckerman, B., Amaro, H., Frank, D., Kayne, H., Sorenson, J., Mitchell, J., Parker, S., Morelock, S., & Timperi, R. (1986). Maternal marijuana use and neonatal outcome: Uncertainty posed by self reports. *American Journal of Public Health, 76*(6), 667-669.

Hurley, D. (1991). Women, alcohol, and incest: An analytic review. *Journal of Studies on Alcohol, 52*(3), 253-268.

Iowa Intervention Project. (2000). *Nursing interventions classification (NIC)* (J. C. McCloskey & G. M. Bulechek, Eds.; 3rd ed.). St Louis: Mosby-Year Book.

Iowa Outcomes Project. (2000). *Nursing outcomes classification (NOC)* (M. Johnson, M. Maas, & S. Moorhead, Eds.; 2nd ed.). St. Louis, MO: Mosby-Year Book.

Jack, L. (1993, Spring). Addictions. *Graduate Nurse,* 26-29.

Kandall, S. R. (1997). *Substance and shadow: Women and addiction in the United States.* Cambridge, MA: Harvard University Press.

Kandall, S. R., & Chavkin, W. (1992). Illicit drugs in America: History, impact on women and children, and treatment strategies for women. *Hastings Law Journal, 43,* 605-643.

Lanehart, R., Clark, H., Kratochvil, D., Rollings, J. P., & Fidora, A. (1994). Case management of pregnant and parenting female crack and polydrug abusers. *Journal of Substance Abuse, 6*(4), 441-448.

Lief, N. (1985). The drug user as a parent. *International Journal of Addictions, 20,* 63-97.

Levy, S. J., & Rutter, E. (1992). *Children of drug abusers.* New York: Lexington.

Little, B. B., Snell, L. M., Rosenfeld, C. R., Gilstrap, L. C., & Grant, N. F. (1990). Failure to recognize fetal alcohol syndrome in newborn infants. *American Journal of the Diseases of Children, 144*(10), 1143-1146.

Little, R. E., & Wendt, J. K. (1993). The effects of maternal drinking in the reproductive period. An epidemiological review. In E. S. L. Gomberg & T. Nirenberg (Eds.), *Women and substance abuse* (pp. 191-213). Norwood, NJ: Ablex.

Marr, D., & Wenner, A. (1996). Gender specific treatment for chemically dependent women: A rationale for inclusion of vocational services. *Alcoholism Treatment Quarterly, 14,* 21-31.

Mayes, L., Granger, R., Frank, M., Schottenfeld, R., & Bornstein, M. (1993). Neurobehavioral profiles of neonates exposed to cocaine prenatally. *Pediatrics, 91*(4), 778-783.

National Council on Alcoholism and Drug Dependence. (1993). One in nine pregnant women test positive for drugs in California study. *Alcoholism Report, 21*(9), 8-9.

National Institute of Alcohol Abuse and Alcoholism. (1987). *Program strategies for preventing fetal alcohol syndrome and alcohol related birth defects* (DHHS Publication No. ADM 87-1482). Washington, DC: Government Printing Office.

National Institute on Drug Abuse. (1994). *Conference on drug addiction research and the health of women.* Tyson's Corner, VA: Author.

North American Nursing Diagnosis Association. (1999). *Nursing diagnoses: Definitions and classification 1998-1999*. Philadelphia: Author.

Olds, D. L., Henderson, C. R., Jr., & Tatelbaum, R. (1994). Intellectual impairment in children of women who smoke cigarettes during pregnancy. *Pediatrics, 93*(3), 221-226.

Pagliaro, A. M., & Pagliaro, L. A. (1996). *Substance use among children and adolescents*. New York: John Wiley.

Rahdert, E. R. (1996). Treatment for drug-exposed women and their children: Advances in research methodology. In *NIDA Research Monograph Series 165* (DHHS NIH Publication No. 96-3632). Rockville, MD: National Institute on Drug Abuse.

Savage, C. (1996). Screening and detection. In K. M. Allen (Ed.), *Nursing care of the addicted client* (pp. 100-117). Philadelphia: J. B. Lippincott.

Schulte-Hobein, B., Schwartz-Bickenbach, D., Abst, S., Plum, C., & Nau, H. (1992). Cigarette smoke exposure and development of infants throughout the first year of life. *Acta Paediatrica, 81*(6/7), 550-557.

Slutsker, L., Smith, R., Higginson, G., & Fleming, D. (1993). Recognizing illicit drug use by pregnant women: Reports from Oregon birth attendants. *American Journal of Public Health, 83,* 61-64.

Snodgrass, S. R. (1994). Cocaine babies: A result of multiple teratogenic influences. *Journal of Child Neurology, 9*(3), 227-233.

Starn, J., Patterson, K., Bemis, G., Castro, O., & Bemis, P. (1993). Can we encourage substance abusers to seek prenatal care? *MCN: American Journal of Maternal Child Nursing, 18*(3), 148-153.

Steinglass, P. (1987). *The alcoholic family*. New York: Basic Books.

Streissguth, A., Barr, H., Sampson, P., Darby, B., & Martin, D. (1989). IQ at age 4 in relation to maternal alcohol use and smoking during pregnancy. *Developmental Psychology, 25,* 3-11.

Streissguth, A., Darby, B., Barr, H., Smith, I., & Martin, D. (1984). Comparison of drinking and smoking patterns during pregnancy over a six year interval. *American Journal of Obstetrics and Gynecology, 145*(6), 716-724.

Streissguth, A., & LaDue, R. (1985). Psychological and behavioral effects in children prenatally exposed to alcohol. *Alcohol Health & Research World, 10*(2), 6-12.

Sullivan, E. J. (1995). *Nursing care of clients with substance abuse*. St. Louis, MO: C. V. Mosby.

Taylor, A. (1993). *Women drug users*. London: Clarendon.

Tiedje, L. B., & Starn, J. (1996). Intervention model for substance-abusing women. *Image: The Journal of Nursing Scholarship, 28*(2), 113-118.

Udell, B. (1989). Crack cocaine. In Ross Laboratories (Eds.), *Special currents: Cocaine babies* (pp. 6-12). Columbus, OH: Ross Laboratories.

U.S. Department of Health and Human Services. (1991). *Healthy people 2000: National health promotion and disease prevention objectives* (DHHS Publication No. PHS 91-50312). Washington, DC: Government Printing Office.

Wilsnack, S. C., & Wilsnack, R. W. (1993). Epidemiological research on women's drinking: Recent progress and directions for the 1990s. In E. S. L. Gomberg & T. D. Nirenberg (Eds.), *Women and substance abuse* (pp. 62-99). Norwood, NJ: Ablex.

Zuckerman, B., Frank, D., Hingson, R., Amaro, H., Levenson, Z., Kayne, H., Parker, S., Vinci, R., Aboagye, K., Fried, L., Cabral, H., Timperi, R., & Bauchern, H. (1989). Effects of maternal marijuana and cocaine use on fetal growth. *New England Journal of Medicine, 320*(12), 762-768.

15

Grief Work Facilitation

Perinatal Loss

Jane E. Wilkins

Perinatal loss, and the subsequent bereavement process, is a significant life crisis often occurring unexpectedly, giving families little time to prepare. In addition, some social customs and beliefs hinder mourning. For example, following a miscarriage there is often no funeral, no period of mourning, and no outward expression of sympathy (Gardner & Merenstein, 1986). A stillborn baby may not be regarded as a real person, and infant death is often viewed as less significant than the death of an older person (Peppers & Knapp, 1980). The following are additional societal beliefs: (a) it is undesirable for males to express their emotions; (b) there is a limited time for mourning, after which it is no longer appropriate to grieve; and (c) another child compensates for the death of a baby (Rajan, 1994). The suddenness of the loss, lack of understanding, and lack of social acceptance for parental grief cause parents to feel alone and confused by the intensity of their loss.

One of the priority areas for the national health initiative *Healthy People 2000* (U.S. Department of Health and Human Services, 1991) is mental health and mental disorders. The purpose of the initiative is to change behaviors and environments that improve health outcomes. When a baby dies, nurses are able to validate the significance of the loss and encourage healthy bereavement behaviors (Ewton, 1993).

In 1991, the National Center for Health Statistics reported a perinatal mortality rate of 8.7 per 1,000 live births in the United States (Gabbe, Niebyl, & Simpson, 1996). Miscarriage occurs in 10% to 15% of clinically recognized pregnancies (Gabbe et al., 1996, p. 717). Therefore, maternal-child nurses should be prepared to intervene when a perinatal loss occurs.

THEORETICAL FRAMEWORK AND LITERATURE REVIEW

Attachment

One of the strongest of all human ties exists between the parent and child. To comprehend the impact of perinatal loss on the mother and father, it is necessary to understand the parental attachment process. Klaus and Kennell (1982) outlined many events necessary to establish a maternal-infant bond. Planning a pregnancy often begins in childhood and continues through the active decision to become pregnant. Confirmation of the pregnancy is an important milestone, and during the process of acceptance of the pregnancy there may be ambivalent feelings. With fetal movement, the woman begins to view the fetus as an individual separate from herself. The last four events described by Klaus and Kennell—birth, seeing, touching, and caring for the baby—occur almost simultaneously, and motherhood becomes real.

The father experiences an attachment process similar to the mother, but he lags behind because much of his attachment is intellectual during the early months of pregnancy. Full attachment may not occur until after birth when caretaking begins. For the father, the fetus is a mixture of fantasy and reality, but for the mother the reality and sensations of pregnancy support the fantasies (Peppers & Knapp, 1980).

Reva Rubin's study of more than 6,000 women, both cross-sectional and longitudinal subjects, provided data for her research on the maternal experience. The method was hypotheses free and therefore a means of discovery rather than confirmation. Data collected through observations, hospital records, surveys, and interviews were analyzed (Rubin, 1984). Rubin described many adaptation tasks for the mother, but of particular note is the maternal task called "binding-in." During the first trimester of pregnancy, the woman must bind-in to the idea of pregnancy. In the second and third trimesters, the woman is very aware of the baby, and fantasies, wishes, and dreams of the idealized child develop. Binding-in accelerates after delivery when, instead of the oneness of pregnancy, polarization occurs and the woman identifies the baby as a separate entity.

Each pregnancy produces a unique maternal-child relationship independent of any other child (Rubin, 1975). A woman cannot replace this unique relationship with a subsequent pregnancy. According to Rubin, the death of a baby terminates further development and extension of the relationship, but it does not eliminate the bond already achieved. In a subsequent pregnancy, women may resist attachment behaviors and experience increased anxiety throughout the gestation (Armstrong & Hutti, 1998).

Bereavement

Grief is a very painful human experience that Lindemann (1944) describes as a normal psychological and somatic reaction to a distressing situation. Solari-Twadell, Bunkers, Wang, and Snyder (1995) describe loss and bereavement as a unique experience and the capacity to grieve as an important dimension of health. Miscarriage, ectopic pregnancy, stillbirth, or newborn death may trigger a grief response as intense as an adult death (Ewton, 1993). Parental grief is for a person who never had a social being; therefore, parents mourn the loss of hopes, dreams, and their future with the child. Parents may be urged to forget the loss, let go, move on with life, and have other children (Brown, 1991). Thus, extended families and others demonstrate their lack of recognition for the intensity of the parents' grief and the impossibility of replacing one relationship with another.

A woman who terminates a pregnancy for fetal or maternal indication may experience an intense grief response putting her at risk for significant psychological morbidity (Zeanah, Dailey, Rosenblatt, & Saller, 1993). Loss in a multiple pregnancy causes a mixture of conflicting emotions. Parents find themselves celebrating life and mourning death at the same time (Wathen, 1990). Contrary to public opinion, the surviving child does not make up for the loss of the other baby (Limbo & Wheeler, 1986). Women who make a plan for adoption also experience grief and find society discounting their feelings of loss (Gardner & Merenstein, 1986).

The loss of a loved one is psychologically traumatic in the same way that being severely wounded or burned is physiologically traumatic (Engel, 1961). Grief represents a departure from the state of health and well-being. Just as healing after an injury is necessary to restore a homeostatic balance in the physiological realm, time for healing is necessary after a loss to reestablish a psychological state of equilibrium. The adaptation to loss is therefore similar to healing (Engel, 1961). Table 15.1 outlines the complex combination of physical sensations, thoughts, behaviors, and feelings the bereaved experience throughout the mourning

TABLE 15.1   Manifestations of Grief

Physical Sensations	Thoughts	Behaviors	Feelings
Lack of energy	Disbelief	Sleep disturbance	Numbness
Dry mouth	Confusion	Appetite disturbance	Shock
Depersonalization	Preoccupation	Social withdrawal	Sadness
Hollowness in the stomach	Sense of the presence of the deceased	Sighing	Yearning
Tightness in the chest or throat	Visual or auditory hallucinations	Crying	Loneliness
Hypersensitivity to noise		Dreaming of the deceased	Helplessness
Shortness of breath		Searching and calling out for the loved one	Fatigue
Weakness in muscles		Restlessness or overactivity	Emancipation
		Avoiding reminders	Relief
		Treasuring objects	Anger
			Guilt
			Self-reproach
			Anxiety

SOURCE: Worden (1991).

process. In addition, cultural heritage, gender, and the developmental stage of the parents are important factors in grief expression.

Worden (1991) describes four tasks of mourning that the individual must complete for equilibrium reestablishment: (a) to accept the reality of the loss, (b) to experience the pain of grief, (c) to adapt to an environment in which the loved one is missing, and (d) to withdraw emotional energy and invest it in another relationship. The time required to complete the mourning process varies with each individual, and no specific time frame can be established. Mourning finishes when the tasks are complete; throughout life, however, memories of the loved one cause the bereaved to experience episodes of grief reoccurrence.

Incongruent grieving between men and women is common, and data indicate that women display grief more than men (Thomas, Striegel, Dudley, Wilkins, & Gibson, 1997). Men often feel unsupported in their grief because the societal expectation for the male is composure, rational thinker, protector, and counselor for his partner. These differences can lead to bitterness, resentment, marital tension, and communication breakdown (Peppers & Knapp, 1980). Cohesion, adaptability, communication, social support, and relationship satisfaction, however, are variables that ease the stress of perinatal loss (Thomas et al., 1997).

NURSING DIAGNOSIS AND
OUTCOME DETERMINATION

Nursing Diagnosis

Anticipatory Grieving and Dysfunctional Grieving are two nursing diagnoses appropriate for perinatal loss (North American Nursing Diagnosis Association, 1999). Assessment determines the strength of the parents' attachment to the pregnancy and their perception of loss (Brown, 1991). Encourage parents to tell their story while listening carefully for the meaning of loss as the mother and father describe the physical sensations, thoughts, and feelings about their infant (Wheeler, 1994). It is also important to assess coping behaviors, nonverbal communication, support systems, spiritual needs, and the stability of the relationship. Description of past ways of grieving is significant, and attention should be given to parents who have a history of complicated bereavement, lack social or family support, have ambivalent feelings about the pregnancy, or have family members who are very directive and controlling concerning decisions (Brown, 1991).

Nurse-Sensitive Outcomes

Grief Resolution is the outcome that should be determined as the parents complete the tasks of mourning (Iowa Outcomes Project, 2000). Some of the outcome indicators may be recognized during a short hospitalization, whereas other indicators may not be observed for many months. The short-term communication indicators for parents include expressing their feelings, verbalizing the reality of the loss, sharing the loss with significant others, and expressing religious beliefs about death. The long-term indicators include the ability to verbalize acceptance of the loss and discuss unresolved conflicts (Iowa Outcomes Project, 2000). The decision-making indicators are short term and include making choices about attachment and bonding activities and planning or participating in the funeral or other rituals significant to parental or cultural beliefs (Iowa Outcomes Project, 2000). Behavioral indicators that should be evaluated soon after a perinatal loss relate to maintenance of a living environment, maintenance of grooming and hygiene, and adequate nutritional intake. Long-term behavioral indicators are the reporting of an absence of somatic distress, the absence of sleep disturbance, and normal sexual desire

TABLE 15.2   Responding to Grieving Families

Appropriate Responses	Inappropriate Responses
"I am so sorry your baby died."	"You can always have another baby."
"I feel so bad for you."	"At least you have children at home."
"This must be terribly difficult."	"At least the baby died at birth so you didn't get attached."
"What can I do for you?"	"I know how you feel."
"I am here, and I want to listen."	"You have an angel in heaven."
	"There was something wrong with the baby anyway."
	Calling the baby "fetus" or "it"
	Not saying anything

SOURCE: Limbo and Wheeler (1986).

(Iowa Outcomes Project, 2000). Seeking social support and reporting involvement in social activity are social indicators in which, after a period of time, parents should be participating. Long-term emotional indicators include the ability to describe the meaning of loss or death, report of decreased preoccupation with the loss, expression of positive expectations about the future, and progress through the tasks of mourning (Iowa Outcomes Project, 2000).

GRIEF WORK FACILITATION: PERINATAL DEATH

Contact with the parents before delivery or a surgical procedure lays the groundwork for support, opens lines of communication, and establishes rapport with the couple. The emotional trauma caused by the loss of a baby heightens parents' sensitivity to the words and actions of others. Even if parents do not remember all the details of what was said, they will remember how they were made to feel (Wathen, 1990). Initial contact with the parents should always include an expression of sympathy, such as "I am so sorry about your loss." Appropriate and inappropriate responses to parental grief are outlined in Table 15.2 (Limbo & Wheeler, 1986).

Activities that promote communication include (a) availability to listen, (b) talking openly and honestly with the family, and (c) involving both parents in information sharing and decision making. If the parents express guilt or self-blame, the issue is addressed and misconceptions are clarified. Good communication prior to delivery facilitates coping, decreases parental fears, and gives a sense of control back to the parents.

Treat all babies with respect and dignity, whether products of conception or newborns that die. Ask the parents whether they want to see their baby. It is insensitive to show parents the products of conception in a jar of formalin, in a metal basin, or on a paper towel. Instead, place a tiny baby in a bunting, on a soft cloth, or on a blanket. To enhance sensory memory, bathe the baby, apply lotion to the skin, and sprinkle baby powder in the blanket. If possible, dress the baby in a gown, hat, booties, and diaper, and wrap him or her in a warm blanket. It is appropriate to encourage the parents to participate in the bathing and dressing of the baby.

A helpful activity for parents when a baby dies is an opportunity to acknowledge the baby as real, complete the attachment process, and bring closure to the experience. This can be accomplished through seeing, holding, and touching activities (Calhoun, 1994). In addition, parent-infant contact facilitates anticipatory grieving when a neonate is critically ill (Thomas & Cordell, 1983). Provide a private room, and encourage the parents to spend as much time as they need with the baby. If the parents decline, offer the option again a few hours later. This is especially true for women who receive analgesics or anesthesia for delivery. If possible, encourage siblings and other family members to participate in the viewing experience.

Contact with the baby is also important when the baby has anomalies, whether the pregnancy ends spontaneously or was terminated (Zeanah et al., 1993). Discuss the appearance of the baby before parental viewing, focusing on the normal features while sensitively discussing any anomalies (e.g., peeling skin, discoloration, molding of the head, and appearance of birth defects). Parents see with loving eyes and will usually focus on the normal aspects of the baby first and then examine the anomalies. If the parents are reluctant to view their baby, ease parental anxiety by offering a Polaroid picture of the baby prepared for viewing. Parents have the right to see the products of conception after a miscarriage or ectopic pregnancy. Some parents will be receptive to this option, whereas others will not. Therefore, a drawing or model of a fetus may help answer parental questions (Wheeler, 1994).

Naming at any gestational age makes the baby a part of the family and is another tangible reminder of the baby's existence. Refer to the baby by name if one is selected (Brown, 1991). The use of medical terminology (e.g., fetus, abortion, and blighted ovum) is undesirable because these phrases are insensitive to parental feelings and depersonalize the infant.

Encourage parents and extended family to implement any cultural, religious, or social custom they find comforting. Offer the services of a chaplain, who may (a) provide spiritual comfort and support; (b) help parents understand their religious belief about death; and (c) perform blessing, baptism, or naming ceremonies (Limbo & Wheeler, 1986).

Burial is possible for a baby of any gestational age, but regulations vary from state to state. The local funeral director is the best resource to explain ordinances and assist families with arrangements. The nurse must be familiar with hospital guidelines and funeral options, however (e.g., chapel service, graveside service, hospital service, and self-transport). Encourage both parents to plan and participate in the funeral when appropriate. Parents may choose to write all or part of the baby's funeral service, so resource books need to be available to assist the parents with this task.

In most instances, the physician will discuss the option of autopsy. This requires the utmost tact and consideration of the family's feelings and cultural beliefs (Fox, Pillai, Porter, & Gill, 1997). Parents need time to adjust to the reality of the loss before this discussion, and the nurse functions as the parents' advocate at this time. To avoid misunderstanding, ensure that the autopsy discussion includes information about the reason for autopsy, what potentially will be determined by the autopsy, and how and when parents will receive the results of the autopsy.

Offer parents the option of postpartum care in or away from the maternity unit. Being in an environment in which other babies are crying and parents are celebrating the births of babies may be very distressing. For some mothers, however, the postpartum unit may be comforting and provide hope for the future. Allow rooming-in privileges for the father and extended visiting hours for other family members. These activities encourage communication and promote healing. When admitting grieving parents to nonmaternity units, ensure that the staff is oriented to perinatal death intervention and postpartum care.

Tangible mementos validate the baby's existence (Heiman, Yankowitz, & Wilkins, 1997). Determine the baby's weight, length, sex, time of birth, and time of death, and record this information on a certificate of birth for the parents. Obtain footprints and hand prints using standard footprint paper or plaster of paris mold or both. Place the gown, blanket, hat, booties, and diaper worn by the baby in a zip-lock plastic bag to preserve the scent of the baby. Save all the baby's personal care items, such as a comb, tape measure, stuffed toys, infant blood pressure cuff, lotion, and powder. Unless it is against cultural belief, obtain a lock of the baby's hair. After gathering the mementos, place them in a special keepsake box or envelope for the parents to take home. Some parents may not want the mementos gathered, but they may request the keepsakes in the future. Therefore, a system for storing the mementos is necessary, and the parents need information on accessing these items in the future.

The value of 35-mm photographs following a perinatal loss is well documented (Primeau & Recht, 1993). Arrange for photographs of the baby unless it is against the cultural or religious beliefs of the family. For the best photographic result, dress and wrap the baby in a soft blanket and place the baby on a soft surface. Position the baby naturally on the side or tummy, include special mementos such as a stuffed toy, and include family members in the photographs.

Parental guidance needs to be fairly directive (Rybarik, 1996). Both written and verbal information should be specific regarding the type of loss experienced, addressing (a) the characteristics of normal and abnormal grieving, (b) triggers that precipitate feelings of sadness, (c) the difference between male and female patterns of grieving, and (d) reactions of family and friends. Suggestions for dealing with grief include balanced nutrition, adequate fluid intake, regular exercise, avoiding alcohol and smoking, adequate rest, reading or writing about loss, avoidance of major decisions, accepting help when offered, and maintaining spiritual activities (Heath & Gensch, 1994). Many excellent resources are available from the organizations listed in Table 15.3.

Sibling grief is a special concern for parents. Attempts to protect children often isolate and exclude them from this important family event (Gardner & Merenstein, 1986). Children understand at an intuitive level that something is wrong, and they pick up on parental behavior. Siblings need to know what is happening, to participate in seeing the baby, to know what to expect, and to participate in the funeral (Walker, 1993). The child's ability to comprehend the meaning of death, however, varies with age and intellectual development (Finke, Birenbaum, & Chand, 1994). Provide families with written and verbal information about age-appropriate sibling grief. Topics to include are the children's concept of death, fears and behaviors, words to use when talking about death, how to clarify misconceptions, and how children act out their feelings in writing, drawing, or play.

Spend time directly with the extended family to discuss their thoughts and feelings and to clarify misconceptions. Suggest that the extended family be available to listen, attend the funeral, provide child care, furnish a meal, help with errands or housework, remember the baby's due date and birthday, and give a remembrance gift (Limbo & Wheeler, 1986).

An extended period of psychological support and intervention decreases depression symptoms in women who experience perinatal loss (Carrera et al., 1998). Support groups are a valuable source of assistance to bereaved parents (Gardner & Merenstein, 1986). Some parents will need this type of help immediately, whereas others may seek this type of support months after the loss. Provide the parents with the name of a support group leader and meeting information, and discuss the benefits of

TABLE 15.3   Bereavement Resources

Centering Corporation
1532 North Saddle Creek Road
Omaha, NE 68104

Wintergreen Press
4105 Oak Street
Long Lake, MN 55356

Rainbow Connection
477 Hannah Branch Road
Burnsville, NC 28714

Center for Loss in Multiple Birth
CLIMB, Inc.
Jeane Kollantai
P.O. Box 1064
Palmer, AK 99645

National SHARE Office
St. Joseph Health Center
300 First Capitol Drive
St. Charles, MO 63301

A Place to Remember
DeRuyter-Nelson Publications, Inc.
1885 University Avenue, Suite 110
St. Paul, MN 55104

For Teen Moms Only
P.O. Box 962
Frankfort, IL 60423

Pineapple Press
P.O. Box 312
St. Johns, MI 48879

Center for Loss and Life Transition
3735 Bows Road
Fort Collins, CO 80526

Pregnancy and Infant Loss Center
1421 East Wayzata Boulevard, Suite 40
Wayzata, MN 55391

Bereavement Services/RTS
Gundersen Lutheran Medical Center
1910 South Avenue
LaCrosse, WI 54601

The Compassionate Friends, Inc.
National Office
P.O. Box 3696
Oak Brook, IL 60522

The Sometimes Line
P.O. Box 638
Greene, IA 50636

Pen-Parents
P.O. Box 8738
Reno, NV 89507

support groups. Other advocacy systems include bereavement newsletters, community mental health resources, and one-to-one parent support.

Follow-up care is available to families with a normal baby, and the bereaved parent desires and needs the same attention (Klingbeil, 1986). Phone calls within 3 weeks, at 4 to 6 months, near the due date, and on the anniversary of the loss assist parents with the grief process (Heath & Gensch, 1994). This activity requires coordination, education, and guidance for the nursing staff involved. The objectives for a follow-up call are to (a) provide a listening ear, (b) allow the parents time to tell their story and share their feelings, (c) receive or review information, (d) make referrals to local perinatal bereavement support groups, (e) clarify misconceptions, and (f) validate parental feelings. Appropriate referrals to mental health facilities should be arranged if potential dysfunctional grief patterns are noted. A follow-up program moves grief work facilitation outside the realm of the acute care or hospital setting (Klingbeil, 1986).

Several weeks after the loss of a baby, a grief conference may be arranged. The goals of the grief conference are to answer questions, review autopsy and test results, discuss information related to a subsequent pregnancy, provide emotional support, provide an opportunity to evaluate the parents' progress through the grief process, implement additional interventions, and make referrals based on parental needs (Health & Gensch, 1994). Parents have the right to decide whom they would like present at the grief conference (e.g., primary care nurse, physician, social worker, chaplain, grief counselor, or all these). The nurse may facilitate the organization of this conference and attend as an advocate for the family.

INTERVENTION APPLICATION

A. S., a 28-year-old who has had four pregnancies with only two live births (gravida 4 and para 2), at 20.5 weeks gestation was referred to the fetal diagnosis and treatment unit because a routine ultrasound was suggestive of anencephaly. Grief Work Facilitation began after the nursing diagnoses Anticipatory Grieving and Potential for Dysfunctional Grief were established. The communication outcome of establishing rapport and good communication was accomplished through listening, talking openly, and involving both parents in the assessment process. The grave nature of the baby's condition was explained, questions were answered, prognosis was discussed, and emotional support was provided. After this extended session, the couple decided for personal and religious reasons that pregnancy termination was not an option.

At subsequent visits, the nurse initiated more activities to prepare the parents for the birth of their baby. Options were discussed and written information shared concerning viewing, seeing and holding, naming, religious rituals, funeral options, autopsy, mementos and photographs, sibling grief, and support groups. Near the time of delivery, the Decision Making outcomes were complete. The birth plan was established, and all the preliminary arrangements were made.

At 38 weeks, after a 9-hour labor, A. S. delivered a stillborn female who died during an unmonitored labor. All the parents' wishes were honored after the delivery. The family was followed with cards and phone calls that gave an additional opportunity to provide guidance, review information, and clarify misconceptions. A grief conference was arranged 8 weeks following the loss. The couple was counseled about the final diagnosis, risk to future pregnancies, and management of subsequent pregnancies. At this time, the nurse evaluated progress toward appropriate behavioral and social outcomes.

A. S. and her husband demonstrated progress toward the emotional outcome of describing meaning to their loss when A. S. wrote,

> Our baby was far from perfect and had many bruises and open sores. We felt she was just as beautiful as our other two children were at birth. Thank you for treating our baby with so much dignity and respect. You helped our experience to be a positive one. The way we were treated, along with our "perfect little angel," has meant more to us than you will ever know. She was never treated as a baby with deformities, but as a baby, "our baby," who tragically died before birth. Thank you so much for the unconditional love, compassion, and respect many of you gave.

Indicators were present to suggest that progress was being made toward Grief Resolution (Iowa Outcomes Project, 2000).

RESEARCH AND PRACTICE IMPLICATIONS

Research

Limited research is available on nursing interventions and their effects on the grief process. Research that evaluates the effect of intervention on grief resolution and makes recommendations for improved care is necessary. Several significant questions need to be answered, including (a) the effect of the intervention on the grief experience, (b) how the grief experience improved with the use of the intervention, and (c) what differences in grief resolution were noted in individuals who did not choose specific activities.

Many studies have been conducted on the use of support groups by parents, but research conducted with families who did not choose this option is important for comparison. Limited research is available concerning the effect of pregnancy loss on a subsequent pregnancy. Research questions to be answered include the following: (a) What is the nature of attachment in a subsequent pregnancy? (b) Does grief affect the attachment to subsequent children? (c) Is there an optimal interval between the loss and the next attempt to conceive? and (d) Does the loss affect the pregnancy experience in subsequent childbearing? In the past decade, fathers have assumed more involvement in pregnancy and greater parenting responsibilities. Additional research is needed concerning paternal involvement in perinatal loss to determine the most effective intervention to address paternal bereavement. Grief Work Facilitation: Perinatal Loss needs to be tested with randomized clinical trials initially. Then, comparative studies to differentiate effects across populations need to be conducted.

Practice Implications

Development of a perinatal loss critical path assists health professionals in planning an intervention. It also ensures continuity of care, completeness, and documentation. Specific protocols must accompany the critical path providing guidelines for management of specific types of loss. In an atmosphere of budgetary constraint, decreased hospital stay, and a shift to outpatient service, comprehensive programs are even more important to grief resolution. Intervention is initiated at the point of service. Collaboration with community health professionals, however, transfers care outside the realm of acute care and ensures continuity throughout the grief experience.

The role of the nurse is to give parents permission to grieve in their own way and to accept their unique differences. The nurse anticipates the family's need to hold on to memories and have tangible mementos, involves family members, and allows the family to choose activities specific to their unique needs. Listening to and being with the family at this moment in their personal history is meaningful to the parents and a growth experience for the nurse.

REFERENCES

Armstrong, D., & Hutti, M. (1998). Pregnancy after perinatal loss: The relationship between anxiety and prenatal attachment. *Journal of Obstetric, Gynecologic, and Neonatal Nursing, 27*(2), 183-189.

Brown, Y. (1991). Perinatal death and grieving. *Canadian Nurse, 87*(8), 26-29.

Calhoun, L. K. (1994). Parents' perceptions of nursing support following neonatal loss. *Journal of Perinatal and Neonatal Nursing, 8*(2), 57-66.

Carrera, L., Diez-Domingo, J., Montanana, V., Monleon Sancho, J., Minguez, J., & Monleon, J. (1998). Depression in women suffering perinatal loss. *International Journal of Gynaecology & Obstetrics, 62*(2), 149-153.

Engel, G. L. (1961). Is grief a disease? A challenge for medical research. *Psychosomatic Medicine, 23*, 18-22.

Ewton, D. S. (1993). A perinatal loss follow-up guide for primary care. *Nurse Practitioner, 18*(12), 30-36.

Finke, L. M., Birenbaum, L. K., & Chand, N. (1994). Two weeks post-death report by parents of siblings' grieving experience. *Journal of Child and Adolescent Psychiatric/Mental Health Nursing, 7*(4), 17-25.

Fox, R., Pillai, M., Porter, H., & Gill, G. (1997). The management of late fetal death: A guide to comprehensive care. *British Journal of Obstetrics and Gynaecology, 104*, 4-10.

Gabbe, S. G., Niebyl, J. R., & Simpson, J. L. (Eds.). (1996). *Obstetrics: Normal and problem pregnancies* (3rd ed.). New York: Churchill Livingstone.

Gardner, S. L., & Merenstein, G. B. (1986). Perinatal grief and loss: An overview. *Neonatal Network, 5*(2), 7-15.

Heath, L. S., & Gensch, B. R. (Eds.). (1994). *RTS counselor training manual* (3rd ed.). LaCrosse, WI: RTS Bereavement Services.

Heiman, J., Yankowitz, J., & Wilkins, J. (1997). Grief support programs: Patients' use of services following the loss of a desired pregnancy and degree of implementation in academic centers. *American Journal of Perinatology, 14*(10), 587-591.

Iowa Outcomes Project. (2000). *Nursing outcomes classification (NOC)* (M. Johnson, M. Maas, & S. Moorhead, Eds.; 2nd ed.). St. Louis, MO: Mosby-Year Book.

Klaus, M. H., & Kennell, J. H. (1982). *Parent-infant bonding.* St. Louis, MO: C. V. Mosby.

Klingbeil, C. G. (1986). Extended nursing care after a perinatal loss: Theoretical implications. *Neonatal Network, 5*(3), 21-28.

Limbo, R. K., & Wheeler, S. R. (1986). *When a baby dies: A handbook for healing and helping.* LaCrosse, WI: RTS Bereavement Services.

Lindemann, E. (1944). Symptomology and management of adult grief. *American Journal of Psychiatry, 101,* 141-148.

North American Nursing Diagnosis Association. (1999). *Nursing diagnoses: Definitions and classification 1995-1996.* Philadelphia: Author.

Peppers, L. G., & Knapp, R. J. (1980). *Motherhood and mourning: Perinatal death.* New York: Praeger.

Primeau, M. R., & Recht, C. K. (1993). Professional bereavement photographs: One aspect of a perinatal bereavement program. *Journal of Obstetric, Gynecologic, and Neonatal Nursing, 23,* 22-25.

Rajan, L. (1994). Social isolation and support in pregnancy loss. *Health Visitor, 67*(3), 97-101.

Rubin, R. (1975). Maternal tasks in pregnancy. *Maternal Child Nursing Journal, 4*(3), 143-153.

Rubin, R. (1984). *Maternal identity and the maternal experience.* New York: Springer.

Rybarik, F. (1996). Ask the experts: What communication skills are most helpful with families grieving a perinatal loss? How can I express my concern while providing appropriate care? *AWHONN Voice, 4*(6), 4.

Solari-Twadell, P. A., Bunkers, S. S., Wang, C., & Snyder, D. (1995). The pinwheel model of bereavement. *Image: The Journal of Nursing Scholarship, 27*(4), 323-326.

Thomas, N., & Cordell, A. S. (1983). The dying infant: Aiding parents in the detachment process. *Pediatric Nursing, 9*(5), 355-357.

Thomas, V., Striegel, P., Dudley, D., Wilkins, J., & Gibson, D. (1997). Parental grief of a perinatal loss: A comparison of individual and relationship variables. *Journal of Personal and Interpersonal Loss, 2,* 167-187.

U.S. Department of Health and Human Services. (1991). *Healthy people 2000: National health promotion and disease prevention objectives* (DHHS Publication No. PHS 91-50312). Washington, DC: Government Printing Office.

Walker, C. L. (1993). Sibling bereavement and grief responses. *Journal of Pediatric Nursing, 8*(5), 325-334.

Wathen, N. C. (1990). Perinatal bereavement. *British Journal of Obstetrics and Gynaecology, 97,* 759-761.

Wheeler, S. R. (1994). Psychosocial needs of women during miscarriage or ectopic pregnancy. *AORN Journal, 60*(2), 221-231.

Worden, J. W. (1991). *Grief counseling and grief therapy.* New York: Springer.

Zeanah, C. H., Dailey, J. V., Rosenblatt, M. J., & Saller, D. N. (1993). Do women grieve after terminating pregnancies because of fetal anomalies? A controlled investigation. *Obstetrics and Gynecology, 82*(2), 270-275.

PART II

Interventions for Child Health Problems

The families of children with illnesses or disabilities have a major role in the care of their children in the home and community. Nurses assist families in preparing them for their unique role in managing the illness while maintaining a sense of normalcy in their everyday lives. This process can be facilitated with the nursing interventions Normalization Promotion, Sibling Adaptation Counseling, and Friendship Promotion. For hospitalized children, the interventions Preparation for Hospitalization, Surgery, and Procedures; Therapeutic Play; and Distraction provide nurses with tools to assist children and families to cope with the pain and uncertainty they face in this potentially threatening environment.

One of the major contributions nurses can make to families who have a child with a chronic condition or disability is case management. Many families receive services from a wide variety of professionals in a host of different settings, from the acute care hospital to the ambulatory clinic and the schools in which their children spend much of their waking hours. Nurses are prepared to coordinate the many services used by families, thus maximizing the use of available resources, eliminating duplication, and preventing families from being lost in the large bureaucratic health care structure.

Nurses in ambulatory, school, and community settings need a wide range of interventions to treat and prevent problems in children and families. Some of the interventions that are useful in these settings include Bowel Incontinence Care: Encopresis, Behavior Modification, and Self-Mutilation Prevention. The interventions in Part II are designed to assist nurses in providing interventions for children with health problems. It is hoped that these interventions will stimulate nurses to design other creative and innovative interventions for this population.

16

Case Management

Deborah K. Bahe

During the past 30 years, there has been a dramatic decrease in the number of deaths of children from acute infectious diseases and congenital anomalies. In contrast, the number of children living with chronic and complex morbidities has increased (Felice & Friedman, 1997; Haynie & Palfrey, 1997; Liptak & Myers, 1997). Among these new childhood morbidities are chronic illnesses, physical disabilities, mental disabilities, and psychosocial and behavioral disorders. It is estimated that 10% to 40% of children have a chronic health problem (Juszczak & Schneider, 1997), whereas an estimated 31% of children under age 18 have more than one chronic condition (Newacheck & Taylor, 1992). From 5% to 10% of all children have a physical disability (Liptak & Myers, 1997), whereas 12% to 22% of all children suffer from some type of mental, emotional, or behavioral disorder (Adelman, Taylor, Bradley, & Lewis, 1997). Children with these chronic conditions are frequently termed "children with special health care needs" (Liptak & Myers, 1997).

According to *Healthy People 2000* (U.S. Department of Health and Human Services [USDHHS], 1991), children with special health care needs have an accentuated need for health promotion and disease prevention efforts because they are at a higher risk for developing future problems than is the general population of children. Health promotion and disease prevention require accessibility to health care and continuity and coordination of a variety of health, educational, and social services

(USDDHS, 1991). Goldsmith (1992) noted that as chronic illness has replaced acute infections as the most significant health problem, the "fit" between health care needs and the health services framework has worsened significantly. Traditional health care continues to be built around acute illness services and is episodic in delivery and categorical in focus (Wiener & Cohen, 1997). Most children who have chronic health concerns need comprehensive, coordinated, and continual care, but they are vulnerable to reductions in needed care because their families face challenges securing those services (Kretz & Pantos, 1996; Smith, Layne, & Garell, 1994). Because of these challenges, U.S. Surgeon General C. Everett Koop (1987) called for the development of systems of care for children with special health care needs and their families that are family centered, community based, and coordinated. Zander (1988b) observed that systems, structures, tools, and roles need to be redesigned to better fit the demands of today's health care clients. According to Falk and Bower (1994), care must be holistic in nature and integrate psychosocial, emotional, and spiritual needs along with physiological needs. Care for some populations needs to be managed over the health-illness continuum for quality and cost outcomes.

One response to the need for restructuring and redesigning the client care delivery system has evolved in the form of case management (Jones, 1994). Case management represents an attempt to reduce the fragmented maze of care and to create a more seamless experience for the nation's at-risk, underserved, and vulnerable populations who have varying and often multiple social, physiological, and psychological needs (Falik et al., 1993).

THEORETICAL FRAMEWORK AND LITERATURE REVIEW

There are several definitions of case management. The Case Management Society of America (1994) defines *case management* as a "collaborative process which assesses, plans, implements, coordinates, monitors, and evaluates options and services to meet an individual's health needs through communications and available resources to promote quality and cost-effective outcomes" (p. 60). The Center for Case Management (1992) defines case management as a clinical system that focuses on the accountability of an identified individual or group for coordinating a client's care (or group of clients) across a continuum of care. Case management facilitates the achievement of quality clinical and financial outcomes by negotiating, procuring, and coordinating services and resources needed by the client and family. It individualizes care according to many variables, or factors, including ethnicity.

The American Nurses' Association (1988) defines nursing case management as a health care delivery process that aims to provide quality health care, enhance quality of life, diminish fragmentation, and contain costs (Mahn & Spross, 1996). Newman (1995) describes case management as a health care delivery process intended to ensure that a client's service needs are met through the provision of quality care in the most appropriate setting, ensuring continuity of care across a continuum of health services from preventive to tertiary care. She views nursing case management as an expanded version of the nursing process, addressing the complexities of multidimensional needs in a holistic manner.

Historical Background

Early forms of case management originated late in the 19th century in an effort to coordinate public services and conserve public funds with the public sector welfare and human services programs (Falik et al., 1993). In the 1940s, medical case management took root with the reform of the state workers' compensation programs to improve health status and functional abilities. Since the 1950s, case management has been used in the management of psychiatric, social, and mental retardation cases (Newman, 1995). In the 1960s and 1970s, case management drew increasing public attention and became attractive because the rapid growth of categorical social welfare programs was resulting in a fragmented and inefficient service delivery system. By the mid-1980s, nursing case management was being introduced into acute care facilities as a cost-effective human resource strategy for delivering nursing care (Conners, 1996). In the late 1990s, case management continued to evolve in response to the rapid changes in health care and is currently being used in various stages of development in more than half of the hospitals in North America. Within the next decade, it is predicted that all health care professionals will use case management (Conners, 1996).

Models

Managed care is a system of health care coordination and resource utilization designed to optimize quality and cost-effectiveness (Mahn & Spross, 1996; McCloskey & Grace, 1994). Goals of managed care center around quality, collaboration, and cost (Zander, 1988a). Managed care has been the driving force behind several shifts in health care delivery, such as the development of case management. Case management organizes health care to meet specific client outcomes within specific time periods (Lynn-McHale, Fitzpatrick, & Shaffer, 1993). This reorganization of health care services places client needs at the center of all care decisions (Conners, 1996) so that the client receives the care needed when the care is needed—no more, no less, no sooner, or no later (Zander, 1992). Original case management models are frequently illustrated as a triangle including the client, payor, and provider, with the client positioned at the top of the triangle (Glettler & Leen, 1996).

With the focus of health care delivery centering on the client, coordinating multiple provider services and funding sources for some client populations is needed. Case management is designed to do this. Elaborating on the original model, case management can be shown in an expanded model weaving multiple physiological, psychological, social, educational, financial, or all these services into a comprehensive, coordinated, and continuous network of care to the client and family (Bahe, 1997).

Empirical Studies

The effectiveness of case management is still being studied. In 1991, Bigelow and Young found that case-managed clients received more services, they had fewer unmet service needs, their quality of life was greater, and hospital utilization was reduced. Kretz and Pantos (1996) found in their review of studies that case management demonstrated tremendous potential for the innovative management of chronic conditions in avoiding acute exacerbations and costly hospitalizations and in improving the long-term outcomes for clients. Opuni, Smith, Arvey, and Solomon (1994) found that comprehensive community coalitions were effective mechanisms for addressing many of today's teen-age high-risk behaviors and health problems, such as care for pregnant teens and better pregnancy outcomes. Pierce and Freedman (1983) described case management interventions that resulted in reduced hospitalization rates and emergency room visits. Stein and Jessop (1984) reported on the Home Care Project, in which case management resulted in improved psychological adjustment and family satisfaction and fewer instances of mental health problems among mothers.

From the perspective of health costs, a study by the Health Insurance Association of America (Boling, 1996) found that medical rehabilitation and case management paid large fiscal dividends—a 30 to 1 return on their investment. Boling, executive director of Case Management Society of America, commented, "This is certainly terrific news since it confirms that case management is a critical component of health care delivery" (p. 122).

Evaluation of case management also must consider the impact on the family and on the individual client and health costs. The reduction of family burden for families of children with disabilities through case management has been well documented in the literature (Ardito, Botuck, Freeman, & Levy, 1997; Pyke & Apa, 1994). In fact, the role played by case managers has been found to be crucial in providing information and support to families, surpassing the impact of overall service system coverage and quality in determining family satisfaction.

NURSING DIAGNOSIS AND OUTCOME DETERMINATION

Part of the rationale for using case management hinges on complexity rather than acuity of client problems. Children with chronic health concerns often present with complexities in diagnosis, such as multiple nursing and medical diagnoses. An example of multiple nursing diagnoses is a child with a high spinal cord injury who is wheelchair bound and ventilator dependent. This child could have an array of nursing diagnoses, such as Bowel Incontinence, Urinary Incontinence, Impaired Physical Mobility, Impaired Skin Integrity, Ineffective Breathing Pattern, Risk for Aspiration, Bathing/Hygiene Self-Care Deficit, and Social Isolation (North American Nursing Diagnosis Association [NANDA], 1999). The same child may have a family with multiple nursing diagnoses, such as Anxiety, Caregiver Role Strain, Altered Family Processes, Ineffective Family Coping, Fatigue, Grieving, Health-Seeking Behaviors, Parent Role Conflict, and Altered Parenting.

Although children with special health care needs may have multiple diagnoses, they may share many common diagnoses. A widely held generalization is that 85% of the health issues for children with disabilities are common to children who have all chronic conditions (Liptak & Myers, 1997). Those diagnoses may include Impaired Social Interaction, Social Isolation, Risk for Loneliness, Ineffective Individual Coping, Impaired Adjustment, Ineffective Management of Therapeutic Regime, Noncompliance, Health-Seeking Behaviors, Altered Growth and Development, Body Image Disturbance, Self-Esteem Disturbance, Personal Identity Disturbance, Powerlessness, Knowledge Deficit, and Fear (NANDA, 1999). Parents of these children may also share common nursing diagnoses, including Altered Parenting, Risk for Altered Parenting, Risk for Parent-Child Attachment, Altered Family Processes, Care Giver Role Strain, Parent Role Conflict, Family Coping, and Grieving.

General outcomes of case management include improved client health status, enhanced client and family satisfaction, and more appropriate use of resources (Falk & Bower, 1994). By addressing systems, procedures, and roles, case management pulls together multiple intradisciplinary and interdisciplinary diagnoses and integrates multiple interventions into a co-ordinated network of care to achieve desired client and organizational outcomes (Zander, 1994). Beneficiaries of case management include the individual client, the client's family, providers of services, and the health care industry. For the individual client, direct outcomes include a reduction in symptoms, improved functional status, and improved quality of life, whereas an indirect benefit is the lowered risk of secondary complications. For the client's family, direct outcomes of case management could be time and energy savings, reducing emotional and economic stress, and minimizing care coordination confusion and frustrations that can accompany a child with multiple health care needs. An indirect benefit for the family is the preservation of the family unit and the strengthening of the family functioning. Care providers can benefit from case management by having more efficient and effective results from their efforts because of the synergistic effect of improved collaboration and coordination of team members. The health care industry, such as health care organizations and health care payors, can benefit directly from case management by conserving costs and improving the quality of their health care product (Zander, 1994). Financial profits and consumer satisfaction are the indirect benefits of conserving costs and improved quality.

INTERVENTION: CASE MANAGEMENT

Case Management Activities

Bahe (1997) views case management as an umbrella intervention under which other interventions within a discipline and across disciplines can be implemented. No one discipline owns case management (Zander, 1994). It is a collaborative, multidisciplinary intervention. Cardinal activities of case management, according to Mahn and Spross (1996) and Jones (1994), include the assignment of a case manager who manages cases for an episode over time and collaborates with a team sharing the same clients.

Case Managers

Case managers lead the case management process for a client or an assigned population of clients. Case manager activities include assessment of health needs, planning and procuring care, coordinating and implementing a plan of care, and evaluating and monitoring services within the multidisciplinary system. Case managers collaborate with administration, management, and clinical staff for the assigned client or population. They consult internally with other disciplines and departments and participate in developing documentation systems and tools, such as critical paths to monitor clinical and fiscal outcomes. Data and information are collected, analyzed, and shared by the case manager to influence process improvements and support integration of core systems and processes in the care environment, such as those involving the school nurse. According to Newman (1995) and Jones (1994), case managers can also serve as primary providers while assisting the client and family to negotiate the health care system. They teach the client and family self-reliance and self-monitoring while teaching and coaching other caregivers on the health care team about the client's condition and response to treatment. It is their goal to integrate the multidisciplinary services into one high-performance team.

Case managers' clinical knowledge and expertise are critically important to the success of case management (Mahn & Spross, 1996). The process will fail if case managers lack adequate knowledge about the disease process, the goals of or response to treatment, health care finances, and organizational and community resources, or if they do not have expert communication and collaboration skills (Kruger, 1989). Because case managers are responsible for clinical and fiscal outcomes, it is essential that they are educated and experienced in a discipline to assume the high-level clinical and management decision-making role (Kruger, 1989). Successful case management also requires skills in interdisciplinary collaboration and negotiation to facilitate cooperative and collaborative relationships among departments and disciplines (American Organization of Nurse Executives, 1992). A broad interdisciplinary knowledge base is needed. For the previously mentioned reasons, the Case Management Society of America endorses a minimum requirement of a baccalaureate degree for case management certification (Mahn & Spross, 1996).

Critical Paths

Critical paths are central to case management. Critical paths are multidisciplinary guidelines that contribute to quality, continuity, and coordination of care among disciplines by providing closer monitoring of the processes and outcomes and reduce costs by reducing duplication (Hamric, Spross, & Hanson, 1996). Critical paths are tailored to the needs of the child and family. Not all children with special health care needs warrant case management, not all children needing case management need a critical path, and not all critical events in a critical path apply to all cohorts using the critical path (Figure 16.1).

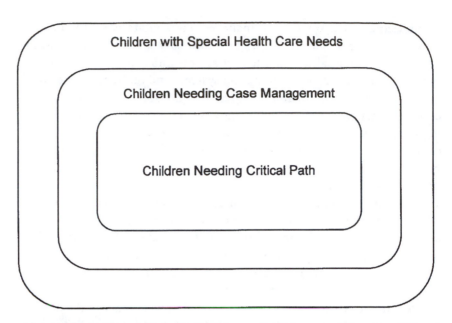

Figure 16.1. Children With Special Needs Needing Case Management and Critical Paths

Critical paths serve as road maps to be used by the case manager in organizing and integrating all levels of care delivered by providers from many disciplines for the case management of commonly encountered conditions in particular clinical areas. Focused on specific client populations or cases, critical paths organize and sequence interventions and the expected outcomes associated with them.

Newman (1995) identified many advantages of critical paths. Critical paths hasten progress through shared goals. They also cultivate understanding, foster teamwork, and facilitate early detection of variance to prevent or minimize unnecessary delays and interruptions in care. By reducing gaps and duplications, critical paths streamline services. Critical paths help clients and their families become more informed and involved so that they become more active participants in care. Outcome comparisons are more apparent, and accountability is improved. Critical paths also increase and enhance case manager visibility and authority. For all these reasons, critical paths are "best practice" tools (Falk & Bower, 1994; Jones, 1994) that have emerged to coordinate care over a health-illness continuum, improve practice and care, contain costs, and conserve resources. Critical paths can also enhance job satisfaction for nurses and improve their position on the health care team (Newman, 1995). Critical Path Development is listed as a nursing intervention in *Nursing Interven-*

tions Classification (Iowa Intervention Project, 2000). Similar models have been called Care Maps or Management Action Plans (Jones, 1994).

Other Implementation Processes

"Microlevel" case management has a scope of services limited to an institution, such as an acute care center (Brault & Kissinger, 1991). Single episodes of care are called "episodic clinical case management," which focuses more on those with an acute illness such as open-heart surgery clients (Mahn & Spross, 1996). Here, the case manager is responsible from preadmission to postdischarge. In episodic clinical case management, the nurse case manager maintains a relationship with the client, monitors the client's daily progress, and provides education and discharge planning services to the client and family. The case manager does not provide direct clinical care. Most clients needing case management in an acute care setting are referred to case management services during their inpatient admission because of high-risk profile criteria. The referrals often come from acute care nursing staff, although they can originate from any part of the system, including physicians, social service, payors, or community organizations. When the client is admitted into the case management program, a case manager is assigned.

"Macrolevel" case management includes a broader scope of services, crosses service settings, and is mostly community based (Brault & Kissinger, 1991). The focus of community-based case management is on maximizing health, whereas the target populations are those with chronic health concerns warranting long-term client relationships. In community-based case management, case managers with varying clinical backgrounds are employed to partner with a wide range of clients with chronic health problems over time and across settings to promote greater self-care. The case manager–client relationship and case management activities extend from the time the client is enrolled into the case management program to the termination of the relationship (Mahn & Spross, 1996).

Intensity of services is directly related to identified client need and is modified to meet changing client conditions. When case management services are no longer required, clients may be put on inactive status, discharged, or transferred to another provider. Case managers do not duplicate services provided elsewhere in the system (Falk & Bower, 1994). In providing services to clients and their families, a case manager performs the following core activities: (a) assesses and monitors the health status of the client, (b) screens for common health problems, (c) teaches self-reliance, (d) teaches self-monitoring, (e) obtains community-based support, (f) coordinates access to needed health services, (g) makes referrals to other health care providers, (h) manages nursing care, (i) facilitates short-term and long-term planning for health management, (j) coordinates other care, (k) brokers services, (l) assists clients to negotiate the health care system, and (m) serves as a primary provider. The following section presents a case study exhibiting community-based case management and the core activities of a case manager.

INTERVENTION APPLICATION

Nathan, a first grader in an elementary school, was making poor progress in almost all academic areas. He could not stay focused on any subject longer than 30 seconds unless his teacher stood beside him to constantly redirect him. Socially, he had few friends because he was impulsive and had difficulty waiting his turn, keeping quiet, and keeping his hands and feet to himself. At home, he constantly picked fights with his siblings, rarely followed through with chores, and would not sit through a meal or settle down to sleep at an appropriate bedtime. Nathan's mother was a single parent who worked at a minimum-wage job in a nursing home. Nathan's father, who dropped out of school in the 10th grade and was unemployed, was not involved with his son. Nathan had a sister in second grade and a 3-year-old brother attending Head Start.

Nathan's teacher was frustrated. She believed that she was spending so much of her time helping him that the other 22 first graders in her class did not get the help they deserved. Despite all the time she spent helping him, Nathan was not doing well in reading, writing, or math. Her frustration with Nathan was intensifying because his misbehavior in class was escalating and disrupting the rest of the students. Although Nathan had a good attitude about school, his teacher feared that he might soon become discouraged and not like school or himself.

Nathan's mother was frustrated. She admitted coming home from work drained of the physical and emotional energy needed to meet the many demands of her young active family. She had few family members or friends for support. Her income was barely above the poverty line, she did not have a telephone, and her car was not dependable. Although Nathan's mother did have health insurance for herself from her employer, she did not take out coverage for her children because the insurance premium would take most of her paycheck. Furthermore, she was also overqualified for the government's Medicaid program. Family life at home was chaotic, with Nathan's mother screaming at the children, the children screaming at each other, the children running and fighting, and the house being in disarray. She found routine, consistency, or follow through next to impossible with her work schedule. Other parents in the neighborhood would not let their children play with Nathan and blamed his mother for not disciplining and supervising her son. Nathan's mother had enough issues to deal with, but now she was being told that there were problems with Nathan at school.

When Nathan's classroom difficulties surfaced, Nathan's school nurse offered to serve as case manager. She believed that she was in the best position to serve in this role because of her close and continual contact with Nathan and his teacher, her position on the school's multidisciplinary Local Education Agency and Area Education Agency team, her familiarity with the primary care providers in the community, her awareness of specialists and specialty clinics in the area, her knowledge and interest in attention deficit hyperactivity disorder (ADHD), and her awareness of funding sources. The tool she used to guide her through this case management process was an ADHD Critical Path (Table 16.1). This critical path evolved over time from past multidisciplinary team proceedings. Following is the sequence of events followed by the ADHD Critical Path that parallel the core activities of a case manager discussed previously.

Nathan was screened for numerous possibilities that could interfere with his attention. Nathan's school nurse screened for common health problems such as hearing and vision deficits, acute and chronic illnesses, metabolic disorders (e.g., hyperthyroidism), neurological problems (e.g., seizures), allergies, medication effects, lack of sleep, and poor nutrition by performing a health assessment on Nathan. To screen for any developmental or environmental issues affecting Nathan's behavior and learning, she obtained a developmental and health history from his mother. To identify any behavioral concerns at home, she asked Nathan's mother to fill out a behavior rating scale on him. Nathan's teacher was asked to fill out several behavior-rating scales to screen him for ADHD and any other comorbid or secondary conditions. The nursing diagnosis of Altered Growth and Development was made (NANDA, 1999).

Self-reliance and self-monitoring were taught by Nathan's school counselor, who worked with him one-on-one to improve his attention span, patience, and organizational skills. She also worked with him in small groups to improve his social skills. The school counselor, the special education teacher, and the school social worker collaborated and then suggested some new classroom strategies for Nathan's teacher to try. Effectiveness of these interventions was monitored using a behavior monitoring form (Table 16.2). The school social worker met with Nathan's mother and gave her some suggestions to improve Nathan's behavior at home. Nathan's mother was loaned a video from the school on discipline to take home and view. Nathan's behavioral screenings suggested the pos-

TABLE 16.1 Comprehensive School Health Critical Path for Suspected ADHD

Case Manager _____
Phone _____

Student _____	*Address* _____	*BD* _____ *Grade* _____	*School* _____
Parent _____	*Address* _____	*Home Phone* _____	*Work Phone* _____
Parent _____	*Address* _____	*Home Phone* _____	*Work Phone* _____

Team	*Stage I*	*Stage II*	*Stage III*	*Stage IV*	*Stage V*	*Stage VI*	*Outcomes*
Classroom teacher	Concern ____ I-plan ____ Parent alerted ____						Attention 1 2 3 4 5 Impulsivity 1 2 3 4 5 Hyperactivity 1 2 3 4 5
Other teacher _____	Refer to: _____						Attention 1 2 3 4 5 Impulsivity 1 2 3 4 5 Hyperactivity 1 2 3 4 5
School counselor _____ _____		Observation _____ Interventions _____ _____					
School nurse _____		Teacher BRS: _____ ACTERs _____ Ned Owens _____ Outcome _____ Health assess _____ Parents: Contacted _____ BRS _____ History _____ Release _____ Booklet _____ Video _____ CHADD _____				Med _____ Dose _____ Time _____ IHP _____ Monitor/mo. _____ 504 _____	

TABLE 16.1 Continued

Team	Stage I	Stage II	Stage III	Stage IV	Stage V	Stage VI	Outcomes
Psychologist			Refer _____ Eval _____ Findings _____				Attention 1 2 3 4 5 Impulsivity 1 2 3 4 5 Hyperactivity 1 2 3 4 5
Social worker			Refer _____ Intervention				Attention 1 2 3 4 5 Impulsivity 1 2 3 4 5 Hyperactivity 1 2 3 4 5
Primary care				Refer _____ PE _____ Labs _____ Dx _____ Rx _____			Attention 1 2 3 4 5 Impulsivity 1 2 3 4 5 Hyperactivity 1 2 3 4 5
Specialist					Refer _____ Dx _____ Rx _____ Dx _____ Rx _____ Dx _____ Rx _____		Attention 1 2 3 4 5 Impulsivity 1 2 3 4 5 Hyperactivity 1 2 3 4 5

TABLE 16.2 Comprehensive School Health Behavior Monitoring

Name _____ Year _____ Grade _____ Class _____ Teacher _____

Attention	Impulsivity	Hyperactivity	Work Completion	Organization Skills	Oppositional	Social Skills	Academics
5-good	5-no problem	5-no problem	5-good	5-good	5-no problem	5-good	5-good
4-	4-	4-	4-	4-	4-	4-	4-
3-fair	3-concern	3-concern	3-fair	3-fair	3-concern	3-fair	3-fair
2-	2-	2-	2-	2-	2-	2-	2-
1-poor	1-problem	1-problem	1-poor	1-poor	1-problem	1-poor	1-poor

Date _____
Med _____
Dose _____
Times _____
Wt _____ Ht _____
BP _____
Other _____
Narrative:

Score _____

Attention	Impulsivity	Hyperactivity	Work Completion	Organization Skills	Oppositional	Social Skills	Academics
5-good	5-no problem	5-no problem	5-good	5-good	5-no problem	5-good	5-good
4-	4-	4-	4-	4-	4-	4-	4-
3-fair	3-concern	3-concern	3-fair	3-fair	3-concern	3-fair	3-fair
2-	2-	2-	2-	2-	2-	2-	2-
1-poor	1-problem	1-problem	1-poor	1-poor	1-problem	1-poor	1-poor

Date _____
Med _____
Dose _____
Times _____
Wt _____ Ht _____
BP _____
Other _____
Narrative:

Score _____

Attention	Impulsivity	Hyperactivity	Work Completion	Organization Skills	Oppositional	Social Skills	Academics
5-good	5-no problem	5-no problem	5-good	5-good	5-no problem	5-good	5-good
4-	4-	4-	4-	4-	4-	4-	4-
3-fair	3-concern	3-concern	3-fair	3-fair	3-concern	3-fair	3-fair
2-	2-	2-	2-	2-	2-	2-	2-
1-poor	1-problem	1-problem	1-poor	1-poor	1-problem	1-poor	1-poor

Date _____
Med _____
Dose _____
Times _____
Wt _____ Ht _____
BP _____
Other _____
Narrative:

Score _____

TABLE 16.2 Continued

Name _____ Year _____ Grade _____ Class _____ Teacher _____

	Attention	Impulsivity	Hyperactivity	Work Completion	Organization Skills	Oppositional	Social Skills	Academics
Date _____	5-good	5-no problem	5-no problem	5-good	5-good	5-no problem	5-good	5-good
Med _____	4-	4-	4-	4-	4-	4-	4-	4-
Dose _____	3-fair	3-concern	3-concern	3-fair	3-fair	3-concern	3-fair	3-fair
Times _____	2-	2-	2-	2-	2-	2-	2-	2-
Wt ___ Ht ___	1-poor	1-problem	1-problem	1-poor	1-poor	1-problem	1-poor	1-poor
BP _____								
Other _____								
Narrative:								Score _____

	Attention	Impulsivity	Hyperactivity	Work Completion	Organization Skills	Oppositional	Social Skills	Academics
Date _____	5-good	5-no problem	5-no problem	5-good	5-good	5-no problem	5-good	5-good
Med _____	4-	4-	4-	4-	4-	4-	4-	4-
Dose _____	3-fair	3-concern	3-concern	3-fair	3-fair	3-concern	3-fair	3-fair
Times _____	2-	2-	2-	2-	2-	2-	2-	2-
Wt ___ Ht ___	1-poor	1-problem	1-problem	1-poor	1-poor	1-problem	1-poor	1-poor
BP _____								
Other _____								
Narrative:								Score _____

sibility of ADHD. Because of these indications and because she was interested in learning more about it, Nathan's mother was given a booklet on ADHD.

Community-based support was obtained. Nathan's mother was encouraged to participate in an 11-week parenting course offered in the community that included a class for parents and a class for children. She was also encouraged to join the local Children With Attention Deficit Disorder support group to learn more about attention deficit, how to deal with it, and to gain the support of other parents who were in similar situations.

Access to other needed services was coordinated. When there were questions regarding Nathan's cognitive ability, Nathan's school nurse was able to oversee the referral for educational testing by the school psychologist.

Referral to other health care providers was made. Nathan's psychological testing revealed that he had the cognitive ability to do schoolwork, and the psychologist's observation of Nathan supported the possibility of ADHD. Because ADHD is a medical diagnosis, Nathan's school nurse made a referral to Nathan's primary care provider. For this referral, she gathered all the assessments, screenings, interventions, and outcomes obtained at school and completed the referral package with a cover letter. Nathan's mother then took him and the referral package to his medical appointment.

Nathan's health care at school was managed by his school nurse. After reviewing the reports from school, Nathan's primary care provider prescribed a 1-month trial of medication. During this medication trial, his school nurse closely monitored the medication's effectiveness by weekly behavior rating scales. The medication's side effects, such as appetite suppression and weight loss, were monitored closely, and the medication times were adjusted to minimize these effects. After the 1-month trial and monitoring, the results were shared with Nathan's primary care provider. Because the original dose of medication showed partial effectiveness, Nathan's medication dosage was increased. Results from this increased dosage showed even better outcomes of decreased symptoms, with indicators supporting positive growth and Child Development: Middle Childhood (6-11 years) (Iowa Outcomes Project, 2000).

Nathan's school did not have a school-based health clinic. If it did have one, a nurse practitioner, a physician's assistant, or a physician could have served as Nathan's case manager while also delivering primary care to him. Nathan's school nurse served as his community-based case manager to ensure a seamless network of continual care. She collaborated with many individuals and coordinated many services to facilitate optimal outcomes for Nathan and his family.

RESEARCH AND PRACTICE IMPLICATIONS

Research Implications

Whereas the development and clarification of case management is still in its early stages, research validating the effectiveness of case management is in even earlier stages. Rubin (1992), Falik et al. (1993), and Hale (1995) found research evaluating case management to be weak and inconclusive. Rubin believed that the efficacy of case management has been "prematurely empirically demonstrated" (p. 139), that outcome studies reflected diversity and ambiguity in how case management was conceptualized and implemented, and that there were problems in the research methodologies used. Falik and colleagues (1993) found there to be little, if any, research on how to measure the effects of case management on clients or to isolate the contribution of case management to changes in a client's health status or general well-being. Hale's (1995) review of the literature revealed only a small number of publications describing some kind of case management evaluations or research studies, and most had small samples and were methodologically so weak that it was impossible to determine if the results were valid.

More rigorous research is needed to support the effectiveness of case management. A few prerequisites are needed to help improve the quality of case management research. A major issue is the lack of a standard conceptual and operational definition of case management, which is needed if the intervention is to be explicated and tested. Outcomes need to be standardized to facilitate measurement. Nursing already has a head start in developing these standardized outcome measures, which are presented in *Nursing Outcomes Classification* (Iowa Outcomes Project, 2000). These outcomes not only reflect nursing diagnoses and nursing interventions but also can be shared across disciplines to address client aggregates, families, organizations, and communities. By standardizing client outcomes, the measurement of health care system's effectiveness can be documented and improved.

To date, the majority of evaluation studies have measured fiscal, quality of life, satisfaction, and symptom control outcomes of case management. No studies were found that (a) showed the long-term effectiveness of case management in reducing secondary complications, (b) evaluated the multidisciplinary team's satisfaction with the case management process or the team's use of a critical path as a tool, (c) correlated the skills of the case manager to the effectiveness of case management, or (d) compared other interventions to the intervention of case management. The only other similar interventions to case management were called care coordination and continuity of care. It is apparent that there is a need for case management research as it relates to the care of children with chronic health care needs and their families.

Clinical Practice Implications

Case management offers nurses the opportunity to assume a greater degree of autonomy and leadership. Current trends support the need for more case management of children with special health care needs. Case management in the community, especially in the school setting, can offer a unique opportunity for nurses to practice health protection and health promotion for at-risk children and their families.

Case management has evolved out of need, and five trends continue to support the use of case management. First, the number of children with complex and chronic health care needs appears to be increasing. Another trend is the increase of parents in the workforce, leaving them with less time, energy, and fortitude to seek out and coordinate multiple services for their child. Because case management serves to conserve financial resources, the soaring costs and limited funds of health care comprise the third trend supporting the use of case management. Fourth, providers are increasingly assuming the financial risks for client outcomes, and case management helps to ensure effective outcomes. Last, the health care industry, like other industries, is subscribing to Demming's total quality management/continuous quality improvement philosophy of improving the quality of its product while at the same time lowering the cost of production (Jones, 1994). Nursing case management and continuous quality improvement are linked in philosophy and purpose (Cesta, 1993).

There are four trends supporting community-based case management. The first is the recent emphasis on health promotion and disease prevention. Case management promotes health in community settings rather than acute or medical settings. Also, the payor views the community setting as a more economical, convenient, and user-friendly setting than costly acute care settings. Furthermore, there is a shift away from the medical dominance and medical model toward alternative health care models and providers. In case management, care providers are equal colleagues on the health care team, and there is no dominance of one discipline. Another trend is for more nursing case management. Nurses are gaining increasing visibility as intelligent, autonomous, and competent practitioners and leaders in health care. Advanced practice nurses have skills and competencies that qualify them as case managers, and they facilitate the development of trust among colleagues on the health care team.

There are a few trends that are opening the doors for school nurses to serve as case managers for children with special health care needs. As a result of Public Law (PL) 94-142 and PL 504 more than 10 years ago and, recently, PL 99-457 and PL 101-476 (Individuals With Disabilities Education Act), children with special needs are required by law to have equal access to education in public schools. As a result, many medically fragile and chronically ill children are mainstreamed into regular education classrooms that in the past were hospitalized, institutionalized, or assigned to special schools or classrooms. Because schools must modify and adapt to safely and effectively accommodate these children, school nurses are ideally located and suited to oversee the process and function as their case manager. School nurses have four advantages to case managing the school-age child that no other provider can offer. First, school nurses are strategically located proximal to large populations of children attending school. Second, school nurses can offer continuity of care on a day-to-day, week-to-week, month-to-month, and year-to-year basis. Third, school nurses are in close contact and can easily collaborate with key players and coordinate necessary health services. Finally, there is a trend toward year-round schools and schools offering day care and preschool programs that would further improve early access, identification, and continuity of care to special needs children by school nurses.

This chapter describes Case Management as an important nursing intervention to promote the health and well-being of children and their families. Many children have chronic and complex needs that warrant multiple and long-term services. For several reasons, access, coordination, and continuity of these multiple services can be ineffective. Multidisciplinary case management, led by a nurse case manager, is an important nursing intervention to assist children and their families in accessing and receiving comprehensive, coordinated, and continuous health services.

REFERENCES

Adelman, H. S., Taylor, L., Bradley, B., & Lewis, K. (1997). Mental health in schools: Expanded opportunities for school nurses. *Journal of School Nursing, 13*(3), 6-12.

American Nurses' Association. (1988). *Nursing case management.* Kansas City, MO: Author.

American Organization of Nurse Executives. (1992). *Role and functions of the hospital nurse manager.* Chicago: Author.

Ardito, M., Botuck, S., Freeman, S. E., & Levy, J. M. (1997). Delivering home-based case management to families with children with mental retardation and developmental disabilities. *Journal of Case Management, 6*(2), 56-61.

Bahe, D. (1997). *Case management.* Unpublished master's degree project. The University of Iowa, Iowa City.

Bigelow, D. A., & Young, D. J. (1991). Effectiveness of case management program. *Community Mental Health Journal, 27*(2), 115-123.

Boling, J. H. (1996). Study finds CM pays big dividends. *Case Management Advisor, 7*(9), 122-127.

Brault, G. L., & Kissinger, L. D. (1991). Case management: Ambiguous at best. *Journal of Pediatric Health Care, 5*(4), 179-183.

Case Management Society of America. (1994). CMSA proposes standards of practice. *Case Manager, 5,* 59-70.

Center for Case Management. (1992). *Case management definition.* South Natick, MA: Author.

Cesta, T. (1993). The link between continuous quality improvement and case management. *Journal of Nursing Administration, 23*(6), 55-61.

Conners, K. (1996). Managed care and case management. *Australian Nursing Journal, 3*(10), 32-34.

Falik, M., Lipson, D., Lewis-Idema, D., Ulmer, C., Kaplan, K., Robinson, G., Hickey, E., & Veiga, R. (1993). Case management for special populations, moving beyond categorical distinctions. *Journal of Case Management, 2*(2), 39-45.

Falk, C. D., & Bower, K. A. (1994). Managing care across department, organization, and setting boundaries. In K. Kelly & M. Maas (Eds.), *Health care rationing, dilemma and paradox* (pp. 161-176). St. Louis, MO: Mosby-Year Book.

Felice, M. E., & Friedman, S. B. (1997). The ill child. In R. A. Hoekelman, S. B. Friedman, N. M. Nelson, H. M. Seidel, & M. L. Weitzman (Eds.), *Primary pediatric care* (3rd ed., pp. 287-297). St. Louis, MO: Mosby-Year Book.

Glettler, E., & Leen, M. G. (1996). The advanced practice nurse as case manager. *Journal of Case Management, 5*(3), 121-126.

Goldsmith, J. (1992). The reshaping of healthcare. *Healthcare Forum Journal, 35*(3), 19-27.

Hale, C. (1995). Research issues in case management. *Nursing Standard, 9*(44), 29-32.

Hamric, A. B., Spross, J. A., & Hanson, C. M. (Eds.). (1996). *Advanced nursing practice.* Philadelphia: W. B. Saunders.

Haynie, M., & Palfrey, J. S. (1997). Children assisted by medical technology. In R. A. Hoekelman, S. B. Friedman, N. M. Nelson, H. M. Seidel, & M. L. Weitzman (Eds.), *Primary pediatric care* (3rd ed., pp. 413-415). St. Louis, MO: Mosby-Year Book.

Iowa Intervention Project. (2000). *Nursing interventions classification (NIC)* (J. C. McCloskey & G. M. Bulechek, Eds.; 3rd ed.). St. Louis, MO: Mosby-Year Book.

Iowa Outcomes Project. (2000). *Nursing outcomes classification (NOC)* (M. Johnson, M. Maas, & S. Moorhead, Eds.; 2nd ed.). St. Louis, MO: Mosby-Year Book.

Jones, K. R. (1994). Restructuring health care services. In K. Kelly & M. Maas (Eds.), *Health care rationing* (pp. 127-146). St. Louis, MO: C. V. Mosby.

Juszczak, L. J., & Schneider, M. B. (1997). The chronically ill and disabled child in school. In R. A. Hoekelman, S. B. Friedman, N. M. Nelson, H. M. Seidel, & M. L. Weitzman (Eds.), *Primary pediatric care* (3rd ed., pp. 437-439). St. Louis, MO: Mosby-Year Book.

Koop, C. E. (1987). *Surgeon general's report: Children with special health care needs: Campaign 87: Commitment to family-centered coordinated care for children with special health care needs* (DHHS Publication No. HRS/D/MC 87/2). Washington, DC: Public Health Service.

Kretz, S. E., & Pantos, B. S. (1996). Cost savings and clinical improvement through disease management. *Journal of Case Management, 5*(4), 173-175.

Kruger, N. R. (1989). Case management: Is it a delivery system for my organization? *Aspen Advisor for Nurse Executives, 4*(10), 4-5, 8.

Liptak, G. S., & Myers, B. A. (1997). Physical disability and chronic illness. In R. A. Hoekelman, S. B. Friedman, N. M. Nelson, H. M. Seidel, & M. L. Weitzman (Eds.), *Pediatric primary care* (3rd ed., pp. 405-407). St. Louis, MO: Mosby-Year Book.

Lynn-McHale, D. J., Fitzpatrick, E. R., & Shaffer, R. B. (1993). Case management: Development of a model. *Clinical Nurse Specialist, 7*(6), 299-307.

Mahn, V. A., & Spross, J. A. (1996). Nurse case management as an advanced practice role. In A. B. Hamric, J. A. Spross, & C. M. Hanson (Eds.), *Advanced nursing practice* (pp. 445-464). Philadelphia: W. B. Saunders.

McCloskey, J. C., & Grace, H. K. (1994). Change creates opportunities. In J. C. McCloskey & H. K. Grace (Eds.), *Current issues in nursing* (p. 209). St. Louis, MO: Mosby-Year Book.

Newacheck, P. W., & Taylor, W. R. (1992). Childhood chronic illness: Prevalence, severity, and impact. *American Journal of Public Health, 82,* 364-371.

Newman, B. (1995). Enhancing patient care: Case management and critical pathways. *Australian Journal of Advanced Nursing, 13,* 16-24.

North American Nursing Diagnosis Association. (1999). *Nursing diagnoses: Definitions and classification 1999-2000.* Philadelphia: Author.

Opuni, K. A., Smith, P. B., Arvey, H., & Solomon, C. (1994). The northeast adolescent project: A collaborative effort to address teen-age pregnancy in Houston, Texas. *Journal of School Health, 64*(5), 212-214.

Pierce, P. M., & Freedman, S. A. (1983). The REACH project: An innovative health delivery model for medically dependent children. *Children's Health Care, 12,* 86-89.

Pyke, J., & Apa, J. (1994). Evaluating a case management service: A family perspective. *Journal of Case Management, 3,* 21-26.

Rubin, A. (1992). Is case management effective for people with serious mental illness? A research review. *Health & Social Work, 17*(2), 138-150.

Smith, K., Layne, M., & Garell, D. (1994). The impact of care coordination on children with special health care needs. *Children's Health Care, 23*(4), 251-266.

Stein, R. E. K., & Jessop, D. J. (1984). Does pediatric home care make a difference for children with chronic illness? Findings from the pediatric ambulatory care treatment study. *Pediatrics, 73*(6), 845-853.

U.S. Department of Health and Human Services. (1991). *Healthy people 2000: National health promotion and disease prevention objectives* (DHHS Publication No. PHS 91-50312). Washington, DC: Government Printing Office.

Weiner, D. E., & Cohen, M. I. (1997). Challenges of delivering healthcare to adolescents. In R. A. Hoekelman, S. B. Friedman, N. M. Nelson, H. M. Seidel, &

prepare children and their families for these experiences by virtue of their education and access to children in a variety of settings.

The overall purpose of preparing children and families for health care experiences is to provide them with knowledge and skills that will enable them to successfully negotiate a stressful experience. Psychological preparation has been defined as a planned strategy used with a child or his or her family to reduce anxiety related to medical procedures, decrease pain, accelerate the healing process, and assist the child in coping with a procedure (Saile, Burgmeier, & Schmidt, 1988). Yap (1988) describes four purposes of preparation for both parents and children: (a) transmit information to decrease stress by increasing cognitive control and decreasing uncertainty; (b) encourage emotional expression so that feelings can be recognized and validated and to provide social support that will buffer stress; (c) develop trust; and (d) teach coping strategies, such as relaxation, self-talk, and imagery.

Nurses have developed a variety of interventions that are used in everyday practice to reduce anxiety and distress of children before and during health care experiences. Most interventions are classified into two categories: (a) those that involve preparation of the child for unexpected events that will occur during hospitalization, surgery, and procedures and (b) those that enable distraction during these experiences and provide the child some measure of control. The purpose of this chapter is to present a model that describes the processes and outcome variables related to preparation of children for hospitalization, surgery, and procedures (Figure 17.1). This model can be used by nurses in practice, researchers studying the effectiveness of these interventions in a variety of settings, and nursing students who will be learning and implementing these interventions.

LITERATURE REVIEW

Overall, the empirical literature examining the effects of preparation of children for stressful health care experiences is not theoretically driven. More than half of the investigators presented no theoretical framework, whereas the other half used a variety of frameworks, including stress and coping, developmental, and anxiety contagion. Table 17.1 provides a listing of frameworks used by researchers to guide their studies of the effectiveness of preparation of children and families for stressful medical procedures.

The literature on preparation of children for stressful health care experiences spans four decades. This chapter focuses on the research literature during the years 1987 to 1999. This is not an exhaustive review but

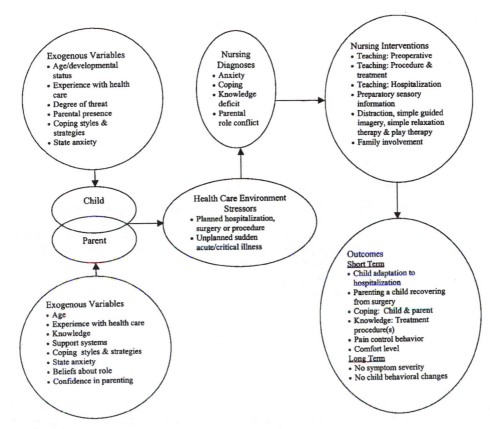

Figure 17.1. Broome and Huth Preparation Model

rather a selection of the current state of research that highlights preparatory methods used with children or parents or both for hospitalization and surgery. More than 25 studies were reviewed. The majority (94%) of studies used quantitative methods and comprised both quasi-experimental and descriptive designs. The type of intervention used organizes the discussions of these studies here.

Preparatory Sensory Information

Procedural information describes routines and events during hospitalization or surgery, whereas sensory information provides children with the sensations they will see, hear, smell, or feel (Lynch, 1994). Research suggests that these two informational approaches are more effective when they are combined (Thompson, 1986). Hospital tours provide an avenue of preparation for children and parents and are frequently given in an attempt to transmit sensory and procedural information and emotional support. In addition, play during preparation programs provides an op-

TABLE 17.1 Theoretical Frameworks in Reviewed Literature

Theory	Theory Intention	Selected Examples
Stress and coping	If child appraises a health care encounter as stressful, he or she will use coping strategies (actual skills or behaviors used to react to perceived stressor that can be added, deleted, or changed) to reduce anxiety and distress (Lazarus & Folkman, 1984; Ryan-Wenger, 1996).	Young children use behavioral strategies and behavioral distraction. School-age children and adolescents use distraction and cognitive distraction (Ryan-Wenger, 1996).
Development (cognitive)	Piaget's (1969) theory describes how the child interacts with the environment to develop cognitive abilities and negotiate and adapt to new experiences.	For children younger than 8 years of age, there is increased distress during procedures, increased anxiety, and increased posthospital upset (Broome et al., 1992; Saile et al., 1988).
Emotional contagion	Emotionally upset parents can transmit anxiety to their children through verbal and nonverbal behavior (Bates & Broome, 1986; Melnyk, 1995).	There is a significantly proactive relationship between child and parent anxiety (Ellerton & Merriam, 1994), or no relationship at all (Campbell et al., 1995).

portunity for the child to safely rehearse alternative ways of responding to stressful situations and to express fears and anxieties with a supportive health care professional (Bates & Broome, 1986).

In the research reviewed, preparation programs included sensory and procedural information provided via written materials, audiovisuals, or a combination of techniques. Combinations of techniques generally included reading a book, a hospital tour, directed or undirected play, a slide or videotape presentation, computer instruction, demonstration of equipment, and a question-and-answer period. Children ranged in age from 2 to 18 years. The majority of studies evaluated preparation programs for the child alone (Nelson & Allen, 1999; Schmidt, 1990), the child and parent (Kotzer, Coy, & LeClaire, 1998; Mansson, Fredrikzon, & Rosberg, 1992), or those offered at different times of the day (Kennedy & Riddle, 1989). These studies showed no significant differences between the groups on a variety of dependent measures, such as anxiety, knowledge, fear, behavioral distress, posthospital upset, pain-related behaviors, self-report of pain, use of hospital equipment, and physiologic measures of stress. Other investigators, however, reported significant differences between children and parents on some physiologic measures of stress, self-reports of anxiety, and emotional distress in those attending their preparation programs and those that did not (Edwinson, Arnbjornsson, & Ekman, 1988; Lynch, 1994).

Several of the studies in the procedural literature also provided information, although the methods used to transmit the information varied. Mediums to transmit the information included videotapes with a basic versus an advanced level of instruction (Rasnake & Linscheid, 1989), puppet therapy for children experiencing a fingerstick during health examinations (Broome & Endsley, 1987), a computerized hospitalization preparation program (Nelson & Allen, 1999), and discussion groups concerning the upcoming procedure (Fegley, 1988). In general, preparation did decrease medical fears or distress and increase cooperation during procedures, although younger children responded with greater levels of distress in the majority of the treatment conditions.

Cognitive-Behavioral Therapies

Cognitive-behavioral models assert that by gaining new knowledge and skills individuals change cognition, behavior, mood, or motivation (Persons, 1989). Specific coping skills such as simple guided imagery, in conjunction with behavioral strategies such as relaxation, attempt to modify thought processes to reduce anxiety or fear. Modeling is a behavioral method of preparation for anxiety reduction in children and parents that uses peer or puppet modeling of a threatening situation through videotape or slides (Melamed & Ridley-Johnson, 1988). This vicarious situation provides the child an opportunity to encounter the situation without fear (mastery model) or to adapt to the fearful situation (coping model) with support (Bates & Broome, 1986). Coping skills are frequently used in combination with modeling and include relaxation, distracting imagery, comforting self-talk, or all three. Providing children with an age-appropriate coping skill encourages them to use cognitive techniques to master fearful or painful events (Lambert, 1999).

Many investigators explored preparing the child-parent dyad using a variety of cognitive-behavioral techniques. For example, information, coping skills, peer modeling, a tour, and play were used in different combinations as cognitive-behavioral interventions in the studies reviewed. A variety of preparation techniques were incorporated into the interventions, such as parental presence or nonpresence (Faust, Olson, & Rodriguez, 1991), peer or adult narration (Pinto & Hollandsworth, 1989), and child coping skills alone or in conjunction with parent coping skills (Robinson & Kobayashi, 1991). All the cognitive-behavioral intervention studies involved preparation of children and parents for surgery. In the cognitive-behavioral investigations, children ranged in age from 2 to 15 years.

Positive outcomes of reduced child anxiety or upset (Campbell, Kirkpatrick, Berry, & Lamberti, 1995; Ellerton & Merriam, 1994; Faust et al., 1991), increased cooperation, and improved posthospital adjustment (Campbell et al., 1995) were demonstrated in the cognitive-behavioral intervention studies. Additional outcome variables included reduced sweating and heart rate (Faust et al., 1991), increased functional health status (Campbell et al., 1995), increased recovery time, and reductions in overall medical costs (Pinto & Hollandsworth, 1989). Parental presence during the intervention reduced parental anxiety (Ellerton & Merriam, 1994) and palmar sweat (Pinto & Hollandsworth, 1989), and it increased perceived competence in caring for the child in the hospital and at home (Campbell et al., 1995).

Most of the research testing the effects of cognitive-behavioral strategies can be found in the procedure literature. In general, the strongest empirical support in the literature has been found for teaching children how to use cognitive-behavioral techniques. Techniques such as simple distraction, simple imagery, and relaxation enhance a child's sense of control and decrease his or her anxiety and stress response during a procedure (Broome, Lillis, & Smith, 1989; Broome, Rehwaldt, & Fogg, 1998; Saile et al., 1988). Use of a cognitive-behavioral intervention, such as distraction, is an effective method in reducing sensory and affective components. Even for very painful procedures, such as lumbar punctures and bone marrow aspirations, cognitive-behavioral techniques have been found to be effective for children who are experiencing these procedures repeatedly over time (Broome, Lillis, McGahee, & Bates, 1992; Broome et al., 1998; Reeb & Bush, 1997). In subpopulations of children (e.g., children with cancer), these techniques have been found to be even more effective than pharmacologic agents (oral Valium) and standard preparation using only cognitive approaches (Rape & Bush, 1994).

Several authors have found that distraction techniques are also useful for children experiencing "minor" stressful procedures, such as venipuncture and intravenous device insertions. Broome and Endsley (1987) used puppets to prepare preschoolers for an immunization and examined their behavior and pulse rates before and after the procedure. There were no significant differences between treatment and control groups, although the treatment group did evidence less distress and arousal on pre- to post measures. These authors recommended recording physiologic parameters on an ongoing basis and using behavioral measures more specific to pain distress. Vessey, Carlson, and McGill (1994) used a kaleidoscope with young children (4 to 7 years old) experiencing venipuncture and reported significantly lower behavioral distress and pain reports in those using the distraction technique. In conclusion, cognitive-behavioral strategies appear to be useful for most children experiencing stressful health care experiences.

Family Involvement

Preparation can provide highly anxious parents with ways to help their children cope with hospitalization, surgery, and procedures (Melamed & Ridley-Johnson, 1988). The premise of providing the parents with information and support is to reduce their feelings of anxiety and discomfort, thereby reducing the child's anxiety (Bates & Broome, 1986; Thompson, 1986) and increasing participation in their child's care (Melynk, 1994). A home-based, parent-directed pain management program with a day surgery sample resulted in children missing one less school day and higher parent satisfaction compared to parents who were given standard preoperative instructions (Seid & Varni, 1999). No differences were found between the groups, however, for the number of phone calls or office visits to the physicians for postoperative concerns and additional prescriptions filled for analgesic medication.

A study in which mothers received child behavioral or parental role audiotaped information reported greater knowledge, lower anxiety, greater participation, and less posthospital anxiety for these mothers compared to mothers in the control group (Melnyk, 1994). Children of mothers who received information displayed significantly less negative behavioral change than those of the control group. This study occurred in an acute care setting with mothers of toddlers and preschoolers admitted for unplanned hospitalization. The exploration of exogenous variables, such as parental coping styles and strategies and their impact on preparation interventions, will advance nursing research and clinical practice.

A variety of studies have been conducted on the effects of parental presence on children during procedures, including dental treatment, immunizations, venipuncture, lumbar punctures, and bone marrow aspirations. In general, studies have found that only younger children respond to the presence of their parent with more distress behaviors, whereas parent presence had little effect on children 5 years of age and older (Broome & Endsley, 1989a; Thompson, 1986). The effects of maternal anxiety and behavior on children during both immunizations (Broome & Endsley, 1989b) and lumbar punctures (Blount, Landolf-Fritsche, Powers, & Sturges, 1991; Naber, Halstead, Broome, & Rehwaldt, 1995) showed that higher levels of maternal anxiety, reassurance, and shaming and ignoring the child were associated with higher levels of behavioral distress.

In these studies, however, children responded to coaching or verbal and nonverbal cues by the parent, especially related to distraction activities. Interestingly, these studies on parental presence and involvement did not necessarily examine directly how preparation influenced the parent's or child's behavior. In fact, no study was found that directly examined how preparation of the parents affected how they felt, behaved, or interacted with their child during the procedure.

Health professionals and parents differ in their acceptance of parental presence during painful procedures (Bauchner, Vinci, & Waring, 1991). In one study, 66% of emergency department physicians and nurses preferred that parents be present during lacerations, but only 14% wanted parents present for lumbar punctures (Bauchner et al., 1991). Another study of 250 parents in an emergency room reported that 80% of parents said they wanted to be present when their child experienced a venipuncture (Bauchner, Vinci, & Waring, 1989). Of those who did not want to be present, half stated that they were too afraid and thought it would hurt their child. Parents wanted to be present because they thought their child wanted them in the room, they wanted to know what the physician was doing, and they wanted to help calm their child. The physician had asked less than half of the parents that chose to stay. The results of this study suggest that health professionals influence the actions of parents and impact their decision to stay with and support their child during a procedure. Health professionals need to examine their own beliefs and attitudes about parent participation.

In conclusion, previous research and literature concluded that psychological preparation for hospitalization, surgery, and procedures is beneficial for some children and their parents, whereas for others preparation may not be the most important factor in their hospital or illness experience. Considering the availability of information through mass media and the reforms that have occurred in pediatric health care during the past decade (i.e., parent rooming-in, reduced parent separation during procedures, use of child life programs, and burgeoning ambulatory services), preparatory efforts may not be needed by all children and parents. Eradication of this service, however, places the entire responsibility for preparation on parents, who may be anxious and have uncertain expectations about hospitalization and their role (Ellerton & Merriam, 1994; Pinto & Hollandsworth, 1989). Ethical and legal obligations also influence health care professionals' decision to provide information about hospitalization, surgery, and procedures. Thus, to effectively meet the needs of parents, to support them and continue to operationalize precepts of family-centered care, health professionals must continue to develop and test new models of preparation and determine their feasibility in today's health care arena.

ASSESSMENT AND OUTCOMES

When children, parents, and nurses interact during a health care experience, it is the responsibility of the nurse to identify relevant nursing diagnoses that will guide the interventions chosen to support them. The outcomes resulting from these interventions should be evaluated using data across settings (Table 17.2).

INTERVENTION

The Nursing Interventions Classification (Iowa Intervention Project, 2000) lists five interventions that support preparation of the child during stressful health care experiences: (a) Teaching: Preoperative; (b) Teaching: Procedure/Treatment; (c) Preparatory Sensory Information; (d) Cognitive-Behavioral Interventions: Distraction, Simple Guided Imagery, Simple Relaxation Therapy and Therapeutic Play; and (e) Family Involvement. Table 17.2 describes the nursing activities and outcomes for Therapeutic Play interventions.

INTERVENTION APPLICATION

Marcus Hall, a 5-year-old, is scheduled for a presurgical evaluation before his tonsillectomy and adenoidectomy (T & A). Marcus was diagnosed with sickle cell disease (SCD) as a newborn but has only been hospitalized three times since diagnosis. Marcus is an only child and lives with both his parents. Mr. Hall also has SCD and is very supportive and involved in his son's care. During Marcus's last hospitalization for vasoocclusive crisis 6 months ago, he was introduced to cognitive-behavioral strategies through the use of a relaxation-imagery audiotape (Broome, 1994) and encouraged to use it at home. During the preoperative interview, Marcus tells the nurse he is scared of needles and has never had an operation. Mr. Hall expresses concern about managing his child at home after surgery. On the basis of the assessment data, the nursing diagnoses of Anxiety, Knowledge Deficit, and Parental Role Conflict were made (North American Nursing Diagnosis Association, 1999).

Preparation for hospitalization, surgery, and procedures was initiated. In an attempt to facilitate psychological preparation of the Hall family prior to surgery, the nurse offered them an opportunity to view video-

TABLE 17.2 Nursing Interventions: Selected Activities, Methods, and Outcomes

Nursing Intervention[a]	Potential Nursing Diagnoses[b]	Nurse Activities[a]	Methods	Nursing Outcomes
Teaching: Preoperative				
Assisting a child or parent to understand and mentally prepare for surgery and the postoperative recovery period	• Anxiety • Ineffective Individual Coping • Knowledge Deficit • Parental Role Conflict	Prepare for procedure or treatment: provide information (e.g., sensory, procedural, and participatory) about event and postevent; assess prior experience; teach participatory skills	Play sessions, tours, coping skills training, and modeling through media such as videotapes and puppet shows	Child Adaptation to Hospitalization (Iowa Outcomes Project, 2000, p. 153-4) Coping: Child and Parent Pain Control (Iowa Outcomes Project, 2000, p. 326) Comfort Level (Iowa Outcomes Project, 2000, p. 173) Symptom Severity (Iowa Outcomes Project, 2000, p. 420) No Child Behavioral Changes
Teaching: Procedural/Treatment				
Preparing a child or parent to understand and mentally prepare for a prescribed procedure or treatment		Preoperative activities: provide information on postoperative routines; instruct in pain control and postoperative treatments		Knowledge: Treatment Procedure(s) (Iowa Outcomes Project, 2000, p. 293)
Preparatory Sensory Information				
Describing both the subjective and objective physical sensations associated with an upcoming stressful health care procedure or treatment	• Anxiety • Ineffective Individual Coping • Knowledge Deficit • Parental Role Conflict	Sensory interventions: concrete, developmentally based, and emotionally supportive sensory and procedural information	Play sessions, tours, coping skills training, and modeling through media such as videotapes and puppet shows	Child Adaptation to Hospitalization (Iowa Outcomes Project, 2000, pp. 153-4) Coping: Parent and Child Knowledge: Treatment Procedure(s) (Iowa Outcomes Project, 2000, p. 293) Comfort Level (Iowa Outcomes Project, 2000, p. 173) Symptom Severity (Iowa Outcomes Project, 2000, p. 420) No Child Behavioral Changes

TABLE 17.2 *Continued*

Nursing Intervention[a]	Potential Nursing Diagnoses[b]	Nurse Activities[a]	Methods	Nursing Outcomes
Cognitive-Behavioral Interventions				
Simple guided imagery and distraction used before, during, and after a procedure, hospitalization, or surgery to assist the child to cope with anxiety, fear, or pain	• Anxiety • Ineffective Individual Coping • Knowledge Deficit • Fear • Pain	Specific strategy: assess and provide individualized technique based on age, past coping, preferences, and ability to participate; instruct on use of strategy alone or combined with others and encourage practice of technique before needed Play therapy: age-appropriate, safe, and stimulating equipment; observations and misconceptions during child's play	Modeling, coping skills training, and undirected or directed play sessions; distraction, imagery, and relaxation taught by one-on-one, videotape, audiotape, or all three	Child Adaptation to Hospitalization (Iowa Outcomes Project, 2000, p. 112) Coping: child Pain control behavior Comfort Level (Iowa Outcomes Project, 1997, p. 128) No Symptom Severity (Iowa Outcomes Project, 2000, p. 420) No Child Behavioral Changes
Family Involvement Facilitating family participation in the emotional and physical care of the child	• Anxiety • Parental Role Conflict • Knowledge Deficit	Assess child's and family's ability to implement treatment plan, resources available to family, desired level of participation, and understanding of illness and plan for care; provide information and educate family about care needed and options for support services; reassessment of family's ability to perform care, burden experienced, and use of support services	Parental prehospital programs, video- or audiotaped instructions or both, policies encouraging parental stay, teaching parents to carry out simple physical care	Coping: child and parent Comfort Level (Iowa Outcomes Project, 2000, p. 173) Knowledge: Treatment Procedure(s) (Iowa Outcomes Project, 2000, p. 293) No Child Behavioral Changes

a. From the Iowa Intervention Project (2000).

b. From the North American Nursing Diagnosis Association (1999).

tapes of the short-stay experience and parental pain management. The child in the video acted as a coping model by displaying initial anxiety, overcoming the anxiety, and coping with stressful events of the hospitalization and surgical experience. The video incorporated procedural and sensory information as well as coping skills (relaxation and simple guided imagery). The Halls then viewed a pain management videotape designed to teach pain assessment and management to parents caring for their child at home after a minor surgical procedure. The nurse suggested that Marcus practice relaxation and imagery with the audiotape he had at home and bring it with him on the day of surgery.

On admission for surgery, Marcus told the nurse about his relaxation-imagery audiotape and stated, "It helps me feel better when I'm scared or have pain." His parents wanted to view the videotape again, but they preferred watching it after Marcus returned from surgery since they would feel more relaxed. Marcus asked to listen to the relaxation-imagery audiotape approximately 30 minutes after he returned to the short stay unit (SSU). While Marcus listened to the audiotape, his parents watched the pain management videotape. Marcus and his family were discharged 4 hours after his return to the SSU.

A follow-up phone call the next day indicated that Marcus was drinking fluids and eating small amounts of soft foods. Mr. Hall also reported that Marcus periodically reported a slightly sore throat (2 on a 0-5 faces scale); he was giving him pain medication every 3 or 4 hours, however, as suggested in the pain management video. Further discussion revealed that Marcus was sleeping well and playing quietly. Mr. Hall told the nurse that the pain management video helped him and Mrs. Hall feel confident about caring for Marcus at home after surgery.

The case scenario of the Hall family illustrates the use of three of the four nursing diagnoses presented in the preparation model (Figure 17.1). For example, Mr. and Mrs. Hall and Marcus identified their anxieties and knowledge deficits in relation to surgery and posthospital home care. Mr. Hall also identified his feeling of inadequacy in providing care for his son at home after ambulatory surgery. The diagnosis of Ineffective Individual Coping was not made because the family verbalized their concerns and knowledge limitations related to surgery and home care.

All six of the nursing interventions displayed in the Broome and Huth Model were represented in the case study and employed across a continuum of care. Consider the cognitive behavioral interventions of simple relaxation and guided imagery that were presented to Marcus in the preparation video and reinforced with the relaxation-imagery audiotape at home before and after surgery. The nurse was able to evaluate both short- and long-term outcomes of the interventions during a follow-up phone call the next day. Mr. Hall identified comfort and confidence in parenting his son as he recovered from surgery, knowledge regarding treatment procedures, and the ability to cope with caring for Marcus at home. The outcomes of Pain Control (Iowa Outcomes Classification, 2000, p. 326), Comfort Level (p. 173), No Symptom Severity, and no behavioral changes were reflected in Marcus taking pain medication, drinking, eating, sleeping, and playing.

IMPLICATIONS FOR RESEARCH AND PRACTICE

In some studies, preparation for stressful medical experiences has been demonstrated to be effective in reducing anxiety and behavioral stress; in others, it is clear that these effects depend on a variety of factors, such as age of the child, the type of health care experience, and parental anxiety and behavior. This indicates a need for additional research that is more rigorously controlled. Methodological concerns include small sample size, self-selected samples, confounding of treatments, sketchy descriptions of the techniques, and lack of controls for age, gender, previous hospitalization, severity of illness, or type of procedure. Outcome variables, such as fear and posthospital behavior, were measured using a variety of instruments, with little consistency in the tools among studies. In contrast to sensory and procedural programs, the majority of studies reviewed on the use of cognitive-behavioral preparation programs with children or parents or both indicate significantly supportive results. The use of multiple preparation strategies, however, has been criticized because it is difficult to interpret data that support a particular strategy (Broome, 1998; Yap, 1988).

Additional research on preparation programs that use informational or cognitive-behavioral strategies or both is needed. For example, research that explores the need for preparation of children and parents with previous hospital or surgery experience and the parents' role in preparation of their child would help explicate preparation variables in the current health care milieu. Additional research should also focus on the child with a chronic condition, compliance with preparation programs, cost benefits of preparation programs, optimal preparation times, and preparation methods for children of all ages in a variety of health care settings.

Several family information programs have successfully increased maternal knowledge and reduced state anxiety as well as increased parental support and participation in child care during hospitalization and at home. Parent information programs that are provided at a time when parents are most receptive to the information (i.e., at home after discharge), however, need further exploration. Studies are needed that explore the influence of parental variables such as coping style, age, and experience with health care on a variety of preparation interventions and their outcomes.

The presence and involvement of a parent during medical experiences is reassuring to most children. Many health professionals, however, have observed that children often seem more distressed when their parents are present and infer the child is experiencing more distress than if the parents were absent. Children often use active coping behaviors that health professionals call distress to signal parents to help them. Some things parents do during procedures are more helpful than others, and it is the responsibility of the health professional to teach parents how to be most supportive to their child. These "parenting behaviors" do not come naturally, although some parents learn useful strategies from trial and error. Parents should always be prepared for a procedure before observing it—a strategy commonly used by nurses (Brennan, 1994). A graphic, concise description from the nurse or physician will help the parent make a decision about whether to be present or not and help the parent to think about how to best time interactions with the child during the procedure.

The nurse or physician must also support the parent in keeping on track with the strategies. Sometimes, parents get tired, frightened, or anxious and need to be coached. Usually, they recover very quickly with the support of those around them. This support will allow the child to master his or her feelings of fear, assist the parent in feeling good about being a supportive parent, and decrease the overall stress on health professionals, who dislike hurting a child. It is only through teamwork between the health professionals, parent, and child that stressful health care experiences can become an experience to be mastered and not feared (Bar-Mor, 1997).

REFERENCES

Bar-Mor, G. (1997). Preparation of children for surgery and invasive procedures: Milestones on the way to success. *Journal of Pediatric Nursing, 12*(4), 252-255.

Bates, T. A., & Broome, M. (1986). Preparation of children for hospitalization and surgery: A review of the literature. *Journal of Pediatric Nursing, 1*(4), 230-239.

Bauchner, H., Vinci, R., & Waring, C. (1989). Pediatric procedures: Do parents want to stay? *Pediatrics, 84*(5), 907-909.

Bauchner, H., Vinci, R., & Waring, C. (1991). Parental presence during procedures in an emergency room: Results from 50 operations. *Pediatrics, 87*(4), 544-548.

Blount, R., Landolf-Fritsche, B., Powers, S., & Sturges, J. (1991). Differences between high and low coping children and between parent and staff behaviors during painful procedures. *Journal of Pediatric Psychology, 16*(6), 795-809.

Brennan, A. (1994). Caring for children during procedures: A review of the literature. *Pediatric Nursing, 20*(5), 451-458.

Broome, M. (1994). *To tame the hurting thing: Relaxation and imagery for children.* Birmingham: University of Alabama.

Broome, M. (1998). Research on acutely ill children: Implications for practice, research, and education. In M. Broome, K. Knafl, K. Pridham, & S. Feetham (Eds.), *Children and families in health and illness: The state of nursing science* (pp. 163-176). Thousand Oaks, CA: Sage.

Broome, M., & Endsley, R. (1987). Group preparation of children as a moderator of child response to pain. *Western Journal of Nursing Research, 9*(4), 484-502.

Broome, M., & Endsley, R. (1989a). Maternal presence, childrearing practices and child response to an injection. *Research in Nursing and Health, 12*(4), 229-235.

Broome, M., & Endsley, R. (1989b). Parent and child reactions to an immunization. *Pain, 37,* 85-92.

Broome, M., Lillis, P., McGahee, T., & Bates, T. (1992). The use of distraction and imagery with children during painful procedures. *Oncology Nursing Forum, 19*(3), 499-502.

Broome, M., Lillis, P., & Smith, M. (1989). Pain interventions with children: A meta-analysis of the research. *Nursing Research, 38*(3), 154-158.

Broome, M. E., Rehwaldt, M., & Fogg, L. (1998). Relationships between cognitive behavioral techniques, temperament, observed distress, and pain reports in children and adolescents during lumbar puncture. *Journal of Pediatric Nursing, 13,* 48-54.

Campbell, L. A., Kirkpatrick, S. E., Berry, C. C., & Lamberti, J. J. (1995). Preparing children with congenital heart disease for cardiac surgery. *Journal of Pediatric Psychology, 20*(3), 313-328.

Edwinson, M., Arnbjornsson, E., & Ekman, R. (1988). Psychologic preparation program for children undergoing acute appendectomy. *Pediatrics, 82,* 30-36.

Ellerton, M., & Merriam, C. (1994). Preparing children and families psychologically for day surgery: An evaluation. *Journal of Advanced Nursing, 19*(6), 1057-1062.

Faust, J., Olson, R., & Rodriguez, H. (1991). Same-day surgery preparation: Reduction of pediatric patient arousal and distress through participant modeling. *Journal of Consulting and Clinical Psychology, 59*(3), 475-478.

Fegley, B. (1988). Preparing children for radiologic procedures: Contingent versus noncontingent instruction. *Research in Nursing and Health, 11,* 3-9.

Iowa Intervention Project. (2000). *Nursing interventions classification (NIC)* (J. C. McCloskey & G. M. Bulechek, Eds.; 3rd ed.). St. Louis, MO: Mosby-Year Book.

Iowa Outcomes Project. (2000). *Nursing outcomes classification (NOC)* (M. Johnson, M. Maas, & S. Moorhead, Eds.; 2nd ed.). St. Louis, MO: Mosby-Year Book.

Kennedy, C. M., & Riddle, I. I. (1989). The influence of the timing of preparation on the anxiety of preschool children experiencing surgery. *MCN: American Journal of Maternal Child Nursing, 18*(2), 117-132.

Kotzer, A. M., Coy, J., & LeClaire, A. D. (1998). The effectiveness of a standardized educational program for children using patient-controlled analgesia. *Journal of the Society of Pediatric Nurses, 3*(3), 117-126.

Lambert, S. A. (1999). Distraction, imagery, and hypnosis: Techniques for management of children's pain. *Journal of Child and Family Nursing, 2,* 5-15.

Lazarus, R. S., & Folkman, S. (1984). *Stress, appraisal and coping.* New York: Springer.

Lynch, M. (1994). Preparing children for day surgery. *Children's Health Care,* 23(2), 75-85.

Mansson, M. E., Fredrikzon, B., & Rosberg, B. (1992). Comparison of preparation and narcotic sedative premedication in children undergoing surgery. *Pediatric Nursing,* 18(4), 337-342.

Melamed, B. G., & Ridley-Johnson, R. (1988). Psychological preparation of families for hospitalization. *Developmental and Behavioral Pediatrics,* 9(2), 96-102.

Melnyk, B. M. (1994). Coping with unplanned childhood hospitalization: Effects of informational interventions on mothers and children. *Nursing Research, 43,* 50-55.

Melnyk, B. M. (1995). Parental coping with childhood hospitalization: A theoretical framework to guide research and clinical interventions. *MCN: American Journal of Maternal Child Nursing,* 23(4), 123-131.

Naber, S., Halstead, L., Broome, M., & Rehwaldt, M. (1995) Communication and control: Parent, child and health professional interactions during painful procedures. *Comprehensive Issues in Pediatric Nursing,* 18(2), 79-90.

Nelson, C. C., & Allen, J. (1999). Reduction of healthy children's fears related to hospitalization and medical procedures: The effectiveness of multimedia computer instruction in pediatric psychology. *Children's Health Care, 28,* 1-13.

North American Nursing Diagnosis Association. (1999). *Nursing diagnoses: Definitions and classification 1999-2000.* Philadelphia: Author.

Persons, J. B. (1989). *Cognitive therapy in practice: A case formulation approach.* New York: Norton.

Piaget, J. (1969). *The theory of stages in cognitive development.* New York: McGraw-Hill.

Pinto, R. P., & Hollandsworth, J. G. (1989). Using videotape modeling to prepare children psychologically for surgery: Influence of parents and costs versus benefits of providing preparation services. *Health Psychology, 8,* 79-85.

Rape, R., & Bush, J. (1994). Psychological preparation for pediatric oncology patients undergoing painful procedures: A methodological critique of the research. *Children's Health Care, 23,* 51-67.

Rasnake, L., & Linschied, T. (1989). Anxiety reduction in children receiving medical care: Developmental considerations. *Developmental and Behavioral Pediatrics, 10*(4), 160-175.

Reeb, R., & Bush, J. (1997). Preprocedural psychological preparation in pediatric oncology: A process-oriented intervention study. *Children's Health Care,* 25(4), 265-280.

Robinson, P. J., & Kobayashi, K. (1991). Development and evaluation of a presurgical preparation program. *Journal of Pediatric Psychology, 16*(2), 193-212.

Ryan-Wenger, N. (1996). Children, coping and the stress of illness: A synthesis of the research. *Journal of the Society of Pediatric Nurses, 1*(3), 126-138.

Saile, H., Burgmeier, R., & Schmidt, L. (1988). A meta-analysis of studies on psychological preparation of children facing medical procedures. *Psychology and Health, 2*(2), 107-132.

Schmidt, C. K. (1990). Pre-operative preparation: Effects on immediate pre-operative behavior, post-operative behavior and recovery in children having same-day surgery. MCN: *American Journal of Maternal Child Nursing, 19*(4), 321-330.

Seid, M., & Varni, J. W. (1999). Pediatric day surgery outcomes management: The role of preoperative anxiety and a home pain management protocol. *Journal of Clinical Outcomes Management, 6*(2), 24-30.

Thompson, R. H. (1986). Where we stand: Twenty years of research on pediatric hospitalization and health care. *Children's Health Care, 14*(3), 200-210.

Vessey, J. A., Carlson, K. L., & McGill, J. (1994). Use of distraction with children during an acute pain experience. *Nursing Research, 43*(6), 369-372.

Yap, J. N. (1988). A critical review of pediatric preoperative preparation procedures: Processes, outcomes, and future directions. *Journal of Applied Developmental Psychology, 9*(4), 359-389.

18

Therapeutic Play

Mary E. Tiedeman

Kathleen A. Simon

Stephanie Clatworthy

Play is an essential component of childhood. It promotes physical, cognitive, emotional, and social development and helps children learn to cope in their reality (Abbott, 1990; DelPo & Frick, 1988; Doverty, 1992; Russ, 1998). When deprived of mechanisms for play, children are deprived of an opportunity for healthy growth and development (LeVieux-Anglin & Sawyer, 1993) and the ability to communicate and cope effectively to promote adaptation.

Play promotes the emotional well-being of children (Vessey & Mahon, 1990; Ziegler & Prior, 1994), which is consistent with the goals of *Healthy People 2000* (U.S. Department of Health and Human Services, 1991). *Healthy People 2000* identifies environmental conditions and stresses as factors influencing mental health. The document suggests that psychosocial interventions can improve psychological well-being during stressful life conditions by helping decrease stressors or helping increase the capacity of the individual to cope or both. Therapeutic play has the ability to meet this need in children and is an appropriate intervention when they are experiencing stressful situations (Tiedeman, Simon, & Clatworthy, 1990).

THEORETICAL FRAMEWORK

Conceptual Framework

Children experience life events that may produce stress and require coping, for example, school entry, hospitalization, and illness. Behavioral and emotional responses of children to these events are a concern of professionals interested in promoting the mental health and optimal development of children.

Whether or not a given event is stressful depends on the perceptions of each individual child. Through a process of cognitive appraisal, the event is evaluated in relation to its significance for well-being, the demands of the situation, and available coping resources and options. An event is stressful when perceived to be significant for well-being with demands taxing or exceeding resources. These perceptions may result in a child experiencing anxiety or fear or both (Lazarus & Folkman, 1984), which can lead to illness or hinder return to health.

Age or developmental level and past experience influence cognitive appraisal, thus affecting children's perceptions. Perceptions are dependent on cognitive development, which does not reach maturity until adolescence or beyond. Coping behaviors are learned (Aguilera & Messick, 1986) and therefore dependent on past experience. Because of cognitive immaturity and limited experience with stressful events, children are more likely than adults to perceive situations or events as exceeding their resources (Lazarus & Folkman, 1984). The conceptual framework is illustrated in Figure 18.1.

Therapeutic Play

Play becomes therapeutic when it is goal directed and guided for the purpose of enhancing physical and psychological well-being. Therapeutic play uses play as a language for children to communicate thoughts and feelings. By exploring their perceptions and facilitating the intake of new information, therapeutic play assists children to become knowledgeable about their reality. Therapeutic play gives children the opportunity to try new coping strategies in the play arena with the support and play language provided by an adult. Therapeutic play is an appropriate and effec-

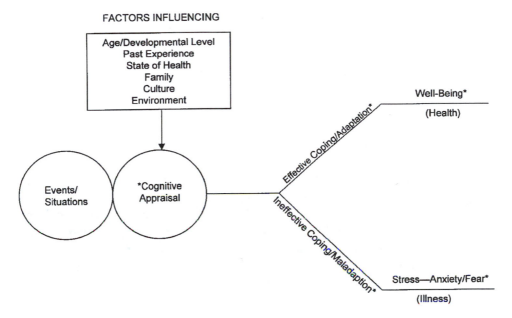

Figure 18.1. Relationship of Variables in Conceptual Framework.
*Therapeutic Play Influences Outcome to Alleviate Stress and Promote Well-Being

tive intervention for assisting children in various life situations to mobilize their resources and to reappraise the situation in a manner that alters the balance between demands and resources in a positive direction (LeVieux-Anglin & Sawyer, 1993; Russ, 1998; Tiedeman et al., 1990; Vessey & Mahon, 1990; Ziegler & Prior, 1994).

Types of Therapeutic Play

Vessey and Mahon (1990) identified these three types of therapeutic play: (a) emotional outlet, (b) instructional, and (c) physiologically enhancing. Each type of therapeutic play has a different purpose or goal. Emotional outlet play may be used both diagnostically and prescriptively, and it is designed to help children gain mastery over potentially emotionally damaging experiences. Instructional play is designed to provide children with information about life situations. Increased knowledge may help children cope more effectively and has the potential to decrease anxiety and fear (Ellerton, Caty, & Ritchie, 1985). Play, that enhances the physiological state, is designed to maintain or improve physical health. Through the use of play, children may more readily accept interventions directed toward their physiological well-being.

Therapeutic Play Modalities

There are two schools of thought regarding therapeutic play that reflect a splitting of therapeutic play modalities: nondirective and directive. Nondirective therapeutic play is child directed. The child is provided with a variety of toys and has responsibility for selecting the materials and content of play and for initiating and controlling the pace of play. The adult is a participant observer who understands the language of play and is educated in the use of play as a therapeutic modality. The adult is sensitive to and accepting of feelings expressed through play and verbalizations and reflects the feelings back to children to assist them in understanding the feelings. Although play is child directed, an adult may structure the environment and materials to provide opportunity for a particular play activity that may encourage the child to act out a stressful situation. The nondirective approach requires regular play sessions and children who are actively interacting with their environment (Axline, 1969; Chambers, 1993; DelPo & Frick, 1988; Rasmussen & Cunningham, 1995; Tiedeman et al., 1990).

Directive therapeutic play is adult directed. The adult has responsibility for the materials, content, and theme of play, and the adult guides and interprets the play (Chambers, 1993; DelPo & Frick, 1988; Rasmussen & Cunningham, 1995). The directive approach is appropriate when children are withdrawn or overwhelmed by their environment or when there is limited time to prepare them for the event. In the directive approach, the adult "reaches in" and "grabs hold" of children to pull them forward (Tiedeman et al., 1990).

Therapeutic Play Categories

Whether directive or nondirective, therapeutic play encompasses the following basic categories: (a) role or fantasy play, (b) expressive play, and (c) aggressive play (Tiedeman et al., 1990). In role play, children can take on various roles and play out feelings and concerns in fantasy, providing an escape from reality, distance from self (which allows feelings and concerns to be put away from self [distanced] and expressed in other ways, e.g., role play and fantasy; this provides safety for expressing feelings and concerns because they need not be directly "owned" by the individual expressing them), and safety for expressing feelings. Role or fantasy play supports acting out of life stresses and enhances the ability to learn new forms of behavior (Tiedeman et al., 1990; Ziegler & Prior, 1994).

Expressive play allows for expression of feelings and concerns without words. Aggressive play provides children opportunity for release and communication of emotions such as anger and frustration in a safe and acceptable manner, and it provides opportunity for regrouping of inner resources to foster coping and learning (Tiedeman et al., 1990).

In summary, therapeutic play offers a nonverbal, alternative means of expressing and dealing with emotions. Use of therapeutic play allows health care professionals to gain insight into feelings, perceptions, and needs of children. Furthermore, children can use the language of play to assist them in learning new behavior and coping. Thus, therapeutic play can facilitate the growth, development, and well-being of children in stressful situations.

NURSING DIAGNOSIS AND OUTCOME DETERMINATION

Assessment and Nursing Diagnosis

Assessing children's thoughts and perceptions is difficult because they cannot always verbalize what they are feeling. Children do not have the cognitive and language skills to say they are experiencing anger, anxiety, or fear, and they are more likely to express feelings in actions or behaviors. Behaviors indicative of fear and anxiety include agitation, avoidance of caregivers, active resistance to treatments or procedures, and regressive behaviors such as bed-wetting. Emotional distress (e.g., crying) is another indicator of fear and anxiety (Ziegler & Prior, 1994). In addition to observation of behavior, a variety of approaches, such as play, art, storytelling or bibliotherapy, and puppets, may be used to gain insight into children's perceptions and feelings. These approaches depend less on verbal abilities and allow for expression of feelings indirectly in fantasy, thereby providing some distance and making it easier to express feelings (Clatworthy, Simon, & Tiedeman, 1999a, 1999b; Tiedeman et al., 1990).

The various assessment strategies provide the nurse with data to support nursing diagnoses. Defining characteristics of each diagnosis assist in categorization of data; defining characteristics serve only as guidelines, however. Defining characteristics, as defined by the North American Nursing Diagnosis Association (NANDA, 1999), focus on verbal, behavioral, and physiological signs and symptoms and may be incomplete or at times inappropriate for children. For example, children may express anxiety by the characteristics of their drawings, but they may not verbalize apprehension, fear, or concern directly.

Two appropriate nursing diagnoses are Fear and Anxiety. Fear produces a feeling of dread and is the appropriate nursing diagnosis when the source of perceived threat or danger to self can be identified. Anxiety is the appropriate diagnosis when the source of the threat is unknown and the children become overexcited or shaky and seem worried. Another diagnosis is Ineffective Individual Coping, which occurs when adaptive behaviors and problem-solving abilities of an individual are not sufficient to meet the demands of a situation (NANDA, 1999). Ineffective coping may lead to emotions such as anxiety, fear, and anger (Lazarus & Folkman, 1984). It is also possible to use therapeutic play in dealing with other nursing diagnoses, such as Body Image Disturbance, Self-Esteem Disturbance, Powerlessness, Knowledge Deficit, Altered Family Processes, and Impaired Social Interaction (NANDA, 1999).

Nurse-Sensitive Outcomes

Assessment data provide the basis for child-specific outcome criteria. Outcome criteria are determined by identifying desired changes in defining characteristics that supported the initial nursing diagnosis. Outcomes provide indicators of the individual's ability to control anxiety or fear or both, indicating effects of the intervention. Indicators for the Nursing Outcomes Classification (NOC) outcomes of Anxiety Control and Fear Control demonstrate considerable overlap. Examples of indicators for Anxiety Control include maintaining role performance (such as role in school) and social relationships. Examples of Fear Control include planning coping strategies for fearful or stressful situations (Iowa Outcomes Project, 2000). With children, these indicators may be evaluated in a variety of ways, including using previously identified assessment techniques. For example, children may reveal planned coping strategies through their stories or role play. Other indicators may be evaluated more directly, such as maintenance of role performance, which may be determined by children's performance of activities of daily living.

INTERVENTION: THERAPEUTIC PLAY

Therapeutic play is a goal-directed activity between child and nurse that uses the language of play to assist children to communicate their perceptions of the world and to help them master the environment (Tiedeman et al., 1990).

Before preparing for therapeutic play, one needs to consider the knowledge and skills of the person using therapeutic play. The nurse with expertise in child development, communication with children, and use of play as a therapeutic modality will be best prepared to use this intervention (DelPo & Frick, 1988). In addition, knowledge of the psychotherapeutic process is important for using emotional outlet therapeutic play to help children cope with stressful events. It is also necessary to have full knowledge of the child's situation and previous experience with stressful situations (Tiedeman et al., 1990).

In preparing for therapeutic play, play media are selected in accordance with the specific purpose of the therapeutic play and the real or perceived needs and developmental level of the children. There are some general guidelines for selecting play materials. Play media should allow for all categories of therapeutic play: role play, expressive play, and aggressive play (Axline, 1969; Moustakas, 1953; Tiedeman et al., 1990). Toys for role or fantasy play include family dolls, animal families, and puppets. Puppets should include family and animal puppets as well as soft, cuddly puppets, such as a dog or bunny, and angry and aggressive puppets, such as a lion or bear. Additional toys for role or fantasy play include baby doll and baby bottle, doll house with furniture, and items for dress-up. Animal families are useful for role play because they provide distance from self. Children who are not ready to "play out" their feelings using family dolls may be able to do so using the animal family. Baby bottles and dolls that can be cuddled, fed, and bathed allow children to play out behaviors and feelings related to their need to be taken care of by another.

With hospitalized children, play media for role play need to include materials related to the hospital, specific treatments, and diagnostic procedures (Tiedeman et al., 1990; Ziegler & Prior, 1994). Toys for hospital role play include hospital gown and pajamas, surgical attire, laboratory coats, and doctor and nurse dolls. Items of hospital equipment suitable for hospital role play include blood pressure cuffs, stethoscopes, bandages, tape, needles, and syringes. Intravenous poles, stretchers, and beds may also be useful in hospital role play. When real equipment is not available or use of it is not feasible, make-believe or miniature equipment will serve the purpose. When needles and syringes are used, individual supervision of the activity is essential.

Expressive play, such as art, requires little physical energy, which makes it useful with children whose energy and activity may be limited. Items for expressive play include crayons, paints, finger paints, paper, paste, and scissors. Items used for expressive play are familiar to children, so they may be more willing to engage in play with these materials.

Punching bags, balls, targets, cars and trucks, Play-Dough, clay, beanbags, paddle balls, and blocks are appropriate items for aggressive play. Play media that facilitate aggressive play allow children to push, throw, and punch without harm to self, others, or the environment.

When selecting toys for the individual child, several factors need to be considered. Toys should be appropriate for the age and developmental level of the child. Whereas toys appropriate for children of a younger age may be more effective with the child experiencing stress-related regression, use of toys appropriate for children of an older age and developmental level might frustrate the child and hinder the therapeutic process. Furthermore, toys selected need to be safe, and children must be able to use them in the given environment.

Establishment of a warm, caring relationship with a feeling of permissiveness that gives children a chance to express their feelings is necessary for implementation of therapeutic play. To establish such a relationship, the nurse must be accepting, avoid expressing approval and disapproval, and listen to the feelings expressed. It is important to remember that words and actions may be defending mechanisms; the feelings behind the words and actions are expressed in a variety of ways and are most likely the true message being communicated. The repetitive nature of an action, words, or play should be noted to aid in identification of feelings. As in all communication, validation, reflection, and mutual exploration are essential. This process allows for a diagnostic conclusion and appropriate nursing intervention (Axline, 1969; Moustakas, 1953; Tiedeman et al., 1990).

To engage in therapeutic play with children, a contract that sets limits with each child is essential. This contract should include what is expected of the child and the time that will be spent in play. Guidelines or limits foster a feeling of trust and security for children, facilitating an environment conducive to expression of feelings. It is best to establish only those limitations that are necessary to anchor play sessions to the world of reality and avoid confusion, guilt, and insecurity (Axline, 1969; Moustakas, 1953; Tiedeman et al., 1990). Basic expectations include no hurting of self or others, no damage to toys, and toys remain with the nurse. In addition, the contract needs to be comfortable to the child and nurse and must be open to renegotiation.

It is essential that the nurse validates with children that it is okay to talk about feelings, that all children have them. It should be clear to children that it is safe to share feelings with the nurse and that what is shared in therapeutic play will be private (Axline, 1969; Moustakas, 1953). Should feelings, needs, or concerns be revealed that need to be shared with parents or other professionals, the nurse is advised to share this need with the child and incorporate the child into collaboration with parents or other professionals. This will maintain the trusting relationship and mutual respect.

Therapeutic play also requires a special relationship with the toys to promote optimal effectiveness of therapeutic play. Therefore, the toys should not be left with the child between play sessions. In addition, when play occurs unsupervised, misconceptions may not be identified and may remain (Tiedeman et al., 1990). An example is a school-age boy admitted for a tonsillectomy who was asked to draw a picture of what was wrong with him. He drew a red "X" on each hand and when asked about the picture said "my mama said if I played with it, it would be cut off." Activities to correct perceptions were needed and given.

Stages of Therapeutic Play

Implementation of the process of therapeutic play involves three basic stages: assessment, intervention, and termination. The assessment stage is an integral part of the therapeutic process and is distinct from the initial assessment that led to the decision to implement therapeutic play. During the assessment stage, the nurse and child are assessing one another. Children will explore the environment, toys, and nature of the contract; for example, they may ask "Can I really play with the toys any way I want?" It is during the assessment stage that children may test the limits that have been set—for example, by verbally threatening to harm self or the nurse. During this stage, children may give brief glimpses of their feelings, which then need to be reflected and verified.

When using a nondirective approach during the assessment stage, children are provided with all the play equipment. Most children rapidly explore all the toys, and the majority begin to interact in a given area of play. This approach allows children to express all their concerns. When using a directive approach, the nurse selects the play materials to foster the expression of feelings related to a given situation. For example, the nurse may select art or puppet play.

During the intervention stage, therapeutic play continues to focus on perceptions and feelings. The most painful feelings are demonstrated by a series of repeated play activities that begin to create a pattern and help identify and resolve feelings. Either a nondirective or a directive approach may be used during the intervention stage.

The following example illustrates play activities and interactions during the intervention stage using a nondirective approach. A 9-year-old boy with osteomyelitis was hospitalized for intravenous antibiotic therapy. At admission, he was talkative, cheerful, and cooperative. The following day, however, it was reported that he had broken his roommate's thumb and seriously bitten the intern who had been attempting to restart his intravenous (IV) infusion. A decision was made to use therapeutic play in an attempt to avoid taking the child to the operating room to restart his IV under general anesthetic. The nurse play therapist presented the child with a variety of toys, from which he chose a giant teddy bear. During the play session, he proceeded to pound violently on the teddy bear saying "I hate you, I hate you. Why did you die?" When asked who died, he said, "my dad." Additional exploration revealed that the child felt he was being punished by God for not successfully carrying out his responsibility as "the man of the family" now that his father was dead. He was angry because he had been trying very hard to fulfill his perceived responsibility. Following this interaction, the child was able to talk with the nurse about having his IV restarted. The child was given control of the procedure with guidelines set by the nurse, and he chose to use bean bags, which he could throw during the procedure. Nondirective therapeutic play allowed the IV to be restarted without the aid of a general anesthetic.

A directive approach may be useful to help focus expression of feelings and perceptions, provide information, and clarify misconceptions in a more timely manner. The following example illustrates the use of the directive approach. An 8-year-old boy was injured in an accident while riding his bicycle on a forbidden road. He sustained bilateral fractured femurs, a fracture of the right humerus, and a subdural hematoma. After regaining consciousness, the child was nonverbal, although his eyes followed the movements of people in his environment. The plan was to institutionalize him because of presumed severe brain damage. After several unsuccessful attempts at nondirective therapeutic play, a directive approach using bibliotherapy was tried. The nurse play therapist told the child a story about a bird who broke his wing when he flew away against his mother's instructions. The bird was so afraid that he would be punished by his mother that he never peeped again. The nurse play therapist then asked the child, "Did that ever happen to you?" The child began to cry and on further inquiry answered "yes" and told the nurse play therapist his story. The child continued to recover from his injuries and was discharged to home with no evidence of permanent brain damage.

The closure or end of the play session(s) follows the process of resolution or termination, the final stage of any therapeutic relationship. As children communicate feelings within the therapeutic relationship, they are able to deal with and resolve those feelings. This resolution may be indicated by a willingness to discontinue play session(s). One child finally drew a picture of her whole family, presented it to the therapist, and announced "Thanks, I don't need you any more" and promptly left the room.

During the final stage, children may return to behaviors similar to those exhibited during the beginning of the therapeutic play process. During this stage, children will explore many things but nothing in-depth. It is a way of bringing closure to the feelings and self that were exposed. At this time, the nurse must reaffirm what has been said and provide support for the child.

The initial contract between child and nurse indicates the duration and number of play sessions. Knowing play sessions will end at a specified time helps children move toward resolution and termination because they know they have a limited amount of time to deal with their feelings. At the end of the contracted time, the nurse and child may renegotiate for more play sessions if conflicts have not been resolved or if new needs have been identified.

Therapeutic Play With Hospitalized Children

Some adaptation of therapeutic methods may be needed in hospital settings. Play sessions may need to be conducted in a variety of settings, such as the child's room, the playroom, a conference room, the cafeteria, or wherever some space and privacy are available. Thus, equipment should be portable. Privacy is an important consideration that takes on additional significance in the hospital, in which children may perceive that no one can be trusted and that no place is safe. In such a situation, it is imperative that therapeutic play time be protected and that no treatment, doctors, or other distressing interruptions are allowed.

Therapeutic play must be adapted based on the realities of children's physical health, including discomfort or activity restrictions. In addition, the establishment of a therapeutic relationship within the hospital may require a greater degree of structure and more limits to provide children with needed security.

COMPARISON WITH NURSING INTERVENTIONS CLASSIFICATION

There is remarkable similarity between the definitions of therapeutic play and Play Therapy provided by Nursing Interventions Classification (NIC) and our definition. NIC defines *Therapeutic Play* as the "purposeful and directive use of toys or other materials to assist children in communicating their perception and knowledge of their world and to help in gaining mastery of their environment" (Iowa Intervention Project, 2000, p. 664). We define *therapeutic play* as a goal-directed activity between the child and nurse that uses the language of play to assist children communicate their perceptions of the world and to help in mastering the environment. There is one important difference in the definitions. NIC defines therapeutic play as directive, whereas our definition encompasses both directive and nondirective modalities.

An additional comparison of the intervention therapeutic play as described by NIC and us reveals differences in how the intervention is classified and the diagnoses for which it is considered an appropriate intervention. According to NIC, Therapeutic Play is classified in the Behavioral domain under the classes of Communication Enhancement and Behavioral Therapy. The primary diagnoses for which NIC considers therapeutic play an appropriate intervention are Diversional Activity Deficit and Activity Intolerance. Some additional diagnoses identified by NIC include Knowledge Deficit, Ineffective Denial, Pain, and Impaired Environmental Interpretation Syndrome (Iowa Intervention Project, 2000). We classify therapeutic play within the Behavioral domain under the classes of Communication Enhancement, Coping Assistance, Psychological Comfort Promotion, and Patient Education. The primary nursing diagnoses for which we consider Therapeutic Play an appropriate intervention are Anxiety, Fear, and Ineffective Individual Coping. Additional diagnoses identified by us include Body Image Disturbance, Self-Esteem Disturbance, Powerlessness, Knowledge Deficit, Altered Family Processes, and Impaired Social Interaction (NANDA, 1999).

INTERVENTION APPLICATION

Michael, a 10-year-old boy with Crohn's disease, was the youngest of four children in a female-dominated household. He lived with his mother, three adolescent sisters, and a father who was a poor male role model. Michael experienced repeated, lengthy hospitalizations for treatment of his disease, with total parenteral nutrition and surgeries to remove portions of his bowel. Michael was quiet, withdrawn, and would not talk, although at times he displayed outbursts of anger. Michael also experienced nightmares and nighttime enuresis. In addition, Michael was doing failing work in school and had no friends.

Nursing diagnoses for Michael included Ineffective Coping, Anxiety, and Fear as well as Powerlessness and Self-Esteem Disturbance related to lack of a positive male role model. A combination of a nondirective and directive approach was selected to encourage Michael to talk about his feelings. The intervention Therapeutic Play was initiated. In his initial play sessions, Michael engaged in aggressive play, expressing anger through the use of Play-Dough and darts. Michael's play was precise, intense, and forceful.

As the play sessions continued, Michael engaged in "hospital" play, acting out surgeries in which every patient died. When asked why everyone died, he stated, "That's just the way it is." Directive hospital role play was used by the nurse play therapist to further explore Michael's anxieties and fears related to hospitalization and surgery and also to assist him in learning new coping behaviors. In subsequent play sessions, Michael continued to engage in hospital play, but he acted out surgeries in which all patients got well.

As Michael dealt with his feelings related to his hospitalization and illness, the focus of his play sessions switched to family life and school issues. Through his therapeutic play sessions, Michael revealed problems that resulted in the recommendation for family therapy. As family therapy helped to resolve some of the issues, Michael's condition improved. Michael's nightmares and nighttime enuresis stopped, he was doing well in school, and he was active in 4-H. In addition, the symptoms of Crohn's disease disappeared. Outcome indicators for Anxiety Control and Fear Control supported the effectiveness of Therapeutic Play.

RESEARCH AND PRACTICE IMPLICATIONS

Research Support and Needed Validation

Clinical research testing therapeutic play has been limited. Several researchers have found therapeutic play to be useful in reducing anxiety and fear in hospitalized children (Clatworthy, 1981; Rae, Worchel, Upchurch, Sanner, & Daniel, 1989). The results of a study by Fosson, Martin, and Haley (1990) suggested that therapeutic play was beneficial in dealing with anxiety in hospitalized children, although the results were not statistically significant. In addition, Saucier (1989) found therapeutic play to have a positive effect on personal and social development of abused children, whereas Kot, Landreth, and Giordano (1998) found beneficial effects from therapeutic play with children who had witnessed domestic violence. Other studies provided evidence of the value of therapeutic play in preparing children for surgery and procedures (Ellerton et al., 1985; Ellerton & Merriam, 1994; Zahr, 1998), including preparation of sibling bone marrow donors (Shama, 1998).

Additional research can expand our knowledge of therapeutic play as a nursing intervention for children and adolescents experiencing stressful life situations. Research is needed to more rapidly identify children most in need of therapeutic play and to determine which approaches to therapeutic play are most effective with specific groups of children. Although research has demonstrated the usefulness of therapeutic play in reducing fear and anxiety, more research is needed to determine the impact of this reduction on outcomes such as length of hospital stay and follow-up health care. Research is also needed to support or refute the cost-effectiveness of therapeutic play.

Clinical Use of Therapeutic Play

Therapeutic play can be conducted in any setting in which there is a commitment to this intervention and in which time, space, toys, and personnel are made available. A large space is not needed, and toys for conducting therapeutic play can be portable and transported from site to site. Appropriate settings for therapeutic play include inpatient units, intensive care units, outpatient clinics, physicians' offices, outpatient surgery, schools, and children's homes. Therapeutic play can be incorporated into routine care and does not require additional time.

Therapeutic Play and the Changing Health Care Environment

Changes have occurred and continue to occur in the health care environment. Changes have involved policies, admission trends, and types of illnesses (Bolig, 1990). For example, hospital stays are shorter, children in inpatient settings have higher acuity illness, and more care is being provided in ambulatory or outpatient settings and the home (Bolig, 1990; Wilson, 1988). Technological developments and increased knowledge about treating many conditions have led to long-term survival of children who previously would have succumbed to their illness. Many of these children are medically or technologically dependent or both (Wilson, 1988) and must deal with the stressors of this dependency along with their normal growth and developmental needs. In addition, there is increasing emphasis on cost containment, which mandates that we demonstrate not only the efficacy of an intervention but also its efficiency and cost-effectiveness.

These changes have implications for the use of therapeutic play as a nursing intervention. Shorter length of hospital stays and increased delivery of care in an ambulatory or outpatient setting mean limited time for nursing interventions, including psychosocial interventions such as therapeutic play. With limited time for intervention, directive therapeutic play may be the more appropriate and effective approach (Tiedeman et al., 1990). Increased illness acuity levels of children in hospitals and increased numbers of medically and technology-dependent children may mean a change in approach to therapeutic play. These children may have decreased energy and physical abilities for engaging in therapeutic play, thus necessitating modifications in which the nurse or play therapist plays for the child (Wilson, 1988).

The various settings may pose a challenge to the implementation of therapeutic play as a nursing intervention. Modifications in both environment and approach to therapeutic play may be needed. The need for therapeutic play remains the same, but new methods of delivery need to be developed. Despite the challenges of providing therapeutic play within the changing health care environment, it is important that we meet these challenges and not only continue therapeutic play but also expand it by providing this important nursing intervention to all children experiencing stressful situations.

REFERENCES

Abbott, K. (1990). Therapeutic use of play in the psychological preparation of pre-school children undergoing cardiac surgery. *Issues in Comprehensive Pediatric Nursing, 13*(4), 265-277.

Aguilera, D. C., & Messick, J. M. (1986). *Crisis intervention: Theory and methodology* (5th ed.). St. Louis, MO: C. V. Mosby.

Axline, V. M. (1969). *Play therapy.* New York: Ballantine.

Bolig, R. (1990). Play in health care settings: A challenge for the 1990s. *Children's Health Care: Journal of the Association for the Care of Children's Health, 19*(4), 229-233.

Chambers, M. A. (1993). Play as therapy for the hospitalized child. *Journal of Clinical Nursing, 2*(6), 349-354.

Clatworthy, S. (1981). Therapeutic play: Effects on hospitalized children. *Children's Health Care: Journal of the Association for the Care of Children's Health, 9*(4), 108-113.

Clatworthy, S., Simon, K., & Tiedeman, M. (1999a). Child drawing: Hospital— An instrument designed to measure the emotional status of hospitalized school-aged children. *Journal of Pediatric Nursing, 14,* 2-9.

Clatworthy, S., Simon, K., & Tiedeman, M. E. (1999b). Child drawing: Hospital manual. *Journal of Pediatric Nursing, 14,* 10-18.

DelPo, E. Z., & Frick, S. B. (1988). Directed and nondirected play as therapeutic modalities. *Children's Health Care: Journal of the Association for the Care of Children's Health, 16*(4), 261-267.

Doverty, N. (1992). Therapeutic use of play in hospital. *British Journal of Nursing, 1*(2), 77-81.

Ellerton, M. L., Caty, S., & Ritchie, J. A. (1985). Helping young children master intrusive procedures through play. *Children's Health Care: Journal of the Association for the Care of Children's Health, 13*(4), 167-173.

Ellerton, M. L., & Merriam, C. (1994). Preparing children and families psychologically for day surgery: An evaluation. *Journal of Advanced Nursing, 19*(6), 1057-1062.

Fosson, A., Martin, J., & Haley, J. (1990). Anxiety among hospitalized latency-age children. *Developmental and Behavioral Pediatrics, 11*(6), 324-327.

Iowa Intervention Project. (2000). *Nursing interventions classification (NIC)* (J. McCloskey & G. Bulechek, Eds.; 3rd ed.). St. Louis, MO: Mosby-Year Book.

Iowa Outcomes Project. (2000). *Nursing outcomes classification (NOC)* (M. Johnson, M. Maas, S. Moorhead, Eds.; 2nd ed.). St. Louis, MO: Mosby-Year Book.

Kot, S., Landreth, G. L., & Giordano, M. (1998). Intensive child-centered play therapy with child witnesses of domestic violence. *International Journal of Play Therapy, 7*(2), 17-36.

Lazarus, R. S., & Folkman, S. (1984). *Stress, appraisal, and coping.* New York: Springer.

LeVieux-Anglin, L., & Sawyer, E. H. (1993). Incorporating play interventions into nursing care. *Pediatric Nursing, 19*(5), 459-463.

Moustakas, C. E. (1953). *Children in play therapy.* New York: McGraw-Hill.

North American Nursing Diagnosis Association. (1999). *Nursing diagnosis: Definitions and classification 1999-2000.* Philadelphia: Author.

Rae, W. A., Worchel, F. F., Upchurch, J., Sanner, J. H., & Daniel, C. A. (1989). The psychosocial impact of play on hospitalized children. *Journal of Pediatric Psychology, 14*(4), 617-627.

Rasmussen, L. A., & Cunningham, C. (1995). Focused play therapy and non-directive play therapy: Can they be integrated? *Journal of Child Sexual Abuse, 4,* 1-20.

Russ, S. W. (1998). Play, creativity, and adaptive functioning: Implications for play interventions. *Journal of Clinical Child Psychology, 27*(4), 469-480.

Saucier, B. (1989). The effects of play therapy on developmental achievement levels of abused children. *Pediatric Nursing, 15,* 27-30.

Shama, W. I. (1998). The experience and preparation of pediatric sibling bone marrow donors. *Social Work in Health Care, 27,* 89-99.

Tiedeman, M. E., Simon, K. A., & Clatworthy, S. (1990). Communication through therapeutic play. In M. J. Craft & J. A. Denehy (Eds.), *Nursing interventions for infants and children* (pp. 93-110). Philadelphia: W. B. Saunders.

U.S. Department of Health and Human Services. (1991). *Healthy people 2000: National health promotion and disease prevention objectives* (DHHS Publication No. PHS 91-50213). Washington, DC: Government Printing Office.

Vessey, J. A., & Mahon, M. M. (1990). Therapeutic play and the hospitalized child. *Journal of Pediatric Nursing, 5*(5), 328-333.

Wilson, J. M. (1988). Future of play in health care settings. *Children's Health Care: Journal of the Association for the Care of Children's Health, 16*(3), 231-237.

Zahr, L. K. (1998). Therapeutic play for hospitalized preschoolers in Lebanon. *Pediatric Nursing, 23*(5), 449-454.

Ziegler, D. B., & Prior, M. M. (1994). Preparation for surgery and adjustment to hospitalization. *Nursing Clinics of North America, 29*(4), 655-669.

19

Distraction

Charmaine Kleiber

A majority of independent nursing practice is the planning for and provision of pain management interventions. Pharmacological interventions for minimizing pain in children have been well described in documents such as the Agency for Health Care Policy and Research (AHCPR, 1992) guideline, *Acute Pain Management in Infants, Children, and Adolescents*. The guideline falls short, however, in describing nonpharmacological interventions for pain management. It suggests that nonpharmacological techniques should be individualized for each child and can be used either alone or in conjunction with medication to achieve the desired effect, but thorough descriptions of nonpharmacological strategies are absent.

Use of nonpharmacological techniques is one of the suggested activities under the Pain Management intervention in the Nursing Interventions Classification (NIC) (Iowa Intervention Project, 2000). Examples of nonpharmacological techniques are distraction, relaxation, guided imagery, music therapy, play therapy, activity therapy, acupressure, hot and cold application, biofeedback, transcutaneous electric nerve stimulation, hypnosis, and massage. Unfortunately, most of the techniques listed cannot be performed without special training beyond basic nursing preparation. Distraction is an intervention nurses can use in their routine practice without additional education. Effective use of distraction, however, requires an understanding of how the intervention should be used, for whom it should be used, and how it should be modified to meet individual needs.

THEORETICAL FRAMEWORK
AND REVIEW OF THE LITERATURE

Distraction is a class of cognitive coping strategies that divert attention from a noxious stimulus through passively redirecting the subject's attention or by actively involving the subject in the performance of a diversional task (Fernandez, 1986). Thus, distraction involves the "cognition," expectancies, or appraisals of an individual and results in a modification of the individual's behavior. According to McCaul and Malott (1984), two assumptions accompany the theory: (a) pain perception is partially a cognitively controlled process and (b) distraction consumes part of an individual's finite attentional capabilities, leaving less attention available to perceive pain. Focused attention is always incomplete, however, and the intensity of the pain may overwhelm an individual's cognitive capabilities to focus on something other than the pain. Therefore, distraction techniques should be used for situations in which the predicted pain is mild to moderate and the experience is brief.

McGrath (1994) suggests distraction is effective because it directly interferes with neuronal activity associated with pain. Basing her theory on studies in humans and animals, she postulates that distraction does not merely divert children's attention from pain but actually reduces the amount of neuronal activity caused by noxious stimuli. The gate control theory of pain (Melzack & Wall, 1965; Wall, 1978) states that pain is modulated by a gating mechanism that opens and closes nerve impulses to the brain. Cognitive processes, such as attention to the noxious, influence the gating mechanism. Thus, distraction can be a powerful intervention in decreasing the amount of pain perceived by the brain.

Distraction can be defined as either passive or active attention diversion (Fernandez, 1986). Examples of passive diversions are talking to the child about anything that will keep the child's attention away from the procedure, such as mechanical toys, picture books, cartoons, and music. Active diversions engage the child's participation in a physical or mental activity. Examples of active diversions are party blowers, kaleidoscopes, imagining fun and exciting things or quiet and relaxing scenes, pop-up books, blowing bubbles, looking for hidden objects in the room, and doing mental mathematics.

In Fernandez's (1986) review, the use of imagery is considered to be a form of distraction. With imagery, the participant's imagination is the source of distraction. Some researchers have tried to differentiate the effects of nonimaginal and imaginal distraction. Kuttner, Bowman, and Teasdale (1988) found that children 3 to 7 years of age involved in an intense, absorbing imaginative process with a therapist had less distress and pain-related behavior during bone marrow aspiration than did children receiving distraction with external props, such as hand puppets and pop-up books. For children ages 7 to 10 years, imaginal and nonimaginal distraction techniques seemed to be equally effective. Devine and Spanos (1990) tested the effects of imaginal distraction, nonimaginal distraction, imaginal reinterpretation, and nonimaginal reinterpretation with 96 adults during exposures to cold pressor pain. All the interventions were successful in decreasing perceived pain. The particularly informative finding of this study is that subjects' absorption in the strategy explained a significant portion of the unique variance in pain reduction. According to this study with adults, the subject's depth of involvement in the intervention is key to the intervention's success. This research indicates that it is very important to find the distractor that most completely captures the child's full attention. Because children have extremely varied interests and capacities for attention, nurses must tailor distraction interventions to meet the needs of individuals rather than limiting interventions to imposed categories of imaginal or nonimaginal distraction. Most researchers have used combinations of nonimaginal and imaginal activities to test the effects of distraction.

Studies on the effects of distraction are sometimes difficult to interpret because many studies used very small sample sizes and lack statistical power. Meta-analysis is a statistical technique that permits researchers to combine small studies to calculate an average effect for the intervention of interest. Broome, Lillis, and Smith (1989) examined the effects of several different types of pain interventions, including distraction, and found them to be significantly related to behavioral, self-report, and physiological outcome measures. Kleiber and Harper (1999) combined all available studies on distraction into a meta-analysis to determine the effects of distraction on young children's pain and distress. Nineteen studies representing a total sample of 535 children were included in the analysis. The conclusion was that distraction has a modest positive effect ($.33 \pm .17$) on children's distress behavior, such as crying, whimpering, or fighting, and a larger but more variable positive effect ($.62 \pm .42$) on children's self-report of pain. A subanalysis restricted to 268 subjects between the ages of 3 and 7 years who were having injections as part of well child care revealed an average effect size of $.47$ ($\pm.26$). This shows that even controlling for age and type of procedure, the effect of distraction on self-reported pain is quite variable.

The results of these meta-analyses show that using distraction with children during medical procedures will reduce the amount of observed behavioral distress for most children. The magnitude of the benefit will vary from child to child. The effect of distraction on children's self-reported pain associated with medical procedures is less clear. For some children, distraction seems to decrease the amount of self-reported pain, but unknown moderator variables influence the effects. Possible variables that might influence the effects of distraction on pain are inconsistencies in the distraction intervention, variations in the characteristics of the children, or variations in the persons delivering the intervention.

The interactive model of acute child distress described by Blount and colleagues (1992) predicts mutually influential parent and child interaction during painful procedures. For example, child distress behavior prompts the parent to act. Certain parent behaviors will in turn influence the child to exhibit more or less distress. Thus, there is a feedback loop established between parent and child behavior.

The evidence of the effectiveness of parent participation in distraction intervention is mixed. Several descriptive studies of parent and child behavior during painful procedures reveal a relationship between the use of distraction and reduced child behavioral distress (Blount, Sturges, & Powers, 1990; Bush & Cockrell, 1987; Manne et al., 1992). This finding is not consistent, however. Jacobsen and colleagues (1990) found that children whose parents used distraction were more distressed. Experimental manipulation of parents' behavior during children's medical procedures has also resulted in mixed findings. Studies by Blount, Bachanas, et al. (1992), Broome, Lillis, McGahee, and Bates (1992), and Manne et al. (1990) indicate that parents can be effective coaches for their children during procedures, but these positive results were not confirmed by others (O'Laughlin & Ridley-Johnson, 1995; Smith, Barabasz, & Barabasz, 1996). More needs to be learned about parents delivering distraction interventions.

NURSING DIAGNOSIS AND OUTCOMES

The primary nursing diagnosis that would trigger the use of distraction is pain in children (North American Nursing Diagnosis Association [NANDA], 1999). Sometimes, it is difficult to determine when children are in pain, especially before children develop adequate language to describe their feelings. Eland (1988) suggests that asking "Is this child in pain?" will not always lead to the correct conclusion. The correct question to ask is "Why would this child not be pain?" Any procedure that stretches, cuts, punctures, pulls, or in any other way displaces or injures tissue can be expected to cause some degree of discomfort. Even procedures that require simple immobilization, such as computed tomography scan or magnetic resonance imaging, can be perceived as uncomfortable or painful by the patient. The philosophy suggested in the AHCPR (1992) guideline for pain management in children is useful in guiding practice: Pain is whatever the patient says it is, and professionals have the obligation to treat and prevent pain. The following is one of the first questions a nurse should ask when assessing a child: "Is there any reason to believe that this child might be experiencing pain?"

The main patient outcome that should be tracked with the use of distraction is Pain Level. According to the Iowa Outcomes Project (2000), indicators of Pain Level include self-report of pain and behavioral and physiologic signs of pain (p. 226). A full discussion of pain measurement in children is beyond the scope of this chapter. This area is filled with uncertainty because young children may not be able to conceptualize "amount" or "intensity" of pain perceptions. Also, young children might confuse the emotions of fear and anxiety with sensations of pain. Nurses have to find a way to measure the effectiveness of their pain-reducing interventions, however. Multidimensional individualized evaluation is needed to produce valid data for judging the effectiveness of the Distraction intervention.

Some tools for self-report of pain level can be used with very young children and there are several, such as the OUCHER (Beyer & Aradine, 1988) and FACES (Wong & Baker, 1988), that are easy to use in clinical practice. The validity and reliability of these instruments have been described elsewhere (Karoly, 1991). When using self-report tools, it is important to establish a baseline rating for each child if possible. Ask the child to rate pain when you expect the child has no pain. Then ask the child to describe a painful situation (e.g., the scraping of a knee) and to rate the amount of pain remembered. This process gives a general idea of how the child perceives the concept of pain and the rating scale.

Observations of pain-related behavior can also be used as indicators of pain level. Most observational tools have been developed for research purposes and are too unwieldy to use in the clinical setting. Simplified checklists can be formed for the practice arena. Some behaviors, taken in context, can fairly reliably be taken as indicators of pain, such as screaming, crying, flailing, moaning, whimpering, and whining. Some children, however, use these behaviors as coping mechanisms to block out other sensations. By asking the parent about previous experiences with procedures, the clinician should be able to make a judgment about the meaning of pain-related behavior. Again, because of the complex nature of pain and the difficulties in measuring pain in children, it is very important to use measurements from several different sources: child's report if possible, parent report of history, and observations of the child's behavior.

The Nursing Outcomes Classification (Iowa Outcomes Project, 2000) outcome Pain Control Behavior is the flip-side of distress-related behavior. For the distraction intervention, the child behavior of interest is paying attention to the distractor. Again, a simple scale can be used in the clinical setting to evaluate the effectiveness of the distraction intervention. Did the child attend to the distractors most of the time, part of the time, or not at all? Was it easy, somewhat difficult, moderately difficult, or very difficult for the nurse to maintain the child's attention? In the clinical setting, the nurse has to be creative and flexible in developing and testing useful outcome measures.

INTERVENTION: DISTRACTION

The NIC definition of *Distraction* is "purposeful focusing of attention away from undesirable sensations" (Iowa Intervention Project, 2000, p. 259). Distraction activities are cross-referenced with the interventions Anxiety Reduction, Pain Management, and Teaching: Procedure/Treatment. Thus, the choice of distraction as an intervention to help children through painful procedures is supported.

The developmental level of the child must be considered when forming pain management plans. More pain and behavioral distress are associated with young age. The toddler and preschooler age groups are particularly at risk for having negative experiences with medical procedures. Specific age-appropriate distraction techniques are listed in Table 19.1.

As stated previously, children vary tremendously in their perceptions of and responses to pain. Individualization of the intervention is key to its success. The distraction has to be powerful and interesting enough to hold the child's attention. Although using distraction sounds deceptively simple, it takes a great deal of creativity and energy to make it effective. Issues that must be considered in the individualization of the pain management plan are the child's developmental level; the child's previous experience with painful situations, including what interventions were successful in the past; the nature of the procedure and the expected level of pain and distress; the child's coping style; the medical condition of the child; the parents' preference for interventions; and the time available for preparation.

It is very important to include the use of nonpharmacological techniques to control pain and distress in children who are likely to experience repeated procedures. There is no evidence that children habituate to repeated procedures and feel less pain or distress over time (Dahlquist et al., 1986; Katz, Kellerman, & Siegel, 1980; Manne, Bakeman, Jacobsen, & Redd, 1993). Indeed, a potent predictor of child distress is the quality of previous experiences with medical procedures (Dahlquist et al., 1986). It is not the quantity of previous experiences but the child's degree of distress with previous experiences that predicts future distress. Children who have illnesses or injuries requiring repeated procedures should be targeted for formalized pain management plans that can be carried out at

TABLE 19.1   Age-Specific Distraction Techniques

Techniques/Objects	Infant	Toddler	Preschooler	School Age	Adolescent
Rapid rocking	X				
Patting	X				
Stroking	X				
Sucking	X				
Cuddling	X				
Positioning	X				
Mobiles	X				
Objects that change color or shape	X				
Small stuffed toys	X	X			
Bubble blowing by adults	X	X			
Nursery rhymes		X			
Finger or hand games (e. g., pat-a-cake)		X	X		
Pop-up books		X	X		
Puppets		X	X		
Elements of surprise		X	X		
Singing songs		X	X		
Speaking to the child through a stuffed toy		X	X		
Storytelling		X	X	X	
Bubble blowing by child		X	X	X	X
Music	X	X	X	X	X
Counting			X	X	X
Whistles, pinwheels, feathers			X	X	X
Magic wands, water wheels, hand-held toys			X	X	X
Pretend situations such as a favorite place, television fantasies			X	X	X
Pretend roles			X	X	
Visual fixation				X	X
Hidden-picture books				X	X
Audiotaped stories			X	X	
Conversation					X

each procedure. The importance of this planning is made clear by recent evidence linking adult fear, pain, and behavior during medical procedures to adverse medical experiences in childhood (Pate, Blount, Cohen, & Smith, 1996).

A convenient format for individualizing a plan for using distraction has been developed by Robin Ostedgaard, who is a Child Life Therapy staff member at The University of Iowa Hospitals and Clinics. Prior to a procedure, a health care professional talks with the parent and child about preferences for pain management interventions, including pharmacological and nonpharmacological treatments. The parents are asked about the child's previous response to painful procedures, including what was helpful and what was not helpful. A particular course of action is decided on, and a specific person is designated as the child's coach for the procedure. If the parent is comfortable in the coaching role and wants to participate, the parent acts as the primary support person throughout the procedure. A clinically useful subjective scale was developed to track the child's response to the intervention. A health professional rates the child's behavior as (a) relaxed, talking; (b) minimal protest; (c) distressed; or (d) inconsolable. After piloting the scale for several months, the child life therapists suggested the children's behavior should be rated for three different phases of the procedure rather than for the procedure as a whole. They found that children's behavior frequently varies across phases of the procedure. Now there is one rating for the preparatory phase (before the uncomfortable part of the procedure), another rating for the painful part of the procedure, and a final rating for the child's behavior after the procedure is completed. The individualized planning form includes space for describing the specific distraction techniques used during the procedure, such as the child's favorite visual image or the child's preference for specific pop-up books. By using the plan as a documentation tool, it is easy for nurses to review the child's response to interventions and to modify the plan for future use.

The nurse must make a judgment about the use of pharmacological and nonpharmacological interventions to attain the best pain relief possible for the individual patient. Distraction alone might not be powerful enough to sufficiently decrease pain during procedures such as bone marrow aspiration, but it may be very effective for other procedures such as venipuncture. The use of anxiety-reducing medication can interfere with the child's ability to attend to the distraction intervention, but that does not mean that distraction should not be used. It can still have an additive effect in reducing child distress.

INTERVENTION APPLICATION

Molly Brown is a 4-year-old girl with vesicoureteral reflux scheduled for a voiding cystourethrogram (VCUG). Molly's medical problems began when she was approximately 1 year old. She developed recurrent urinary tract infections, and ureteral reflux was discovered at her first VCUG. Molly has been followed with renal scans and VCUGs every 6 months since her diagnosis. A peripheral intravenous is started when renal scans are done, and a urinary catheter is placed for VCUGs. She is currently returning to the clinic for her seventh episode of invasive medical procedures.

Brenda, Molly's nurse, reviews Molly's medical record and finds that, as usual, there is no mention of Molly's behavior during the previous procedures. She approaches Molly and her mother in the waiting room to assess the situation. While Molly is busy playing with the toys in the children's area, she questions Ms. Brown about Molly's previous experiences. Ms. Brown says Molly's tolerance of the procedures has been getting progressively worse. At her last appointment, she screamed through the entire visit. Ms. Brown was so upset with her daughter's distress that she had to leave the room, which made her feel like she had abandoned her child in a time of need. Brenda asked Ms. Brown about Molly's general temperament and things that really seemed to get Molly's attention, for instance, on a long car trip. Ms. Brown reported that Molly was a very active and inquisitive child. She was usually a patient traveler, easy to direct toward different things when she got bored. She especially liked being read to and coloring. Brenda decides to use a distraction intervention (Iowa Intervention Project, 2000) to help Molly cope with the mild to moderate acute pain (NANDA, 1999) expected during urinary catheterization. She tells Ms. Brown that there are a variety of interesting books and objects to play with in the treatment room, and every effort will be made to make Molly comfortable during the procedure. She encourages Ms. Brown to stay with Molly today and asks her to be the main coach for Molly in keeping her distracted from the procedure. When Brenda approaches Molly in the waiting room, she pulls a small stuffed animal from her lab coat pocket and says, "Molly, I have a friend who wants to meet you! This is Scruffles." Brenda goes on to talk to Molly through the stuffed animal, telling her she knows a trick that will make time in the treatment room go more quickly. There are lots of fun things to do and look at in the treatment room, and her mom will be there to help her choose what to do. Also, she will get to choose a prize sticker when she is done.

Brenda has ensured that the treatment room is completely set up before Molly enters. No scary instruments are in sight. When Molly is seated on the exam table, Brenda pulls out a tray full of pop-up books, bubbles, party blowers, and touch toys. She asks Ms. Brown to help Molly select things from the tray with which to play. So far, Molly is calm and cooperative. When another nurses enters the room to assist with the catheter placement, Molly begins to whine and cling to her mother. Brenda introduces the new nurse and tells Molly she is a special nurse with special skills. She pulls Scruffles out of her pocket again and asks him to talk to

Molly. By talking to Molly through the stuffed toy, Brenda adds a magical quality to her communication. Toddlers and preschoolers often respond very positively to this. By this point, Ms. Brown has become comfortable enough to guide Molly's attention to some of the pop-up books. Brenda and her coworker quickly and calmly prepare Molly for the catheter insertion. Throughout the cleansing routine, Brenda briefly mentions unusual sensations that Molly will feel, such as coolness or touch, but she redirects Molly's attention back to her mother's storybook immediately.

Insertion of a urinary catheter is painful for many children. For Molly, it is best to use the most intense distractor possible to help her maintain her behavioral control. In her experience, Brenda has noticed that having children participate in diversions that include some sort of breath control, such as blowing through party blowers, pretending to blow out flashlights, playing a train "choo-choo" game, or blowing bubbles, is very helpful during the painful parts of procedures. Brenda asks Molly if she likes to blow bubbles. When she says yes, Brenda directs Ms. Brown to take out the bottle of bubbles and have Molly try to blow as many little tiny bubbles into the air as she can. As Molly blows, the catheter is inserted easily because her muscles are relaxed. Molly cries out with pain as the catheter slips into the bladder, but the pain is short-lived, and Molly is easily redirected to blow bubbles into Brenda's face. They both laugh.

Molly has been able to maintain calm behavior throughout most of the procedure with her mother's help. Indicators for Pain Control behavior were apparent. This is a large improvement from her previous experiences, when the attitude of the adults in the treatment room was "Let's just get it over with." Ms. Brown has also benefited from this experience. She feels more confident in her abilities to help her child through difficult times. She also has a renewed appreciation for the special qualities of pediatric nurses who know how to work well with children.

RESEARCH AND PRACTICE IMPLICATIONS

Distraction is an attractive intervention for nurses to use with children undergoing painful procedures because it is relatively easy to use and it can be done with little preparation of the patient. Research has shown that distraction techniques reduce self-reported pain and observed distress behavior in many children. It appears that the appeal of the diversion—its ability to hold the child's attention—is an important factor in the success of the intervention.

One of the problems encountered when using and studying the effects of distraction is the extreme variability between children in their reactions to both medical procedures and the distraction intervention. Clinicians who work with children can attest to the fact some children scream and flail throughout seemingly minor procedures, paying no attention at all to the efforts of adults to distract them. Other children lay quietly without any adult intervention, even at times when pain is likely to be present. Researchers need to develop predictive criteria identifying children who need more than simple distraction to help with pain and behavior control. When screening criteria are available, children can be appropriately referred for more intensive cognitive or behavioral therapy, such as hypnosis, desensitization, modeling, and operant conditioning.

One factor that shows promise as a predictor of perceived pain and distress behavior is temperament. Temperament is the innate behavioral style of an individual. Pain researchers have found a relationship between behavioral distress during painful procedures and difficult temperament indicators (Lee & White-Traut, 1996; Schechter, Bernstein, Beck, Hart, & Scherzer, 1991; Young & Fu, 1988). The relationship between child temperament and response to cognitive interventions such as distraction has not been thoroughly explored.

Distraction is a simple, low-cost, low-risk intervention that offers real benefits to children during painful procedures. The research clearly indicates that most children will be less distressed during medical procedures when distraction is used, and some children will even report less procedure-related pain. Quick and accurate medical tests are more achievable when children are calm and cooperative. Also, the stress level of the staff decreases when children are composed. Involving parents in the delivery of the distraction intervention is a way to extend the number of adults who are skilled at helping the child during the procedure. It is also a way to empower the parent and enhance satisfaction with care. An additional benefit to teaching distraction skills to parents is that they can use these skills in any setting, making them partners-in-healing with all providers who care for their children.

All child health care institutions should have a pain management policy that clearly directs the use of nonpharmacological techniques such as distraction to help children during medical procedures. Distracting a child's attention from a medical procedure is no longer just "a nice thing to do" when someone happens to remember to do it. Parents and children should expect state-of-the-art care from pediatric nurses, which includes using distraction to assist children whenever possible.

REFERENCES

Agency for Health Care Policy and Research (AHCPR). (1992). *Acute pain management in infants, children and adolescents: Operative and medical proce-*

dures. Quick reference guide for clinicians (DHHS Publication No. AHCPR 92-0019). Silver Spring, MD: AHCPR Clearinghouse.

Beyer, J. E., & Aradine, C. R. (1988). Convergent and discriminant validity of a self-report measure of pain intensity for children. *Children's Health Care, 16,* 274-282.

Blount, R. L., Bachanas, P. J., Powers, S. W., Cotter, M. C., Franklin, A., Chaplin, W., Mayfield, J., Henderson, M., & Blount, S. D. (1992). Training children to cope and parents to coach them during routine immunizations: Effects on child, parent, and staff behaviors. *Behavior Therapy, 23,* 689-705.

Blount, R. L., Sturges, J. W., & Powers, S. W. (1990). Analysis of child and adult behavioral variations by phase of medical procedure. *Behavior Therapy, 21,* 33-48.

Broome, M. E., Lillis, P. P., McGahee, T. W., & Bates, T. (1992). The use of distraction and imagery with children during painful procedures. *Oncology Nursing Forum, 19,* 499-502.

Broome, M. E., Lillis, P. P., & Smith, M. C. (1989). Pain interventions with children: A meta-analysis of the research. *Nursing Research, 38*(3), 154-158.

Bush, J. P., & Cockrell, C. S. (1987). Maternal factors predicting parenting behaviors in the pediatric clinic. *Journal of Pediatric Psychology, 12,* 505-518.

Dahlquist, L. M., Gil, K. M., Armstrong, F. D., DeLawyer, D. D., Greene, P., & Wuori, D. (1986). Preparing children for medical examinations: The importance of previous medical experience. *Health Psychology, 5,* 249-259.

Devine, D. P., & Spanos, N. P. (1990). Effectiveness of maximally different cognitive strategies and expectancy in attenuation of reported pain. *Journal of Personality and Social Psychology, 58,* 672-678.

Eland, J. M. (1988). Pharmacologic management of acute and chronic pediatric pain. *Issues in Comprehensive Pediatric Nursing, 11,* 93-111.

Fernandez, E. (1986). A classification system of cognitive coping strategies for pain. *Pain, 26,* 141-151.

Iowa Intervention Project. (2000). *Nursing interventions classification (NIC)* (J. C. McCloskey & G. M. Bulechek, Eds.; 3rd ed.). St., Louis, MO: Mosby-Year Book.

Iowa Outcomes Project. (2000). *Nursing outcomes classification (NOC)* (M. Johnson, M. Maas, & S. Moorhead, Eds.; 2nd ed.). St. Louis, MO: Mosby-Year Book.

Jacobsen, P. B., Manne, S. L., Gorfinkle, K., Schorr, O., Rapkin, B., & Redd, W. (1990). Analysis of child and parent behavior during painful medical procedures. *Health Psychology, 9,* 559-576.

Karoly, P. (1991). Assessment of pediatric pain. In J. P. Bush & S. W. Harkins (Eds.), *Children in pain.* New York: Springer-Verlag.

Katz, E., Kellerman, J., & Siegel, S. (1980). Behavioral distress in children with cancer undergoing medical procedures: Developmental considerations. *Journal of Consulting and Clinical Psychology, 48,* 356-365.

Kleiber, C., & Harper, D. (1999). The effects of distraction on child distress and pain during medical procedures: A meta-analysis. *Nursing Research, 48,* 44-49.

Kuttner, L., Bowman, M., & Teasdale, M. (1988). Psychological treatment of distress, pain, and anxiety for young children with cancer. *Journal of Developmental and Behavioral Pediatrics, 9,* 374-381.

Lee, L. W., & White-Traut, R. C. (1996). The role of temperament in pediatric pain response. *Issues in Comprehensive Pediatric Nursing, 19,* 49-63.

Manne, S. L., Bakeman, R., Jacobsen, P. B., Gorfinkle, K., Bernstein, D., & Redd, W. H. (1992). Adult-child interaction during invasive medical procedures. *Health Psychology, 11,* 241-249.

Manne, S. L., Bakeman, R., Jacobsen, P. B., & Redd, W. H. (1993). Children's coping during invasive medical procedures. *Behavior Therapy, 24,* 143-158.

Manne, S. L., Redd, W. H., Jacobsen, P. B., Gorfinkle, K., Schorr, O., & Rapkin, B. (1990). Behavioral intervention to reduce child and parent distress during venipuncture. *Journal of Consulting and Clinical Psychology, 58,* 565-572.

McCaul, K., & Malott, J. (1984). Distraction and coping with pain. *Psychological Bulletin, 95,* 516-533.

McGrath, P. A. (1994). Psychological aspects of pain perception. *Archives of Oral Biology, 39,* 55s-62s.

Melzack, R., & Wall, P. D. (1965). Pain mechanisms: A new theory. *Science, 150,* 971-979.

North American Nursing Diagnosis Association. (1999). *Nursing diagnoses: Definitions and classification 1995-1996.* Philadelphia: Author.

O'Laughlin, E., & Ridley-Johnson, R. (1995). Maternal presence during children's routine immunizations: The effect of mother as observer in reducing child distress. *Children's Health Care, 24,* 175-191.

Pate, J. T., Blount, R. L., Cohen, L. L., & Smith, A. J. (1996). Childhood medical experience and temperament as predictors of adult functioning in medical situations. *Children's Health Care, 25,* 281-298.

Schechter, N. L., Bernstein, B. A., Beck, A., Hart, L., & Scherzer, L. (1991). Individual differences in children's response to pain: Role of temperament and parental characteristics. *Pediatrics, 87,* 171-177.

Smith, J., Barabasz, A., & Barabasz, M. (1996). Comparison of hypnosis and distraction in severely ill children undergoing painful medical procedures. *Journal of Counseling Psychology, 43,* 187-195.

Wall, P. D. (1978). The gate control theory of pain mechanisms. A re-examination and re-statement. *Brain, 101,* 1-18.

Wong, D., & Baker, C. (1988). Pain in children: Comparison of assessment scales. *Pediatric Nursing, 14,* 9-17.

Young, M. R., & Fu, V. R. (1988). Influence of play and temperament on the young child's response to pain. *Children's Health Care, 18,* 209-217.

20

Sibling Adaptation Counseling

Martha Craft-Rosenberg

Stress is a part of life, and learning to cope with stress in a manner that leads to positive adaptation is an important skill for children (Garmezy & Rutter, 1983). Illness in children is a stressful event that requires coping and adaptation in all family members, including siblings of the ill child (Craft, 1985; Craft, Wyatt, & Sandell, 1985; Kleiber, Montgomery, & Craft-Rosenberg, 1995; Knafl, Cavallari, & Dixon, 1988; Simon, 1993; Stewart, Stein, Forrest, & Clark, 1992). When children experience illness, their siblings usually experience a great deal of change. Perhaps the most significant change is their relationship with their parents, who are understandably focused emotionally on the ill child (Craft, 1985; Cuskelly & Gunn, 1993; Williams, Lorenzo, & Borja, 1993). Parents might be preoccupied, and they are usually required to be absent from their healthy children for both brief and lengthy intervals. Thus, siblings can be left in the care of other adults, contributing to a lack of physical or emotional access to their parents. Furthermore, expectations of siblings are sometimes changed to include increased household responsibilities, leaving less time for school and social activities (Cuskelly & Gunn, 1993; Williams et al., 1993).

Reports in the literature and observations from clinical practice as a clinical nursing specialist prompted me to begin a program of research on responses in siblings of ill and hospitalized children in 1978 to determine responses and variables related to responses. This research was intended to identify siblings at risk for adverse responses and to identify variables that could be manipulated through intervention to assist siblings. The program of research included the development, testing, and refinement of an instrument to assess sibling responses and the conduct of several studies investigating variables influencing sibling response. Two multivariate studies were used to first specify and then test a model showing a causal pattern of constructs influencing responses in siblings of hospitalized children. This model identified variables that could be altered in a nursing intervention to promote positive sibling adaptation. Although this model was developed using data from siblings of ill and hospitalized children, these data are very similar to data from siblings of ill children in general (Cuskelly & Gunn, 1993; Heffernan & Zanelli, 1997; Williams et al., 1993). Therefore, the intervention to be discussed is intended for siblings of ill children. The purpose of this chapter is to describe the Sibling Adaptation Counseling intervention, which was developed from multivariate research and a tested model to facilitate sibling coping and positive adaptation.

THEORETICAL FRAMEWORK AND LITERATURE REVIEW

Theories

The three theories used for research on siblings of ill children were a physiological perspective, the General Adaptation Syndrome proposed by Selye (1956), and the work on coping by Lazarus and Folkman (1984). From a physiological perspective, a stressful event is perceived by the sensory system, interpreted by the cerebral cortex, and integrated via the limbic system. Stressors that are perceived as threatening cause stimulation of the posterior hypothalamus and an immediate response of the autonomic nervous system via neural pathways. Stimulation of the adrenal medulla releases catecholamines, which affect end-organs in a manner similar to direct sympathetic stimulation. In addition, almost any type of stress will cause an immediate and marked increase in adrenocorticotropic hormone (ACTH) secretion by the anterior pituitary gland that is then followed within minutes by an increased adrenocortical secretion of cortisol (Guyton, 1986). Selye (1956) presented the General Adaptation Syndrome as an explanatory theoretical framework to describe the role of the endocrine axes during chronic stress. According to his theory, the adrenocortical response is the most critical during the "alarm" phase,

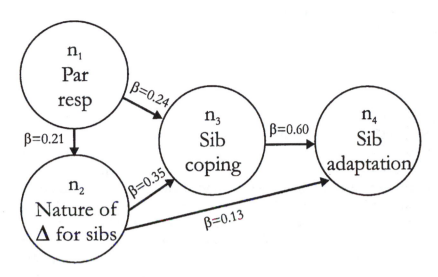

Figure 20.1. Sibling Coping and Adaptation: Final Model With Four Constructs

with the somatotropic axis taking priority during the "state of resistance" as the body attempts to maintain homeostasis. A "state of exhaustion" exists if the stressor persists because energy to maintain homeostasis is depleted. All axes are highly activated during the state of exhaustion, and permanent damage to the circulatory, digestive, immune, and cardiovascular system may result.

Lazarus and Folkman (1984) described coping as a process in which constantly changing cognitive and behavioral efforts are used to manage specific external or internal demands or both that are appraised as taxing or exceeding the resources of the individual. The coping process has been described as a two-stage process in which individuals first conduct a "primary" appraisal to appraise danger and threat and then a "secondary" appraisal to determine the extent to which any particular action will relieve the danger (Lazarus & Folkman, 1984). The two classes of variables are thought to determine the process of secondary appraisal, including (a) the ambiguity of the threat and (b) the determinants of coping, such as viability of resources and situational constraints. Emotion-focused coping and problem-solving coping processes have been identified by Lazarus and Folkman. The processes can be facilitated through intervention. Thus, intervention activities to provide information should decrease threat ambiguity and assist in problem solving. Additional intervention activities to foster expression of feelings for siblings should be helpful in emotion-focused coping. I view these coping processes as mediators for the influence of stress on siblings (Figure 20.1).

Empirical Literature
and Model Development

The empirical literature indicates that siblings of ill children experience many changes that have the potential to influence responses. These changes include relationships, responsibilities, and roles. The sibling relationship with the ill child and parents has been shown to be influenced by stress and separation. Also, the role in siblings has been reported to be altered with the possibility of changes in place of residence, care providers, and responsibilities. Their role in the community has been found to be altered because neighbors, teachers, and friends treat them differently (Craft & Wyatt, 1986; Craft et al., 1985; Knafl & Dixon, 1983). In addition, fear of acquiring the illness of the hospitalized child, uncertainty, a sense of vulnerability and isolation, and fear of emotional abandonment have been reported (Cairns, Clark, Smith, & Lansky, 1979; Craft, 1986; Craft & Craft, 1989; Craft & Wyatt, 1986; Craft et al., 1985; Minagawa, 1997). Furthermore, the jealousy experienced by siblings or even a fear that they could have been responsible for the illness in some way have been found to increase sibling stress. Siblings also have been found to keep silent due to guilt in contributing to already existing parental concerns (Cairns et al., 1979; Heffernan & Zanelli, 1997; Spinetta, 1981; Walker, 1990).

These changes for siblings have been found to produce some changes in feelings and behavior (Craft, 1986; Craft & Craft, 1989; Craft & Wyatt, 1986; Craft et al., 1985; Heffernan & Zanelli, 1997; McKeever, 1983). Some researchers have reported positive effects on siblings, such as maturity of attitudes and behavior (Iles, 1979; Kruger, Shauver, & Jones, 1980; Minagawa, 1997; Simeonsson & Bailey, 1986; Taylor, 1980). In addition, negative effects have been reported, such as losses perceived in the relationship with the affected child, difficulty with the presence of parent substitutes (Iles, 1979), decreased family communication, family role changes, and increasing expectations of siblings (Heffernan & Zanelli, 1997; McKeever, 1983). The measurement of effects has differed in reported studies, however, which has made their interpretation difficult. Only a few studies have used control group comparisons. Importantly, many researchers have used parent perception and report as the measure of sibling effects rather than using the primary data source—the siblings. The views of parents and siblings have been found to differ (Craft & Craft, 1989; Heffernan & Zanelli, 1997).

Sibling responses are influenced by family characteristics and relationships, the nature of the threat, changes occurring in their roles and life patterns, and resources or support systems available. The variables are numerous and complex. Selected variables have been studied under the following constructs: (a) family socioeconomic class, (b) sibling–ill child relationship, (c) perceived nature of the threat, (d) nature of changes for siblings, and (e) assistance and support provided for the sibling (Craft-Rosenberg, 1997). Family socioeconomic class, as measured by the education and occupation of parents, has been studied because family income alters available resources and has been shown to influence parental anxiety (McCollum, 1975). In addition, the education or occupation of the mother has been found to be related to sibling anxiety (Craft et al., 1985). The meaning of the relationship of mother's education and occupation on sibling anxiety is unclear, but it may be related to maternal sensitivity toward the effects of this event on siblings and maternal motivation to assist them through increased communication. The sibling–ill child relationship has been shown to be associated with the degree of perceived threat (Craft et al., 1985). Although this relationship is very difficult to measure, developmental psychologists have studied gender comparison and age difference as relationship determinants (Dunn, 1983; Dunn & Munn, 1985; Dunn & Shatz, 1989). Dunn (1983), however, noted that age difference, gender comparison, and ordinal distance have been studied as determinants of sibling relationships, probably due to the ease in measurement of these variables. Because sibling relationships are self-perceived, I used self-report data. Siblings were asked if they were "friends," "good friends," or "best friends" of the child who was hospitalized. Siblings who stated that they were the best friend of the hospitalized child had significantly higher adverse effects as measured by the Perceived Change Scale (PCS) (Craft & Wyatt, 1986; Craft et al., 1985). The perceived nature of the threat for siblings was studied by examining the influence of the hospitalized child's type of illness, the length of illness, and sibling age. Prior data on responses of siblings of children hospitalized with acute, chronic, and progressive illness have shown that siblings have significantly higher scores on the PCS when the diagnosis is new as opposed to a previously diagnosed illness or condition. Also, siblings scored significantly higher on the PCS when their brother or sister had a progressive or life-threatening illness (Craft, 1985; Craft et al., 1985). These data are similar to those of other investigators. Spinetta (1981) found that siblings of children with cancer scored significantly lower in overall adaptation on the criterion measures used in his research than did the children ill with cancer. Furthermore, Cairns and associates (1979) found striking similarities between children with cancer and their healthy siblings in the areas of social isolation, a sense of vulnerability to illness, injury, and self-esteem. Heffernan and Zanelli (1997) found that siblings had trouble sleeping, complained of headaches, and fought more. For the child with a progressive illness, the family faces years of uncertainty about the eventual out-come of the illness, and the status of siblings has been an underestimated area of concern (Carr-Gregg & White, 1987; Mott, 1990). Thus, both the type of illness and the length of diagnosis influence sibling responses. The risk of sibling adverse response is less with acute illnesses and than with chronic illnesses (Craft, 1985).

Sibling age is related to cognitive function and ability to perceive events. Using the Piagetian theory, school-age siblings have understand-ing limited to concrete tasks, and they have difficulty with hypothetical reasoning divorced from experience, which is possible for older siblings (Piaget & Inhelder, 1969). In addition, school-age children lack under-standing of how changes in one variable can be compensated for by changes in another. These characteristics support the need for careful, concrete explanations for school-age siblings and more abstract explana-tions for adolescent siblings (Siegel, 1987). In addition, a poor concept of time in younger siblings can contribute to the negative effects of parental separation. Craft found that the younger siblings reported significantly more stress-related changes than older siblings (Craft, 1985, 1986; Craft & Craft, 1989; Craft & Wyatt, 1986; Craft et al., 1985). This finding is similar with that of Knafl and Dixon (1983), who reported that negative responses in siblings of pediatric patients clustered in those siblings in the 4 to 11 years of age range. The nature of changes experienced by siblings is large and diverse. One major change is separation from the ill child. An-other change is separation from parents, which can be interpreted by sib-lings as a loss of love, rejection, emotional abandonment, or punishment. It is easy to see, then, how separation from parents can intensify sibling ri-valry, with siblings feeling jealousy about the attention given to the hospi-talized child and then a sense of guilt about their feelings. Other new emo-tions for siblings are magical or unrealistic fears of getting the illness themselves. Craft (1985, 1986) found that 50% of siblings studied are fearful of getting the illness of the hospitalized child. These new emotions are often intensified by changes in place of residence when parents must use care providers who cannot come to the home (Craft et al., 1985; Knafl & Dixon, 1983). Similarly, feelings of vulnerability, uncertainty, and emotional abandonment are further heightened by parental use of care providers who siblings do not know and who change frequently. The changing authority figures and changing expectations of the authority fig-ures contribute to the stress of the total experience. One of the most influ-ential factors for adverse effects in siblings is perceived parenting changes. Siblings who reported changes in their parents' supervision, emotional availability, and anger were found to have significantly higher scores on the PCS, indicating a higher stress response (Craft, 1985).

Assistance and Support Provided

The nature of sibling explanation is the one type of assistance related significantly to sibling response as measured by the PCS. It is important for parents to communicate with siblings about the illness and to encourage sibling expression of feelings regarding the illness (Canam, 1987). If parents are unable to do so, nurses must do it. Those siblings characterizing their explanation of events as being open have reported significantly fewer adverse responses (Craft & Wyatt, 1986; Craft et al., 1985). The testing of interventions to assist siblings is just beginning, however. I hope that by the end of the next decade, nurses will have identified other nursing interventions in addition to sibling explanation that are effective in reducing adverse sibling responses.

Craft-Rosenberg (1997) specified a model developed from a multivariate study of 100 siblings of hospitalized children and then tested it using LISREL with a data set from the study of 120 siblings of hospitalized children. The original model included constructs of family socioeconomic class, sibling–ill child relationship, perceived nature of the threat, parent response, nature of changes for siblings, sibling assistance, sibling coping, and sibling adaptation. The number of constructs was reduced to four after analysis of LISREL (Figure 20.1), showing a direct relationship between the nature of change for siblings and sibling adaptation (Craft-Rosenberg, 1997). Therefore, the intervention presented later is directed toward change and promoting normalcy for siblings. These findings concur with the work of Knafl (1982), Knafl and Dixon (1983), Knafl et al. (1988), and Heffernan and Zanelli, (1997).

In summary, sibling responses include physiological, cognitive, and emotional processes that can be modified by nursing intervention. Siblings of hospitalized children who are at the greatest risk for adverse stress effects are younger, report a fear of getting the illness, are brothers or sisters of a child with a new diagnosis, are brothers and sisters of a child who has an illness that is thought to be progressive or terminal, perceive their parents as treating them much differently, have received little information about their ill brother or sister, and whose caretakers and residences change.

ASSESSMENT

Both siblings and parents reported that siblings experienced changes in feelings and sleeping. These changes can be viewed as a response measure for siblings and have been developed into a PCS that can be used as an assessment measure by both parents and nurses. The content for scale items was based on Selye's adaptation theory. The items include self-observable changes reported in his early book (Selye, 1956, pp. 73-118).

The PCS has been used to study the effects of pediatric illness and hospitalization in more than 400 siblings in several studies (Craft, 1986, 1993; Craft & Wyatt, 1986; Craft et al., 1985). The 12-item PCS was developed to determine directional sibling self-perceived physiological and behavioral changes. Siblings were asked if the item topics were occurring to a greater extent (more), to the same extent (same), or to a lesser extent (less) than was the case before the hospitalization of a brother or sister. For example, on one item a sibling would be asked if he or she was getting nervous "more," the "same," or "less" during the time that the brother or sister was in the hospital. Other scale items address (a) getting mad or angry; (b) trouble thinking or concentrating; (c) difficulty sleeping; (d) fighting or arguing with other children; (e) having nightmares; (f) biting nails; (g) desire to be alone; (h) desire to be with parents; (i) feeling sad or unhappy; (j) health perception, or "Are you feeling more, the same, or less healthy?"; and (k) food intake.

The items are scored by assigning the number 1 to each reported stress-related change. For example, a report of more trouble sleeping will receive a score of 1 because this behavior is clearly stress related. For some behaviors, however, either an increase or a decrease represent a stress-related response. Thus, reports of both "more" and "less" would receive a score of 1 for the items of "Desire to be alone," "Desire to be with parents," and "Food intake." Furthermore, a response of feeling less healthy would receive a score of 1. The PCS was developed for a wide age range and has been studied using two age groups or age cohorts. The first age group was school-age siblings, and the second age group was adolescent siblings. Data supporting the psychometric strength of the PCS have been reported elsewhere (Craft, 1986). Factor analysis of the scale by Craft and Oppliger identified the five major factors accounting for the majority (67%) of variance in reported responses for both age cohorts: (a) uncertainty, (b) sorrow, (c) helplessness and frustration, (d) preoccupation, and (e) conflict. These responses are consistent with the reports in the literature on stress, and findings of other authors, such as Iles (1979), Kramer (1981), and Walker (1990). Although some health professionals question the reliability and validity of reports from children less than 10 years of age, the findings from this analysis have supported their reliability and validity. That is, the findings were almost identical for both the younger and the older age cohorts with regard to the variance accounted for by every scale item, which means that the two age groups of siblings were experiencing and reporting similar perceptions. Thus, the usefulness of the PCS for the younger group of siblings clinically and in research has been supported by these data. Furthermore, preschool-aged siblings have been studied using the PCS with parent report. The data have been found to be similar (Montgomery, 1988). Siblings should be assessed by both parents and nurses to determine the number and extent of sibling changes in feelings and behavior to detect a need for intervention (Gallo, Breitmayer, Knafl, & Zoeller, 1991; Thompson, 1994).

DIAGNOSIS AND OUTCOMES

The changes in sibling feelings and behaviors included in the PCS are consistent with the defining characteristics of the North American Nursing Diagnosis Association (NANDA, 1999) diagnosis of Ineffective Individual Coping. The extent to which this NANDA diagnosis has been validated on children is unknown, however. Furthermore, the feelings and behaviors listed in the PCS are more specific than the defining characteristics for the NANDA diagnosis for Ineffective Individual Coping, and they would probably be more helpful to both parents and nurses in determining the coping and adaptation of siblings.

Actions to manage stressors that tax an individual's resources or coping (Iowa Outcomes Project, 2000) act as mediators for the return to baseline for all the indicators listed in the PCS. That is, if a sibling is having trouble concentrating at school, one desired outcome is that the sibling would return to baseline concentration. Similarly, if a sibling had been feeling more nervous and was having trouble sleeping, desired outcomes would be that the feelings of nervousness decreased and the normal sleeping pattern returned.

INTERVENTION: SIBLING ADAPTATION COUNSELING

Sibling Adaptation Counseling is an intervention that provides guidance for parents to help their well children use problem-focused and emotion-focused coping as they adapt their lives to changing circumstances (Gradoville, Craft-Rosenberg, Denehy, & Gagan, 1995; Lazarus & Folkman, 1984). Research findings by myself and others (Gallo et al., 1991; Martinson, Gilliss, Colaizzo, Freeman, & Bossert, 1990; Walker, 1990) indicate that siblings need information, a sense of emotional connectedness with their parents and their ill brother or sister, and help with change management.

Information sharing may be difficult for parents. In ongoing research, data have shown that parents experience stress and must deal with their own feelings (Kleiber et al., 1995). Also, they may not know what they should tell their other children or how to tell them. Craft, Cohen, Titler,

338 CHILD HEALTH PROBLEMS

and DeHammer (1993) found that many adults believe or possess a myth that children are too young to understand and therefore do not need to know what is happening to an ill family member. This myth or misinformation is compounded by attempts of family members to protect one another during an acute illness of a family member (Titler, Cohen, & Craft, 1991). Thus, parents may believe that siblings are too young to understand or they want to protect them or both. Similarly, siblings may not talk to anyone about their fears and worries because they do not want to add to their parents' burdens (Cairns et al., 1979). Therefore, nurses should take the initiative to encourage parents to be open in providing information to siblings (Adams, Peveler, Stein, & Dunger, 1991; Faux, 1991). When parents have concerns about the approach to use in talking with siblings, nurses can provide them with guidance in using developmentally appropriate strategies using words that are understood by children.

The methods parents choose to talk with siblings may differ, but the content needs to include an open discussion of the condition of the ill child and the meaning the condition has for the lives of the siblings and their family. All possible concerns need to be introduced by parents, especially worries about death (Havermans & Eiser, 1994). The ill child's diagnosis and illness management are the general topics for discussion. Information about doctor or clinic visits; hospital stays; laboratory, X-ray, and every other type of data should be provided on an ongoing basis. Furthermore, siblings should be told that they did not cause the illness. In addition, they should be reassured that they are not likely to get the illness themselves if that is the situation. If there is a chance that they may get the illness, such as in the case of diabetes, parents should inform them of monitoring possibilities so that siblings work with their parents to monitor themselves. Siblings should have opportunities to talk about implications of the disease, especially worries about death (Havermans & Eiser, 1994). Although most health professionals (Spinetta, 1981) agree that it is best for parents to discuss these issues with siblings of hospitalized children, parents may be psychologically immobilized at certain periods and unable to meet sibling informational needs. It is during these periods that nurses must directly implement activities with information to assist with siblings. Opportunities for nurses to intervene directly with siblings occur during hospital stays if the ill child is hospitalized and during clinic visits or nurse visits to the home. If the affected child does need hospitalization, visitation provides opportunities to share information on what is happening with the ill child. Siblings can see, feel, and touch the ill child as well as observe what the ill child is experiencing. Nurses can capture each learning opportunity and teach siblings about the condition and care of their ill brother or sister. For siblings less than 7 years of age, visitation is essential because of the inability of children this age to use abstract thinking and to gain information from verbal or written explanations (Carandang, Folkins, Hines, & Steward, 1979; Dorn, 1984). Younger siblings need information-sharing activities, such as activities with dolls and puppets, to explain what is happening with their ill brother or sister. However, younger siblings may be sent to the playroom and distracted with play when they visit as opposed to learning when they visit (Craft & Craft, 1989). Ironically, I have observed that younger siblings who are most in need of information sharing are often least likely to get it. Frequently, they are ignored because many adults consider them too young to understand about the condition and care of their ill brother or sister. This dilemma could be overcome with the development of a younger sibling orientation and information protocols for use in acute care settings (Montgomery, 1988; Montgomery, Kleiber, Nicholson, & Craft-Rosenberg, 1997). Regardless of sibling age, preparation for visiting the hospital is recommended to ensure that each sibling visit provides a learning opportunity. Importantly, each contact with the ill sibling and parent promotes a sense of needed connectedness for siblings.

Parenting styles are patterns of parent supervision and expectations, limit setting, affection, and emotional connectedness with which children live and become comfortable. They are usually predictable in families and seem to provide children with a sense of security. It is easy to see, however, how these styles could be altered when parents are experiencing extreme stress. Parental stress and related anxiety are likely to contribute to preoccupation and emotional distancing, increased irritability, and a change in parental expectations of sibling behavior (Craft, 1985; Dyson, Edgar, & Crnic, 1989). Nurses can assist parents to maintain their parenting styles in two ways. First, nurses can help parents reduce their stress through the use of sound communication skills and the provision of informational and emotional support. Second, they can counsel parents on the importance of maintaining parental expectations for siblings. For example, if siblings have always been expected to do their homework before watching television, this expectation should continue, and parents can inquire about this issue when they call home. In addition, parents should be urged to share verbal expressions of affection with siblings whenever possible.

Communication between parents and siblings is crucial. Telephone calls, letters, and notes are meaningful even to the youngest children when parents must be absent. Similarly, tape-recorded voices or voices reading favorite stories bring a sense of continuity and reassurance to siblings. Similarly, families who have video cameras can benefit by recording both events in the hospital and events in the home to share experiences when hospitalization of the ill child is required. All these activities are directed toward maintaining the same attachment and emotional connectedness of siblings with their parents and hospitalized brother or sister, and these strategies can be suggested by nurses to parents. The last area of intervention is change management. Major changes in residence and in care providers need to be prevented whenever possible. It is best for siblings to stay in their own home and have a consistent care provider who is a family member or long-term friend who is trusted by siblings when parents must be absent. If it is impossible for parents to leave siblings at home, then they should have one place of residence, as opposed to several, and the care provider should still be consistent. Because children spend much of their life in school, the experiences and relationships there can play a major role in providing normalcy and security for siblings. In fact, an ideal situation is one in which a school nurse referral would be made automatically whenever a child is hospitalized so that school personnel would be on the alert for cues of adverse sibling responses. Other referral options include family clergy and community mental health centers.

INTERVENTION APPLICATION

Amy was a 6-year-old who had a baby brother (Ted) with congenital heart disease. Ted was quite ill and needed to go to the emergency room, physician's office, and even to be hospitalized quite often. During one trip to the clinic, Amy's parents expressed concern to their cardiology nurse that Amy was experiencing one health problem after another. In addition, she was eating a great deal, seemed to be "hyper," and was having trouble sleeping. Whenever one of the parents sat down, she climbed into his or her lap. They both stated that they did not have the knowledge or the extra energy to deal with Amy's problems when their energies were being used to cope with Ted's illness. On the basis of these reported changes in feelings and behaviors identified on the PCS, the nurse acknowledged that Amy was exhibiting ineffective coping from the many changes occurring in her life. These changes included a new baby brother, a new baby brother who was ill, perceived changes in parenting, changes in caretakers when Ted needed hospitalization, and even changes in residence if the hospitalization was long, in which case Amy stayed with a neighbor. The nurse validated parental report about changes in feelings and behaviors with Amy. Amy reported more changes than the parents reported and scored higher on the PCS than the nurse expected. The nurse then asked Amy what was the worst part about having a baby brother who was ill. Amy responded that it was "Having to pretend I am sick and take all of that medicine. It is so yuk!" The answer to the question of why Amy was having repeated illnesses was that Amy was pretending to be ill for parental attention. The Sibling Adaptation Counseling intervention was implemented with the parents through a personal counseling session followed by a tape recording for them to take home. Follow-up telephone calls were used by the nurse to reinforce learning by the parents.

Two months later, Amy was not taking any medications even though the condition of her brother was becoming more life threatening. She was "back to normal," according to her parents, in terms of ability to concentrate, ability to play with other children, and with regard to her sleeping and eating patterns. Also, she did not insist on sitting on her parents' laps whenever they were in the room. These behaviors are consistent with the indicators for Coping (Iowa Outcomes Project, 2000).

RESEARCH AND PRACTICE IMPLICATIONS

The intervention presented in this chapter has been tested. The following pilot study can assist others who wish to extend the research. The Sibling Adaptation Counseling intervention was tested in a quasi-experimental study with eight siblings of children recently diagnosed with cancer who were randomly assigned to control and experimental groups (Gradoville, 1995; Gradoville et al., 1995). The four siblings in the control group received customary family counseling, and the four siblings in the experimental group received the Sibling Adaptation Counseling intervention. Siblings were 8 to 12 years of age and closest in age to that of the ill child. Dependent variable measures included the PCS (Craft, 1985), Revised Children's Manifest Anxiety Scale (RCMAS) (Reynolds & Richmond, 1992), Child Behavior Checklist (CBCL) (Achenbach, 1991), and urinary and salivary cortisol levels, both obtained on sibling arousal in the morning. Salivary measures were obtained by asking siblings to put a cotton swab in their mouth for 1 or 2 minutes. Selected extraneous variables were measured by the Hollingshead Four Factor Index of Social Position (Hollingshead, 1975), State-Trait Anxiety Inventory (Spielberger, 1973), Norbeck's Social Support Questionnaire (Norbeck, 1982), Feetham Family Functioning Survey (Feetham, 1988), and Stress Inventory-Life Event Scale (Chandler, 1981). Data were collected in both a private and a public hospital for five measurement points during a period of 9 weeks to measure changes in response to stress.

The data showed significantly lower scores in the control group on the PCS at 7 days and significantly lower scores at 14 days for the RCMAS. Significantly higher scores occurred from baseline through 7 days on the measure of salivary cortisol in the control group ($t = -21.00$). Within the experimental group, significantly higher scores were found for the total competence in the CBCL, $t(3) = -3.00$, $p < .05$, and significantly lower scores were found from 7 to 14 days, $t(2) = 5.99$, $p < .05$. Extraneous variable scores were comparable on all measures except state and trait anxiety. There was a statistically significant difference between groups on the measure of trait anxiety at 14 days, $t(5) = 2.24$, $p < .05$, and state anxiety at baseline (7 days), $t(3) = 2.45$, $p < .05$, and at 14 to 21 days, $t(3) = 3.57$, $p < .05$, with both state and trait measures being significantly higher for parents of the experimental group.

This pilot research by my colleagues and I demonstrated that it is possible to study sibling responses using a randomized clinical trail using physiological measures for dependent variables. Furthermore, these preliminary results suggest sibling adaptation counseling might make a difference that can be supported with empirical evidence. A larger study is needed, however, and is currently being planned. This study is one of many that are needed to investigate the effectiveness of interventions to ameliorate adverse effects for siblings of ill children. These studies are difficult because they should be multivariate due to the complexity of the problem and longitudinal to determine intervention effects over time. Such complex and resource-intensive studies require funding. To many in the health sciences, however, the welfare of siblings is of lesser importance than other funding priorities. It is possible that the national sensitivity for the need for prevention may increase attention toward interventions such as Sibling Adaptation Counseling.

In the meantime, nurses who practice in every setting have numerous opportunities to assess siblings and counsel parents using this intervention. Every sibling should be assessed using the brief PCS. Furthermore, siblings need all the information that is given to parents, and siblings need to be included in the care of the ill child. The lives of siblings need to be as normal as possible, with efforts made to increase their sense of competence and mastery.

In summary, empirical research on sibling responses for more than a decade led me to specify and test a model to identify causal influences on sibling responses to develop an intervention that promotes positive adaptation. In this chapter, the resulting intervention and the pilot testing of the intervention have been discussed. There are still many unknown variables influencing sibling adaptation to the experience of an ill brother or sister, and more research is needed on these influences and interventions to ameliorate negative influences (Minagawa, 1997; Sahler et al., 1997; Thompson, 1994; Williams et al., 1997). More research is being planned. Readers are encouraged to be active in sharing their experiences with the use of this intervention. More important, readers are encouraged to be active in assisting this population of children to deal with a difficult life event so that it becomes a growth-promoting experience for them and for their families. Illness in a brother or sister may be a question of vulnerability or resilience (Leonard, 1991). It is the responsibility of the nurse to make it a question of resilience.

REFERENCES

Achenbach, T. M. (1991). *Manual for child behavior checklist for ages 4-18 and 1001 profile.* Burlington: University of Vermont, Department of Psychiatry.

Adams, R., Peveler, R. C., Stein, A., & Dunger, D. B. (1991). Siblings of children with diabetes: Involvement, understanding and adaptation. *Diabetic Medicine, 8*(9), 855-859.

Cairns, N. U., Clark, G. M., Smith, S. F., & Lansky, S. B. (1979). Adaptation of siblings to childhood malignancy. *Journal of Pediatrics, 95*(3), 484-487.

Canam, C. (1987). Coping with feelings: Chronically ill children and their families. *Nursing Papers/Perspectives in Nursing, 19*(3), 9-21.

Carandang, M. L. A., Folkins, C. H., Hines, P. A., & Steward, M. S. (1979). The role of cognitive level and sibling illness in children's conceptualizations of illness. *American Journal of Orthopsychiatry, 49*(3), 474-481.

Carr-Gregg, M., & White, L. (1987). Siblings of pediatric cancer patients: A population at risk. *Medical and Pediatric Oncology, 15*(2), 62-68.

Chandler, L. A. (1981). The source of stress inventory. *Psychology in the Schools, 18*(2), 164-168.

Craft, M. (1985). Responses in siblings of hospitalized children (Doctoral dissertation, University of Iowa, 1985). *Dissertation Abstracts International, 87,* 6040B.

Craft, M. J. (1986). Responses in school-aged siblings of hospitalized children: Validation of self-report data. *Children's Health Care, 14*(5), 272-280.

Craft, M. J. (1993). Siblings of hospitalized children: Assessment and intervention. *Journal of Pediatric Nursing, 8*(5), 289-296.

Craft, M. J., Cohen, M., Titler, M., & DeHammer, M. (1993). Experiences in children of critically ill parents: A time of emotional disruption and need for support. *Critical Care Nurse Quarterly, 16*(3), 64-71.

Craft, M. J., & Craft, J. L. (1989). Responses in siblings of hospitalized children: A comparison of sibling and parent perception. *Children's Health Care, 18,* 42-49.

Craft, M. J., & Wyatt, N. (1986). Effect of visitation upon siblings of hospitalized children. *Maternal Child Nursing Journal, 15,* 47-59.

Craft, M. J., Wyatt, N., & Sandell, B. (1985). Feeling and behavior changes in siblings of hospitalized children. *Clinical Pediatrics, 24*(7), 374-378.

Craft-Rosenberg, M. J. (2000). *Sibling adaptation model.* Manuscript in review.

Cuskelly, M., & Gunn, P. (1993). Maternal reports of behavior of siblings of children with Down syndrome. *American Journal on Mental Retardation, 97*(5), 521-529.

Dorn, L. D. (1984). Children's concepts of illness: Clinical applications. *Pediatric Nursing, 10*(5), 325-327.

Dunn, J. (1983). Sibling relationships in early childhood. *Child Development, 54*(3), 787-811.

Dunn, J., & Munn, P. (1985). Becoming a family member: Family conflict and the development of social understanding in the second year. *Child Development, 56*(2), 480-492.

Dunn, J., & Shatz, M. (1989). Becoming a conversationalist despite (or because of) having an older sibling. *Child Development, 60*(2), 399-410.

Dyson, L., Edgar, E., & Crnic, K. (1989). Psychological predictors of adjustment by siblings of developmentally disabled children. *American Journal of Mental Retardation, 94*(3), 292-302.

Faux, S. A. (1991). Sibling relationships in families with congenitally impaired children. *Journal of Pediatric Nursing, 6*(3), 175-183.

Feetham, S. L. (1988). *Feetham Family Functioning Survey.* Washington, DC: Children's Hospital National Medical Center.

Gallo, A. M., Breitmayer, B. J., Knafl, K. A., & Zoeller, L. H. (1991). Well siblings of children with chronic illness: Parents' reports of their psychological adjustment. *Pediatric Nursing, 18,* 23-27.

Garmezy, N., & Rutter, M. (1983). *Stress, coping, and development in children.* New York: McGraw-Hill.

Gradoville, K. (1995). *Sibling adaptation counseling: A pilot study.* Unpublished thesis, University of Iowa, Iowa City.

Gradoville, K., Craft-Rosenberg, M. J., Denehy, J., & Gagan, M. J. (1995). Adaptation counseling for siblings of children with cancer. *Current Issues Affecting Office Based Pediatric Nurses, 6*(2), 1-6.

Guyton, A. C. (1986). *Textbook of medical physiology.* Philadelphia: W. B. Saunders.

Havermans, T., & Eiser, C. (1994). Siblings of a child with cancer. *Child: Care, Health and Development, 20*(5), 309-322.

Heffernan, S. M., & Zanelli, A. S. (1997). Behavior changes exhibited by siblings of pediatric oncology patients: A comparison between maternal and sibling descriptions. *Journal of Pediatric Oncology Nursing, 14,* 3-14.

Hollingshead, A. B. (1975). *Four Factor Index for Social Position.* New Haven, CT: Yale University, Department of Sociology.

Iles, P. J. (1979). Children with cancer: Healthy siblings' perspectives during the illness experience. *Cancer Nursing, 2*(5), 371-377.

Iowa Outcomes Project. (2000). *Nursing outcomes classification (NOC)* (M. Johnson, M. Maas, & S. Moorhead, Eds.; 2nd ed.). St. Louis, MO: Mosby-Year book.

Kleiber, C., Montgomery, L. A., & Craft-Rosenberg, M. J. (1995). Information needs of the siblings of critically ill children. *Children's Health Care, 24,* 47-60.

Knafl, K. A. (1982). Parents' views of the responses of sibling to pediatric hospitalization. *Research in Nursing and Health, 5,* 13-20.

Knafl, K. A., Cavallari, K. A., & Dixon, D. M. (1988). *Pediatric hospitalization: Family and nurse perspectives.* Boston: Scott, Foresman.

Knafl, K. A., & Dixon, D. M. (1983). The role of siblings during pediatric hospitalization. *Issues in Comprehensive Pediatric Nursing, 6,* 13-22.

Kramer, R. F. (1981). Living with childhood cancer: Healthy siblings. Perspective. *Issues in Comprehensive Pediatric Nursing, 5*(3), 155-165.

Kruger, S., Shauver, M., & Jones, L. (1980). Reactions of families the child with cystic fibrosis. *Image: The Journal of Nursing Scholarship, 12*(3), 72-74.

Lazarus, R. S., & Folkman, S. (1984). *Stress, appraisal, and coping.* New York: Springer.

Leonard, B. J. (1991). Siblings of chronically ill children. *Pediatric Annals, 20*(9), 501-506.

Martinson, I. M., Gilliss, C., Colaizzo, D. C., Freeman, M., & Bossert, E. (1990). Impact of childhood cancer on healthy school-age siblings. *Cancer Nursing, 13*(3), 1183-1990.

McCollum, A. (1975). *Coping with prolonged health impairment in your child.* Boston: Little, Brown.

McKeever, P. (1983). Siblings of chronically ill children: A literature review with implications for research and practice. *American Journal of Orthopsychiatry, 53*(2), 209-218.

Minagawa, M. (1997). Sibling relationships of Japanese children with diabetes. *Journal of Pediatric Nursing, 12*(5), 311-316.

Montgomery, L. A. (1988). *Responses in preschool siblings of ill children.* Unpublished thesis, University of Iowa, Iowa City.

Montgomery, L. A., Kleiber, C., Nicholson, A., & Craft-Rosenberg, M. J. (1997). A research-based sibling visitation program for the neonatal ICU. *Critical Care Nurse, 17*(2), 29-35.

Mott, M. G. (1990). A child with cancer: A family in crisis. *British Medical Journal, 301*(6744), 133-134.

Norbeck, J. S. (1982). *Norbeck Social Support Questionnaire.* San Francisco: University of California, San Francisco.

North American Nursing Diagnosis Association. (1999). *Nursing diagnoses: Definitions and classification 1999-2000.* Philadelphia: Author.

Piaget, J., & Inhelder, B. (1969). *The psychology of the child.* New York: Basic Books.

Reynolds, C. R., & Richmond, B. O. (1992). *Revised children's manifest anxiety scale manual.* Los Angeles: Western Psychological Services.

Sahler, O. J., Roghmann, K. J., Mulhern, R. K., Carpenter, P. J., Sargent, J. R., Copeland, D. R., Barbarin, O. A., Zeltzer, L. K., & Dolgin, M. J. (1997). Sibling adaptation to childhood cancer collaborative study: The association of sibling adaptation with maternal well-being, physical health, and resource use. *Journal of Developmental & Behavioral Pediatrics, 18*(4), 233-243.

Selye, H. (1956). *The stress of life.* New York: McGraw-Hill.

Siegel, M. G. (1987). *Psychological testing from early childhood through adolescence.* Madison, CT: International Universities Press.

Simeonsson, R. J., & Bailey, D. B. (1986). Siblings of handicapped children. In J. J. Gallagher & P. M. Vietze (Eds.), *Families of handicapped persons* (pp. 46-64). Baltimore, MD: Brooks.

Simon, K. (1993). Perceived stress of nonhospitalized children during the hospitalization of a sibling. *Journal of Pediatric Nursing, 8*(5), 298-304.

Spielberger, C. D. (1973). *State-Trait Anxiety Inventory for Children: Preliminary manual.* Palo Alto, CA: Consulting Psychologists Press.

Spinetta, J. J. (1981). The siblings of the child with cancer. In J. J. Spinetta & P. Deasy-Spinetta (Eds.), *Living with childhood cancer* (pp. 133-142). St. Louis, MO: C. V. Mosby.

Stewart, D. A., Stein, A., Forrest, G. C., & Clark, D. M. (1992). Psychosocial adjustment in siblings of children with chronic life-threatening illness: A research note. *Journal of Child Psychology and Psychiatry, 33*(4), 779-784.

Taylor, S. (1980). The effects of chronic childhood illnesses upon well siblings. *Maternal Child Nursing Journal, 9*(2), 109-116.

Thompson, A. B. (1994). The psychosocial adjustment of well sibling of chronically ill children. *Children's Health Care, 23*(3), 211-226.

Titler, M., Cohen, M., & Craft, M. J. (1991). The impact of adult critical care hospitalization: Perceptions of patients, spouses, children, and nurses. *Heart & Lung, 20*(2), 174-182.

Walker, C. (1990). Siblings of children with cancer. *Oncology Nursing Forum, 17*(3), 355-360.

Williams, P. D., Hanson, R., Ridder, L., Liebergern, A., Olson, F., Barnard, M. U., & Tobin-Rommelhart, S. (1997). Outcomes of a nursing intervention for siblings of chronically ill children: A pilot study. *Journal of the Society of Pediatric Nurses, 2*(3), 127-137.

Williams, P. D., Lorenzo, F. D., & Borja, M. (1993). Pediatric chronic illness: Effects on siblings and mothers. *Maternal Child Nursing Journal, 21*(4), 11-21.

21

Visitation Facilitation

Anita Nicholson

Critical care hospitalization of a family member often occurs suddenly, leaving families in a state of crisis. Illness in one family member can disrupt the functioning of the entire family system (Guidubaldi & Clemenshaw, 1985; McKeever, 1983; von Bertalanffy, 1968). Children experience stress and behavioral changes in response to the illness of a loved one (Craft, 1986, 1993; Craft, Wyatt, & Sandell, 1985). Although there has been considerable research on methods to meet needs of adults in families, little emphasis has been placed on children and helping them cope with the stress of a critically ill family member.

Critical care nurses need to implement interventions that meet the needs of children of critically ill patients. Visitation Facilitation in critical care units (CCUs) by nurses is an intervention designed to meet these needs. Children have not routinely been allowed to visit CCUs because of a concern regarding the epidemiological risk of exposing patients to infection. There are no data to support this concern, however (Kowba & Schwirian, 1985; Umphenour, 1980; Wranesh, 1982). Another common reason for failure to allow children to visit CCUs is the fear of adverse emotional effects on the child. Data from the two studies implemented on facilitating child visitation in CCUs, however, have shown no harm to the children (Nicholson et al., 1993; Titler et al., 2000).

Healthy People 2000 (U.S. Department of Health and Human Services, 1991) advocates the promotion of mental health by focusing on

347

decreasing stressors and increasing the capacity of families to cope with stress. Interventions are needed to improve the family well-being during stressful life events and promote family support systems. The Visitation Facilitation intervention was developed to address these needs. The goal of Visitation Facilitation is to help family members, including children, cope with the stress of a critically ill loved one. The intervention fosters family support to ameliorate the adverse emotional effects family members and children experience. The purpose of this chapter is to review the Visitation Facilitation intervention and suggest successful implementation activities for nurses. The impact of the intervention on children and family members will be discussed.

THEORETICAL FRAMEWORK AND LITERATURE REVIEW

Family systems, stress, and coping theories provide the theoretical perspective for preparing children to visit a sick family member (Cannon, 1914; Lazarus, 1966; Lazarus & Folkman 1984; Selye, 1956; von Bertalanffy, 1968). Families are viewed as dynamic open systems composed of individual subsystems (family members such as parents or children) who interact with one another and the health care system in an attempt to maintain homeostasis and health of their members (Craft & Willadsen, 1992). Craft and Willadsen (1992) define *family* as

> a societal context of two or more people characterized by mutual attachment, caring, long-term commitment, and responsibility to provide individual growth, supportive relationships, health of members and of the unit, and maintenance of the organization and system during constant individual, family, and societal change. (p. 519)

Changes in one subsystem, such as parents, have an impact on the other subsystems and the functioning of the family (Feetham, 1984). Nurses must consider the impact of an illness on all family members and treat a patient within the family context to provide family-centered care (Craft & Willadsen, 1992).

Families commonly appraise the critical illness of a loved one as a stressful event. Lazarus and Folkman (1984) define *coping* as constantly changing cognitive and behavioral efforts to manage specific external and internal demands that are appraised as exceeding the individual's resources. *Coping* refers to psychological and behavioral activities used to overcome external or internal demands and conflicts (Lazarus, 1966). Individual family members react to the stressor of a critical illness with a wide variety of behavioral and emotional responses to maintain some degree of homeostasis. Family members of the critically ill often experience feelings of being overwhelmed, vulnerable, and helpless (Daley, 1984; Molter, 1979; Titler, Cohen, & Craft, 1991). When the coping responses are limited, the external stressful event can lead to an interpersonal crisis as well (Lazarus, 1966; Lazarus & Folkman, 1984). The behavioral and emotional responses illicited by the crisis of critical illness of a loved one will vary depending on the role of the family member and the interaction among the individuals in the family. Many factors, including these feelings, coupled with limited coping responses can lead to interpersonal crises.

Families provide the critically ill member with physical and psychological support, comfort, and reassurance. Families also have specific needs that include the need to see the patient and the need for information, support, and decreased anxiety (Jamerson et al., 1996; Molter, 1979). Data from studies on restricted visitation have shown that family members experience increased hostility, anger, and fears (Bedsworth & Molen, 1982; Halm, 1990; Titler, Cohen, & Craft, 1991). These emotions were commonly directed at the nursing staff and contributed to strained nurse-family interactions (Bedsworth & Molen, 1982; Titler et al., 1991). Nurses play an important role in supporting visitation practices to help meet needs of patients and family members and to provide the family and patient with some measure of control (Brannon & Gailey, 1990; Heater, 1985; Krapohl, 1995). Visitation policies vary from hospital to hospital regarding guidelines, age restriction, visiting times, and locations within the hospital setting (Kirchhoff, 1982; Titler, 1995; Titler & Walsh, 1992), but there is an increasing awareness of the importance of allowing children to visit their relatives in the CCU (Nicholson et al., 1993; Smith, 1998; Titler et al., 2000). Young children who are denied hospital visitation privileges can develop distorted perceptions of reality. They may, in fact, develop misconceptions and fantasies about the ill family member that are more distressing than the actual reality (Shuler & Reich, 1982; Titler et al., 1991).

A qualitative research study on the impact of adult critical care hospitalization on children revealed that parents shielded their children from visiting a parent in the critical care unit. Children were able to accurately describe what was happening to the hospitalized parent in accurate terms despite this protective posture, however (Titler et al., 1991). A common adult assumption is that children cannot cope with crises such as illness or poor prognosis of a family member, and children should be protected by lack of information. Empirical data do not support this assumption, however (Shuler & Reich, 1982; Titler et al., 1991). This study was followed by two others on child Visitation Facilitation in the CCUs.

The first study examined the behavioral and emotional responses of children and nonhospitalized family members to facilitate child visitation in the CCU setting in a quasi-experimental study (Nicholson et al., 1993). Twenty families participated—10 families in a restricted and 10 families in a facilitated visitation group. The children in the latter group received systematic facilitation and supervision during visitation to a critically ill adult family member in a surgical CCU and provision of emotional support before, during, and after the visitation. Children in the facilitated visitation group experienced a greater reduction ($t = 4.0$, $df = 18$, $p = .0004$) in negative behavioral and emotional changes as measured by the Child-Perceived Change Scale (Craft, 1985) when compared with those in the restricted visitation group.

A second study, replicated the study by Nicholson et al. (1993), used a larger sample size (Titler et al., 2000). Fifty-two families participated—30 families in a restricted and 22 families in a facilitated visitation group. Children in the facilitated visitation group did not have a greater reduction in behavioral and emotional responses compared to children in the restricted visitation group. The findings showed the behavioral and emotional responses of the children in both the restricted and the facilitated visitation groups decreased over time. Although the facilitated child visitation intervention was not found to decrease behavioral and emotional responses, an important finding of this study was that the children did not experience adverse behavioral and emotional responses from visiting their loved one in the CCU. Also, a significant treatment by time effect ($F = 6.33$, $p = .01$) was found on the Revised Children's Manifest Anxiety Scale, Social Concern/Concentration score (Reynolds & Richmond, 1985). Children receiving the Visitation Facilitation intervention had a greater decline in their score compared to children in the restricted visitation group. The findings suggest that children who visited in the CCU experienced improved concentration and had fewer social concerns, such as how others perceived them. The findings from both studies suggest that child visitation in the CCUs was not harmful to the child and may have been beneficial in helping the child cope with the critical illness of a loved one. Additional replication studies in this area are needed with larger sample sizes.

Children whose loved ones are critically ill have many unique needs that often go unnoticed and unmet due to the stress of the family (Baker, Nieswidomy, & Arnold, 1988). The parents' concern at the time of crisis is focused on the ill family member, leading them to be less aware of the needs and feeling of the child (Craft, 1979, 1986, 1993; Craft & Wyatt, 1986; Craft et al., 1985). Children often feel guilty for the illness of the loved one. Parents need to explain to children that they had nothing to do with the illness. Children also may fear getting the same illness; therefore, children need open lines of communication with the parents about the ill family member and honest dialogue on the likelihood that the children could get the illness (Craft, 1979, 1986; Craft & Wyatt, 1986).

Preparing young children for a stressful situation requires more than a simple explanation because of their immature verbal and comprehension skills. Helpful methods in giving young children information include the use of play, puppets, storybooks, and pictures (Baker et al., 1988; Ferguson, 1979). If children are able to visit the loved one, preparation for what to expect at the hospital and the appearance of the patient is needed. It is helpful for children to know what will be seen, heard, smelled, and felt. In addition, encouragement of expression of feelings is healthy for children and important before and after visitation (Baker et al., 1988; Craft & Wyatt, 1986; Johnson, 1994). Research is advocating the use of open, honest communication with children to assist them in coping with the illness of a family member. Child visitation provides a realistic experience concerning hospitalization, and it opens the door for communication (Craft & Wyatt, 1986; Shuler & Reich, 1982; Titler et al., 1991). Health care professionals need to explain to parents that changes in their child's behavior are common and very understandable. Nurses need to guide parents toward interventions to help their child cope with the illness of a loved one.

NURSING DIAGNOSIS AND OUTCOME DETERMINATION

Several nursing diagnoses might trigger the intervention Visitation Facilitation of children in adult CCUs, including Altered Family Processes, Ineffective Family Coping, Knowledge Deficit, Anxiety, Fear, Hopelessness, and Anticipatory Grieving (North American Nursing Diagnosis Association [NANDA], 1999). Outcomes of the first three nursing diagnoses will be discussed in detail.

The situational crisis and stressor of a critical illness of an adult family member can be overwhelming to a family and lead to altered family processes. The desired outcome of Visitation Facilitation is to help the family members return to their prior level of family functioning to meet their physical and emotional needs.

Ineffective Family Coping can occur during the crisis of a critically ill loved one. Family members can become so overwhelmed with the stressor of the critical illness that their coping mechanisms fail. Important Nursing Outcomes Classification (NOC) indicators of Coping that apply to family members of the critically ill include (a) identifying effective coping patterns, (b) seeking information concerning illness and treatment, (c) using available social support, and (d) using effective coping strategies (Iowa Outcomes Project, 2000). The desired outcome is to help family members return to their prior level of family coping.

of extraneous items, and shielding the patient housed in an open bay unit from other patients.

The child and NHAFM are assisted by the nurse to wash hands and prepare for visiting. Preparation might include the wearing of a mask or gown or both depending on institutional epidemiological recommendations. The nurse accompanies the child and NHAFM and remains present during the visit. The nurse is present to answer questions about the patient's appearance and the lights and sounds of the equipment. Children are commonly very inquisitive about the equipment, flashing lights, and buzzers. The nurse explains the alarms and how the equipment is helping the patient. The CCU environment can be less frightening to children if they know how the equipment is helping their loved one. The nurse monitors the responses of the patient and child and facilitates conversation. Commonly, after the child's questions are answered by the nurse, the parents take over and continue to facilitate the interaction between the patient and child. Most visits last between 10 and 20 minutes.

After the visit, the nurse meets with the child and NHAFM to talk about the visit using the following questions: Tell me about your visit, what did you feel? Do you have any questions? and Would you like to visit again? Nurses evaluate the child's verbal and nonverbal responses. If the child appears stressed and the nurse feels professionally unable to deal with the response, the nurse may call on additional resources, such as clinical nursing specialists, child development specialists, psychiatric nurses, hospital psychologists, or social workers, to assist with further debriefing and follow-up.

The nurse encourages the NHAFM to talk about the visit with the child after they leave. The child may be more willing to express his or her feelings in private. The nurse also provides the NHAFM with additional recommendations for ongoing support such as maintaining normality by keeping similar routines, habits, and rituals and being truthful and honest about the loved one's condition. The follow-up after the visit takes approximately 10 minutes.

Nursing staff wanting to use Visitation Facilitation may wish to make "child visitation cue cards." A set of cue cards summarizing the intervention, including the steps of the previsit, the visit, and the postvisit, is helpful to prevent omission of important information. Photographs of a CCU bedside and equipment (such as ventilator, cardiac monitors, and intravenous pumps) are helpful to show children during a previsit what they will see in the unit. Developmental level cue cards that briefly outline the developmental tasks and typical behaviors that children display when under stress are helpful so that the nursing staff will know what to say to children of different ages. For example, for the 5- to 10-year-old group, the cue cards remind the nursing staff that the key developmental task is industry versus inferiority. A typical behavior demonstrated is withdrawal, and a useful strategy is to provide the child with accurate, honest information and encourage expression of feelings. The cue cards and photographs can be attached to a key ring and placed on a shelf at the nurse's station with health screening forms.

If the child does not wish to visit, it is important that the nursing staff provide family members with other interventions to support the child. Some ideas include planning special activities with the child; providing consistent caretakers for the child in the child's home if possible; giving honest, simple updates about the loved one's condition on a regular basis; using commercially prepared or unit-designed coloring books or photo books that explain critical illness to the child; and encouraging the child to send photos, colored pictures, audiotapes, and other personal items to be available at the loved one's bedside (Montgomery, 1988).

INTERVENTION APPLICATION

Visitation Facilitation was implemented in the surgical intensive care unit (SICU), which was a research site for the two studies (Nicholson et al., 1993; Titler et al., 2000). Sarah was an 8-year-old who participated in the intervention. Sarah's father, Joe, was in a traumatic motorcycle accident 24 hours ago. The suddenness of the accident contributed to the diagnoses of Anxiety and Fear (NANDA, 1999). The nurse contacted Sarah and her mother, Mary, in the waiting room. The SICU had restricted child visitation; therefore, when the opportunity arose for Sarah to visit her father, she was very excited to participate in the Visitation Facilitation intervention. A time was scheduled for Sarah to visit her father. Prior to the visit, the nurse talked with Sarah and her mother to obtain background information on what Sarah knew about her father's injuries so that her needs could best be met. Sarah had been well informed by her mother about her father's accident and injuries. She knew he had many broken bones and was on a breathing machine.

The nurse talked privately with Mary about any behavioral changes noted in Sarah. Mary reported Sarah appeared much more emotional, restless, and irritable since her father's accident. The nurse explained to Mary that her behavior was "normal" and that visiting a loved one in the CCU can open many feelings and emotions. It would be normal for Sarah to feel sad and cry when she sees her father. While the nurse was visiting with Mary and Sarah, other nurses were preparing Joe's bedside by straightening the linens and closing the curtains to other patient beds. Joe's condition was stable, and he wanted Sarah to visit.

At the time of the visit, the nurse talked with Sarah in more detail about the visit. Sarah was very excited to see her father and missed him very much. She verbalized feeling "sad and sorry" that he was hurt. Sarah had never been in a hospital before, so the nurse used simple terms and pictures to explain what she would see and hear during the visit. For example, Joe was on a ventilator and the nurse explained, "This is a machine to help your dad breathe for a short time until he can breathe on his own again." She explained to Sarah that this machine makes many beeping and buzzing sounds. The nurse also used a picture to simply explain the oral endotracheal tube and why her father would temporarily not be able to talk. The nurse and Sarah worked on writing out some yes-no questions that she would ask him. The nurse also explained her father's appearance. Joe had experienced facial trauma with severe swelling and bruising on his forehead, eyes, and cheeks. She explained to Sarah that the bruising and swelling would last 3 or 4 weeks, and then his face would return to normal because none of the bones in it were broken.

Sarah's health screening survey was completed, and the nurse assisted her with washing hands before they entered the SICU. Sarah held her mother's hand as they walked up to Joe's bedside. Sarah eagerly grabbed her father's hand and said, "I love you and miss you dad! Please get better fast." Joe smiled through the oral endotracheal tube. His eyes sparkled seeing his daughter. During the first few minutes, Sarah was inquisitive about all the equipment she had seen in the pictures. She wanted to be reassured that the flashing lights and buzzers were okay. The nurse reexplained the alarms and some of the equipment. Once she was more comfortable with her surroundings, she talked to her father about the kids she had met in the waiting room and how she liked eating in the cafeteria. The visit lasted approximately 15 minutes. Joe wrote Sarah a note, "I love you, come see me again soon."

Afterwards, Sarah was grinning from ear to ear about visiting her father. She was very happy to see him and could not wait unit the next visit. Sarah talked about how good it was to see him, and that after seeing him she knew he would be okay. She also verbalized relief that the swelling in his face would decrease, but he did not look as bad as she thought he would look. The nurse encouraged Mary to continue to talk with Sarah about the visit and her feelings. She praised Mary for keeping Sarah well informed of her father's condition and sharing information that was helping Sarah to reach the indicators of anxiety control and fear control. Sarah appeared to be coping well with her father's accident.

RESEARCH AND PRACTICE IMPLICATIONS

Replication studies are needed on the child Visitation Facilitation intervention in CCUs. The studies were implemented at a large tertiary health care center in the Midwest. Replication of this study is needed in small and large hospitals throughout the United States to sample diverse populations with varied cultures, races, and socioeconomic status. A majority of the research data were obtained from the SICU. Other critical care settings should also be used as data collection sites, such as medical, cardiovascular, and pediatric units, to demonstrate the effectiveness of the intervention in these settings. Follow-up study on the psychological effects of the intervention is needed to determine the long-term effects. Home interviews regarding the effects of the intervention would be helpful to determine how the child and family members are coping. Also, additional research is needed to examine the behavioral, emotional, and physiological effects of the intervention on patients.

Many families during the research studies verbalized the importance of their children visiting in the CCU and that Visitation Facilitation was very helpful. Children received important, age-appropriate information about their loved ones and actually got to see them in the critical care environment. The intervention helped the children get a more accurate view of the situation by informing them of the patient's condition. The intervention was simple and systematic in preparing children to visit in the CCU to help the family unit work through the crisis of the critical illness. It is an intervention that can and should be implemented in any setting to assist children and their families.

REFERENCES

Baker, C., Nieswidomy, R., & Arnold, W. (1988). Nursing interventions for children with a parent in the intensive care unit. *Heart & Lung, 17,* 441-446.

Bedsworth, I., & Molen, M. (1982). Psychological stress in spouses of patients with myocardial infarction. *Heart & Lung, 11*(5), 450-456.

Brannon, A., & Gailey, A. (1990). Visitation in the ICU: From "rules" to contracts. *Nursing Management, 21,* 64-65.

Cannon, W. (1914). The emergency functions of the adrenal medulla in pain or in the major emotions. *American Journal of Physiology, 33,* 356-377.

Craft, M. J. (1979). Help for the family's neglected other child. *MCN: American Journal of Maternal Child Nursing, 4,* 297-300.

Craft, M. J. (1985). *Perceived Change Scale (child and parent forms).* Iowa City: University of Iowa, College of Nursing.

Craft, M. J. (1986). Validation of responses reported by school-aged siblings of hospitalized children. *Children's Health Care, 15,* 6-13.

Craft, M. J. (1993). Siblings of hospitalized children: Assessment and intervention. *Journal of Pediatric Nursing, 8*(5), 289-297.

Craft, M. J., & Willadsen, J. (1992). Nursing interventions related to family. *Nursing Clinics of North America, 27,* 517-541.

Craft, M. J., & Wyatt, N. (1986). Effect of visitation upon siblings of hospitalized children. *Maternal Child Nursing Journal, 15,* 47-59.

Craft, M. J., Wyatt, N., & Sandell, B. (1985). Behavior and feeling changes in siblings of hospitalized children. *Clinical Pediatrics, 24,* 374-378.

Daley, L. (1984). The perceived immediate needs of families with relatives in the intensive care setting. *Heart & Lung, 13*(3), 231-237.

Feetham, S. (1984). Family research: Issues and directions for nursing. In H. Werley & J. Fitzpatrick (Eds.), *Annual review of nursing research* (pp. 3-27). New York: Springer.

Ferguson, B. F. (1979). Preparing young children for hospitalization: A comparison of two methods. *Pediatrics, 64*(5), 656-664.

Guidubaldi, J., & Clemenshaw, H. (1985). Divorce, family health, and child adjustment. *Family Relations, 34,* 35-41.

Halm, M. (1990). The effect of support groups on anxiety of family members during critical illness. *Heart & Lung, 19,* 62-71.

Heater, B. (1985). Nursing responsibilities in changing visiting restrictions in the intensive care unit. *Heart & Lung, 14*(2), 181-186.

Iowa Intervention Project. (2000). *Nursing interventions classification (NIC)* (J. C. McCloskey & G. Bulechek, Eds.; 3rd ed.). St. Louis, MO: Mosby-Year Book.

Iowa Outcomes Project. (2000). *Nursing outcomes classification (NOC)* (M. Johnson, M. Maas, & S. Moorhead, Eds.; 2nd ed.). St. Louis, MO: Mosby-Year Book.

Jamerson, P., Scheibmeir, M., Bott, M., Crighton, F., Hinton, R., & Cobb, A. (1996). The experiences of families with a relative in the intensive care unit. *Heart & Lung, 25*(6), 467-474.

Johnson, D. (1994). Preparing children for visiting parents in the adult ICU. *Dimensions of Critical Care Nursing, 13*(3), 152-165.

Kirchhoff, K. (1982). Visiting policies for patients with myocardial infarctions—A national survey. *Heart & Lung, 11*(6), 571-576.

Kowba, M., & Schwirian, P. (1985). Direct sibling contact and bacterial colonization in newborns. *Journal of Obstetric, Gynecologic, and Neonatal Nursing, 14,* 412-417.

Krapohl, G. L. (1995). Visiting hours in the adult intensive care unit: Using research to develop a system that works. *Dimensions of Critical Care Nursing, 14*(5), 245-258.

Lazarus, R. (1966). *Psychological stress and the coping process.* New York: McGraw-Hill.

Lazarus, R., & Folkman, S. (1984). *Stress, appraisal and coping.* New York: Springer.

McKeever, P. (1983). Siblings of chronically ill children: A literature review with implications for research and practice. *American Journal of Orthopsychiatry, 53,* 209-217.

Molter, N. (1979). Needs of relatives of critically ill patients; A descriptive study. *Heart & Lung, 6*(3), 332-339.

Montgomery, L. A. (1988). *Response in preschool children to the hospitalization of a newborn sibling.* Unpublished master's thesis, University of Iowa, College of Nursing, Iowa City.

Nicholson, A. C., Titler, M., Montgomery, L. A., Kleiber, C., Craft, M. J., Halm, M., Buckwalter, K., & Johnson, S. (1993). Effects of child visitation in adult critical care units: A pilot study. *Heart & Lung, 22,* 36-45.

North American Nursing Diagnosis Association. (1999). *Nursing diagnoses: Definitions and classifications 1999-2000.* Philadelphia: Author.

Reynolds, C., & Richmond, B. (1985). *Revised Children's Manifest Anxiety Scale manual.* Los Angeles: Western Psychological Services.

Selye, H. (1956). *The stress of life.* New York: McGraw-Hill.

Shuler, S., & Reich, C. (1982). Sibling visitation in pediatric hospitalization: Policies, opinions, issues. *Children's Health Care, 11,* 54-60.

Smith, M. B. E. (1998). A study of facilities for siblings on the neonatal unit: Enhancing family care. *Journal of Neonatal Nursing, 4*(5), 18-22.

Titler, M. (1995). Changing visiting practices in critical care units. *Medical Surgical Nursing, 4,* 65-68.

Titler, M., Cohen, M., & Craft, M. J. (1991). Impact of critical hospitalization: Perceptions of patients, spouses, children and nurses. *Heart & Lung, 20*(2), 174-181.

Titler, M., Nicholson, A., Halm, M., Montgomery, L. A., Kleiber, C., Craft, M. J., Buckwalter, K., & Johnson, S. (2000). *Effects of child visitation in adult critical care units.* Unpublished manuscript.

Titler, M., & Walsh, S. (1992). Visiting critically ill adults. *Family Issues in Critical Care, 4*(4), 623-632.

Umphenour, H. (1980). Bacterial colonization in neonates with sibling visitation. *Journal of Obstetric, Gynecologic, and Neonatal Nursing, 9,* 73-75.

U.S. Department of Health and Human Services. (1991). *Healthy people 2000: National health promotion and disease prevention objectives* (DHHS Publication No. PHS 91-50312). Washington DC: Government Printing Office.

von Bertalanffy, L. (1968). *General systems theory: Foundation, development, application.* New York: George Braziller.

Wranesh, B. (1982). The effect of sibling visitation on bacterial colonization rates in neonates. *Journal of Obstetric, Gynecologic, and Neonatal Nursing, 11,* 211-213.

Forming friendships may be especially difficult for children who are disabled or chronically ill (Short, & Noll, 1998; Yude, Goodman, & McConachie, 1998). The physical needs or abilities of disabled or ill children often preclude their attendance at places where they can meet and interact with potential friends. When disabled or chronically ill children do engage in peer interactions, the situations are often scripted, less spontaneous, and less conducive to developing true friendship (Pflederer, 1990). In many cases, children who have an infirmity are organized into play or peer groups that center around the infirmity, such as camps for children with diabetes, and not around their distinct personality characteristics. Although these encounters are valuable (Bluebond-Langner, Perkel, & Goertzel, 1991), they are not representative of the reality of the children's lives. Because the development of social competence is highly related to the opportunities and ability to engage in intimate social interactions from infancy to adulthood, these opportunities should be as plentiful and diverse as possible (Hartup, 1996). Friendship Promotion is an intervention that can be used to decrease social isolation and increase social competence and self-worth.

LITERATURE REVIEW

Social competence, self-esteem, and friendships are inextricably entwined (Rose & Asher, 1999; Zarbatany, Van-Brunschot, Meadow, & Pepper, 1996). Coleman and Lindsay (1992) noted that "self-esteem is greatly enhanced by the peer acceptance often stemming from well-developed social skills" (p. 552). *Social competence* has been defined as "children's abilities to (a) seek out peers and initiate/sustain positive interactions with them . . . (b) form affiliative ties or relationships with peers . . . and (c) avoid debilitating peer-related emotional states . . . and peer relationships" (Ladd & Le Sieur, 1995, p. 378). Emphasizing the importance that peer relations, acceptance, and friendships have for children, Grey (1990) observed that "resilient children are characterized as having strong feelings of competence and having a network of relatives and friends who provide basic affirmation and support. They are central to children's concepts of who they are and what they can do successfully" (p. 309). Likewise, Berndt and Keefe (1995) documented the positive effect of friendships on school adjustment during adolescence. The formation of friendships depends on the child's developmental capacity and ability to commit resources to the relationship (Caroline, 1993). Because only a small number of the many social interactions in which a child engages evolve into friendships, the child needs as many opportunities to make friends as possible (Pflederer, 1990, p. 201).

Research has documented the important role parents play in their children's social competence (Howes, Hamilton, & Philipsen, 1998). Early attachment positively and strongly correlates with later ability to form friendships (Freitag, Belsky, Grossman, Grossmann, & Scheuerer-Englisch, 1996; Ladd & LeSieur, 1995). Once thought of as separate systems, the family and peer systems are now viewed as complimentary and interdependent (Gauze, Bukowski, Aquan-Assee, & Sippola, 1996). It is possible, especially for a child with a disability, that the first friend a child will have is a sibling or a parent (Dunn & McGuire, 1992). The parent may be the child's first confidante and the first individual who likes the child because of his or her personality characteristics regardless of the disability. Field, Land, Yando, and Bendell (1995) found that intimacy with parents, especially mothers, was positively correlated with self-esteem, lower reported risk taking, lower depression, and more positive peer relations. Rigby (1993) noted, "In general, positive attitude and relations with family and parents were associated, as expected, with children's tendencies to act prosocially and not to engage in bullying behavior" (p. 510).

Four parental roles that directly influence peer relationships and friendship development are designer, mediator, supervisor, and consultant (Ladd & Le Sieur 1995; Ladd, Le Sieur, & Profilet, 1993). As designers, parents choose which neighborhood to live in, which schools the child will attend, and in which religious and extracurricular activities the child participates. In a recent study of adolescents with acquired spinal cord injury, Sawain and Marshall (1992) found that the number and quality of peer interactions were directly related to the number of friends acquired, and children of parents who provided few opportunities for peer involvement were less socially competent than their peers. Because parents of school-age and early adolescent age children often dictate the amount of time that children spend with their peer group and the circumstances in which these encounters occur, knowledge of the child's abilities at any particular point in time is necessary so that appropriate activities can be designed and proper supervision given. Supervision that is age or developmentally inappropriate is detrimental both to the child's ability to make friends and to the child's engagement in appropriate peer activities.

The mediator and consultant role of the parent helps the child learn the appropriate interactions or behaviors necessary to create and maintain friendships. Grey (1990) noted that parents can "teach them how to make friends with their peers, neighbors, and others in the community so that they have many people with whom they share affection and who will support them when they are having difficulties" (p. 309). It is relatively easy, in the best of circumstances, for children and adolescents who have no altered health status to feel alienated or cut off from their peer group. For children and adolescents who have differences due to their health status or who spend much of their time away from peers, the feelings of alienation can be overwhelming. Parents can step in and redirect children's friendships or educate children about the facets of friendship (Coleman & Lindsay, 1992). Children whose parents are ignorant of their child's friendships or social competence in the area of friendship formation are at a social disadvantage.

Indirect influences on peer relations and friendship development include parental, economic, and marital stress. Personal and marital stress diverts emotional resources and time and keeps parents from engaging in more child-centered behaviors. For instance, Compas and Williams (1990) found that parental stresses, especially daily hassles, were more pronounced in single mothers than in their married counterparts, and this interfered with the social life of their children. Parental, marital, and economic stresses are also more pronounced in families with an ill or disabled child, which may affect the family's ability to cope with the demands of a child's social development.

NURSING DIAGNOSIS AND OUTCOME DETERMINATION

A basic component of health promotion for all children, regardless of age or ability, is to determine the amount and the quality of social interaction obtained within and without the family system. Nursing diagnoses that might alert the nurse to the need for the intervention of Friendship Promotion include Loneliness, Altered Growth and Development, Impaired Social Interaction, Social Isolation, Altered Family Coping, and Altered Parenting (North American Nursing Diagnosis Association, 1999). To determine if the intervention is appropriate, the nurse should assess the quality of interactions within the family. Are parents able to model friendships and be friends with their children? How do siblings get along? Are the siblings friendly with each other? Do the siblings share with and depend on each other? Outside activities should be assessed for their potential to provide friendship opportunities. Interaction is important. If the child is always the observer, always on the sideline with no real role in the activity, the probability for meaningful interaction with peers is decreased.

Questions about day care, preschool, and school are very important. Does the child like school? Does the child receive invitations to peers' homes? Does the child invite peers to his or her home? Does the child have friends? How many? What do the friends like to do together? The particular location of social contacts is less important than their nature. The critical factors are the attendance of peers and the opportunity to engage in meaningful, reciprocal encounters. If a child seems to have limited peer social contacts with whom sharing occurs, the nursing intervention of Friendship Promotion should be considered.

Children should be assessed independently of the parents, if possible, so that every opportunity is given for the child to articulate feelings of loneliness or social isolation. Indicators include expressions of being excluded or separate from their peer group, lack of belonging, being misunderstood, dissatisfaction with social circumstances and with close relationships, lack of interaction with peers, or lack of people the child can call on for help or assistance.

The Nursing Outcomes Classification (NOC) includes many outcomes that are relevant in measuring the effectiveness of Friendship Promotion (Iowa Outcomes Project, 2000). Self-Esteem, Social Interaction Skills, Social Involvement, and Social Support provide indicators appropriate for children and families that measure feelings about themselves, the ability to effectively interact with others, involvement with friends and community, and use of support from others. These outcomes and their associated indicators give nurses the framework to quantitatively measure changes in children and families over time.

For younger children, the outcome of Friendship Promotion is primarily for the child to obtain friendship opportunities. Secondarily, outcomes should include the ability to follow rules, to share willingly and spontaneously, and to engage cooperatively and appropriately with selected peers and others. Often, preschool children can tell you if they have friends, who their special friends are, and how they interact with these peers.

The outcomes of this intervention for school-age children include the ability to play in groups, the development of close or best friendships, and identification with a same-sex peer group. Two related outcome indicators for school-age children are the display of self-confidence and the ability to perform as well as possible in school. These children should be able to express their number of friends and the intensity of individual friendships. School-age children should express a feeling for belonging to a peer group and that they do not feel isolated or misunderstood by their peers.

For adolescents, the outcomes are the appropriate use of interaction skills, the ability to resolve conflicts appropriately, good relationships with same-sex and opposite-sex peers, the ability to develop intimate friendships, and the ability to perform as well as possible in school and other situations. Outcome indicators include reports of emotional assistance by others, reports of a confidant relationship, knowing who to turn to for help, and evidence that the child or adolescent calls on peers for help when needed.

FRIENDSHIP PROMOTION

The activities related to this intervention are multifaceted. Nurses should be very knowledgeable about community resources, activities, and attitudes. Chronically ill or disabled children often have opportunities to participate in activities such as swimming, little league, theatre groups, summer camps, and the electronic superhighway, depending on their ability and interest. Nurses also need to be knowledgeable about the specific disorder or illness afflicting the children so that appropriate activities can be recommended, such as swimming for asthmatic children and electronic mail for hearing- or speech-impaired children. Parents need to be educated about the capabilities of the child at any given time to identify adaptations needed to accommodate the child's limitations in the social setting. It may be necessary for the nurse to model appropriate behavior so that parents can refocus on the child's abilities rather than on the child's disability in a social setting.

The health care team needs to be aware of the future potential of the chronically ill or disabled child so that appropriate activities can be suggested that will lead to increased social interaction with peers in the present and in the future. Nurses can promote activities that will decrease the time spent away from the normal childhood environment and increase the time spent in social interaction with peers. In addition, nurses should encourage specific parental activities, such as (a) creating safe, well-defined spaces and plentiful opportunities for the child to interact with his or her peers in activities appropriate to developmental level and ability, emphasizing that most activities can be provided, with modifications, to the disabled child; (b) assisting the child with sharing and taking turns and fostering cooperation between child and peers by role modeling interaction skills; (c) providing alternative opportunities for peer interaction when children cannot physically be present because of hospitalizations or home care. For example, most schools have Internet connections, making this type of peer interaction more common and acceptable, and many nonprofit groups donate computers to disabled persons so that they can have access to the electronic network; (d) deemphasizing the uniqueness of the child's condition, which will help decrease the child's feeling of alienation or "differentness" from his or her peers; (e) making changes that will decrease reminders of the child's special needs and avoid potential embarrassment of the child in social situations; and (f) having the same expectations of social competence from the chronically ill or disabled child as they have from their other children.

Nurses can work with families to encourage children to try new activities and to challenge their existing abilities. When children feel competent, they are more likely to engage in social interaction with peers.

Children can also be challenged to participate in school and community activities to the best of their developmental and ability level. Finally, the nurse should monitor the family situation and determine barriers to providing opportunities for friendship attainment. If any problems are identified, the nurse should make appropriate referrals. This is particularly important if the family is undergoing inordinate amounts of stress, and this stress is interfering with normal family functioning or causing alterations in parenting. Consultation with team members caring for the family, and with the child, parents, and siblings, is important so that a concerted effort may be made in regard to relieving stress and improving family and parental functioning. If financial difficulties are interfering with Friendship Promotion—for example, there is not enough money to enroll a child in community programs, camps, or other activities that will provide peer interactions—then the nurse should be able to refer to appropriate community resources that may alleviate or ameliorate this burden. Also, referrals to social services can be very helpful for families of children with chronic illnesses or disabilities so that needed acute and preventive care can be acquired at the least possible cost to the family.

INTERVENTION APPLICATION

Jaime Jones is a 10-year-old girl with newly diagnosed insulin-dependent diabetes. She has recently moved to this town of 200,000 people with her mother, father, and two older brothers (ages 12 and 15). Jaime has not yet started attending her new school or had time to join in community activities, such as soccer, little league, or swimming (which she loves). This diagnosis comes as a shock to Mr. and Mrs. Jones. There is no family history of diabetes, and the children have always been in good health. The two older children have never been hospitalized or had any serious illnesses. Mr. Jones seems especially worried and anxious about Jaime and voices concern that she will have an insulin reaction when no one is around to help her. As the care coordinator for Jaime and her family, Ms. Smith wants to ensure that Jaime receives good medical care and maintains her compliance with the medical regime. Ms. Smith recognizes that Jaime's peer group is and will be influential in her life and knows that positive peer friendships and support are essential to helping Jaime maintain a healthy lifestyle throughout her school-age and adolescent years.

Ms. Smith completes a family assessment of the Joneses. Questions about family roles, communication, and affective and socialization functions are pursued and the Jones's social support system within the new and previous communities is assessed. Jaime is questioned about her friends, her relationship with her parents and her brothers, and her likes and dislikes with regard to activities and food.

Ms. Smith's assessment of the Jones family and of Jaime leads to many nursing diagnoses, including Potential for Altered Family Processes; Family Coping, Compromised; Loneliness (Jaime's distance from her old friends and her lack of new friendships); Alteration in Social Support; and Risk for Impaired Social Interaction. Ms. Smith decides that the intervention of Friendship Promotion is appropriate for this family in general and Jaime in particular.

Proactively, Ms. Smith schedules two team conferences with Jaime, Mr. and Mrs. Jones, Jaime's brothers, the physician, and the medical social worker 3 days apart. At the first conference, the medical facts and regime are articulated; Jaime and her family are given all the facts about insulin-dependent diabetes, the treatment, and the complications—insulin reaction and shock and diabetic coma. The family is also made aware of various support groups within the community, the support that social services can provide, and the option of counseling. A dietician is asked to consult with Jaime and her parents to discuss how the dietary restrictions can be minimized and deemphasized. Jaime and her parents are given suggestions on how to tell her teachers and her peers about her need to take insulin shots and the importance of normal physical activity.

At the second team conference, questions from the previous conference are answered, and the possible social implications of Jaime's diagnoses are discussed. The need for normal social interaction is stressed. Ms. Smith tells Jaime it is important that she maintain her friendships from her previous hometown by phone or mail. Mr. and Mrs. Jones are encouraged to let Jaime engage in peer activities as usual. Community activities and the supervision needed for such activities are discussed. Ms. Smith encouraged Jaime to continue with her swimming and soccer and discussed with the family how to best maintain insulin levels while vigorously exercising. Mr. and Mrs. Jones were encouraged to maintain the normal family activities and routines; they are asked to list barriers to maintaining this routine. Jaime was given names of other children her age with insulin-dependent diabetes who could be contacted for help and advice. A follow-up team conference was scheduled in 4 weeks to determine how she and her family were coping with her illness and to determine how Jaime's social life was progressing.

RESEARCH AND PRACTICE IMPLICATIONS

There has been much research in the past decade on the formation of friendships and peer interactions with children and adolescents who do not have disabilities or chronic illnesses, but little research in this area has been done with children and adolescents who have chronic illnesses or disabilities. It is not known if the processes are different or similar. Both qualitative and quantitative research are needed to assist in understanding the basic processes by which friendships are formed and the way in which friends might be used to support activities necessary to maintain functional status. Research is also necessary to identify the determinants of forming friendships with particular peers. Variables influencing friendship formation have not been identified for healthy children. Importantly, the characteristics of children with no disability or chronic illness that lead them to befriend a disabled or chronically ill child are still to be determined and tested. In this era of computer technology, individuals often lack understanding about how to form or maintain friendships that are not predicated on mutual physical nearness, such as telephone or e-mail.

Friendship is something most take for granted. Whether a best friend is a sibling, a spouse, or an unrelated but highly valued person, however, most individuals would have a difficult time imagining how they would get through the bad times, or who they would share the good times with, if friends did not exist. Likewise, one may not even be aware of how or why that level of friendship developed. Many of the friendship-promoting activities that most take for granted are denied to the child with a disability or with a chronic illness. Understanding that the conditions for friendship to develop need to be nurtured and exploited is a main concern of nurses who work with chronically ill or disabled children, whether that work occurs in a hospital, a community setting, or a school. The assessment that needs to occur to intervene effectively and efficiently is fairly straightforward, but it takes time from other valuable activities. Knowing that friends and peers provide necessary social support and are necessary for mental health and hopefulness will help nurses to devote appropriate time and energy to Friendship Promotion.

REFERENCES

Bagwell, C. L., Newcomb, A. F., & Bukowski, W. M. (1998). Preadolescent friendship and peer rejection as predictors of adult adjustment. *Child Development, 69,* 140-153.

Berndt, T. J., & Keefe, K. (1995). Friends' influence on adolescents' adjustment to school. *Child Development, 66,* 1312-1329.

Bluebond-Langner, M., Perkel, D., & Goertzel, T. (1991). Pediatric cancer patients' peer relationships: The impact of an oncology camp experience. *Journal of Psychosocial Oncology, 9*(2), 67-80.

Caroline, H. A. (1993). Explorations of close friendships: A concept analysis. *Archives of Psychiatric Nursing, 7*(4), 236-243.

Coleman, W. L., & Lindsay, R. L. (1992). Interpersonal disabilities: Social skills deficits in older children and adolescents. *Pediatric Clinics of North America, 39*(3), 551-567.

Compas, B. E., & Williams, R. A. (1990). Stress, coping, and adjustment in mothers and young adolescents in single- and two-parent families. *American Journal of Community Psychology, 18*(4), 525-545.

Dunn, J., & McGuire, S. (1992). Sibling and peer relationships in childhood. *Journal of Child Psychology and Psychiatry, 33,* 67-105.

Field, T., Lang, C., Yando, R., & Bendell, D. (1995). Adolescents' intimacy with parents and friends. *Adolescence, 30*(117), 133-140.

Freitag, M. K., Belsky, J., Grossman, K., Grossmann, K. E., & Scheuerer-Englisch, H. (1996). Continuity in parent-child relationships from infancy to middle childhood and relations with friendship competence. *Child Development, 67,* 1437-1454.

Gauze, C., Bukowski, W. M., Aquan-Assee, J., & Sippola, L. K. (1996). Interactions between family environment and friendship and associations with self-perceived well-being during early adolescence. *Child Development, 67*(5), 2201-2216.

Grey, M. (1990). Helping children cope with stress. *Journal of Pediatric Health Care, 4*(6), 309-310.

Hartup, W. W. (1996). The company they keep: Friendships and their developmental significance. *Child Development, 67,* 1-13.

Hawkins, J. M. (Ed.). (1986). *The Oxford reference dictionary.* Oxford, UK: Clarendon.

Hodges, E. V., Boivin, M., Vitaro, F., & Bukowski, W. M. (1999). The power of friendship: Protection against an escalating cycle of peer victimization. *Developmental Psychology, 35,* 94-101.

Howes, C., Hamilton, C. E., & Philipsen, L. C. (1998). Stability and continuity of child-caregiver and child-peer relationships. *Child Development, 69*(2), 418-426.

Iowa Outcomes Project. (2000). *Nursing outcomes classification (NOC)* (M. Johnson, M. Maas, & S. Moorhead, Eds.; 2nd ed.). St. Louis, MO: Mosby-Year Book.

Ladd, G. W., & Le Sieur, K. D. (1995). Parents and children's peer relationships. In M. H. Bornstein (Ed.), *Handbook of parenting: Vol. 4. Applied and practical parenting* (pp. 377-410). Hillsdale, NJ: Lawrence Erlbaum.

Ladd, G. W., Le Sieur, K. D., & Profilet, S. M. (1993). Direct parental influences of young children's peer relations. In S. Duck (Ed.), *Learning about relationships* (pp. 152-183). London: Sage.

Mulderij, K. J. (1997). Peer relations and friendship in physically disabled children. *Child Care and Health Development, 23*(5), 379-389.

North American Nursing Diagnosis Association. (1999). *Nursing diagnoses: Definitions and classification 1999-2000.* Philadelphia: Author.

Pflederer, D. (1990). Using friends as a social support system for children. In M. J. Craft & J. A. Denehy (Eds.), *Nursing interventions for infants and children* (pp. 201-212). Philadelphia: W. B. Saunders.

Rigby, K. (1993). School children's perceptions of their families and parents as a function of peer relations. *Journal of Genetic Psychology, 154*(4), 501-513.

Rose, A. J., & Asher, S. R. (1999). Children's goals and strategies in response to conflicts within a friendship. *Developmental Psychology, 35,* 69-79.

Ross, L. (1981). The intuitive scientist formulation and its developmental implications. In J. H. Flavell & L. Ross (Eds.), *Social cognitive development: Frontiers and possible futures.* Cambridge, UK: Cambridge University Press.

Sawain, K. J., & Marshall, J. (1992). Developmental competence in adolescents with an acquired disability. *Rehabilitation Nursing Research, 1,* 41-50.

Stoneman, Z. (1993). Children: Social competence, friendships, and adaptive behavior. *Current Opinion in Psychiatry, 6*(5), 615-622.

Yude, C., Goodman, R., & McConachie, H. (1998). Peer problems of children with hemiplegia in mainstream primary schools. *Journal of Child Psychology and Psychiatry and Allied Disciplines, 39*(4), 533-541.

Zarbatany, L., Van-Brunschot, M., Meadow, K., & Pepper, S. (1996). Effects of friendship and gender on peer group entry. *Child Development, 67*(5), 2287-2300.

23

Normalization Promotion

Kathleen A. Knafl

Janet A. Deatrick

Adrienne Kirby

Childhood chronic conditions present families and individual family members with multiple challenges. Typically, parents are expected to master new, often sophisticated, medical information and complex treatment regimens. Moreover, they are expected to do so in such a way that managing the condition is incorporated into the usual flow of everyday life rather than becoming a dominant focus of either the family's or the child's life. Corbin and Strauss (1988) discussed how life with a chronic condition entails three types of interrelated work: illness, everyday, and biographical. Whereas illness work focuses on the treatment regimen and interactions with health care professionals, everyday work entails efforts to continue usual activities. Biographical work focuses on constructing a meaningful life for one's self and family. Everyday and biographical work point to the importance for families of viewing the chronic condition in a way that sustains a positive view of the child and family as well as the importance of developing illness management strategies and family routines that contribute to optimal family functioning. There is considerable evidence that many families rise to the challenges of childhood chronic conditions and create a life for the ill child and the family that is experienced as both normal and satisfying (Austin, 1991; Knafl & Deatrick, 1986; Leff & Walizer, 1992).

During the past 30 years, research and firsthand accounts of family response to childhood chronic conditions have drawn on the concept of normalization to convey the way in which many families respond to childhood chronic illness and disability. Recently, nurse researchers have directed their attention to refining the concept of normalization and systematically evaluating interventions that promote the normalization of family life in the context of childhood chronic conditions (Craft & Willadsen, 1992; Knafl & Deatrick, 1986; Robinson, 1993). The purpose of this chapter is to provide a critical overview of the literature on normalization and offer guidelines for assessing and intervening to promote the normalization efforts of families. In addition, a case study is provided to illustrate the use of the nursing intervention of Normalization Promotion for a family experiencing difficulty in managing a child's chronic condition.

THEORETICAL FOUNDATION

In her article on normalization of family life in the context of a chronic condition, Robinson (1993) maintains that "normalization has proven to be both a theoretically and clinically pertinent concept" (p. 6). Theoretically, the concept contributes to the understanding of a family's efforts to manage a chronic condition. For example, parents' willingness to forego certain aspects of the treatment regimen often are more understandable when viewed through a normalization as opposed to a compliance lens. The perspective of normalization can help providers understand the goals parents may be attempting to achieve in altering a prescribed treatment regimen. Moreover, normalization provides a framework that can give direction to clinical interventions. The clinician who understands the family's goal to normalize life in the context of a chronic condition can work collaboratively with that family to modify and individualize the treatment regimen in a way that maximizes control of the condition while minimizing disruption to the child's and family's life.

The concept of normalization has emerged and evolved as the result of numerous studies addressing how families respond to childhood chronic conditions. In recent years, several authors have synthesized this research in an effort to clarify and continue the development of the concept. Knafl and Deatrick (1986) provided an historical overview of the concept, tracing its roots to an early study by Schwartz (1957) of wives of men with serious mental illness and research by Davis (1963) on families in which a child had polio. On the basis of the literature and using formal concept analysis techniques, Knafl and Deatrick (1986) identified the following defining criteria for normalization:

- Acknowledge existence of impairment.
- Define family life as essentially normal.
- Define social consequences of situation as minimal.
- Engage in behaviors designed to demonstrate essential normalcy of family to others.

Their initial review identified 11 articles that addressed the concept and distinguished normalization from other family responses to chronic childhood conditions such as disassociation and denial.

In a recent reanalysis of the concept, Deatrick, Knafl, and Murphy-Moore (1999) identified 26 research-based articles addressing normalization that had been published since their original analysis. The review of these articles served to further clarify the concept and resulted in the following revised criteria:

- Acknowledge the condition and its potential to threaten lifestyle.
- Adapt normalcy lens for defining child and family.
- Engage in parenting behaviors and family routines that are consistent with normalcy lens.
- Develop a treatment regimen that is consistent with normalcy lens.
- Interact with others based on view of the child and family as normal.

These revised criteria emphasize that normalization is a process grounded in the interplay between parents' definition of the situation (i.e., the lens they use for viewing their child and family life) and their deliberate efforts to engage in normal parenting and family life activities. In their reanalysis, Deatrick, Knafl, and Murphy-Moore (1999) also discussed the distinct but interrelated aspects of normalization as a goal that shapes behaviors, activities directed toward that goal, and the outcome of such activities. Different authors have tended to direct their attention to one or the other of these aspects of the concept, with relatively little attention given to their interrelationship.

Robinson's (1993) and Mays's (1997) research has been particularly useful in tracing the process through which families move from a problem-focused to a normalcy-focused view of their situation. Robinson detailed "how the story of life 'as normal' is constructed, how the story is lived, the impact that health care professionals exert on the story process, and the consequences of the story in terms of costs and benefits" (p. 9). May discusses how the family's previous lifestyle serves as a benchmark for judging the success of its normalization efforts. Robinson's efforts to describe both the positive and negative aspects of normalization and the role of health care professionals in initiating and sustaining a family's normalization efforts make her work especially relevant clinically.

The Family Management Style (FMS) framework developed by Knafl and Deatrick (1990) and other research on normalization have distinguished adaptation difficulties that are grounded in how families define their situation from those that are grounded in the family's management strategies. On the basis of a study of 63 families in which a child had a chronic illness, Knafl, Breitmayer, Gallo, and Zoeller (1996) described a variety of styles families used in their efforts to adapt to a child's chronic illness and found that normalization was characteristic of some but not all styles. Clarke-Steffen (1993, 1997) described the difficulties of adhering to the treatment regimen experienced by parents of very young children with insulin-dependent diabetes, and Bossert, Holaday, Harkins, and Turner-Henson (1990) found that parents sometimes experienced tremendous difficulty providing normal experiences and activities for their child with a chronic illness. Although the families in these studies continued to function reasonably well in terms of meeting members' physical and emotional needs, they nonetheless reported problems linked to the chronic condition and were open to interventions that would promote a more normalized family life.

Other authors have identified the limits of parents' ability to normalize family life (Clarke-Steffen, 1993, 1997; Cohen, 1993; Seideman & Kleine, 1995). Cohen described the uncertainty and difficulties that often surround the diagnostic period of a child's illness and obviate attempts at normalization. Similarly, Clarke-Steffen's (1993, 1997) and Hatton, Canam, Thorne, and Hughes's (1995) work suggest that the challenges of certain illness situations (e.g., cancer and very young children with diabetes) contribute to parents viewing normalization as an impossible goal. Similarly, Cohen and Clarke-Steffen described how even in these extremely difficult situations parents developed new "normal" routines; however, they were routines that parents viewed as setting the family apart from other families. Seideman and Kleine (1995) developed a theory of transformed parenting to convey the family life of parents of children with developmental delay and mental retardation. They identified "striving for normalcy" as an ongoing struggle for parents who wanted their family to participate in the same activities as families with normal, healthy children. In contrast, Ablon (1988), in a study of families with dwarf children, found that the work of normalization decreased over time as parents "determined that their child could lead a 'normal' life" (p. 137). Studies such as these offer useful insights into those factors or situations that inhibit or promote normalization.

Other authors discussed the ways in which health care providers or school personnel can sometimes inhibit a family's ability to live a normal life when a member has a chronic condition (Jerrett, 1994; Robinson, 1993; Turner-Henson, Holaday, Corser, Ogletree, & Swan, 1994; Williams, 1994). Robinson argued that "families often experience the negative judgments of health care professionals who see their normalizing practices as evidence of denial. The problem saturated perspective leads us to try to disrupt the practices that support normalization" (p. 20). Jerrett found that parents of children with juvenile arthritis often had differing views from those of health care providers regarding their child's illness and their own ability to manage the illness, and these differing views "increased conflict and confusion for them, and served to highlight their sense of isolation" (p. 1053).

School professionals also can pose threats to parents' normalization efforts. Williams (1994) reported that mothers of girls with precocious puberty or Turner syndrome often had to invest considerable time and effort into ensuring that school personnel had an adequate understanding of their daughters' condition. Mothers viewed teachers' failure to understand the unique needs of these children as impeding parental efforts to provide a normal childhood for their children. Difficulties with the school system typically were grounded in teachers' and administrators' lack of understanding regarding the nature and special requirements of the condition or problems with adhering to the treatment regimen during school hours. A survey of parents' perceptions of the discrimination experienced by their school-age children with chronic illnesses revealed that school-related problems accounted for 55% of the perceived discriminatory situations (Turner-Henson et al., 1994). Parents most often reported discrimination related to physical education classes, unwillingness to provide for the child's special care, and exclusion from school activities and trips. These findings suggest that an important component of normalization promotion is working with families and other systems to address the sources and outcomes of discriminatory practices.

Given the volume of research, combined with major efforts to synthesize the work in the field, it is appropriate and timely that nurses direct their attention to further elaborating the clinical implications of this well-developed concept. Efforts to date to specify the defining characteristics of the concept and to elucidate how families normalize life in the context of childhood chronic conditions provide the theoretical and empirical grounding for assessment and intervention to promote normalization.

NURSING DIAGNOSIS AND
OUTCOME DETERMINATION

Normalization promotion is appropriate when there is evidence that a child with a chronic condition or the family unit is having difficulty adapting to the situation. The need for normalization promotion can stem from diverse sources of difficulty, and several nursing diagnoses, either singly or in combination, indicate that interventions to promote normalization would be appropriate. These diagnoses include Altered Parenting, Altered Family Process, Ineffective Family Coping: Compromised, and Family Coping: Potential for Growth (North American Nursing Diagnosis Association [NANDA], 1999). With more severe problems and families that are judged to be severely dysfunctional, however, nursing interventions targeting normalization promotion may be inadequate. Families with a nursing diagnosis of Ineffective Family Coping: Disabling may require referral for family counseling or therapy.

The themes and subthemes that comprise the management styles identified by Knafl et al. (1996) can be used to direct assessment efforts by providing a set of topics to be discussed during the course of assessing the family's response to the chronic condition and its impact on family life. The authors identified major defining, managing, and outcome themes and subthemes that characterized how families responded to childhood chronic illness. Table 23.1 lists these themes. Although the major themes, such as child identity and illness view, represent common aspects of the illness experience for all families, the subthemes reflect the range of variation across families with regard to a particular theme. To craft appropriate interventions, it is essential to know if coping difficulties are linked to altered parenting behaviors that have resulted from parents viewing their child's identity as no longer normal or if coping difficulties are the result of a reactive management approach that leads to constant disruptions in the family's usual routine. The content of these themes and subthemes is described elsewhere (Knafl et al., 1996).

In addition to the direction provided by the FMS framework, there are numerous structured instruments for assessing family functioning and parenting behavior, some of which are specific to families who are coping with chronic conditions. Sawin and Harrigan (1995) did an excellent job of summarizing and critically evaluating these instruments. Although many of the instruments have been developed for research purposes rather than clinical practice, they offer important insights into assessing family response to a variety of health care challenges. The more well-developed instruments that Sawin and Harrigan discuss would be appropriate for assessing family response to chronic conditions. The instruments include the Feetham Family Functioning Scale (Feetham, 1991), the Family Apgar (Smilkstein, 1978), and the Family Assessment Device (Epstein, Baldwin, & Bishop, 1983). Ideally, the assessment of the family would include a combination of open-ended questions based on the family management style framework and structured measures that have been carefully selected to take into account the family's characteristics and the constraints of the practice setting.

These same assessment protocols could also help set appropriate outcome goals. As defined by the Nursing Outcomes Classification (Iowa Outcomes Project, 2000), Parenting entails "provision of an environment that promotes optimum growth and development of dependent children" (p. 332). The literature, however, suggests that some parents have difficulty viewing their child with a chronic condition as a normal child. For these parents, target outcomes could focus on providing for the child's special needs while still directing adequate attention to cognitive, social, and emotional growth and using appropriate discipline. Alternatively, other parents have difficulty as a result of a reactive management approach that fails to anticipate illness-related problems and incorporate the treatment regimen into the usual schedule of family life. Target outcomes for these families could focus on routinization of the treatment regimen and adaptation of the family's usual schedule to accommodate the child's special needs. In either case, the goal would be a more normalized family life. The previously discussed defining characteristics of normalization provide criteria for determining if this outcome has been achieved and the relative changes made by the family.

INTERVENTION: NORMALIZATION PROMOTION

In working with families to devise activities that promote normalization and effective coping and parenting, it is important to incorporate current knowledge about effective ways for health care providers in general and nurses in particular to work with families. The faculty of the family nursing unit (FNU) of the University of Calgary continue to have a leading role in developing intervention approaches that contribute to families' abilities to meet the challenges of chronic illness (Wright & Leahey, 1994). The FNU is based on the assumption that the family-nurse relationship is nonhierarchical and reciprocal, recognizes the expertise of the family and the nurse, recognizes the unique resources and strengths of the family and the nurse, and provides feedback on several different relationship levels (Leahey & Harper-Jacques, 1996).

In addition to the general guidelines for working with families provided by clinicians and researchers associated with the FNU, the developers of the Nursing Interventions Classification (NIC) (Iowa Intervention

TABLE 23.1 Defining, Managing, and Consequence Themes and Subthemes

Themes	Subthemes
Defining themes	
Child identity	
Parental views of the child and his or her capabilities	Normal
	Problem
	Tragic
Illness view	
Parental understanding and beliefs about the child's illness, including both technical understanding and subjective evaluation	Life goes on
	Ominous
	Hateful
	Uninformed
Self view	
Ill child's perception of own health in comparison to peers	More healthy
	Equally healthy
	Less healthy
Managing themes	
Parenting philosophy	
Parental goals, strategies, and behaviors linked to caring for a child with a chronic illness	Accommodative
	Sheltering
	Minimizing
	Inconsistent
Management mind-set	
Parental views of ease or difficulty of carrying out the treatment regimen and their ability to manage effectively	Confident
	Burdened
	Inadequate
	Observer
Management approach	
Parental orientation to illness management and their associated behaviors	Proactive
	Reactive
	Complaint
	Uninvolved
Self-care behaviors	
Ill child's participation in the treatment regimen, including behaviors and perceptions of abilities	Competent
	Deficient
	Unconventional

TABLE 23.1 *Continued*

Themes	Subthemes
Consequence themes	
Parental mutuality	
Parental views on the degree to which they hold shared or complementary perceptions of situation and approach to managing	Present Absent
Foreground	
Parental views on the extent to which the illness is a dominant focus of family life	Yes No
Future dread	
Parental belief that their family's and child's future well-being is seriously jeopardized as a result of the illness	Present Absent
Child consequences	
Ill child's perception of how the illness touches own daily life	No big deal Intrusive Worry

Reprinted with the permission of W. B. Saunders Company from the *Journal of Pediatric Nursing, 11,* 317.

Project, 2000) identified specific nursing activities that can promote normalization in families with a child with a chronic condition. NIC defines *Normalization Promotion* as "assisting parents and other family members of children with chronic illness or disabilities in providing normal life experiences for their children and families" (p. 473). Of the 24 normalization promotion activities listed, 2 are directed at how parents define their child (assist the family to view the affected child as a child first rather than a chronically ill or disabled individual and deemphasize the uniqueness of the child's condition).

Many studies indicate that following an initial period of adjustment during which parents focus on the illness and mastering the treatment regimen, they eventually come to view their child with a chronic condition as an essentially normal individual who happens to have a chronic illness (Jerrett, 1994; Knafl & Deatrick, 1986; Robinson, 1993). Robinson described this as a shift from a story of life as problem focused to a story of life "as normal." She noted that the shift could come as the result of a conscious decision to view one's situation as normal, often entailed reframing of the situation and involved "making choices or discriminating between data that are to be included in the construction and data that are not to be included" (p. 12). In their study of children with developmental delays or mental retardation, Seideman and Kleine (1995) found that parents also used many cognitive strategies, including guarding hope, downward comparisons, and redefining the situation, that contributed to a positive view of the situation and enhanced their ability to lead a satisfying family life.

When assessment reveals that the parents are focusing on the child's illness or disability, the nurse can play a pivotal role in helping them to see the many ways in which their child is still normal. This activity can be especially meaningful during the time immediately following the diagnosis when parents may be struggling to understand the implications of the condition for their child's and the family's life. The sometimes pivotal role of the nurse in shaping the meaning of diagnosis for the family was illustrated by Van Riper and Selder's (1989) descriptions of the importance that mothers attributed to nurses' reactions to and treatment of their newborns with Down syndrome. Depending on the reaction, nurses could enhance or detract from the mother's ability to view her child positively.

The 22 remaining activities described in the NIC intervention Normalization Promotion provide an array of possibilities for helping families manage their situation in a way that promotes a normal childhood for the ill child and a normal family life as well. Although some of the activities directly target the child, others focus on the family unit or on external systems. Activities to help parents provide opportunities for the child to have normal childhood experiences and to avoid potentially embarrassing situations focus on the child. Bossert et al.'s (1990) research provides an excellent example of such activities. They described specific parenting strategies such as altering the prescribed therapeutic regimen that made it possible for the child to participate in valued activities.

Normalization Promotion activities, such as assisting the family to alter the prescribed treatment regimen to fit the family's normal schedule and encouraging the maintenance of family habits, rituals, and routines, contribute to the family's sense of normalcy in the face of a chronic condition. The continuation of activities such as vacations and traditional family celebrations signifies a continuity of life before and after the chronic condition and provides tangible evidence to the family that it is the same (normal) family it was in the past. If assessment reveals the family is distressed by what it views as dramatic alterations in its usual routine or by its perceived inability to sustain usual "special events," it signals a need to intervene and explore possibilities for adapting the treatment regimen to the family's unique situation and preferences. Situations such as this provide an excellent opportunity for the nurse to work collaboratively with parents to balance their efforts to ensure their child's special needs are met with their efforts to sustain a normal family life. For example, one mother in Knafl et al.'s (1996) study of families with a child with chronic illness discussed how she and the nurse worked together to adapt the child's treatment regimen to make it possible for the girl to attend sleepovers with her friends. Other parents talked about how health care providers helped them anticipate and plan for possible illness-related problems so that their child would not be singled out in school and other public settings.

Sometimes, systems or groups outside the family, such as the school system or those who run extracurricular activities, pose a threat to a normal childhood or family life. For example, a family in the Knafl, Breitmayer, Gallo, and Zoeller (1994) study reported that the daughter's school initially expected the girl to resign her membership on the tennis team following her diagnosis of lupus. Tennis was a major focus of the girl's life, and for her and her family the prospect of no longer being on the team symbolized that she no longer was normal. In this case, the parents expressed their concerns to their physician, who helped them modify the treatment regimen and devise a plan of action for convincing school officials that their daughter could and should continue to play tennis. In situations such as this, Normalization Promotion activities such as communicating information about the child's condition to ensure safe supervision and engagement in school programs and identifying adaptations needed to accommodate the child's limitations can contribute to a more normal situation for the child and family. When the school is hesitant to let a child with a chronic condition continue on a sports team, health care professionals can work with the parents to develop strategies that make continued participation possible.

An important consideration to keep in mind when working with families to promote normalization is the extent to which family members, especially parents, identify normalization as a goal. When normalization is the goal, activities typically are directed at developing management behaviors that balance the demands of the treatment regimen with the parents' desire to continue a normal life for their child and family. In some families, however, a normal childhood and family life are not viewed as an attainable goal by parents. In these instances, activities are most likely to be directed first to how the family defines its situation, with subsequent activities targeting illness management. Activities to change the family's definition of its situation, especially a definition of some duration, require extreme tact and sensitivity on the part of the nurse. As noted by Anderson (1986), striving for a normal life in the face of chronic condition may be a uniquely Western goal. In her comparative study of Anglo-Canadian families and recently immigrated Chinese families, she found that Chinese families had "not assimilated the ideology of normalization of the chronically ill child in the same way that white middle-class families have assimilated this ideology" (p. 1280). The Chinese families valued comforting the child and promoting contentment over normalization. Anderson's work, like that of Wright and Leahey (1994), underscores the importance of acknowledging and respecting the family's belief system even when trying to influence the nature of those beliefs.

INTERVENTION APPLICATION

Ellen Becker is an 11-year-old girl who has had insulin-dependent diabetes for 2 years. In general, both she and her family have adapted extremely well to her condition. Both parents were eager to learn everything they could about their daughter's illness and mastered the treatment regimen with relative ease. Over time, Ellen had taken increasing responsibility for testing her blood sugar levels and giving her own insulin injections. There are two other children in the Becker family, an older sister and a younger brother, and the parents described their lives as essentially unaffected by their sister's diabetes.

The parents described family life as having returned to near normal following the initial shock of the diagnosis. Nonetheless, the nurse at the diabetic treatment center noted some new concerns on the part of both Ellen and her parents during a routine checkup. As usual, the parents described Ellen as "doing well" and "a real nice kid." Their comments were supported by information about excellent grades and peer relationships and Ellen's own description of her many friends and activities and her delight at starting middle school.

At the same time, the parents described their shock and dismay over Ellen's recent refusal to test her blood sugar. Further probing by the nurse revealed that Ellen had been reporting excellent blood sugar levels to her parents even though she had not been doing her daily tests. The situation revealed itself when Ellen had a severe hypoglycemic reaction that resulted in a trip to the emergency room. The nurse interpreted the fact that both parents had come to the routine visit, when usually either one or the other did, as an indication of how distressed they were by the situation. Ellen's mother reported, "This has really thrown us for a loop," and her father described frequent battles with Ellen, who resented her parents' renewed efforts to monitor her treatment regimen. In contrast to how diabetes had been managed in the past, both Ellen and her parents described diabetes as the current focus of family life. Ellen's mother said, "I can't help obsessing about this," and her father noted, "I think it's all we talk about now. Sometimes I really dread walking in the front door at night."

Through this interaction, the nurse was able to assess that the family was having difficulty coping with Ellen's recent change in behavior. This led to the nursing diagnosis of Ineffective Family Coping: Compromised (NANDA, 1999). As described later, the intervention for this diagnosis, Normalization Promotion, included communicating with Ellen and her parents individually to obtain a better understanding of the situation. Second, together the family and nurse developed an acceptable compromise on managing the diabetes.

The nurse chose to meet individually with Ellen and her parents. In each case, she sympathized with the frustration they were experiencing. With the parents, she helped them reframe the situation as a normal, developmental incident. For Ellen, the nurse listened attentively to concerns about growing up with a chronic illness and noted that her parents' heightened vigilance may have been the result of normal parental concern. When the family reconvened, the nurse introduced the possibility that they try to work out a compromise solution that would be agreeable both to Ellen and to her parents. Ellen expressed the basis for her behavior, saying "I just get sick of having diabetes. Some days I just want to get up and not think about it." Ellen's father asked, "Is it absolutely essential that she test her blood sugar everyday?" Responding to these remarks, the nurse introduced the possibility of less frequent testing. After additional discussion, the family agreed to a provisional solution regarding the type of insulin Ellen would take and how often she would monitor her blood sugar. The arrangement was for 2 or 3 months so that Ellen could get a break from her diabetes. Ellen promised to adhere to the provisional plan for testing and to report the results to her parents. The following week, the nurse called the family, and Ellen's mother reported, "Things have really calmed down around here. I can't believe we didn't think of something like that sooner." At Ellen's next routine visit, the nurse suggested it was probably time to go back to her previous treatment regimen.

The expected outcome for normalization was achieved. The family agreed on a compromise and implemented it in the home setting. Ellen and her parents learned to effectively cope with a situation involving diabetes and reported a return to their normal family life. At this point, an appropriate new nursing diagnosis would be Family Coping: Potential for Growth (NANDA, 1999). As Ellen continues to mature, similar situations of conflict may arise with her diabetes management. Together with the nurse, they can anticipate such situations and work together to transition more smoothly, with less conflict, thereby promoting normalization in the family.

RESEARCH AND PRACTICE IMPLICATIONS

Families typically strive to manage chronic conditions in a way that promotes normalcy for both the child and the family, a goal that is supported by professionals. Although many families are able to adapt their usual routines to the demands of the chronic condition, others experience ongoing or periodic difficulty in sustaining a normalized family life and turn to health care professionals to help them achieve optimal adaptation. The concept of normalization is well developed and provides direction to health care providers' efforts to help families minimize the negative impact of a chronic condition on both the child and the family.

The literature on normalization has identified varying types of threats to sustaining a normal family life when a child has a chronic condition, and an understanding of these can guide assessment efforts. Difficulties may be grounded in the parents' definition of the situation or in their approach to managing the treatment regimen; they may focus on the child or the family system as a whole. Before appropriate interventions can be implemented, both the nurse and the family must understand the nature and source of normalization problems.

The effective use of Normalization Promotion as an intervention requires collaborative problem solving between family members and nurses that takes advantage of the unique expertise and resources of each (Leahey & Harper-Jacques, 1996). It is also useful to keep in mind that the nurse's style of interacting with families can be as important as the content of the interaction. Robinson (1994, 1996) found that family members attributed tremendous importance to the nurse's interaction style. Although the professionals she studied viewed effective interventions as those that lead to targeted outcomes, family members linked desirable outcomes to the quality of their interactions with professionals rather than to specific intervention activities. Her work reminds us of the importance of grounding any intervention in a style of interaction that respects and takes into account the family's beliefs and goals.

Although considerable research has been done on how chronic conditions can pose a threat to normal family life and the ways in which families address the challenges of chronic conditions to create a normal family life, there are still aspects of normalization that are relatively unexplored. Little is known about the interactive processes that occur between family members and nurses that contribute to normalization. In particular, it would be useful to know how nurses can work with families during the time of the diagnosis to promote normalcy from the onset of the condition. It would also be useful to understand more about those families who view normalization as a desirable but unattainable goal and the role nurses could play in working with them to improve their situation and cross-cultural variations in how normalization is viewed. Additional research will no doubt contribute to the further refinement of the concept. This refinement can be enhanced through empirical testing with children who have chronic conditions and their families. In the meantime, Normalization Promotion continues to be an appropriate intervention for helping many families effectively meet the multiple challenges of childhood chronic conditions.

REFERENCES

Ablon, J. (1988). *Living with difference: Families with dwarf children*. New York: Praeger.

Anderson, J. (1986). Ethnicity and illness experience: Ideological structures and the health care system. *Social Science and Medicine, 22*(11), 1277-1283.

Austin, J. (1991). Family adaptation to a child's chronic illness. In J. Fitzpatrick, R. Tauton, & A. Jacox (Eds.), *Annual review of nursing research* (pp. 103-120). New York: Springer.

Bossert, E., Holaday, B., Harkins, A., & Turner-Henson, A. (1990). Strategies of normalization used by parents of chronically ill school age children. *Journal of Child Psychiatric Nursing, 3*(2), 57-61.

Clarke-Steffen, L. (1993). A model of family transition to living with childhood cancer. *Cancer Practice, 1,* 285-292.

Clarke-Steffen, L. (1997). Reconstructing reality: Family strategies for managing childhood cancer. *Journal of Pediatric Nursing, 12,* 278-287.

Cohen, M. H. (1993). The unknown and the unknowable—Managing sustained uncertainty. *Western Journal of Nursing Research, 15,* 77-96.

Corbin, J., & Strauss, A. (1988). *Unending work and care: Managing chronic illness at home*. San Francisco: Jossey-Bass.

Craft, M. J., & Willadsen, J. (1992). Interventions related to family. *Nursing Clinics of North America, 27,* 517-540.

Davis, F. (1963). *Passage through crisis: Polio victims and their families*. Indianapolis, IN: Bobbs-Merrill.

Deatrick, J. A., Knafl, K. A., & Murphy-Moore, C. (1999). Clarifying the concept of normalization. *Image: The Journal of Nursing Scholarship, 31,* 209-214.

Epstein, N. B., Baldwin, L. M., & Bishop, D. S. (1983). The McMaster Family Assessment Device. *Journal of Marital and Family Therapy, 9*(12), 171-180.

Feetham, S. (1991). *Feetham Family Functioning Survey manual*. Chicago: University of Illinois.

Hatton, D., Canam, C., Thorne, S., & Hughes, A. M. (1995). Parents' perceptions of caring for an infant or toddler with diabetes. *Journal of Advanced Nursing, 22, 569-577.*

Iowa Intervention Project. (2000). *Nursing interventions classification (NIC)* (McCloskey, J. C. & G. M. Bulechek, Eds.; 3rd ed.). St. Louis, MO: Mosby-Year Book.

Iowa Outcomes Project. (2000). *Nursing outcomes classification (NOC)* (M. Johnson, M. Maas, & S. Moorhead, Eds.; 2nd ed.). St. Louis, MO: Mosby-Year Book.

Jerrett, M. D. (1994). Parents' experience of coming to know the care of a chronically ill child. *Journal of Advanced Nursing, 19,* 1050-1056.

Knafl, K., Breitmayer, B., Gallo, A., & Zoeller, L. (1994). *Final report: How families define and manage a child's chronic illness*. Washington, DC: National Institute of Nursing Research.

Knafl, K., Breitmayer, B., Gallo, A., & Zoeller, L. (1996). Family response to childhood chronic illness: Description of management styles. *Journal of Pediatric Nursing, 11,* 315-326.

Knafl, K. A., & Deatrick, J. A. (1986). How families manage chronic conditions: An analysis of the concept of normalization. *Research in Nursing and Health, 9,* 215-222.

Knafl, K. A., & Deatrick, J. A. (1990). Family management style: Concept analysis and development. *Journal of Pediatric Nursing, 5,* 4-14.

Leahey, M., & Harper-Jacques, S. (1996). Family-nurse relationships: Core assumptions and clinical implications. *Journal of Family Nursing, 2,* 131-151.

Leff, P., & Walizer, E. (1992). *Building the healing partnership: Parents, professionals, and children with chronic illnesses and disabilities.* Cambridge, MA: Brookline.

May, K. (1997). Searching for normalcy: Mothers' caregiving for low weight infants. *Pediatric Nursing, 23,* 17-20.

North American Nursing Diagnosis Association. (1999). *Nursing diagnoses: Definitions and classification 1999-2000.* Philadelphia: Author.

Robinson, C. A. (1993). Managing life with a chronic condition: The story of normalization. *Qualitative Health Research, 3,* 7-28.

Robinson, C. A. (1994). Nursing interventions with families: A demand or an invitation to change? *Journal of Advanced Nursing, 19,* 897-904.

Robinson, C. A. (1996). Health care relationships revisited. *Journal of Family Nursing, 2,* 152-173.

Sawin, K., & Harrigan, M. (1995). *Measures of family functioning for research and practice.* New York: Springer.

Schwartz, C. (1957). Perspectives on deviance—Wives' definitions of their husbands' mental illness. *Psychiatry, 20,* 275-291.

Seideman, R., & Kleine, P. (1995). Theory of transformed parenting: Parenting a child with developmental delay/mental retardation. *Nursing Research, 44,* 38-44.

Smilkstein, G. (1978). The Family Apgar: A proposal for a family function test and its use by physicians. *Journal of Family Practice, 6,* 1231-1239.

Turner-Henson, A., Holaday, B., Corser, N., Ogletree, G., & Swan, J. (1994). The experiences of discrimination: Challenges for chronically ill children. *Pediatric Nursing, 20,* 571-577.

Van Riper, M., & Selder, F. (1989). Parental response to the birth of a child with Down syndrome. *Loss, Grief and Care: A Journal of Professional Practice, 3,* 59-75.

Williams, J. K. (1994). Parenting a daughter with precocious puberty or Turner syndrome. *Journal of Pediatric Health Care, 9*(3), 109-114.

Wright, L. M., & Leahey, M. (1994). *Nurses and families: A guide to family assessment and intervention* (2nd ed.). Philadelphia: F. A. Davis.

24

Feeding Behavior Modification

Kirsten Sueppel Hanrahan

Feeding a young child can and should be a rewarding experience for both the parent and the child. As the child develops, the feeding relationship changes but should continue to be mutually gratifying. When something happens to alter the parent, the child, or the feeding relationship, feeding problems can occur. As a result, both participants may be deprived of gratification from the feeding process. This can further develop into a variety of problems from increased parental stress to delays in growth and development (Cooper et al., 1995). It is important to recognize the significance of feeding problems and plan interventions that support the parent and the child. Feeding Behavior Modification is an intervention developed to provide nurses with activities to facilitate a positive feeding experience.

Feeding behaviors are the actions and reactions of both parent and child to the process of giving and taking nourishment. Feeding behaviors rely on reciprocal cues from parent to child and child to parent. *Feeding problems* are defined as those behaviors that interfere or interrupt the mutually satisfying process and progression of giving and taking nourishment. Examples of problem behaviors are having temper tantrums, food rejection, and rumination. The etiology of feeding problems is most likely a combination of child, caretaker, and environmental factors. Characteristics of the child, such as prematurity, colic, chronic or acute illness, anatomical and structural defects, malabsorption, or neurological impairments, may lead to feeding problems. Problems can also be related to the caregiver, such as poor or inappropriate feeding techniques, mismatched temperament, and physical or mental impairments. Factors in the environment, such as aversive oral stimulation, hospitalization, or inadequate resources, can also contribute to feeding problems.

A spectrum of feeding problems exists. Feeding problems are experienced by most parents and children at some point in the first years of life. Most problems are transient, easily resolved with simple management techniques, and benign in nature. Even simple feeding problems, however, can escalate into later difficulties with nutrition, dental development, speech development, and social and emotional relationships (Christophersen & Hall, 1978). Children diagnosed as "failure to thrive" may have feeding problems, including eating skimpier, less regular meals; poorer response to food; decreased caloric intake; and other behavioral disturbances in the areas of sleep, elimination, autoerotic, and self-harming behaviors (Pollitt & Eichler, 1976). Feeding behaviors learned in early childhood shape the future for adult eating patterns, both healthy and problematic.

The intervention Feeding Behavior Modification and its related activities are intended for a variety of children experiencing a spectrum of feeding problems. It can be used for a premature infant who experienced a great deal of aversive oral stimulation and must learn to accept oral feedings, or it might be used as anticipatory guidance for the parent of a toddler who is becoming increasingly selective in food choices. Although the differentiation of organic and nonorganic failure to thrive is important for understanding feeding problems, the interventions used to treat these problems, including Feeding Behavior Modification, may be similar. A child with failure to thrive due to cystic fibrosis might benefit from some of the same nursing activities (e.g., offering small frequent meals) as those for the child with failure to thrive due to poor parenting skills. The same activities might also benefit a child not diagnosed as failure to thrive but demonstrating normal finicky toddler eating patterns. The key is individualizing the intervention to the problem. Given the spectrum of feeding problems and etiologies, it should be understood that this intervention varies in intensity from a few simple nursing activities to complex behavioral techniques. Use of the intervention with complex behavioral cases may necessitate advanced practice nursing and involvement of a multidisciplinary team.

Feeding involves complex interaction. Feeding problems seldom have a single cause and therefore may present as developmental, nutritional, or behavioral problems (Palmer, Thompson, & Linscheid, 1975). This chapter examines three components of feeding: oral motor development, nutrition, and behavior. The focus is on the major perspective of this chapter—behavior. When recognizing feeding problems as a distinct clinical entity, however, nurses must assess each component of feeding to plan successful intervention (Frappier, Marino, & Shishmanian, 1987).

Oral Motor Development

In normal full-term infants, feeding skills are present at birth and develop in an orderly fashion. With each stage of development, there are changes in the child's anatomy, movements, and functions required for feeding (Frappier et al., 1987). Developmental transitions mark critical times when the child is ready for dietary progression in terms of new foods, textures, and particle size. Readiness is communicated through behavioral cues demonstrated by the child and received by the parent. Thus, both the parent and the child play an active role in the developmental process (Bosma, 1986). When feedings are not advanced during critical developmental times, the transitions are more difficult (Blackman & Nelson, 1987).

As the central nervous system matures, the child goes through developmental changes in preparation for advancing feedings. As early as the second trimester, sucking behavior is acquired and swallowing occurs, preparing the infant for suckle feeding at term (Bosma, 1986). The suckle feeding pattern persists for the first 5 or 6 months of life. By this time, the child has developed the oral motor skills needed for spoon feeding. Chewing movements appear at approximately 6 months with increased strength and coordination of oral muscles and the beginning eruptions of teeth (Frappier et al., 1987). During this time, food types, textures, and particle size should advance. By 1 year, the child demonstrates increased needs for independence and can be weaned from suckle feedings and begin experimenting with self-feeding (Christophersen & Hall, 1978). By 3 to 6 years, chewing is fully developed (Bosma, 1986).

Health problems, resulting from congenital anomalies, renal disease, chronic lung disease, congestive heart failure, neurological impairment, or malabsorption, can result in aversive experiences with feeding, prolong the advancement of feedings, and result in feeding problems (Blackman & Nelson, 1987; Dunbar, Jarvis, & Breyer, 1991; Handen, Mandell, &

Russo, 1986). Mismanagement of feeding by the parent, including inconsistency, prolonged feeding by the parent, late introduction of textured foods, or inappropriate diet selection, can also result in feeding difficulties (Christophersen & Hall, 1978). Blackman and Nelson (1987) report that poor feeding skills are sometimes linked with crying, fighting, gagging, or vomiting when food is placed in the child's mouth. Such behaviors frighten parents and professionals trying to assist in transition feedings and can have a spiraling effect leading to greater feeding and behavioral problems.

Delayed or problematic transitions are sometimes related to oral motor dysfunction (sucking, chewing, and swallowing difficulties). Reilly, Skuse, Wolke, and Stevenson (1999) found that 20% of children with failure to thrive were not referred for further evaluation, and diagnosis of oral motor dysfunction was missed. They concluded that a substantial number of children diagnosed with failure to thrive due to no known organic cause have significant oral motor dysfunction. It is important to include identification and treatment for oral motor dysfunction as part of behavioral intervention.

Psychology of Nutrition

During the early years of life, nutritional requirements are the greatest. Both total caloric intake and distribution of calories are important (Frappier et al., 1987). Lipsitt, Crook, and Booth (1985) contend that although physiological sustenance is important, the psychology of nutrition cannot be ignored. They state two facts: (a) The child relies completely on a social relationship with the parent for his or her nutritional requirements and (b) feeding interactions are determinate of other interactions and subsequent feeding behaviors. Bosma (1986) states that the dietary patterns and preferences learned early are maintained throughout life. Sustained poor nutrition is also of concern because nutritional factors are known to influence health (Frappier et al., 1987). Thus, behavior, nutrition, and health are interrelated.

Behavior

The feeding process is more than simply giving and receiving food. It is a complex set of behaviors. Feeding affects other behaviors, and other behaviors affect feeding (Lipsitt et al., 1985). In treating feeding problems, the emphasis is shifting away from treating the symptoms to an understanding of the circumstances in which these behaviors are developed, maintained, and changed. Feeding behaviors do not occur in isolation but are related to other behaviors and the environment.

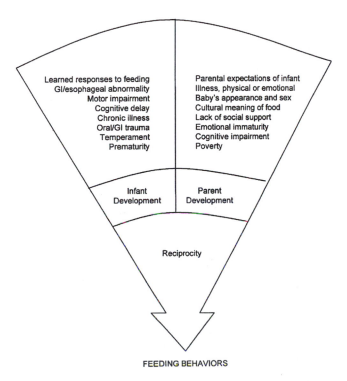

Figure 24.1. Factors Contributing to Infant Feeding Behaviors (Reproduced with permission from Frappier et al., 1987)

Frappier and others (1987) use a three-tiered model to conceptualize the behavioral component of feeding (Figure 24.1). The first tier is reciprocity, the effects that the feeder and child have on each other. The effects can be either positive, providing gratification to both members, or negative, leading to feeding and interaction problems. The second tier is individual development of the child and feeder. Both the child and the feeder are seen as initially immature in their ability to give and receive feeding cues. Over time, the child and feeder will advance in their ability to give and receive feeding cues. When feeding behaviors of the child and feeder progress in unison, there is likely to be positive reciprocity. When the feeder or child does not develop appropriately, however, they may be unable to progress and give or receive cues that advance feeding behaviors and provide gratification. The result is altered feeding interaction, which alters feeding behaviors. Tier three encompasses a broad range of physical, psychosocial, and environmental variables that affect the feeder's and the child's ability to give and receive cues. Child influences include, but are not limited to, learned responses, physical abnormalities, oral trauma, temperament, cognitive ability, and maturity. Feeder variables include parenting expectations, illness, child's appearance, gender, social support, income, and cognitive ability. Many of the reasons for feeding problems occur at tier three, and any variable that affects the development of the feeder or child ultimately affects feeding behavior (Frappier et al., 1987). When the child is difficult to feed or the feeder responds inconsistently or inappropriately to the child, negative cycles of interaction and behavior become established.

Summary

The primary components that influence feeding are oral motor development, nutrition, and behavior. Each requires an interaction pattern that should be gratifying to both the parent and the child. It is a reciprocal process, however, that is dependent on the skills and characteristics of each. Nurses can use their knowledge of the feeding components to plan comprehensive care that addresses each of these factors and promotes positive feeding interaction.

NURSING DIAGNOSIS AND OUTCOMES DETERMINATION

Before behavioral assessment and intervention begin, it is important to know about oral motor abilities and limitations and the nutritional status and requirements for the child. Assessment of oral motor development and nutritional requirements is discussed elsewhere (Bottei, 1991). Organic causes of malnourishment must be evaluated and treated as appropriate. None of these factors exist in isolation, however, and therefore it is appropriate that assessments and interventions should overlap regardless of etiologies.

The intensity of behavioral assessment required to evaluate feeding varies with the severity of the problem. Assessment requires a careful history from the parent. It may also include behavioral observations of feeding interaction, feeding diaries, or even intensive behavioral analysis by psychologists to develop an appropriate feeding plan. Wacker, Northup, and Cooper (1992) state that the purpose of behavioral assessment is not to make descriptive diagnosis of a specific feeding problem but rather to prescribe treatment based on the child's interaction in a given environment. Behavior is viewed as a function of both the child and his or her environment; therefore, assessment focuses on specific interactions. Using observational findings, the environment can then be altered to guide and motivate behavioral change. Thus, the treatment is discovered through behavioral assessment, and success is defined by the ability to prescribe effective treatment that produces the desired behavioral outcomes.

The ABC model can be used to guide behavioral assessment (Bijou, Peterson, & Ault, 1968). This model views the child's behavior (B) as a function of antecedent (A) variables and the consequences (C) for the behavior. Observations of feedings require little observer interpretation and produce the most direct assessment of the parent, child, and environment. The feeding problem can be analyzed according to the targeted behaviors for change, what triggers those behaviors, and what consequences could be used to produce and maintain the desired changes (Palmer et al., 1975). Use of these principles and information yielded is valuable for nurses in planning care and implementing behavioral plans.

In addition to providing a basis for their interventions, nurses can use assessment as a measure of baseline behaviors, to quantify behaviors for evaluation, and to set outcome goals. Analysis of the antecedent conditions produces information about the type of directions and foods to which the child is most receptive. Parent behaviors, the consequences of child's behavior, including allowing the child to escape from a direction, providing access to preferred foods and activities, ignoring, reprimanding, guided compliance, time-out, and social responses (positive or negative), can be avoided or encouraged based on the outcome. Nurses can then use information about a child's social and eating behavior to build an environment that encourages positive eating behaviors and socialization.

On the basis of the etiology and defining characteristics of the problem, a variety of nursing diagnoses can be used for feeding interaction. The nutritional component of feeding problems can be identified by the diagnosis *Altered Nutrition: Less Than Body Requirements,* defined as "the state in which an individual experiences an intake of nutrients insufficient to meet metabolic needs" (North American Diagnosis Association [NANDA], 1999, p. 9). This diagnosis is limited to feeding problems that have already resulted in nutritional and health problems.

The diagnosis Altered Growth and Development can be used when the child does not grow or develop or both according to expected norms. This nursing diagnosis is most similar to the medical diagnosis *Failure to Thrive,* which is defined as weight that is below the third or fifth percentile or less than 80% of ideal weight for age based on standardized growth curves (Drotar, 1991). Like Altered Nutrition, Altered Growth and Development is diagnosed after it becomes a significant problem—that is, when growth and performance are already affected. At this point, intervention is needed to treat the problems that exist, but potentially the same intervention could be used preventively.

The nursing diagnoses of *Impaired Swallowing,* "the state in which an individual has decreased ability to voluntarily pass fluids and/or solids from the mouth to the stomach" (NANDA, 1999, p. 98), and *Ineffective*

Infant Feeding Pattern, "the state in which an infant demonstrates an impaired ability to suck or coordinate the suck-swallow response" (p. 68), can be used to describe problems with oral motor development as they are defined by an inability or difficulty with basic mechanisms required for eating. Ineffective Breast-Feeding is appropriate when the child or mother "experiences dissatisfaction or difficulty with the breast-feeding process" (NANDA, 1999, p. 66).

In addition to approved diagnoses, new and more specific diagnoses are being developed, such as Alterations in Maternal Affective Communication, Alterations in Infant Social Responsiveness (Sullivan, 1991), and Feeding Dysfunction (Bottei, 1991). Nurses must select the best diagnoses available to communicate the specific problem.

Desired outcomes for the individual child and caretaker must be determined before intervention begins. Baseline data are essential to quantitatively benchmark the progress. These data might include specific behaviors such as the number of bites taken, the amount of time to complete a feeding, calories ingested, or patient weight. The feeding process can be broken down into specific behaviors. Target behaviors can then be tracked to evaluate progress. Videotaping can be useful not only because behaviors can be specifically quantified at a later time but also because the tapes can be used for teaching parents and other feeders the specific behavioral activities and the child's responses.

Specific outcome goals should be established based on assessment and diagnosis of the individual. Nursing Outcomes Classification outcomes related to feeding problems include Nutritional Status: Nutritional Intake, Growth, Child Development, Parenting, Caregiver-Patient Relationship, and Social Interaction Skills (Iowa Outcomes Project, 1997). Further development of outcomes related to feeding behaviors, such as Reciprocal Feeding Pattern or Feeding Interaction Skills, is needed. Long-term outcomes are more difficult to evaluate, but children need to be monitored for growth and development, school performance, other medical and behavioral problems, and problems with socialization.

INTERVENTION: FEEDING BEHAVIOR MODIFICATION

Nurses use a variety of interventions to promote child growth and development. They integrate knowledge of oral motor development, nutrition, and behavior with effective communication skills to build a holistic plan of care for the child and family. Although other health care professionals have described Feeding Behavior Modification as an intervention, often a holistic plan is absent. For example, the intervention might be more successful when combined with other interventions, such as boosting calories or promoting parenting. Nurses have access to both the child and the family and the knowledge base needed to plan holistic care and coordinate other specialties. Nurses often lack an understanding of feeding behavior modification and the specific activities that are needed to implement this intervention. Chapter 26 will familiarize the reader with behavioral concepts and terminology, whereas this chapter describes the specific application of behavioral principles to feeding problems.

The intervention label Feeding Behavior Modification was selected to best describe the phenomena of interest. The definition of *Feeding Behavior Modification,* "promoting feeding behaviors to optimize health and socialization," was formulated based on the activities and desired outcomes of the intervention. Related interventions developed by the Iowa Intervention Project (2000) are *Behavior Management* ("helping a patient to manage negative behavior" [p. 160]) and *Behavior Modification* ("promotion of a behavioral change" [p. 166]). Conceptually, Feeding Behavior Modification is more consistent with the latter intervention; therefore, similar terminology was chosen. Feeding Behavior Modification was developed as a new intervention because a unique application of activities to feeding problems is required for managing feeding problems.

Activities

The activities used to implement Feeding Behavior Modification are listed in Table 24.1. The list is neither exclusive nor exhaustive, but it includes the essential activities for the intervention. In developing the feeding plan, it is important to set up the antecedent conditions that are most likely to ensure the successful feeding behaviors. Activities that involve the manipulation of the antecedents include involving significant others in the feeding plan, limiting the number of feeders, providing four to six small meals a day, specifying how food is presented, identifying foods to be eaten, and offering new foods with repetition.

Establishing goals that are satisfactory to the parent or primary feeder and the nurse can be achieved by involving significant others in the feeding plan. Cultural patterns and social influences should be carefully considered in determining a feeding plan that will be adapted by the family (Holmes, 1993). The plan can use the parent as the therapist to initiate the behavioral plan (Cooper, Wacker, Sasso, Reimers, & Donn, 1990; Stark, Powers, Jelalian, Rape, & Miller, 1994) or as a reinforcer until behaviors are established and then the intervention is transferred (Palmer et al., 1975). Drotar (1991) advocates for the involvement of not only the mother but also other family members in the treatment plan. Others have demonstrated the success of peers to influence food acceptance and swallowing (Dorow, Williams, McCorkle, & Asnes, 1991). Involvement in the

TABLE 24.1   Feeding Behavior Modification

Definition

Feeding Behavior Modification is the promotion of feeding behaviors to optimize nutrition and socialization.

Activities

Involve significant others in feeding plan.

Limit the number of feeders.

Provide four to six small meals per day.

Specify how food is to be presented.

Identify foods to be eaten.

Offer new foods with repetition.

Monitor child feeding cues.

Give child feeding cues to start, pace, and end meal.

Offer child choices.

Limit mealtime.

Provide diversional activities, if necessary.

Prepare for extinction burst.

Offer differential reinforcement for appropriate and inappropriate behaviors.

Offer preferred foods or activities contingent on behavior, if necessary.

Pair preferred reinforcers with social attention.

Keep a discrete group of reinforcers.

Explain consequences of inappropriate behavior, if necessary.

Use time-out from reinforcement, if necessary.

Use guided compliance, if necessary.

Finish meal with appropriate behavior.

---

treatment plan by multiple persons does not necessitate participation in the actual feeding but might include other roles, such as reinforcement, limiting other distractions, or preparing food. Limiting the number of actual feeders ensures consistency and accuracy in implementing the plan (Handen et al., 1986). It also allows the child and feeder to become familiar with subtle feeding cues.

Providing four to six small meals per day increases the likelihood of success because smaller amounts are required each time. Increased frequency of meals exposes the child to the contingencies more often and allows him or her to learn expected behaviors in a timely manner (Handen et al., 1986). Brown et al. (1995) found that young children decreased their intake when offered higher energy density foods. When energy density was controlled, however, intake increased when they were offered more frequent feedings.

Specifying how food is to be presented allows the feeder to control the feeding environment. Most children are fed in isolated areas to avoid distraction (Handen et al., 1986). Other specifications might include who is present during meals, limiting diversions such as telephones and televisions, ensuring proper positioning at a table or highchair, and proper-sized utensils (Christophersen & Hall, 1978). To ensure portions are realistic and selection is balanced with preferred and nutritional foods, it is important to identify the foods that are to be eaten. This can be achieved by putting only small portions of a few well-balanced foods on the plate at a time. Large portions or too many choices are likely to be overwhelming to the child. Parents often overestimate the amount children need to eat and may need to be educated about appropriate portions (Birch & Fisher, 1995). Smaller proportions are indicated to start with to ensure success is at least possible (Handen et al., 1986).

New foods are most likely to be rejected with the initial exposure. Some foods may require 8 to 10 exposures, which includes tasting the food, before they are accepted (Birch & Fisher, 1995). To increase balance and variety in the diet, new foods need to be offered with repetition and in a neutral manner. Unfamiliar foods gain in children's preference value as a function of repeated presentation and familiarity (Hammer, 1992). One bite of new foods initially should be required, and then serving size can be gradually increased over several meals (Stark et al., 1994).

The feeding plan should also include mechanisms for monitoring and supporting feeding behaviors. This plan allows the nurse and feeder continuous feedback on how well the plan is working. Activities that monitor and support feeding behaviors include monitoring the child's feeding cues; giving the child cues to start, pace, and end the meal; offering the child choices; limiting mealtime; and preparing for extinction burst. Monitoring child feeding cues assists the feeder to identify the child's behavioral cues and respond appropriately. The feeder and child learn the behavioral pattern and can respond appropriately to one another (Frappier et al., 1987). For example, children often lift their chins and open their mouths when they are ready for a bite. The feeder must recognize this cue and give a bite to maintain the behavior. To establish reciprocity, it is important to give the child cues to start, pace, and end the meal. Simple cues, such as presenting food, putting on a bib or napkin, and sitting in a designated chair, may indicate the beginning of the meal. The feeder may open his or her mouth to model and cue the child to open for a bite. Regular prompting or patterned eating (two bites and then drink) may assist with timing. Children with feeding problems may not recognize internal cues of hunger and satiety, but external cues can be offered to assist them with timing of the meal (Birch & Fisher, 1995).

Offering the child choices gives them some control over the feeding. The feeder can manipulate food choices offered to ensure intake is balanced. As long as behaviors are appropriate, many choices are offered. If behaviors are inappropriate, choices are restricted. If the child does not make a choice, then the feeder chooses for the child (Cooper et al., 1995).

Limiting mealtime sets the standard for appropriate behavior (Christo-phersen & Hall, 1978). Brown et al. (1995) found that young infants fed cereal mixture took 15 to 20 minutes to reach satiety. Others recom-mend 20 to 30 minutes for older children. The time may need to be altered depending on the child's development and physical tolerance. Occa-sionally, particularly when the intervention is initiated, feedings may last longer when trying to end the meal with appropriate behavior. In this case, it is important for the feeder to begin to identify cues that the child is full so that the meal can be ended earlier and a battle over the last bite does not occur.

When extreme aversion to feeding is present, providing diversional activities may be indicated to move the focus from the feeding process to socialization. The child is enlisted in conversation or diversional games (such as word games, board games, and coloring) while the feeding pro-cess continues. An initial warm-up period may include making play-related demands before meal-related request or playing with eating uten-sil or toys near the mouth (Cooper et al., 1995). This activity is differenti-ated from distraction in that the feeder remains in control, and feeding is not interrupted.

Health professionals and feeders should be prepared for an initial temporary increase or stability in problematic feeding behaviors after im-plementation of behavioral intervention activities. This phenomenon, called extinction burst, can lead caretakers to believe falsely that the feed-ing plan is failing. Nurses must be aware of this phenomenon and prepare parents for it. Parents should be prepared to use behavioral interventions consistently over time to ensure success (Stark et al., 1994). Consequences of feeding behaviors must also be clearly stated in the feeding plan. These activities define consequences to manipulate behavior. They include offer-ing differential reinforcement, offering preferred foods or activities con-tingent on behavior, pairing reinforcers with social attention, keeping a discrete group of reinforcers, explaining consequences of inappropriate behavior, time-out from reinforcement, guided compliance, and finishing the meal with appropriate behavior.

Differential reinforcement for appropriate and inappropriate behav-iors is used to alter behavioral patterns. Desired behaviors, such as taking bites, chewing food well, and asking for more, are rewarded with social praise, preferred activities, preferred foods, or all three to increase the likelihood they will be repeated. Inappropriate behaviors, such as having temper tantrums, spitting out food, and refusing bites, are completely ig-nored, and attention is only given for appropriate behaviors (Palmer et al., 1975; Stark et al., 1994; Wacker et al., 1992). Offering preferred foods or activities contingent on behavior is similar to differential rein-forcement of behaviors, but the conditions are discussed before the be-havior occurs. The feeder verbalizes what behavior is required to receive the reinforcement (Cooper et al., 1995; Handen et al., 1986; Stark et al., 1994; Wacker et al., 1992)—for example, "If you take a bite of beans, then you can have a drink of chocolate milk."

Pairing preferred reinforcers with social attention enables the feeder to eventually maintain the behaviors with praise instead of preferred foods or activities. The goal is to pair a more powerful reinforcer with a less powerful one, thereby increasing its value so that it can be an effective reinforcer. Social attention, either positive or negative, can be a powerful motivator. Care must be taken to ensure social attention rewards the desired behaviors. The presence of the parent is one way to manipulate social attention and reward the child for appropriate behaviors (Palmer et al., 1975). To increase the probability that the reinforcer will be a powerful motivator, it is important to keep a discrete group of reinforcers. These reinforcers (e.g., preferred foods, special toys, and a high five) are used only during mealtimes. This will assist the child to discriminate between mealtime and other activities (Handen et al., 1986).

Explaining the consequences of inappropriate behavior lets the child know the conditions for behaviors before they occur. When necessary, the feeder delivers the message in a neutral manner; the child can then choose how to behave knowing the consequences of his or her behavior (Handen et al., 1986)—for example, "If you throw your food, you will have to clean it up." When differential reinforcement for negative behavior is inadequate, time-out from reinforcement may be indicated. As a result of inappropriate behaviors, the child is briefly removed (often just turned away) from the feeding situation and returned contingent on appropriate behaviors (Palmer et al., 1975; Wacker et al., 1992). When the child is noncompliant with a request and gains reward from escaping the request, guided compliance may be needed. To avoid allowing the child to escape, he or she is "guided" through the behavior using the least amount of physical force necessary (Wacker et al., 1992). This activity should always be preceded by offering the child a chance to do the activity without help. It is important for teaching the child that escape from eating is not possible and that good things (the reinforcers) happen when he or she eats. Therefore, it is important to finish the meal with appropriate behavior (Cooper et al., 1995; Palmer et al., 1975). Guided compliance should be used only with extreme caution, in consultation with a behavioral psychologist. It is important to keep mealtime pleasant. Some believe that this type of "forced feeding" is not appropriate in any circumstances (Arvedson, 1997) and warn that rewarding or coercing children to eat may limit the child's ability to learn self-controlled eating patterns and reinforce a preference for an unhealthful diet (Birch & Fisher, 1995).

The intervention activities described vary in complexity. Some activities may apply to children in general and not only to children with eating problems (e.g., eating four to six small meals a day). Other activities (such as guided compliance) are more complex and are intended for a select population of problem feeders. When implementing this intervention, it is important to make clear and consistent guidelines but to not overly restrict the child. Only when this fails should a more restrictive plan be implemented. The goal is to achieve a balance in the struggle for autonomy and dependence, which is particularly difficult in the feeding situation (Arvedson, 1997). More complex and restrictive intervention activities often require advanced practice nursing and multidisciplinary team involvement.

INTERVENTION APPLICATION

Jimmy was a 20-month-old who was admitted to the hospital for failure to gain weight. He had been followed in the outpatient clinic during the previous 6 months for failure to thrive (FTT). There was no known organic cause for his FTT, nor were there any clinical indicators for an organic cause. The mother described the child's poor intake, having temper tantrums at mealtimes, and opposition to directions.

Observations of the parent feeding the child revealed that Jimmy initially ate well, taking bites without prompting. He continued eating while the mother, busy preparing a meal, ignored him. After 10 minutes, the child refused more food and began having temper tantrums (whining, crying, kicking, and head banging), and oppositional behavior (turning away from foods offered, yelling at his mother, and saying "no" to all requests) increased. Jimmy also engaged his mother in conversation or ignored requests to avoid eating. Social interactions were positive during the majority of the meal. Behavioral assessment showed that Jimmy was highly responsive to social interaction and motivated to escape requests. The nursing diagnosis Altered Nutrition: Less Than Body Requirements was made based on reports and observations of Jimmy's eating behavior. The outcome Growth (Iowa Outcomes Project, 1997) was selected to monitor progress toward the goal of weight gain.

The intervention Feeding Behavior Modification was instituted with the family. The mother was coached by a psychologist and a nurse to be the feeder and to initiate the feeding plan because of her positive social interactions with Jimmy. The coaches remained with the mother during the initial feedings, one giving directions and demonstrating technique when necessary and the other doing behavioral assessment data collection. Small portions of food were set out in advance, and the child was offered a choice of foods. The mother and coaches used differential reinforcement for appropriate behavior; positive reinforcers (praise, high fives, and kisses) were offered for bites taken. Diversional activities were also used:

As long as Jimmy ate, the television (a preferred activity) remained on; when bites were not taken, the television was shut off. The first meal Jimmy tantrummed less and ate approximately the same amount. The next few meals progressed similarly, with the mother reporting significantly less temper tantrums. Intake, however, was still inadequate, Jimmy was escaping requests, and the it was taking more than 30 minutes to complete the last requested bite.

After 1 week, the team met and the plan was modified to increase the consequences for negative behavior and decrease the probability for escape. When the child was off task, the mother left his side (time-out from reinforcement), and a nurse did the prompting until he took a bite. The mother's continued attention proved to be a strong motivator. Also, the plan became increasingly restrictive if Jimmy tried to escape a request. He was offered a choice of two foods. If he did not choose, the feeder chose for him. The bite was then offered in his vision. If he did not open his mouth, the bite was placed at his lips. If he did not accept the bite, it was pushed off the spoon into his open mouth. Jimmy required no further physical guidance for compliance.

With consistent use of the plan, Jimmy's tantrums became infrequent, his intake improved, he took progressively fewer assisted bites, and he gained weight appropriate for catch-up growth, indicating progress toward the outcome goal. After 7 days, he was discharged. He continued to gain weight at home. Initially, Jimmy and his mother returned for follow-up visits every 2 weeks. When new problem behaviors occurred, such as self-induced vomiting, the mother consulted the psychologist over the phone and the treatment plan was adjusted. Jimmy continued to gain weight and was not rehospitalized for the next 6 months. He continued to return to the clinic every 2 months for follow-up.

RESEARCH AND PRACTICE IMPLICATIONS

Developing and validating an intervention are just the beginning of a process to delineate nursing interventions that improve patient outcomes. Validation of the nursing intervention Feeding Behavior Modification requires two levels of evaluation: (a) the outcome for the individual child and family and (b) outcome of the intervention for populations of children and their families. Evaluation of individual outcomes was previously discussed and is an important part of intervention validation as well. Additional research is needed to validate Feeding Behavior Modification activities in different settings and with various populations. Experimental studies need to be developed to compare outcomes of this intervention to those of other treatments. Evaluation of outcomes needs to include not only short-term but also long-term outcomes. In addition, effectiveness research with evaluation of population aggregates is needed when possible.

The clinical utility of the intervention must also be evaluated by nurses. It needs to be determined that nurses can reliably and consistently carry out the intervention. They must be able to select and appropriately implement intervention activities. The nurse also needs to be able to teach the intervention to family members and evaluate their ability to carry out the feeding plan. Collaboration with other professionals experienced with behavior modification can build the skills and knowledge that nurses need to apply this intervention. In addition, the intervention activities need to be individually evaluated for effectiveness. Further clarification of what activities are most successful, in which situation, and why is essential.

For nurses to carry out an intervention, it must be adapted to the practice setting. Adapting intervention activities to the care plan system is advantageous because it (a) provides nurses with a functional system to plan cares, (b) saves nursing time, and (c) provides a system of monitoring acuity and documenting nursing activities. Nurses must have skills and education to carry out a behavioral feeding plan. They must understand the components of feeding, the characteristics of the target population, and the specific activities of intervention. In addition, skills must be developed through practice with an experienced mentor.

There has been a lack of interventions described in the nursing literature for feeding problems in infants and children. By applying knowledge from other disciplines, nurses can apply nursing principles to children with feeding problems. Nurses are experienced at coordinating a multidisciplinary care plan, spending large amounts of time with the patient, and applying a holistic perspective to care. These skills uniquely qualify nurses to plan, implement, and evaluate the intervention Feeding Behavior Modification.

REFERENCES

Arvedson, J. C. (1997). Behavioral issues and implications with pediatric feeding disorders. *Seminars in Speech and Language, 18,* 51-69.

Bijou, S. W., Peterson, R. F., & Ault, M. H. (1968). A method to integrate descriptive and experimental field studies at the level of data and empirical concepts. *Journal of Applied Behavior Analysis, 1,* 175-191.

Birch, L. L., & Fisher, J. A. (1995). Appetite and eating behavior in children. *Pediatric Clinics of North America, 42*(4), 931-953.

Blackman, J. A., & Nelson, C. L. (1987). Rapid introduction of tube-fed patients. *Journal of Developmental and Behavioral Pediatrics, 8*(2), 63-67.

Bosma, J. F. (1986). Development of feeding. *Clinical Nutrition, 5*(5), 210-218.

Bottei, K. K. (1991). *Validation of the nursing diagnosis "Feeding Dysfunction."* Unpublished master's thesis, University of Iowa, Iowa City.

Brown, K. H., Sanchez-Grinan, M., Perez, F., Peerson, J. M., Ganoza, L., & Stern, J. S. (1995). Effects of dietary energy density and feeding frequency on total daily energy intakes of recovering malnourished children. *American Journal of Clinical Nutrition, 62,* 13-18.

Christophersen, E. R., & Hall, C. L. (1978). Eating patterns and associated problems encountered in normal children. *Issues in Comprehensive Pediatric Nursing, 3,* 1-16.

Cooper, L. J., Wacker, D. P., McComas, J. J., Brown, K., Peck, S. M., Richman, D., Drew, J., Frischmeyer, P., & Millard, T. (1995). Use of component analyses to identify active variables in treatment packages for children with feeding disorders. *Journal of Applied Behavioral Analysis, 28,* 139-153.

Cooper, L. J., Wacker, D. P., Sasso, G. M., Reimers, T. M., & Donn, L. K. (1990). Using parents as therapist to evaluate appropriate behavior of their children: Application to a tertiary diagnostic clinic. *Journal of Applied Behavioral Analysis, 23*(3), 285-296.

Dorow, L., Williams, G., McCorkle, N., & Asnes, R. (1991). Peer-mediated procedures to induce swallowing and food acceptance in young children. *Journal of Applied Behavioral Analysis, 24*(4), 783-790.

Drotar, D. (1991). The family context of nonorganic failure to thrive. *American Journal of Orthopsychiatry, 61,* 23-34.

Dunbar, S. B., Jarvis, A. H., & Breyer, M. (1991). The transition from non-oral to oral feeding in children. *American Journal of Occupational Therapy, 45*(5), 402-408.

Frappier, P. A., Marino, B. L., & Shishmanian, E. (1987). Nursing assessment of infant feeding problems. *Journal of Pediatric Nursing, 2,* 37-44.

Hammer, L. D. (1992). The development of eating behavior in children. *Pediatric Clinics of North America, 39*(3), 379-394.

Handen, B. L., Mandell, F., & Russo, D. C. (1986). Feeding induction in children who refuse to eat. *American Journal of Diseases in Children, 140,* 52-54.

Holmes, S. (1993). Force of habits. *Nursing Times, 89,* 48-50.

Iowa Intervention Project. (2000). *Nursing interventions classification (NIC)* (J. C. McCloskey & G. M. Bulechek, Eds.; 3rd ed.). St. Louis, MO: Mosby-Year Book.

Iowa Outcomes Project. (2000). *Nursing outcomes classification (NOC)* (M. Johnson, M. Maas, & S. Moorhead, Eds.; 2nd ed.). St. Louis, MO: Mosby-Year Book.

Lipsitt, L. P., Crook, C., & Booth, C. A. (1985). The transitional infant: Behavioral development and feeding. *American Journal of Clinical Nutrition, 41*(2), 485-496.

North American Nursing Diagnosis Association. (1999). *Nursing diagnoses: Definitions and classification 1999-2000.* Philadelphia: Author.

Palmer, S., Thompson, R. J., & Linscheid, T. R. (1975). Applied behavior analysis in the treatment of childhood feeding problems. *Developmental Medicine and Child Neurology, 17,* 333-339.

Pollitt, E., & Eichler, A. (1976). Behavioral disturbances among failure to thrive children. *American Journal of Diseases in Children, 130,* 24-29.

Reilly, S. M., Skuse, D. H., Wolke, D., & Stevenson, J. (1999). Oral-motor dysfunction in children who fail to thrive: Organic or non-organic? *Developmental Medicine and Child Neurology, 41*(2), 115-122.

Stark, L. J., Powers, S. W., Jelalian, E., Rape, R. N., & Miller, D. L. (1994). Modifying problematic mealtime interactions of children with cystic fibrosis and their parents via behavioral parent training. *Journal of Pediatric Psychology, 19*(6), 751-768.

Sullivan, B. (1991). Growth-enhancing intervention for non-organic failure to thrive. *Journal of Pediatric Nursing, 6*(4), 236-242.

Wacker, D., Northup, J., & Cooper, L. (1992). Behavioral assessment. In D. E. Greydanus & M. L. Wolraich (Eds.), *Behavioral pediatrics* (pp. 57-68). New York: Springer-Verlag.

25

Bowel Incontinence Care

Encopresis

Susan Poulton

Encopresis is a condition characterized by lack of bowel control with persistent defecation of formed or semiformed stool in underwear, or other inappropriate places, after the age of 4 years in the absence of an obvious organic condition (Levine, 1975). It affects 1.5% to 3% of children (Levine, 1975; Loening-Baucke, 1993). Encopresis is often differentiated as primary and secondary encopresis. Encopresis is called primary or continuous when a child has never been toilet trained for bowel movements. It is called secondary or discontinuous encopresis when a child was completely toilet trained and had no bowel incontinence for a minimum of several months (Levine, 1975). A variety of possible causative and related factors are described in the literature; therefore, a multidisciplinary approach to treatment is highly recommended (Levine, 1975).

The physiology of encopresis can be explained by a process occurring over time when a child does not have regular bowel movements or the bowel does not empty completely on a regular basis. When either irregular bowel movements or incomplete defecation occur, feces build up in the colon and become large, hard, and dry, causing defecation to be potentially painful. Because of the pain associated with defecation, the child often avoids having a bowel movement by withholding the stool, thus increasing the buildup of feces. The child also may complain of abdominal pain related to the stool mass. Liquid feces often leak out around the stool mass, causing soiling. This leakage is often confused with diarrhea. As a result of this buildup of feces, the colon and rectum stretch to the point at which nerve and muscle innervation is disrupted and can cause a condition known as megacolon (Figure 25.1). The stretching and disruption of nerves and muscles decrease the signals sent to the child about the need to have a bowel movement. With decreased signals, the child no longer feels the urge to have a bowel movement and consequently has stool accidents. Also, because the urge to defecate is not apparent, the colon and rectum do not empty completely when stool is expelled. Furthermore, some children with encopresis have abnormal defecation mechanics and actually contract their external anal sphincter instead of relaxing it so that stool can be expelled (Loening-Baucke, Cruikshank, & Savage, 1987). Often, enuresis is an associated symptom, usually related to the distended colon (Levine, 1975).

LITERATURE REVIEW

The literature on encopresis includes various approaches to its treatment and also explores the relationships of multiple factors associated with treatment outcome. Sprague-McRae (1990) proposes an approach to treatment that combines physiological, behavioral, and developmental theories. The ideal treatment is based on the combination of these theories using a multidisciplinary approach. From a physiological perspective, treatment is based on the physiology of the bowel, with the goal of attaining normal bowel function. Medical treatment consists of initial bowel clean-out, the use of laxatives to avoid reimpaction, and retraining the bowel muscles. Other interventions include a high-fiber diet and adequate fluid intake.

From a behavioral perspective, encopresis is viewed as a socially unacceptable behavior that needs to be changed. The behavioral approach is to focus strictly on changing the encopretic behavior of defecating in inappropriate places. The negative behavior is changed by using reinforcers that reward positive behavior and punishment for negative behavior. The goal of behavior modification is for the child to defecate in the toilet. This behavior modification approach has been used both with and without medical treatment.

When viewed from a developmental perspective, encopresis involves the struggle of a child's "holding on and letting go" (Sprague-McRae, 1990, p.11), which can be considered as reflective of Erikson's developmental stage of autonomy versus shame and doubt. These struggles are

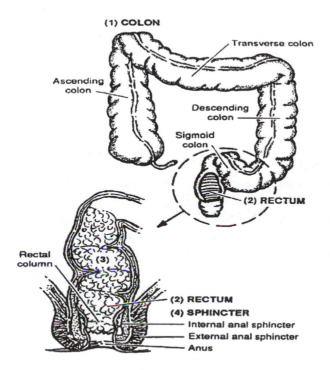

Figure 25.1. The colon: Feces or bowel movements move through the colon (1) on their way to the rectum (2). If these feces are not passed, they will collect into a large mass in the rectum (3). This can cause a condition known as megacolon. More liquid fecal matter will sometimes run down around the solid feces. If the child's sphincter (4) relaxes, this liquid waste may leak enough to soil a child's clothing. This illustration used by permission of University Hospital School, The University of Iowa Hospitals and Clinics, Iowa City, Iowa.

usually predominate between the ages of 18 months and 3 years. For some reason, the child with encopresis may not have resolved these issues because of factors that have contributed to the child's regression to earlier functioning (secondary encopresis) or the child's inability to completely work through this stage of development (primary encopresis). The child may then face a potentially serious developmental crisis. Sprague-McRae explains this in the context of Caplan's crisis theory. When a person is in a state of disequilibrium and unable to control the situation, the situation goes unresolved and eventually becomes a crisis. Factors that can influence equilibrium are the person's perception of the event, availability of a support system, and the person's coping mechanisms. On the basis of this theory, encopresis can be viewed either as the stressor that decreases the child's equilibrium or as an indication of the child's disequilibrium due to other stressors. Therefore, the approach to treatment should include an assessment to determine the child's stressors.

Current Treatments and Outcomes

Encopresis is complex. In most cases, encopresis seems to affect the child's overall health, self-esteem, social functioning, and behavior aspects that are the focus of the majority of the research on encopresis. Some of the classic research done by Levine (1975) differentiated between primary and secondary encopresis in a sample of 102 children. Characteristics of the children in these two groups were compared. One interesting finding was that toilet training was started before 2 years of age for 69% of the children with secondary encopresis compared to 43% of the children with primary encopresis. Levine and Bakow (1976) developed a medical and behavioral treatment plan for 127 children with encopresis: 87% were boys and 39% had primary encopresis. The treatment plan included education about encopresis and an initial bowel clean out with enemas and laxatives. Abdominal x-ray was obtained before and after the clean out to document the presence of stool and need for further clean-out. Once the bowel was cleaned out, a maintenance program was started with the regular use of laxatives, assisting the child to learn how to feel comfortable on the toilet, and retraining the child's intestinal muscles by having the child sit on the toilet for at least 10 minutes at the same time, twice a day, to establish a pattern for defecation.

After 1 year, follow-up of 110 children showed that 51% were cured (defined as having no incontinence of stool or soiling for 6 months), 27% had decreased the number of incontinence episodes to less than one every 2 weeks, 14% showed some improvement, and 8% showed no improvement. There was little difference in the success rate of boys versus girls and little variability in socioeconomic status and parental marital status. Hyperactivity, learning problems, and reading problems were more common in the two groups that showed some improvement or no improvement. In addition, there were more difficulties with early bowel training in these two least successful groups. The group that showed no improvement had more severe constipation and more frequent incontinence initially than the other groups. Signs of depression and social withdrawal were similar throughout the groups, which may be secondary to encopresis. Compliance of all groups was found to be a determining factor of success, but it was noted that this decreased over time as the treatment program seemed to be increasingly less successful. Compliance was improved with additional support, more frequent follow-up, and reassurance that the child and family were doing a good job with the program.

One of the few nursing studies on encopresis (Sprague-McRae, Lamb, & Homer, 1993) compared the use of oral laxatives versus rectal suppositories and enemas for long-term management of encopresis. Initial bowel disimpaction with enemas was completed, followed by implementation of a behavior modification plan and a high-fiber diet. The group was randomly assigned a maintenance program of either a regular dose of an oral laxative or a glycerin suppository when a bowel movement was not obtained with scheduled toilet sitting. An enema was given if the suppository was not effective. Sixty-one children completed treatment, and follow-up was provided for 6 to 12 months. There was no significant difference in response to treatment with the use of oral laxatives compared to the use of rectal suppositories and enemas.

In comparing the characteristics of children who responded to treatment and those who failed treatment, Landman and colleagues found that the success of the child early in the treatment program was not indicative of success at the 1- or 2-year follow-up (Landman, Levine, & Rappaport, 1983). Parental perception of the cause of their child's encopresis was related to the outcome, however. For example, at the follow-up appointment, parents of the treatment-resistant group believed encopresis was caused by emotional and moral factors rather than medical and physical factors, even though the medical and physical factors were emphasized in the educational aspect of the treatment program. Those in the failure group showed decreased school performance, which may be secondary to the persistent encopresis, or the encopresis could be secondary to school difficulties.

Additional research by Landman, Rappaport, Fenton, and Levine (1986) revealed that compared to children with chronic symptoms of abdominal pain, enuresis, and chronic headaches, more children with encopresis experienced low self-esteem, felt less in control of life events, and wanted to change and be different. These results suggest that a relationship exists between encopresis and these negative feelings, but the authors note that it is not known which occurred first, the encopresis or the negative feelings. With the use of the Child Behavior Checklist, a high incidence of maladaptive social functioning and behavior problems was found in a group of 38 children with encopresis compared to the norm per this checklist's standards (Achenbach, 1991; Loening-Baucke et al., 1987).

A purely behavioral approach to treatment was used by Davis, Mitchell, and Marks (1977), who did a pilot study of 11 encopretic children between the ages of 7 and 14 years who were treated with behavior modification. The treatment program focused on teaching the child to identify body cues indicating the need to defecate by having the child sit on the toilet frequently throughout the day during the initial treatment phase and then gradually decreasing this frequency to the point at which the child would only sit on the toilet when he or she felt the urge to defecate. The child was given the responsibility to clean himself or herself if he or she had an accident. The program also focused on helping parents consistently reward continence and discourage incontinence. When the child was no longer soiling, a maintenance program was implemented that consisted of checking the child's underwear at designated times and rewarding him or her if he or she was clean. The results showed that 5 of the children experienced no incontinence at the 5- to 7-month follow-up, 2 had no incontinence at the 2- or 3-month follow-up, and 4 did not respond to the treatment program. Lack of response was attributed to parents' inability to control the child. An overall improvement in the child's general behavior was frequently reported by the parents. The authors concluded that a behavioral approach to encopresis is an option for parents and can easily be done in the home, regardless of other problems with the child or family.

Recent research has combined a medical and behavioral treatment approach. Many studies showed overall behavior improved with successful response to a combined treatment plan that included bowel disimpaction, maintenance laxatives, and behavioral modification (Levine, Mazonson, & Bakow, 1980; Sprague-McRae et al., 1993). Levine and colleagues also found that social withdrawal and aggressive behaviors decreased in all groups, whether or not they responded to treatment.

Another area of research is defecation dynamics, the ability to relax the external anal sphincter during defecation, which can be assessed by the use of anorectal manometry. In two studies by Loening-Baucke and colleagues, results showed that within 1 hour of bowel disimpaction with one or two enemas, 56% ($n = 25$) and 66% ($n = 38$) of children with encopresis were unable to voluntarily defecate rectal balloons filled with 30 to 100 milliliters of water after sitting on the toilet for 5 minutes (Loening-Baucke, 1987; Loening-Baucke et al., 1987). Most were noted to have an abnormal contraction of the external anal sphincter during defecation, which was determined by electromyography testing. With a treatment plan including bowel disimpaction with enemas, maintenance laxatives, high-fiber diet, regular toileting with education in bowel training techniques, and record keeping of bowel movements and soiling, 70% of those who could defecate rectal balloons recovered after 1 year. Regardless of defecation dynamics, those with an abdominal fecal mass on initial exam did not recover after 1 year.

Biofeedback treatment to learn normal defecation dynamics has been used in combination with conventional treatment. Loening-Baucke (1990) found that of 22 children treated with both biofeedback and conventional treatment, 77% had normal defecation dynamics after 7 months compared to only 13% of 19 children treated with conventional treatment alone. A later study, however, showed that biofeedback did not affect long-term outcome. At follow-up (4.1 ± 1.5 years), 62% of the 66 children (49 boys and 17 girls) who received conventional treatment alone had recovered from encopresis. Sixty-three children (48 boys and 15 girls) were treated with biofeedback combined with conventional treatment, but only 50%

of those who learned to relax their external anal sphincter ($n = 50$) had recovered from encopresis (Loening-Baucke, 1995).

In summary, research on encopresis has shown that boys are more often affected than girls, more children with secondary encopresis were attempted to be toilet trained before 2 years of age, and school problems were more prevalent in children who failed to respond to treatment. Compliance was associated with response to treatment but was shown to be very difficult and tended to decrease over time when the treatment program seemed less successful (Landman et al., 1983, 1986; Levine & Bakow, 1976). Initial severity of constipation was not consistently predictive of treatment outcome among the studies (Landman et al., 1983; Levine & Bakow, 1976; Loening-Baucke, 1987). Aggressive, oppositional, and antisocial behaviors decreased in both the behavioral and the medical approach (Davis et al., 1977; Levine et al., 1980; Sprague-McRae et al., 1993). In the studies of defecation dynamics, the combination of biofeedback and conventional treatment proved to be useful in the short term, but it did not improve long-term outcomes compared to conventional treatment alone (Loening-Baucke, 1995). The complexity of encopresis is evident in the literature, which further supports the need for a multidisciplinary approach to treatment based on Sprague-McRae's (1990) model.

NURSING DIAGNOSIS AND OUTCOME DETERMINATION

As noted previously, encopresis is a complicated phenomenon often involving a combination of physiological, behavioral, and developmental factors. When determining a nursing diagnosis to describe the phenomenon and problem area, the nurse must focus on the primary concern that needs to be addressed by the nurse. The main problem is bowel incontinence, which is associated with many of the problems facing the child with encopresis. The related North America Nursing Diagnosis Association (NANDA, 1999) diagnosis for this problem is Bowel Incontinence. Other nursing diagnoses that describe related problems include Constipation, Social Isolation, Ineffective Individual/Family Coping, Self-Esteem Disturbance, Pain, Noncompliance, and Ineffective Management of Therapeutic Regimen: Individual/Families.

The child's response to treatment after a specific length of time is the actual treatment outcome. It is important to establish a way to measure and document that response so the child's success or failure to treatment can be determined and appropriate changes made in the interventions.

Loening-Baucke (1995) defined recovery as having three or more bowel movements per week and no more than two episodes of soiling per month while off laxatives for at least 1 month. This definition may need to be altered depending on the severity of constipation, the developmental age of the child, and other psychosocial or psychological factors.

The Nursing Outcomes Classification lists indicators for the outcome *Bowel Continence,* which is defined as the "control of passage of stool from the bowel" (Iowa Outcomes Project, 2000, p. 126). Many of these indicators can be used to measure and document outcome to the treatment of encopresis. Indicators such as predictable evacuation of stool, diarrhea not present, constipation not present, sphincter tone adequate to control defecation, sphincter innervation functional, identifies urge to defecate, and adequate intake of fluids and fiber are important in measuring the effectiveness of treatment for encopresis.

INTERVENTION:
BOWEL INCONTINENCE CARE: ENCOPRESIS

The Nursing Interventions Classification (NIC) (Iowa Intervention Project, 2000) includes the intervention Bowel Incontinence Care: Encopresis. The specific activities listed offer the nurse many options applicable to the treatment of encopresis. On the basis of a multidisciplinary perspective, the successful treatment of encopresis needs to include careful assessment, bowel clean-out and retraining, education, high-fiber diet with a large amount of fluid intake, motivation for compliance, developmental and behavioral evaluation, individual and family counseling as indicated, and long-term follow-up. These specific activities are included in the intervention Bowel Incontinence Care: Encopresis. Also, the use of other applicable NIC interventions will be included. Ideally, members of other disciplines should be consulted to complete activities in their areas of expertise. Many activities can be completed with collaboration of the nurse and other professionals, whereas some activities are specific nursing activities. This section is intended to give the nurse a foundation for choosing, providing, and delegating the appropriate intervention activities to successfully treat encopresis.

The NIC intervention *Bowel Incontinence Care: Encopresis* is defined as "promotion of bowel continence in children" (Iowa Intervention Project, 2000, p. 187). As previously stated, the first goal of the nurse is to complete a thorough assessment to gather pertinent information so that the appropriate activities can be determined. The first activity is to gather information about toilet training history, duration of encopresis, and attempts made to eliminate the problem. A thorough medical history and family psychosocial profile should also be obtained to rule out all possible causes of encopresis. A thorough physical examination should be done, including abdominal palpation, rectal examination, and sensory and motor examination. The rectal exam may need to be deferred if the child is not cooperative or is uncomfortable with the exam because of previous trauma (i.e., sexual abuse). The child's developmental level should also be assessed to determine if he or she is developmentally ready to successfully accomplish toilet training.

Possible physical causes for constipation and encopresis must be ruled out before proceeding with a structured treatment program. It is important to obtain this information from the parents and medical records. Differential diagnoses, such as Hirschsprung's disease, anorectal anomalies, intestinal pseudo-obstruction, metabolic abnormalities, and other conditions that may cause constipation, should be considered and ruled out (Nowicki & Bishop, 1999). This is done with a thorough physical examination, including a neurological examination and appropriate diagnostic tests. A referral for additional evaluation by a pediatrician or specialist should be made at this time, if necessary, based on any abnormal findings. Abdominal radiographs may be done as part of the initial workup to determine a physical cause for encopresis or to establish a baseline of the child's degree of constipation. An abdominal radiograph may also be done when a child refuses to cooperate with the rectal exam or the child is extremely obese (Loening-Baucke, 1993). The nurse should prepare the child and family for any diagnostic test by informing them of the purpose of the test, any dietary restrictions on bowel "prep," and what will be done during and after the test.

After the diagnostic workup is complete and any physical pathology ruled out, the nurse can proceed with the intervention implementation for encopresis. Intervention activities include patient and family education, which is ongoing and usually begun at the first encounter. The family and child should be taught the physiology of normal defecation and the physiology of the development of constipation and megacolon. It is important that the family understands that encopresis is not the parents' or child's fault, and that soiling is involuntary and "usually without the knowledge of the child" (Loening-Baucke, 1993, p. 1560). The family must also be informed that treatment is long term, at least 6 months, and they need to know that the child may have setbacks during the treatment program.

The next step is disimpaction or bowel clean-out to remove any accumulated stool from the colon and rectum so that bowel retraining can begin. Phosphate enemas are used at 1 ounce per 5 kg in children weighing 20 kg or less, or an adult-sized enema is used for children more than 20 kg (Loening-Baucke, 1993). They are administered by the nurse or parent one or two times per day for 1 to 3 days until clear results are seen. Refer to the NIC intervention Bowel Irrigation (Iowa Intervention Project,

2000) for the appropriate nursing activities to complete the bowel clean-out. During the bowel clean-out, an oral laxative may be used if the child has significant constipation.

After the bowel clean-out is completed, the child needs to start regular toilet sitting two to four times per day, which is necessary to establish a routine for the child and to promote bowel evacuation on a regular basis. The child should sit within 30 minutes after each meal to take advantage of the gastrocolic reflex, which initiates contraction of the intestines, facilitating movement of the stool. Toilet sitting also should be done at bedtime. The child should sit for at least 5 minutes and push with abdominal muscles (Valsalva) to have a bowel movement. Valsalva can be taught by having the child blow bubbles or blow on a noisemaker such as a kazoo. The school nurse, parent, teacher, or other caregiver should facilitate toilet sitting and supervise the child initially.

To prevent the buildup of stool in the bowel, a maintenance laxative, high-fiber diet, and adequate fluid intake are prescribed. Laxative choice and dosage are based on age, weight, severity of constipation, taste, cost to the family, and child's cooperation (Loening-Baucke, 1993). Mineral oil should be used with caution because of the risk of lipid pneumonia if aspirated. Mineral oil may also cause rectal irritation due to leakage and malabsorption of fat-soluble vitamins with long-term use (Lowe & Parks, 1999). Milk of magnesia and Senna are reasonably priced and effective. Laxatives need to be used for several months to years to induce a daily soft bowel movement. Most third-party payors do not routinely cover the cost of laxatives, but many will make an exception to this policy based on the diagnosis and need for long-term use.

After the disimpaction is completed, a high-fiber diet is important because dietary fiber increases the bulk and water content of the stool, resulting in softer stools that are easier to defecate on a more regular basis. The American Academy of Pediatrics (1995) recommends that the minimal dietary fiber intake for children older than 3 years of age should be equal to the child's age plus 5 g per day. Most children do not consume an adequate amount of fiber, and adding fiber to their diets can be a challenge for caregivers. A dietitian may need to be consulted to assess the child's intake and develop dietary guidelines. It is important to determine the child's baseline fiber intake and add to this amount. The best way to do this is to include a variety of foods that are high in fiber. Fruits and vegetables high in fiber are apples, berries, pears, oranges, prunes, broccoli, carrots, corn, peas, potatoes with skins, lettuce, kidney beans, and lentils. Cereals high in fiber include bran and granola. Other sources of fiber are whole wheat breads and oat or wheat bran muffins. Some innovative ways to include fiber in the child's diet are with popsicles made from prune juice, granola bars, and oatmeal with oat or wheat bran added. It will be easier for the child to accept these foods if the whole family eats a highfiber diet. The nurse can help parents learn to read food labels to identify fiber and then to plan healthy meals and snacks.

Adequate fluid intake is also an important component of the treatment plan to promote soft and regular bowel movements. Water is the best source of fluid for the child with encopresis. The child should have free access to water (or juice) both at home and at school. A special cup or bottle can be kept in the refrigerator, in the car, and at the child's desk. If the child cannot keep a drink at school, frequent trips to the water fountain should be encouraged. Refer to NIC interventions Bowel Management and Bowel Training (Iowa Intervention Project, 2000) for other activities appropriate in the long-term management of encopresis.

To assist the child in complying with this difficult treatment modality, there needs to be a reward system. Depending on the child's developmental level, such things as a sticker chart or other positive reward systems can be used to reward compliance with the program, such as sitting on the toilet at the scheduled times, taking the prescribed laxative, drinking adequate fluids, and eating high-fiber foods. For example, the older child could be rewarded with an activity of choice with one parent at the end of a week. A record-keeping system should be established and should include doses of laxatives taken, sitting times, and occurrence and description of bowel movements. A diary could also be used to monitor the child's progress and response to treatment so that appropriate changes can be made in the program. Record keeping should be the responsibility of the school-age child. In other instances, the parent or other caregiver can keep records. The child should be rewarded for cooperation with the program initially and not necessarily for having a bowel movement in the toilet because this is something the child cannot always control. As the program progresses and the bowel muscles become retrained, the child will gain more control over bowel movements and can then be rewarded for bowel movements in the toilet. The child must never be punished or ridiculed for bowel accidents but can be given some responsibility for cleanup if developmentally appropriate. For example, a child functioning at a 6- to 8-year-old level should be able to remove soiled clothing and put on clean clothes. This same child, however, may need help cleaning his or her body. An older child should be able to clean his or her body and rinse out soiled clothing. These responsibilities can be carried out in school if the child has access to a private restroom with a sink, washcloths, and clean clothes.

The treatment program also includes assessing and supporting family dynamics, including attitudes, communication patterns, strengths, and coping abilities. A psychologist or social worker may need to be involved to complete this assessment and provide appropriate interventions. The child needs to work through feelings related to the encopresis, self-esteem, and stress factors in the environment. Therapeutic play by the nurse or psychologist may be helpful in assisting the child to work through feelings.

Another area that needs to be determined is peer relationships. Being accepted by peers is important to children of all ages. Children with encopresis are at risk for rejection by peers because of their condition and the smell related to bowel accidents. The child may be singled out by the peer group as being different and left out of activities, teased, and bullied. This social rejection can affect the child's self-esteem and self-image, which are important elements of well-being and personal growth. It is important for the nurse to monitor the child's relationships with peers and the child's ability to cope with the negative aspects of these relationships (Winkelstein, 1989). The school nurse can educate and alert the school staff about the child's risk for peer rejection and ask the staff to observe interactions between the child and peers, intervene appropriately, and report concerns. The child should also be encouraged to tell his or her parents, the teacher, or nurse if he or she is being teased or bullied. Rather than leave the child to deal with this problem, the adult should help the child develop skills to respond appropriately to teasing or bullying. One approach is to discuss strategies the child can tell the bully to stop the teasing or physical aggression and suggest ways to avoid situations that put the child at risk for teasing. If necessary, the adult may need to confront the bully. An effective way to stop bullying behavior is intervention by an adult authority (Garrity & Baris, 1996).

An additional NIC intervention to consider in the treatment of encopresis is *Self-Care Assistance,* defined as "assisting another to perform activities of daily living" (Iowa Intervention Project, 2000, p. 575). Hygiene practices and motor skills of the child should be assessed. An occupational therapist may need to be consulted to complete this assessment. Often, small amounts of stool found in the child's undergarment is not stool leakage at all but may be due to the child's inability to wipe the perianal area well after a bowel movement. Also, expectations of the parents should be determined. It is important to know if the child is responsible for cleaning up after stool accidents and for doing his or her own laundry. If possible, the nurse, social worker, or psychologist should ask the child how he or she feels about these responsibilities. Parents may need guidance and education so that their expectations are developmentally appropriate for the child. In addition, the child may need supervision, assistance, and education to improve hygiene practices.

Children with encopresis encounter nurses in a variety of settings, including schools, community health clinics, primary care providers' offices, hospitals, and in homes in which nurses visit. Ideally, the nurse will have collaborative relationships with other professionals so that a multidisciplinary treatment plan can be developed for the child. The nursing intervention Bowel Incontinence Care: Encopresis and other related interventions can be accomplished in all practice settings if the nurse and other members of the multidisciplinary team are willing to be flexible. The initial bowel clean-out can be accomplished in the home, school, clinic, or hospital. It can be accomplished by the nurse or other care provider, such as the parent, if appropriate. With careful planning and frequent monitoring, the ongoing bowel management program can also be accomplished in all settings. The bowel management program must be a part of the child's individualized health care plan (IHP) in the school setting. It should be developed as a team, including the child, parents, and school staff. At both school and home, the program can only be successful if teachers and parents are willing to adjust schedules so that the child will be allowed adequate time to comply with the scheduled toileting program, take medications, and be offered adequate fluids. The environment must also include private facilities for toileting and hygiene. The bowel and toileting record should be in an accessible and private place for accurate record keeping. There also needs to be support for carrying out a consistent reward system both at home and in school. Everyone involved in the care of the child must maintain good communication with each other regarding the child's progress. Bowel and toileting records should be sent to the parents and health care providers on a regular basis. The child's IHP should be reviewed with the child's primary health care provider or specialist on a regular basis. One way to accomplish this review is to send a copy of the updated IHP with the child to each clinic visit.

Frequent follow-up and long-term management are crucial to achieving desired outcomes. The nurse should follow-up by phone or visit within 1 week after the bowel disimpaction (O'Rorke, 1995; Sprague-McRae, 1990). Ongoing follow-up should occur every 1 to 12 weeks, depending on the child's situation. Follow-up will be necessary for at least 1 year, but it may need to continue for several years. Frequent follow-up provides the opportunity to review stool records; examine the child; change laxative dose; evaluate any behavioral, psychological, or psychosocial issues; and give ongoing support and encouragement to the child and family. Parents need to have realistic expectations of treatment and should know that relapses may occur. If the child does relapse, the child and family will need the nurse's guidance and support with repeating the bowel disimpaction and reestablishing a regular toileting program.

Frequent follow-up also allows the nurse to monitor the child's progress. Compliance was found to be predictive of treatment outcome and decreased over time as the child was less responsive to treatment (Landman et al., 1983, 1986; Levine & Bakow, 1976). The overall success of the treatment program depends on both the child's ability and willingness to carry out the treatment program and the child's social support system in the family and the school. All interventions, direct and indirect, must focus on the interaction of the child, family, and the environment.

INTERVENTION APPLICATION

When James was admitted to the hospital, he was almost 11 years old with a history of primary encopresis. He lived with his parents and two sisters in a rural area. He was in a regular-education fifth-grade class. His teacher described him as being an average student who was quite social and had no major behavior concerns. He did tend to have difficulty completing assignments and meeting deadlines, however. James had no major medical concerns during infancy or early childhood. His parents attempted to toilet train him at 2½ years of age, but "he never had good bowel control." He began to have problems with constipation when he was 4 years old. He was referred for evaluation of constipation when he was 5½ years of age after his prekindergarten checkup at the well child clinic.

James was seen by several physicians during the next 2 years, but he continued to have problems with constipation, stool incontinence, and stool withholding. He did not have regular follow-up or a multidisciplinary approach to treatment. Laxatives were used, and bowel disimpaction was tried on several occasions. A barium enema and rectal manometry were normal, except the manometry test showed decreased rectal pressures secondary to the stretched colon and disrupted nerve innervation.

Three months later, James was referred to the encopresis clinic at a tertiary care center. Rectal manometry at that time showed decreased rectal sensation, decreased rectal contractility, and abnormal defecation dynamics. Bowel disimpaction was completed with three subsequent phosphate enemas. A regimen of milk of magnesia and Senokot, regular toilet sitting three or four times per day, and a stool chart was recommended. He did well for 10 days after the bowel disimpaction but then missed some laxative doses and soiling and bedwetting increased.

Enemas were often needed to disimpact the bowel at monthly follow-up appointments. James's parents were having difficulty enforcing the toileting program at home. James also refused to rinse his underwear after soiling as requested by his mother. He began to hide his soiled underwear so that his parents would not know how many accidents he was having. Biofeedback training was tried but was unsuccessful.

Due to the failure of outpatient management, James was eventually hospitalized in a multidisciplinary setting for disimpaction and the development of a bowel management program. The pediatric nurse practitioner, who coordinated the treatment program in this setting, made the nursing diagnosis of Bowel Incontinence (NANDA, 1994). In reviewing past medical records, it was determined that all differential diagnoses had been considered; therefore, the intervention Bowel Incontinence Care: Encopresis was initiated (Iowa Intervention Project, 1996). Bowel disimpaction was accomplished during the first 2 days of the admission with an enema two times per day until clear. Milk of magnesia was given during the disimpaction to act as a cathartic from the top of the colon. James was initially resistant to the rectal exam and enemas, but with preparation and an understanding staff he cooperated with the procedures. The bowel management program consisted of regular toilet sitting four times per day for 5 to 10 minutes, learning to Valsalva and relax the external sphincter with defecation, keeping stool charts, a high-fiber diet after the bowel clean-out was completed, increased fluid intake, a positive reward system for compliance, and Senokot every morning. The nurse practitioner and staff nurses provided ongoing education to James and his parents, who had many misunderstandings about encopresis, its causes, and its treatment. His parents believed that they had very little control over the situation and doubted their ability to help James. James became very independent in the program, setting the timer for toilet sitting, taking medications, and documenting stools.

During this hospitalization, psychological evaluation ruled out oppositional defiant disorder that was previously considered by another psychologist. The results, however, suggested that James experienced considerable stress due to his encopresis, school demands, and relations with parents and peers. Self-esteem testing showed that James had a positive outlook regarding his future. Because James had been dealing with his encopresis for a very long time with little success, the importance of a positive reward system was emphasized. To increase compliance with toilet sitting at home, it was suggested that his parents provide a preferred activity for James immediately after toilet sitting, such as playing a card game, and a reward for more long-term compliance that could be documented on the stool charts. James and his parents chose to reward James with $1 at the end of each week of compliance with the program.

James was discharged after 10 days and followed closely by a nurse practitioner on an outpatient basis every 1 or 2 months initially and then every 3 months. James's mother also phoned frequently with questions and progress reports. An Individualized Healthcare Plan (IHP) was developed so that the treatment plan could be carried out in the school setting (Box 25.1). He did well with the program but occasionally experienced soiling in the late afternoon. The family ate dinner after 6:30 p.m., so James usually had an interval of 6 or 7 hours during which he did not sit on the toilet. By changing times to include sitting on the toilet after school at 4:30, the soiling decreased because he often had a bowel movement at this time. Laxative doses had to be changed by the nurse practitioner several times because of loose stools. James learned to drink lots of fluids, keeping his own personal containers of juice and water in the refrigerator. He added bran flakes and whole wheat toast to his breakfast menu, and granola bars became his favorite snack.

Box 25.1: Individualized Health Care Plan

Student name: James   *Birthdate:* 11-29-84

Effective date: 9-1-96   *School:* Wood Elementary

School nurse: Susan Poulton, RN, MSN   *Physician:* Dr. E. Brown

Medical diagnosis: Primary encopresis

Assessment data: 11-year-old, never completely toilet trained for bowel movements. Has been recently hospitalized for encopresis and development of a bowel management program. Has made significant progress since that hospitalization. Has some difficulty organizing and remembering sequence of tasks. Feeling stressed about this ongoing problem, but encouraged by his more recent progress. No other medical concerns.

Nursing diagnosis: Bowel Incontinence related to encopresis (NANDA, 1994, p. 19)

Student outcome goal: Bowel Continence (Iowa Outcomes Project, 1997, p. 89)

1. James will have less than one stool accident per week during this semester.
2. James will cooperatively sit on the toilet for 5 minutes after lunch during this semester.
3. James will independently ask teacher when he needs to use the toilet (at nonscheduled times) or needs to clean himself after soiling during this semester.
4. James will cooperate with requests to remove soiled underwear during this semester.
5. James will drink adequate fluids and eat adequate fiber to have at least one soft bowel movement daily (at home or school) during this semester.

Nursing interventions:

Bowel Incontinence Care: Encopresis (Iowa Intervention Project, 1996, p. 150)

Activities

- Accompany James to the restroom in health office within 30 minutes of eating lunch. (Health aid or teacher)
- Stay with James in the restroom and monitor that he sits on the toilet for at least 5 minutes by setting the timer. (Health aid or teacher)
- If necessary, remind James to fill in bowel record after toileting and when he has accidents. (Health aid or teacher)

Box 25.1: Individualized Health Care Plan

- Notify school nurse if James does not have a bowel movement on the second day. (Health aid or teacher) School nurse will then notify parents.

- On Fridays, make a copy of the bowel record for school nurse, send the original copy home with James, and hang a new chart in the health office for the next week. (Health aid or teacher)

- Assist James with cleaning himself and rinsing underwear when he soils. (Health aid, teacher, or nurse)

- Document on bowel record when James complies with toilet sitting and cleaning messes. (Health aid, teacher, or nurse)

- Offer a prize from the "prize box" in the health office when James receives five checks for compliance. (Health aid, teacher, or nurse)

- Allow James two extra trips to the water fountain during the day. (Teacher)

- Review drinks and high-fiber food in James's lunch from home and amount consumed daily for 2 to 4 weeks. Report to school nurse. Decrease frequency to every 2 or 3 days if no concerns. (Health aid, teacher, or nurse)

- Review progress with James weekly and assess his feelings regarding the bowel management program both at home and at school, parents' support, and peer relations. Discuss any concerns with parents or guidance counselor or both. (Nurse)

Health Care Information Exchange (Iowa Intervention Project, 1996, p. 307)

Activities

- Report to educational team at scheduled IHP meetings. (Nurse)
- Report any changes or problems to team members as appropriate. (Nurse)
- Report to parents, health care providers regularly. (Nurse)
- Review progress toward or attainment of goals regularly. (Nurse)

Evaluation of student outcome goals:

Accomplished

Review dates	Yes	No	Comments:
1) 11-1-96			
2)			
3)			
4)			

Box 25.1: Individualized Health Care Plan

I have read and approve of the above plan for school health care:

Parent signature _____

School nurse signature _____

Physician signature (optional) _____

Date reviewed by the educational team _____

The psychologist and educational consultant also continued to follow James. Prior psychological testing showed that James had average intellectual skill and academic achievement, consistent with school reports. Current testing suggested difficulties related to cognitive organizational processing. James was given extra assistance and support at school in the area of organizational management skills to help him remember assignments and deadlines. He was very positive about his success in school, especially in math. At the most recent follow-up visit with the nurse practitioner, he expressed that he had made 10 good friends, when 1 year prior he could only identify 2 or 3 friends. Now, James can usually feel the urge to defecate and has a soft bowel movement every morning. He continues to take Senokot daily and eat high-fiber foods. He has not had a soiling accident at home in the past 2 weeks or at school in the past 6 months. Indicators showed the outcome of Bowel Continence had been reached (Iowa Outcomes Project, 1997). James is proud of himself and his accomplishments and so are his parents.

NURSING RESEARCH AND PRACTICE IMPLICATIONS

Because of nurses' holistic approach to patient care and positive nurse-patient/family relationship, the nurse can take an active role in prevention of constipation and encopresis by providing careful and ongoing evaluation, anticipatory guidance, and education. For the same reasons, the nurse can also be involved in the treatment plan for encopresis. The nurse is an integral part of the health care team, coordinating care, providing support and continuity to the child and family, assisting the child and family in coping with a difficult situation, and providing ongoing follow-up.

Sprague-McRae et al. (1993) presented the only nursing research published on encopresis management and comparison of historical, demographic, and behavioral characteristics of children with encopresis. There are many nursing articles, however, describing the treatment of encopresis, most from a physiological, behavioral, and developmental approach (Ellett, 1990; O'Rorke, 1995; Papenfus, 1998). Stadtler (1989) describes the role of the pediatric nurse in preventing encopresis through anticipatory guidance and education. Understanding of the contributing factors that lead to constipation and encopresis and knowledge of developmental stages will help identify specific situations that may put any child at risk for developing encopresis.

Sprague-McRae et al. (1993) also emphasize the nurse's role in educating parents. The influence of punishment is unknown. In this study, however, approximately 50% of the 136 families of children with encopresis used some form of punishment during toilet training. Therefore, nurses need to educate parents about appropriate toilet training techniques and expectations. It is important to help parents identify their child's readiness for toilet training so that it is begun at an appropriate time. Signs of readiness include that the child shows an interest in toileting, can hold urine in the bladder for several hours, and is aware of wet and soiled diapers (Chow, Durand, Feldman, & Mills, 1984).

Research is also needed to better identify children at risk for encopresis so that nurses can intervene early to prevent long-term problems. Research is needed to compare the effectiveness of various nursing interventions for encopresis and to compare outcome variability in children with differentiating follow-up. The NIC interventions require testing for effectiveness. Documentation and associated research on the use of NIC interventions in the treatment of encopresis and the outcomes of these interventions are needed.

REFERENCES

Achenbach, T. M. (1991). *Child Behavior Checklist*. Burlington, VT: University Associates in Psychiatry.

American Academy of Pediatrics. (1995). A summary of conference recommendations on dietary fiber in childhood. *Pediatrics, 96*, 1023-1028.

Chow, M. P., Durand, B. A., Feldman, M. N., & Mills, M. A. (1984). *Handbook of pediatric primary care* (2nd ed.). Albany, NY: Delmar.

Davis, H. M., Mitchell, W. S., & Marks, F. M. (1977). A pilot study of encopretic children treated by behavior modification. *Practitioner, 219*, 228-230.

Ellett, M. L. (1990). Constipation/encopresis: A nursing perspective. *Journal of Pediatric Health Care, 4*, 141-146.

Garrity, C., & Baris, M. A. (1996). Bullies and victims: A guide for pediatricians. *Contemporary Pediatrics, 13*(2), 90-92, 97, 102-114.

Iowa Intervention Project. (1996). *Nursing interventions classification (NIC)* (J. C. McCloskey & G. M. Bulechek, Eds.; 2nd ed.). St. Louis, MO: Mosby-Year Book.

Iowa Intervention Project. (2000). *Nursing interventions classification (NIC)* (J. C. McCloskey & G. M. Bulechek, Eds.; 3rd ed.). St. Louis, MO: Mosby-Year Book.

Iowa Outcomes Project. (1997). *Nursing outcomes classification (NOC)* (M. Johnson& M. Maas, Eds.; 2nd ed.). St. Louis, MO: Mosby-Year Book.

Iowa Outcomes Project. (2000). *Nursing outcomes classification (NOC)* (M. Johnson, M. Maas, & S. Moorhead, Eds.; 2nd ed.). St. Louis, MO: Mosby-Year Book.

Landman, G. B., Levine, M. D., & Rappaport, L. (1983). A study of treatment resistance among children referred for encopresis. *Clinical Pediatrics, 23,* 449-452.

Landman, G. B., Rappaport, L., Fenton, T., & Levine, M. D. (1986). Locus of control and self-esteem in children with encopresis. *Journal of Developmental and Behavioral Pediatrics, 7,* 111-113.

Levine, M. D. (1975). Children with encopresis: A descriptive analysis. *Pediatrics, 56,* 412-416.

Levine, M. D., & Bakow, H. (1976). Children with encopresis: A study of treatment outcome. *Pediatrics, 58,* 845-852.

Levine, M. D., Mazonson, P., & Bakow, H. (1980). Behavioral symptom substitution in children cured of encopresis. *American Journal of Diseases of Children, 134,* 663-667.

Loening-Baucke, V. (1987). Factors responsible for persistence of childhood constipation. *Journal of Pediatric Gastroenterology and Nutrition, 6,* 915-922.

Loening-Baucke, V. (1990). Modulation of abnormal defecation dynamics by biofeedback treatment in chronically constipated children with encopresis. *Journal of Pediatrics, 116,* 214-222.

Loening-Baucke, V. (1993). Chronic constipation in children. *Gastroenterology, 105,* 1557-1564.

Loening-Baucke, V. (1995). Biofeedback treatment for chronic constipation and encopresis in childhood: Long-term outcome. *Pediatrics, 96,* 105-110.

Loening-Baucke, V., Cruikshank, B., & Savage, C. (1987). Defecation dynamics and behavior profiles in encopretic children. *Pediatrics, 80,* 672-679.

Lowe, J. R., & Parks, B. R., Jr. (1999). Movers and shakers: A clinician's guide to laxatives. *Pediatric Annals, 28*(5), 307-310.

North American Nursing Diagnosis Association. (1994). *Nursing diagnoses: Definitions and classification 1995-1996.* Philadelphia: Author.

North American Nursing Diagnosis Association. (1999). *Nursing diagnoses: Definitions and classification 1999-2000.* Philadelphia: Author.

Nowicki, M. J., & Bishop, P. R. (1999). Organic causes of constipation in infants and children. *Pediatric Annals, 28*(5), 293-300.

O'Rorke, C. E. (1995). Helping children overcome fecal incontinence. *American Journal of Nursing, 95*(4), 16A-16B, 16D.

Papenfus, H. A. (1998). Encopresis in the school-aged child. *Journal of School Nursing, 14,* 26-31.

Sprague-McRae, J. M. (1990). Encopresis: Developmental, behavioral and physiological considerations for treatment. *Nurse Practitioner, 15*(6), 8-24.

Sprague-McRae, J. M., Lamb, W., & Homer, D. (1993). Encopresis: A study of treatment alternatives and historical and behavioral characteristics. *Nurse Practitioner: American Journal of Primary Health Care, 18*(10), 52-53, 56-57, 59-63.

Stadtler, A. C. (1989). Preventing encopresis. *Pediatric Nursing, 15,* 282-284.

Winkelstein, M. L. (1989). Fostering positive self-concept in the school-age child. *Pediatric Nursing, 15,* 229-233.

26

Behavior Modification

Judith A. Coucouvanis
Ann Marie McCarthy

Nurses encounter a variety of children in pediatric settings who display behaviors that are viewed as disruptive to the adults in their environment: toddlers with frequent temper tantrums, preschoolers who do not comply with parental requests, school-age children with inattentive and hyperactive behavior at home or in school, and adolescents who display oppositional behavior. *Disruptive* is defined as "to throw into disorder" and "to interrupt the normal course or unity of" (*Merriam-Webster's Collegiate Dictionary*, 1993), and *behavior* is defined as "the way in which someone behaves" and "the response of an individual, group, or species to its environment" (p. 103). When the frequency or intensity of a child's response to adult expectations is judged by adults as too high or too low or the behavior is viewed as inappropriate for the child's age, the behavior is labeled disruptive, and behavior modification is required.

A child's disruptive behavior creates unique challenges for parents, teachers, and caregivers. *Healthy People 2000* (U.S. Department of Health and Human Services, 1991) includes the recommendation that learning, behavioral, and emotional problems in children be addressed. Advanced practice nurses and school nurses are in ideal situations to counsel parents and others in the use of behavior modification to manage disruptive behavior. Specialized knowledge and skills are needed to intervene effectively. This chapter presents strategies for modifying disruptive behavior in children. These strategies are adapted from the activities presented in the Behavior Modification intervention from Nursing Interventions Classification (Iowa Intervention Project, 2000). The theoretical framework underlying these strategies along with assessment strategies, related nursing diagnoses, and expected outcomes are also addressed.

THEORETICAL FRAMEWORK AND LITERATURE REVIEW

Currently, there is no one conceptual model that explains behavior so thoroughly that it is universally accepted. The mechanisms that influence behavior are complex, diverse, and multifaceted and vary from individual to individual (Chess & Thomas, 1984). When discussing relevant causative factors of behavior, one might consider the child's personal characteristics of temperament, motivation, and abilities; environmental factors that include parental attitudes and child care practices; early life experiences; and stresses and demands imposed by the school and community. Therefore, recognizing that disruptive behavior evolves from a host of complex factors, the literature review will focus on the behavioral model as the framework from which to intervene when disruptive behavior occurs.

The Behavioral Model

The behavioral model assumes that behavior is acquired and regulated by certain principles of learning. These principles describe the relationships among behavior, antecedent stimuli, and consequences (Bijou, Peterson, & Ault, 1968). This model, referred to as the ABC model, reads as follows:

$$\text{Antecedent stimuli} \rightarrow \text{target behavior} \leftrightarrow \text{consequences}$$
$$\text{A} \qquad\qquad\qquad \text{B} \qquad\qquad \text{C}$$

Antecedent stimuli are those events in the environment that immediately precede the behavior, whereas consequences are those events that follow the behavior. The stimuli that immediately precede the behavior are the cues to perform a certain action. These antecedent stimuli might include a person, command, setting, tone of voice, or event. Stimuli are viewed as having some control over what behaviors occur. Altering the stimuli can affect a change in behavior.

Consequences of a behavior may strengthen, weaken, or have no effect on future occurrences of that behavior. Reinforcing consequences are thought to increase a behavior, whereas those consequences that are punishing are believed to decrease a behavior. To produce an effect, consequences must be contingent on the behavior's occurrence. Reinforcement can be either positive or negative. Positive reinforcement occurs when an event is provided following a behavior, such as providing praise or candy, and as a result the behavior increases. For example, a child is quietly playing with blocks and is joined by a peer who also wants to play with the blocks (antecedent stimuli). The child willingly shares the blocks (behavior). A teacher praises the child for sharing (consequence, positive reinforcement). In subsequent situations, the probability that the child will share is increased. Negative reinforcement occurs when an event is removed or withdrawn following a behavior, such as withdrawing a command, disapproval, or aggression, and as a result the behavior increases. For example, a child is quietly playing with blocks and is joined by a peer who also wants to play with the blocks (antecedent stimuli). The child begins to scream (behavior). The peer walks away (consequence, negative reinforcement, event removed). The child's screaming was negatively reinforced. In subsequent situations, the probability the child will use screaming, an aversive behavior, to escape from sharing is increased.

Consequences that are punishing are believed to decrease future occurrences of that behavior. Punishment can be the introduction of an aversive event, such as a reprimand, or the removal of a positive one, such as losing a privilege (Barkley, 1987). For example, a 12-year-old spending too much time on the telephone and too little time on homework (antecedent stimuli) brings home a math test that she failed (behavior). The parents limit her access to the telephone (consequence, punishment, removal of a positive event). The child's behavior has been punished, and the probability that the child will fail another test is potentially decreased.

When consequences that have been maintaining or reinforcing a behavior are discontinued and a behavior is no longer reinforced by the environment, extinction occurs (Christophersen, 1995). There are two problems with extinction when used to manage disruptive behavior. First, using extinction, a slow and gradual process, may be discouraging for those involved with the child. Second, when a reinforcer is initially removed, the target behavior tends to increase as the child tries to produce the expected response, the reinforcer. Over time, however, because the reinforcing event no longer occurs, the behavior eventually stops.

Another concept important to understanding the impact of Behavior Modification on behavior is schedules of reinforcement—the frequency and pattern of when reinforcers are provided. Schedules of reinforcement can be either continuous or intermittent. Continuous schedules are those in which every occurrence of a behavior is reinforced. In such cases, the desired behavior increases rapidly but does not persevere once the environment suspends reinforcement. Intermittent schedules are those in which periodic reinforcement occurs. These schedules take longer to change behavior; the behavior, however, is more likely to persist. In real life, all behavioral principles are likely to be acting simultaneously in chains of behavior. The same event can be an antecedent stimulus for one behavior and a consequence for another. For example, a mother's smile may be a consequence to the child's touch and an antecedent to the child's kiss. A behavior may also produce both reinforcing and punishing consequences. For example, a child's tantrum may elicit a parent's talking and soothing efforts, which positively reinforce the tantrum behavior; the parent's eventual resort to spanking, however, is a punishing consequence.

NURSING DIAGNOSIS AND OUTCOME DETERMINATION

Most children display disruptive behavior at some time in the normal process of development. For example, a child may have difficulty with toilet training, complying with parental requests, or attending in a structured classroom setting. Although these may be transitory, situational behavioral problems, they can be upsetting to adults in the child's environment. It is often difficult to distinguish between transient, normal, expected developmental responses and long-standing behavior disorders. There are no specific rules to help with this interpretation. More concerning disruptive behavior, however, represents patterns of functioning that often violate ideal or typical standards of normality. Such deviations might involve behavior that is uncharacteristic of the child's age or sex. The frequency, intensity, and persistence of a behavior are also important considerations. A child who exhibits a problem, often to an extreme degree, in multiple situations or more or less continually over a substantial period of time is more likely to be identified as behaviorally disordered (Campbell, 1995). There may be mitigating factors in such judgments, particularly factors such as the occurrence of a highly stressful procedure, a recent change in family structure, or a change in schools.

Disruptive, inappropriate behavior requires modification when it persistently interferes with learning, impedes the promotion of health, consistently interrupts home or school routines, or infringes on the rights of others. Examples of such behavior include excessive motor activity (running, climbing, or fidgeting), poor impulse control (interrupting, destroying property, and aggressive behaviors), noncompliance (acts of defiance and verbal refusals), short attention span, and teasing. Whether the disruptive behavior is the result of a transitory situation or represents a long-standing disorder, nurses often are asked to assess the problem and assist in the development of interventions to decrease the disruptive behavior and foster the development of more appropriate behavior. To intervene, nurses need to assess the disruptive behavior and identify appropriate nursing diagnoses and desired outcomes prior to the development of a comprehensive behavior modification plan.

Assessment

The purposes of behavioral assessment are to identify the targeted disruptive behavior, hypothesize the function the behavior serves, and determine the variables that are maintaining the behavior. To begin to grasp the severity and complexity of any child's disruptive behavior, the nurse must first identify a specific and measurable target behavior. "Hitting," "biting," and "throwing" are all examples of specific target behaviors. There are many functions of disruptive behavior. Common functions include escaping from a nondesired activity (e.g., chores), gaining attention (e.g., from parents), and obtaining desired activities or materials (e.g., a toy). The variables that typically maintain the behavior are antecedent stimuli and consequences in the environment (Wacker, Northup, & Cooper, 1992). Indirect and direct measures are used to determine the antecedent and consequence variables that are maintaining the child's target, disruptive behavior.

Indirect Measures

Indirect measures include review of pertinent academic or medical records, normative behavior checklists, and comprehensive interviews with parents and other caregivers. Records may provide a history of the problem behavior or clues to contributing factors. Normative behavior checklists allow comparisons of the child's behavior with that of other children and, if completed by multiple caregivers, comparisons across settings (e.g., school and home). Checklists commonly used in clinical settings are the parent, teacher, and child versions of the Child Behavior Checklist (Achenbach & Edelbrock, 1985), the Revised Behavior Problem Checklist (Quay & Peterson, 1983), and the Conners Scales (Goyette, Conners, & Ulrich, 1978). Records and checklists may be obtained and reviewed prior to assessment of the child, often allowing the clinician to begin formulating hypotheses. Interviews should clarify the situations in which the disruptive behavior occurs (e.g., home, school, and playground), hypothesize possible antecedent stimuli that trigger the disruptive behavior, and determine the consequences that occur in response to the disruptive behavior.

Direct Measures

Validating one's perceptions of disruptive behavior is accomplished by observing the child and the disruptive behavior in natural settings (Alberto & Troutman, 1995; Wacker et al., 1992). Such direct assessment measures are used for both diagnosis and monitoring the effectiveness of a treatment plan. Direct observations can be carried out in many settings and under a variety of conditions. Typically, either the frequency (how many times the behavior occurs) or the duration (how long the behavior lasts) of the target behavior is recorded during the observation. Some behaviors occur so frequently that it is impossible to count every occurrence. In such instances, time sampling is used. A time of day is selected to observe and record the behavior when it is most likely to occur. The frequency or duration is recorded during the same time each day, usually for varying intervals, with some as brief as a few minutes and others longer, such as 15- to 30-minute intervals. Recording the occurrence of the target behavior before introducing an intervention is called a *baseline measurement*. Baseline measurements are ideally collected for 1 or 2 weeks; the length of time, however, may vary depending on the type and severity of the problem behavior. Ideally, the nurse carries out direct observations, but often this is not possible. A teacher or parent may be directed to collect these data. For example, a teacher might document the percentage of on- or off-task behavior in the classroom, or a parent might keep a sleep diary, recording specific predesignated behaviors.

It is important to remember that behavioral assessment is an ongoing process. After the initial assessment and baseline observations, tentative diagnoses are made and a behavior modification plan is developed. The occurrence of the target behavior should continue to be monitored following the implementation of the intervention. This is the most effective way to determine if the intervention is working and if behavior is changing over time.

Nursing Diagnoses

Nurses working with children displaying disruptive behavior and their families may identify many relevant nursing diagnoses. For families dealing with transitory, developmental, or situational disruptive behavior, there may be few related nursing diagnoses. For other families, particularly those who have a child who displays ongoing disruptive disorders, multiple nursing diagnoses may be appropriate. When a family has a child with disruptive behavior, the behavior may upset the routines of family functioning. Parents may disagree about appropriate discipline approaches, or one parent may withdraw while the other becomes overburdened with the demands of the child's care. Siblings may react in an effort to obtain attention.

Diagnoses focusing on the child that nurses may find appropriate include Ineffective Individual Coping, Impaired Social Interaction, Noncompliance, Altered Thought Processes, Risk for Violence: Self-Directed or Directed at Others, and Anxiety (North American Nursing Diagnosis Association [NANDA], 1999). Each of these diagnoses includes defining characteristics that may be displayed by children with disruptive behavior. Diagnoses focusing on the family include Altered Parenting, Altered Family Processes, Caregiver Role Strain, and Ineffective Family Coping (NANDA, 1999). Families trying to cope with a disruptive child may display characteristics of one or more of these diagnoses.

Outcomes

The primary outcome of behavior modification for children with disruptive behavior is a decrease or cessation of the targeted, disruptive behavior. Frequently, the disruptive behavior is replaced with a more appropriate, acceptable behavior. Secondary outcomes involve the removal or reversal of defining characteristics of related nursing diagnoses following implementation of the intervention. Outcomes from the Nursing Outcomes Classification that might be used to measure the child's progress with behavioral interventions include Adherence Behavior, Aggression Control, Anxiety Control, Caregiver Well-Being, Impulse Control, and Social Interaction Skills (Iowa Outcomes Project, 2000).

INTERVENTION: BEHAVIOR MODIFICATION

Relevant activities from the Nursing Interventions Classification intervention Behavior Modification foster the replacement of disruptive behavior with acceptable alternative behavior (Iowa Intervention Project, 2000). This occurs through the alteration of specified antecedents and consequences. Typically, multiple activities are combined into a treatment package or intervention that meets the child's needs.

Altering Antecedents

Many aspects of the physical environment can positively or negatively influence disruptive behavior. Environmental antecedents, such as noise, crowds, physical activity, cramped spaces, and visual distractions, can all increase disruptive behavior. These antecedents are easily overlooked when considering a specific child's disturbing behavior. Modifying or eliminating these variables, however, may help to reduce the frequency or intensity of many disruptive behaviors (Coucouvanis, 1997). When a child is consistently unable to manage his behavior in a noisy, overstimulating environment, the child will be more successful when either he or she or the source of overstimulation is removed.

Consistent routines and rules can also influence disruptive behavior. For example, the child with hyperactive, impulsive behavior can disrupt an entire classroom unless strategies are implemented to increase structure and provide consistent routines. Hodgdon (1995) recommends creating a daily plan and a weekly or monthly calendar to assist the child. Identifying the sequence of activities through pictures is recommended for the child who cannot tell time or read. Visual cues help the child to predict what is going to happen and encourage organization in the child. In addition, schedules assist the child who has difficulty coping with unforeseen schedule changes or interruptions in activities.

Parents and teachers need reminders that although they are not directly to blame for the disruptive behavior, the way they approach and interact with the child can make the problem better or worse. Disruptive behavior evokes strong emotions. Frustration and intolerance are common reactions to children who are uncooperative, hostile, demanding, and rejecting. Everyone must adopt an attitude that is empathic, supportive, and constructive while remaining calm, matter-of-fact, and reassuring when managing the disruptive behavior.

Verbal communication is the final antecedent that influences disruptive behavior (Blum, Williams, Friman, & Christophersen, 1995). When communicating with children who are disruptive, it is recommended that adults speak calmly, clearly, and simply to ensure their message is heard and processed. Multiple-step directions can be presented one at a time. Occasionally, two- to three-word phrases are most helpful (e.g., "find your coat," "sit down," and "come and eat"). These can be paired with gestures and other visual cues. When giving directives, the individual should be in close proximity to the child. Obtaining the child's attention by clearly establishing eye contact and asking the child to repeat the directive is often helpful. Rules or directives are most likely to be followed when they are stated positively (e.g., "The rule is ride your bike on the sidewalk" instead of "Don't ride your bike on the street") (Carns & Carns, 1994). Directives can be given twice, and then the child is guided to comply. It is best not to argue or bargain about established limits and rules.

Altering Consequences

There are occasions when modifying the environment and effective verbal communication do not eliminate or even sufficiently decrease targeted disruptive behavior. In these situations, the consequences maintaining the disruptive behavior must be changed.

Reinforcing Consequences

Reinforcing consequences maintain and strengthen behavior and can be manipulated to achieve a desired outcome. An event or object is said to be reinforcing if the child will work to obtain access to it (Christophersen, 1995). Reinforcing consequences occur through the use of (a) positive reinforcement, (b) the Premack principle, (c) a token economy, or (d) a contract.

Positive reinforcement is a powerful method of behavior change and is often used to develop alternative, appropriate behavior (Barkley, 1987). It occurs when an event is provided following a behavior that is contingent on the occurrence of the behavior and results in the increased occurrence of the behavior. Reinforcing appropriate behavior begins with defining the desired behavior that is to replace the disruptive behavior. Keeping hands to self, using gentle touch, using self-control, speaking in a quiet voice, or holding mom's hand in the store are examples of desired behaviors. With successful intervention, the frequency of desired behavior will increase while the frequency of the target disruptive behavior decreases.

Choosing a positive reinforcer or reward is essential to developing an intervention program. Social reinforcers, such as attention, enthusiastic praise, a hug, or a smile, can be effective reinforcers. They encourage a child to continue engaging in the acceptable behavior and should be used generously when a behavior program is introduced. Pairing social reinforcers with a tangible reinforcer is even more effective. Frequently, parents comment that their child is not interested or motivated by rewards. With careful questioning about favorite foods and activities as well as how the child spends his or her time, however, a list of rewards can usually be generated. For example, a favorite activity, such as time on the telephone, playing a video game, or playing with a parent, can be chosen as the reward. Access to the designated reward must be limited and be contingent on the occurrence of the desired behavior. It should be given immediately following and every time the desired behavior occurs (Webster-Stratton & Herbert, 1994).

Parents may have concerns about the use of positive reinforcement. They may believe that the child should act appropriately without a reward. They can be reminded that using rewards will accelerate behavior change. For example, adults receive their paychecks contingent on completing their work. Parents may also perceive reinforcement as a form of bribery. They must be helped to understand the differences between bribery and reinforcement. Bribery, frequently used "after the fact," may stop a negative behavior that is already in progress. Bribery, however, places the child in control and does not teach the child appropriate behavior. For example, a child misbehaving in the grocery store who stops only when the parent offers a treat is responding to a bribe. A reinforcement program that is planned in advance keeps the parent in control and teaches acceptable behavior. For example, "When you shop for groceries with me without crying or fussing, you can have a treat when we get to the car."

Second, the Premack principle, more commonly known as "grandma's rule," is an informal use of positive reinforcement. The child is informed that involvement in a desired activity is contingent on the child completing a less desired activity. For example, the statement, "When you eat your dinner, you can have ice cream," uses highly probable behaviors to reinforce low-probability behaviors and is frequently very successful (Clark, 1985).

Third, a token economy is a another form of reinforcing consequence. It uses tokens, coins, or points that have no intrinsic reinforcing properties but take on reinforcing properties when they can be exchanged for items or activities that are reinforcing to the child. Simple earn and exchange systems are useful for children as young as 3 to 5 years of age, whereas more sophisticated systems can be developed for teenagers. The success of a token economy depends on how consistently it is used and the variety of reinforcing activities available to the child (Christophersen, 1995).

Finally, a contract states the relationship between desired future behavior of the child and the reinforcing consequences that the child will receive when those behaviors occur (Carns & Carns, 1994). Contracts can use stars, stickers, checklists, simple statements, or written agreements. The older the child, the more involved the child should be in negotiating the contract. The contract is a positive list of desired behaviors rather than a list of don'ts and includes the responsibilities of both parent and child. The expectations are low and specific so that the child can earn the first reinforcer within 3 days. For younger children, creative, colorful charts can use pictures to identify desired behavior, or the chart can be made in the shape of an animal, airplane, train, or other age-appropriate item. For older children, a written, signed contract clarifies expected behaviors of those involved, decreases conflicts, and may incorporate punishing consequences along with reinforcing consequences. The contract for this chapter's case study is shown in Figure 26.1.

Punishing Consequences

Punishing consequences are frequently used to decrease the frequency of a highly troublesome disruptive behavior such as aggression. There are

Michael's Behavior Plan

	Monday	Tuesday	Wednesday	Thursday	Friday	Saturday	Sunday
I followed directions							
I asked for help							
I asked for a break							
I kept my hands to myself							

When you receive 3 stars for the day you can play a game of chess after dinner.

When you earn all 4 stars for the day you can have a special bedtime story.

Figure 26.1. Example of a Contract

five commonly used punishing consequences: (a) extinction, (b) verbal reprimand, (c) natural consequences, (d) response cost, and (e) time-out.

Extinction is a widely used method of reducing disruptive behavior. With extinction, no reward, including attention, follows the behavior; the behavior is simply ignored. Although easy to describe, ignoring is not easy to implement. It requires that the individual look away from the child; refrain from speaking to, scolding, or touching the child; and keep a muted facial expression whenever the disruptive behavior is observed. By decreasing the supply of attention for disruptive behavior through extinction, the chance the misbehavior will occur again decreases. Tantrums, whining, sulking, and swearing are best ignored. These behaviors, although disruptive, rarely hurt anyone and usually disappear if systematically ignored. Parents and teachers should be forewarned, however, that ignored behaviors often get worse before they get better, and behavior change will be gradual. Ignoring requires a conscientious effort from all individuals who interact with the child. Consistency and cooperation are essential if a behavior is to be ignored immediately and every time it occurs (Christophersen, 1995).

Another punishing consequence involves the presentation of an aversive event, a verbal reprimand, on the occurrence of disruptive behavior. A verbal reprimand includes the use of a loud tone of voice, a verbal statement conveying disapproval, and a clear, direct, and specific command. This is most effective if used with a single child rather than a group of children and if the adult establishes eye contact with the child (Barkley, 1987). Examples of verbal reprimands are "No spitting!" and "No hitting!" A progression to a statement of consequences may or may not be necessary, depending on the child's response.

Natural consequences are those events that naturally follow a behavior unless someone steps in to prevent them. A natural consequence for not wearing gloves on a cold day is having cold hands. Having a broken toy is a natural consequence to purposefully breaking a toy. Arriving late to school is a natural consequence of getting up late in the morning or of slowly getting ready for school. Those who use natural consequences believe children learn to improve their behavior when they are allowed to experience the naturally occurring negative or punishing consequence for their decisions and actions.

When token economies include the removal or loss of previously earned tokens or points, this is termed "response cost." The "cost" is a punishing consequence that follows a predetermined disruptive behavior. For example, a child might earn three tokens for playing nicely with friends for 1 hour but lose two of them when he hits a friend. He "pays" two tokens for hitting. Specific prosocial and target behaviors coupled with their "rewards" and costs are identified. These systems can be effective with school-age children and young teens.

Time-out (TO) is the removal of positive events. Historically, it has meant time-out from reinforcement (Patterson, 1975). The child is moved from a situation that is reinforcing problem behavior to one that is not at all reinforcing (Christophersen, 1992). TO is most appropriate for behavior that cannot be ignored, such as hitting, property destruction, stealing, or noncompliance. It is most effective for children ages 2 to 12 years and for one or two target behaviors at a time. The ideal place for TO is dull, boring, and symbolizes all that is nonreinforcing. It must be free of books, television, toys, and especially people. The length of TO is typically 1 minute for each year of the child's age. Setting a kitchen timer at the beginning of TO clearly signals the end of TO for both parent and child. TO is applied immediately following the misbehavior. The behavior is identified for the child and paired with the word "time-out"—for example, "That's hitting; time-out" or "No spitting; time-out!" Any verbal interactions with the child are brief, to the point, and neutral. To be effective, TO must be used every time the targeted, disruptive behavior occurs. The arrangement for TO is explained to the child before it is used, as suggested. The following is an example of how to explain TO to a child:

I know you have trouble playing nicely with other people. You have problems hitting and kicking other children. I also know you are tired of being scolded. We have a program that will help you practice not hitting or kicking people. First, you will earn one star if you play without hitting or kicking anyone for 30 minutes. Each time you hit or kick, you will lose one star. We will keep track on this chart on the door. When you have earned four stars, you can have a comic book or a special treat. To help with the practice, we are also going to use time-out. Each time you hit or kick someone, we will tell you and then you go to time-out. We will set the timer so that it rings at the end of 5 minutes. You go into the bathroom and wait for it to go off, then you come out.

Some parents encounter difficulties in implementing TO. A child may try to argue or insist on debating the situation once TO has been implemented. This behavior is best ignored, and the adult can state, "For every 15 seconds it takes you to get to TO, you have 1 more minute in TO." The adult ignores the child's arguments except to state, "One minute more, 2 minutes more." If the child does not go into TO after receiving 20 minutes of TO, the child is informed that if he or she does not go into TO within 1 minute, special privileges will be lost for the rest of the day (or there will be some other consequence). The adult waits for 1 more minute and then walks away. Sometimes, a child may kick the door, yell, or cry while in TO. When this occurs, the child is informed that TO will not be over until there is quiet. If a mess is made, the child is told that the room must be cleaned before he or she can leave TO. The child should not be reprimanded when TO is over. When appropriate behavior (sharing and sitting quietly) is displayed, this behavior should be praised.

Often a very effective behavior management strategy with children, TO can also be highly reinforcing. In these instances, TO is perceived by the child as a positive consequence because it is viewed as an escape from an undesirable activity (Coucouvanis, 1997). In such situations, children will deliberately act out to avoid a task. TO may also be perceived as reinforcing when it is the only attention a child receives. To counterbalance these possibilities, one must be very careful to guarantee that a high frequency of reinforcement occurs for desired, appropriate behavior while the child is not in TO.

INTERVENTION APPLICATION

Michael was referred for an evaluation by his first-grade teacher at age 6 because of severe disruptive behavior, including hyperactivity, noncompliance, screaming, and difficulty sustaining attention. He was seen by a local pediatrician, who diagnosed Attention Deficit Hyperactivity Disorder and began treatment with Ritalin (5 mg) in the morning and at noon. Michael's family was referred to the nurse practitioner for behavior management suggestions and parent guidance at the time of the original evaluation. The parents elected to delay meeting with the nurse practitioner, however, and Michael continued to display escalating behavior problems, including aggression. The family then decided to follow through with behavior management and parent training.

Michael came to the clinic accompanied by his parents. The assessment revealed that the parents were both employed full-time, and the mother was the primary caretaker in the home. Michael had severe temper tantrums at home and school whenever something did not go his way or when he could not do exactly as he wanted. He also threw toys, had no sense of danger, and was very active and impulsive. Standardized behavior checklists confirmed that both the parents and the teacher found Michael to be significantly above the norm on activity level, aggression, and impulsivity compared with children his age. Psychological testing was requested by the nurse practitioner to rule out the presence of any learning disabilities. The testing revealed high-average cognitive abilities with superior verbal skills. A learning disability was not identified.

The parents and school staff began collecting baseline data on noncompliance and temper tantrums. Antecedents to temper tantrums appeared to be frustrating events, paint colors getting mixed together, a project not going exactly right, and so on. Consequences to Michael's disruptive behavior were often either obtaining what he wanted or escaping from demands. A classroom observation by the nurse practitioner was arranged. During this observation, Michael demonstrated excellent attention to structured activities, and he followed directions well. He was quite adept at setting up situations to fit his beliefs of how a game should be played or activity should be completed. For example, when he could not find a left-hand glove for sweeping, he traded a right-hand glove with a peer. He was easily frustrated when situations did not go as he directed them, and he became tearful and loud. At one point, he struck a peer. Nursing diagnoses for Michael included Individual Coping, Ineffective and Social Interaction, Impaired. The goals of intervention were to decrease Michael's disruptive behaviors and improve his coping behaviors and social skills. Specific outcomes that were measured were Impulse Control and Social Interaction Skills.

Following this observation, the nurse practitioner developed an intervention that included a behavior modification plan. She spoke with the parents and teaching staff and offered specific management strategies. Structure, clear directions, consistent response to Michael's behavior, positive reinforcement for appropriate behavior, natural consequences, time-out, and a reward chart were all incorporated into a behavior modification plan for Michael that both his parents and teachers could carry out (Barkley, 1987). This positive behavior management program included earning a daily chess game with one of the parents when he successfully used self-control strategies during the day (see Figure 26.1). Ongoing family treatment continued to emphasize compliance training and the appropriate use of structure. Michael's mother began to talk simply and firmly to him, and she became consistent in her use of both positive and negative consequences. The effectiveness of the intervention was measured through indicators for specific outcomes. For the outcome Impulse Control, Michael demonstrated an increase in his ability to identify feelings that led to impulsive behaviors and in his ability to identify the consequence of his impulsive actions. For the outcome Social Interaction Skills, Michael demonstrated more cooperative and less confrontational behavior over time.

RESEARCH AND PRACTICE IMPLICATIONS

Ongoing research is needed in the area of disruptive behavior in children. Assessment strategies need to be refined, with recognition that assessments need to respond to the limitations imposed by managed care. Additional analysis of disruptive behavior might refine the definition and establish norms of disruptive behavior and behavior modification interventions for identified age groups, settings, health status, and developmental levels. Currently, specific research is lacking in these areas. The role of community nurses, including public health nurses, pediatric nurse practitioners, and school nurses, in assessing and managing disruptive behaviors in children needs further clarification. Research on both predictors of disruptive behaviors and prevention of these behaviors would be valuable in decreasing the prevalence of this problem. The role of education programs for parents, children, and teachers on managing specific aspects of disruptive behavior, such as aggressiveness and hyperactivity, needs additional research. Also, comparative study and analyses of various management strategies would further determine the effectiveness of specific interventions.

Although research is needed on the assessment and management of children with disruptive behavior, community nurses need to continue to play an active role in the early identification and management of these children. The move to focus the provision of health care in the community places community nurses at the forefront in providing care to these children and their families. Other health care providers, such as psychologists and psychiatrists who are frequently involved in the care of children with disruptive behaviors, need to recognize the role nurses can play in direct assessments of these children and in the development, implementation, and evaluation of behavior modification interventions.

REFERENCES

Achenbach, T. M., & Edelbrock, C. S. (1985). *Manual for the Revised Child Behavioral Checklist.* Burlington, VT: University Associates in Psychiatry.

Alberto, P. A., & Troutman, A. C. (1995). *Applied behavioral analysis for teachers* (4th ed.). Englewood Cliffs, NJ: Prentice Hall.

Barkley, R. A. (1987). *Defiant children: A clinicians manual for parent training.* New York: Guilford.

Bijou, S. W., Peterson, R. F., & Ault, M. H. (1968). A method to integrate descriptive and experimental field studies at the level of data and empirical concepts. *Journal of Applied Behavior Analysis, 1,* 175-191.

Blum, N. J., Williams, G. E., Friman, P. C., & Christophersen, E. R. (1995). Disciplining young children: The role of verbal instructions and reasoning. *Pediatrics, 96*(2, Pt. 1), 336-341.

Campbell, S. B. (1995). Behavior problems in preschool children: A review of recent research. *Journal of Child Psychology and Psychiatry and Allied Disciplines, 36,* 113-149.

Carns, A. W., & Carns, M. R. (1994). On the scene: Making behavioral contracts successful. *School Counselor, 42*(2), 155-160.

Chess, S., & Thomas, A. (1984). *Origins and evolutions of behavior disorders: From infancy to early adult life.* New York: Brunner/Mazel.

Christophersen, E. R. (1992). Discipline. *Pediatric Clinics of North America, 39*(3), 395-411.

Christophersen, E. R. (1995). Behavioral management: Theory and practice. In S. Parker & B. Zuckerman (Eds.), *Behavioral and developmental pediatrics* (pp. 46-51). New York: Little, Brown.

Clark, L. (1985). *SOS! Help for parents.* Bowling Green, KY: Parents Press.

Coucouvanis, J. A. (1997). Behavioral intervention for children with autism. *Journal of Child and Adolescent Psychiatric Nursing, 10,* 37-44.

Goyette, C. H., Conners, C. K., & Ulrich, R. F. (1978). Normative data on Revised Conners Parent and Teacher Rating Scales. *Journal of Abnormal Child Psychology, 6*(2), 221-236.

Hodgdon, L. A. (1995). *Visual strategies for improving communication.* Troy, MI: Quirk Roberts.

Iowa Intervention Project. (2000). *Nursing interventions classification (NIC)* (J. C. McCloskey & G. M. Bulechek, Eds.; 3rd ed.). St. Louis, MO: Mosby-Year Book.

Iowa Outcomes Project. (1997). *Nursing outcomes classification (NOC)* (M. Johnson, M. Maas, & S. Moorhead, Eds.; 2nd ed.). St. Louis, MO: Mosby-Year Book.

Merriam-Webster's collegiate dictionary (10th ed.). (1993). Springfield, MA: Merriam-Webster.

North American Nursing Diagnosis Association. (2000). *Nursing diagnoses: Definitions and classification 1999-2000.* Philadelphia: Author.

Patterson, G. (1975). *Families.* Champaign, IL: Research Press.

Quay, H. C., & Peterson, D. (1983). *Manual for the Revised Behavior Problem Checklist.* Coral Gables, FL: University of Miami.

U.S. Department of Health and Human Services. (1991). *Healthy people 2000: National health promotion and disease prevention objectives* (DHHS Publication No. PHS 91-50312). Washington, DC: Government Printing Office.

Wacker, D., Northup, J., & Cooper, L. (1992). Behavioral assessment. In D. E. Greydanus & M. L. Wolraich (Eds.), *Behavioral pediatrics* (pp. 57-68). New York: Springer-Verlag.

Webster-Stratton, C., & Herbert, M. (1994). *Troubled families—problem children.* New York: John Wiley.

27

Self-Mutilation Prevention

Jo Ellen Crowe

Catherine Willoughby

Self-mutilation is not a new phenomenon. For centuries, people of various cultures have practiced appearance-altering, self-mutilating behaviors for a variety of reasons. Among young people today, it is not unusual for them to tattoo, pierce, or brand various body parts. Although not necessarily accepted by some people, many of these body alterations can be viewed as culturally acceptable and rarely indicate the need for therapeutic intervention (Sebree & Popkess-Vawter, 1991; Valente, 1991). In some cases, however, young people communicate serious emotional instability by deliberately damaging their bodies with behaviors such as cutting, abrading, or burning skin. These are the situations that require intervention and are especially challenging for health care providers.

In their classic book, *Self-Mutilation: Theory, Research and Treatment,* Walsh and Rosen (1988) describe four types of "self-alteration of physical form" that occur on a spectrum (p. 7). Type I alterations are acceptable in most social groups, reflect no disturbed psychological state, and at most cause only superficial physical damage. These behaviors include ear piercing, cosmetic plastic surgery, small professionally applied tattoos, and nail biting. Type II behaviors do more tissue damage and may reflect a benign psychological state, or they may be associated with some agitation. Behaviors in this group include more extensive body piercing, ritualistic scarring such as that found among some Polynesian and African clans, and large tattoos. This level of body alteration is acceptable only within specific subcultures. The third category reflects some degree of psychic crisis resulting in mild to moderate physical damage that is generally unacceptable in all social groups except possibly among a few like-minded peers. Type III behaviors include wrist and body cutting, self-inflicted burns and tattoos, and wound excoriation. The rare Type IV behaviors, such as autocastration and self-enucleation, are very severe and unaccepted by all social groups. They are usually indicative of psychotic thinking. The focus of this chapter is limited to adolescent use of Type III self-alteration.

LITERATURE REVIEW

There is limited research on self-mutilation in adolescents. Walsh and Rosen (1988) reported the incidence of self-mutilation ranged from 14 to 600 persons per 100,000 population per year, with the wide variation due to imprecise record keeping and definition. Reasons for this behavior are complex. Miller (1994) described many motivations that are classified into the following categories: (a) escape from empty or unreal feelings, (b) relief of tension, (c) expression of feelings, or (d) control over one's own body or reactions of others.

The typical cluster of behaviors associated with self-mutilation in adolescents includes intense and labile affect (mood swings), impulsive behavior, inadequate coping, chaotic and disturbed interpersonal relationships, and unstable self-image or sense of self (Walsh & Rosen, 1988). In the United States, adults with an enduring pattern of this kind of emotional instability are often diagnosed with Borderline Personality Disorder (BPD). The diagnostic features of BPD include "a pervasive pattern of instability of interpersonal relationships, self-image and affect, and marked impulsivity that begins by early adulthood and is present in a variety of contexts" (American Psychiatric Association, 1994, p. 650). It is important to note that these diagnostic features may also be seen in depression, in posttraumatic stress disorder, in attachment or mood disorders, and in normal adolescence. As a general rule, the diagnosis of BPD is not given to children and only rarely to adolescents younger than 18 years of age. Research has shown that BPD features in childhood do not necessarily predict their continuation into late adolescence or adulthood (Lofgren, Bemporad, King, Lindem, & O'Driscoll, 1991). It is imperative to differentiate between symptoms that may likely become a lifelong pattern of coping and those that are part of the transitory characteristics of adolescence.

Walsh and Rosen (1988) studied adolescents in four treatment centers and identified correlations between self-mutilation and variables present in childhood. The two highest correlations were sexual abuse and childhood illness (both $r = .48$), followed closely by group care ($r = .47$) and physical abuse ($r = .44$). Other significant but moderate correlations were found for family violence ($r = .33$), family alcoholism ($r = .33$), and divorce ($r = .31$). All these relationships were significant at the .001 probability level. Correlations significant at the .01 level were foster care ($r = .29$) and surgical repair of physical anomalies ($r = .27$). The two central themes in these data were the childhood experience of seriously disrupted family life and severe or traumatic damage to the body. In adolescents who have no history of abuse or illness and who have grown up in supportive intact families, stressors may be related to perfectionism, stress, and peer expectations.

Walsh and Rosen (1988) also studied the correlations between self-mutilation and other problems experienced by adolescents concurrent with their use of self-mutilation. Significant at the .001 level were correlations with eating disorders ($r = .58$), physical illness ($r = .55$), sexual identity distress ($r = .50$), inattentiveness to appearance ($r = .34$), and recent loss ($r = .33$). Lower correlations significant at the .01 level were peer conflict ($r = .27$), drug abuse ($r = .26$), and alcohol abuse ($r = .26$) (p. 68). The authors describe these young people as having severe problems with self- and body image, tending to hate their bodies in an intense, self-alienating way that may be especially poignant when experiencing puberty or sexual conflict. In addition, their self-mutilation may lead to needed attention from caring individuals who provide medical attention for their self-inflicted wounds or who sympathize and worry about them. These data indicate that certain adolescents may be more prone to self-mutilation due to individual past experiences, but clinical experience shows that these risk factors are not necessarily present in all cases.

NURSING DIAGNOSIS AND OUTCOMES DETERMINATION

Many people, including some professionals, have the perception that self-mutilation is related to suicidal intent or behavior. The available literature does not support this belief. On the basis of their literature review and their research, Walsh and Rosen (1988) concluded that self-mutilation is not an attempt to end one's life but rather is a way of coping with life stressors and frustrations to keep on living. The key to diagnosis and distinguishing between self-mutilation and suicidal behavior lies in personal motivation. Rosen, Walsh, and Rode (1990) define *self-mutilation* as "a self-directed, deliberate, non-life-threatening act of self-harm that leaves a visible mark or injury" (p. 179). A similar definition has been adopted for the purpose of nursing diagnosis.

The North American Nursing Diagnosis Association (NANDA, 1999) defined *Risk of Self-Mutilation* as "a state in which the individual is at risk to perform an act upon the self to injure, not kill, which produces tissue damage and tension relief" (p. 128). Other NANDA nursing diagnoses to consider because of similar or overlapping characteristics include Ineffective Individual Coping, Self-Esteem Disturbance, and Anxiety. All these diagnoses may indicate an increased risk of self-mutilation.

Related nursing outcomes in the Nursing Outcomes Classification (NOC) (Iowa Outcomes Project, 2000) include *Self-Mutilation Restraint,* referring to the physical act of refraining from intentional but nonlethal self-inflicted injury (p. 393); *Coping*—"actions to manage stressors that tax an individual's resources, with indicators such as verbalizes sense of control . . . acceptance of situation . . . need for assistance" (p. 192); *Self-Esteem*—"personal judgment of self-worth, with indicators such as acceptance of self-limitations, and fulfillment of personally significant roles" (p. 391); and *Anxiety Control*—"ability to eliminate or reduce feelings of apprehension and tension from an unidentifiable source" (p. 116). Clearly, the first desired outcome of intervention is for the individual to refrain from self-injury. In addition, the individual's ability to employ more appropriate ways of coping, improving self-esteem, and reducing anxiety are necessary. As with many psychological outcomes, measurement is a challenge. It is often difficult to measure the absence of a symptom and be assured its absence is the direct result of the interventions or of other intervening variables.

INTERVENTION: SELF-MUTILATION PREVENTION

Effective Communication

It is apparent from the available literature that Self-Mutilation Prevention is not a clearly defined area of practice, and health care providers face several challenges. Accurate, ongoing assessment, intervention, and evaluation are necessary to ensure safety. Although self-mutilation has low mortality, it may be associated with other impulsive behaviors that are either intentionally or unintentionally more dangerous. It is possible for a person who uses self-mutilation to become depressed and suicidal.

Determination of risk must guide intervention activities while ensuring safety and promoting more effective coping strategies. Simultaneously, these activities must not inadvertently reinforce and strengthen the self-harm response. Prevention of self-mutilation occurs at two levels—the level of overall psychopathology and the symptom level. The overall psychopathology, of which self-mutilation is a symptom, is treated by a primary therapist who addresses such topics as past trauma, its continuing effects, and other private issues. The symptoms of self-mutilation can be responded to by a variety of professionals or other concerned adults who have the knowledge and ability to tailor their responses for therapeutic effect.

Prevention of self-mutilation in adolescents can best be conceptualized as occurring across the community health continuum of primary, secondary, and tertiary prevention (Stanhope & Lancaster, 1996). Primary prevention includes interacting with and teaching skills to all children and adolescents to promote good coping and decision making and the formation of healthy relationships and self-concept. Even in the absence of mental health training with specific cognitive therapies, nurses can tailor simple personal responses in ways that may discourage the development of self-mutilation in teens with whom they have contact and will promote adaptive responses in those who struggle with self-mutilation.

Secondary prevention involves "detect(ing) disease in the early stages before clinical signs and symptoms manifest" (Stanhope & Lancaster, 1996, p. 214) and includes identifying at-risk adolescents and focusing additional resources and programming on them. Adolescents can be helped to avoid use of self-mutilation by interventions developed with regard to the following key areas: (a) learning to handle personal stress in nonharmful ways; (b) gaining acceptance and respect for one's own body; (c) learning to solve relationship problems through words instead of actions; and (d) viewing oneself as a competent human being, not as sick or damaged.

The specific strategies chosen from those described will depend on the practitioner's background and expertise in mental health nursing. In working with adolescents, identifying these activities as solely for prevention of self-mutilation should be avoided. It is more therapeutic to label any activity as the teaching of appropriate skills and coping strategies. Tertiary prevention with identification of actual self-mutilation should include referral for outside counseling. In the case of self-mutilation, there is often overlap among the three levels of prevention.

As noted previously, a key element of Self-Mutilation Prevention is the awareness and conscious use of effective interactions. Pipher's *Reviving Ophelia: Saving the Selves of Adolescent Girls* (1994) describes many keys to effective communication with adolescents and gives specific ideas for adult responses that communicate healthy values and promote critical thinking and maturity. Although the stated focus is on adolescent girls, many suggestions will be of benefit to boys as well. Specific activities include the following:

- Listen. Ask open-ended questions.
- Resist the urge to offer too much advice. Ask questions that help adolescents sort things out: "What can and can't you control?"
- Encourage flexible thinking and reflection on past successes with problem solving and coping.
- Focus on positive ways to be independent. Note examples they describe but may not recognize as appropriate expression of independence.
- Encourage deliberate, slow, careful decision making.
- Discourage victim talk, self-pity and blaming. It might be done by neutral or absent adult responses to these stories. Encourage "solution-focused stories" and more optimistic talk.
- Try to be a purveyor of hope without resorting to superficial platitudes and without communicating the idea that life can or will be perfect. A more realistic framework is "life can be hard sometimes . . . developing coping strategies is the way to go." It is important to remember, however, that if you know an adolescent is in a terrible situation, it would be insensitive and possibly damaging to be a purveyor of unrealistic hope. This is an important time to contact a resource person for consultation or referral.

Consultation

Adolescents who have serious emotional instability and disordered relationships (who *may* have early BPD symptoms) are more apt to be the ones who present challenges in maintaining healthy relationships despite the best interpersonal communication skills of concerned adults. One cause for concern is if the problems remain severe or even get worse despite appropriate interpersonal responses. In this case, higher-level interventions may be indicated. It also may be indicative of a problem if the adult develops the sense that she or he is the adolescent's only or primary support person. In these cases, consultation with the adolescent's parents or mental health professional, or both, after obtaining written consent, is indicated.

Tertiary prevention is necessary when adolescents use self-mutilation on a regular basis. If an individual's reasons for self-mutilation are identified, nursing activities can be more accurately targeted. This is not a simple matter of picking a goal or explanation from a list, however, and of supposing "if this is what caused it, then doing that will make it go away."

Motivation for self-mutilation is complex, and even if the reasons for one person's self-mutilation could be clearly identified, treatment is difficult and takes time.

Emotional Support

The buildup of intolerable stress can sometimes be prevented by appropriate emotional support. A typical pattern is that the person experiences mounting tension and an irresistible desire to self-mutilate when faced with such stresses as real or potential loss of a relationship, guilt, anger, or self-hatred. After self-mutilation, the individual feels a relief of tension and a return to baseline mood (Barstow, 1995).

Be alert for signs of self-mutilation. Some adolescents will display self-inflicted injuries very openly, but others will go to great lengths to conceal them. If you notice anything that leads you to suspect the behavior occurred, discuss it with another professional and develop a plan for communicating your concern to the adolescent and his or her parent. People who hide their self-mutilation may be troubled and embarrassed about their own behavior and its implications for being "crazy." Be very sensitive to fears and the need for privacy and confidentiality. Be sure, however, to explain that you have no choice but to follow up on anything that is causing them harm.

Problem-Solving and Coping Skills

The inability to plan solutions, defer needs, and act on the basis of long-term consequences is a signal characteristic of many people who engage in self-mutilation. An Australian study found that people who self-mutilate engage in more problem avoidance behaviors and believe they have less control over problem-solving options (Haines, Williams, Brain, & Wilson, 1997). Use cognitive approaches to teach problem-solving and coping skills. Teach adolescents to think of the short- and long-term costs and payoffs of their actions. Then teach and model the steps of effective problem solving. Once learned and practiced, these skills can be called into use for addressing personal problems as an alternative to self-mutilation.

Expression of Feelings

Self-mutilation may be an acting-out behavior. People who mutilate themselves tend to be very action oriented, believing that when something is wrong they have to do something about it, literally and physically. Teach the identification and verbal expression of feelings. Adults are commonly advised to help adolescents "get in touch with their feelings." Adolescents who hurt themselves to send messages about their distress need help learning to *say* what they feel and to *ask for* what they need. Assertiveness training has a role here, as does teaching and practicing "I" statements, such as "I want her to know I'm upset, but I don't want her to think I'm going to kill myself. I'll tell her I'm depressed and that I could use some support. She'll understand if I just tell her. I don't have to communicate it by hurting myself." Help adolescents use language effectively so they can learn the power of words. Young people also need to learn to recognize their self-talk, the messages they give themselves in their thoughts. They can learn to control their thoughts, regulate the intensity of their feelings, and feel pleased with steps toward emotional control—for example, "I can learn to tolerate these feelings. It is a good thing that I am feeling something intensely, but not reacting." Journaling is a useful technique that often assists an adolescent observe and better understand feelings and behavior and the relationship between the two.

Cognitive Restructuring

Walsh and Rosen (1988) define four basic faulty beliefs that therapists must work to correct: (a) "Self-mutilation is acceptable," (b) "One's body and self are disgusting and deserving of punishment," (c) "Action is needed to overcome unpleasant feelings and bring relief," and (d) "Overt action is necessary to communicate feelings to others" (p. 156).

Individual or group cognitive therapy are recommended to help adolescents change thoughts and beliefs that lead to self-mutilation. One belief among this group of teens it that self-mutilation is acceptable. Nurses need to be clear that deliberate self-mutilation is unacceptable for any reason. Take care to convey that it is the self-mutilation that is unacceptable, not the person. It is tricky for an adult to make this point when it overlaps with such fads as body piercing that may be intended as much to cause adult disapproval as to decorate the body. Using the term deliberate self-mutilation will help deglamorize it. Be matter of fact, not punishing or overly critical.

Another faulty belief that teens have is that the body and the self are disgusting and deserving of punishment. Nurses need to consider the messages conveyed about beauty and appearance. There are many issues related to the body that are part of the self-mutilation picture, such as eating disorders, inattentiveness to appearance, sexual identity distress, sexual and physical abuse, illness, and surgeries. Much has been written about media messages on thinness and beauty and the importance placed on appearance by teachers, parents, and others as well as by adolescents. In addition, the complicated outcomes of too-early sexuality and sexual trauma, and the particular vulnerability of adolescents, are crucial as they get to know the adult bodies they will have for the rest of their lives.

Giving direct compliments on appearance actually contributes to the problem; instead, give attention for skills and attributes that are completely unrelated to how one looks. Adults who care and are aware of these issues and committed to creating wholesome, reinforcing environments in which adolescents are valued more for their minds and actions than for how their bodies measure up will help create a climate in which every adolescent can thrive. Groups for exploring issues of personal appearance, sexuality, and relationships will help teens become conscious of these issues and band together to insist on their right to be the people they are with the bodies they have. Again, *Reviving Ophelia: Saving the Selves of Adolescent Girls* (Pipher, 1994) is an excellent resource. Because adolescents tend to be strongly influenced by the opposite sex in group situations, however, they can benefit from sharing some activities and talk with just same-sex peers. In addition, work for school policies to end student-to-student sexual harassment that is prevalent in many schools.

A final perception that is common among teens who self-mutilate is that action is needed to overcome unpleasant feelings, to bring relief, and to communicate feelings to others. Nurses can emphasize the power of thinking and the power of words. Examples of effective interpersonal problem solving and communication can be pointed out wherever they occur—in stories, in school, and in examples from the lives of other adolescents. Nurses can assist adolescents in deciding what to say in difficult situations, help them practice it, and coach them through stressful conversations. The perspective and skill of nurses in finding teachable moments that are part of the adolescent's life are tremendously valuable.

Relationship Skills

In the drama of interpersonal conflict, behaviors that gain a great deal of attention or cause distress, guilt, and anxiety in others are valuable social currency. Using self-mutilation for this purpose may be categorized as "attention-seeking behavior" or "manipulation," but it is not necessarily a deliberate ploy to get what is wanted from others. These tend to be pejorative terms that may be used by some to dismiss the importance of the behavior or to express their own frustration in dealing with it.

Facilitate the development of honest caring relationships without hidden agendas. Often, the adolescent has become accustomed to attention from others only when the adolescent is having trouble, is hurt, or when another person wants something from him or her. A supportive relationship with an adult or mentor, not related to the self-mutilation behavior, can be a useful tool in teaching appropriate relational skills. Give attention lavishly. Keeping the background issues that are behind self-mutilation behavior in mind, it is important to remember that attention-seeking behavior is really attention-needing behavior. Concerned adults should give all the attention they can, but only at the right times and not for the wrong things. The right times are every possible time when the adolescent can be greeted by name with a friendly voice or when he or she can be engaged in a conversation about a positive event or interest. The formal name for this powerful force for positive change is "noncontingent reinforcement."

Impulse Control Training

Some people experience poor affective regulation with dramatic, intense highs and lows in their mood and do not have the ability to regain emotional balance or to moderate extremes of mood to tolerable levels. Teach emotional self-control skills. Stress management, anger control training, and cognitive restructuring all include methods of identifying physical signs of stress, using them to trigger positive self-help strategies, and practicing these coping skills so that they are usable when real troubles occur. An advantage of working with a group of adolescents instead of individual counseling, when possible, is that it keeps the focus on the emotional self-regulation skills that are being taught rather than on discussions of one person's issues and history. These are better handled by the primary therapist. Medication may play an important role. Some people are helped by medication that increases the predictability of their somatic responses to stress, including medication that may regulate the amount of the neurotransmitter serotonin in the system and thus stabilize mood. Suggest that a physician be consulted.

Group Management

Group contagion is a major factor in some settings and among some groups. The issue is well-known to school or treatment facility staff members who have dealt with similar contagions of suicide threats, attempts, and acts or eating disorders. Because adolescents who engage in self-mutilation are likely to have major problems with relationships, their peer groups provide a natural stage for acting out the drama of stormy emotions. Individuals may mutilate themselves to imitate someone they admire, to get others to pay as much attention to them as to another self-mutilator, to outdo others, to demonstrate their desperation, or simply to identify themselves as members of that particular group of people who cut or burn themselves. As Walsh and Rosen (1988) note,

> Deviant groups that center on self-mutilation are appealing for several reasons. The group is seen as highly tolerant of personality and physical flaws; it is untraditional and countercultural in its structure; and members provide strong positive feedback. The deviant group

may be the first one that has made a mutilator feel accepted. To be fully accepted by a group, regardless of its deviance, is very meaningful for such individuals. These are people who are outcasts. Their self-esteem is enhanced by the group, but this esteem is entirely dependent on the continuation of group membership. If the group disbands or a member leaves, the loss of self-esteem is profound. (p. 218)

Dealing with groups of self-mutilators presents essentially the same problems as when trying to deal with gangs. Attempts to split them apart are likely to be met with resistance and greater group cohesion. Instead, try to become a valuable resource to the group—an adult who cares about each one of them and who wants to be with them because of who they are and not because of the self-mutilation they do. Involve the group in some of the consciousness-raising and problem-solving activities mentioned earlier. Help them get involved in positive activities that are less "self-focused" and reward them with schoolwide attention. Attempt to help the followers in the group find new attachments, and attempt to help the leaders define themselves in new ways. Consult with a professional from a mental health or social services agency to determine if he or she thinks it wise and possible to be a resource for the group by starting a coping skills or support group. Orchestrate and provide success opportunities for individuals to help raise their self-esteem. Adolescents are not helped by telling them that they are fine and should feel better about themselves; caring adults help by assisting them to do things well to gain self-confidence and feelings of personal competence and worth. Young people who rely on group membership to feel okay need to experience satisfaction in things they have done essentially on their own. They can be helped by fostering unique interests and talents, finding positive group opportunities such as being on a team as a player or a manager, or by having helping roles or paying jobs.

An excellent resource for all levels of prevention that can be used for individual or group cognitive work is *Clear Thinking—Clearing Dark Thought With New Words and Images: A Program for Teachers and Counseling Professionals* (Nichols, 1996). This book makes the concepts and therapeutic techniques of Beck, Ellis, and other cognitive behavioral therapists fully accessible to children and adolescents. Each chapter can stand alone for short-term, finely focused work teaching specific cognitive skills, or the entire manual can be used as a complete curriculum to support long-term therapy or a long-term skill development class. Cognitive restructuring can be used to help the adolescent view his or her feelings as manageable and not out of control or automatic, resulting in better coping skills.

Another useful resource is *Coping Skills Interventions for Children and Adolescents* (Forman, 1993), which includes a literature review for each skill area and identifies strategies to teach each skill taken from a variety of sources. Many stress scales for children and adolescents are reviewed, followed by descriptions of various interventions to help children and adolescents cope with these stressors.

In addition to the activities previously described, the following nursing interventions noted in the *Nursing Interventions Classification (NIC)* may suggest additional activities: Cognitive Restructuring, Coping Enhancement, Impulse Control Training, Self-Responsibility Facilitation and Anxiety Reduction (Iowa Intervention Project, 2000). The case study presented in the following section illustrates some of the recommended nursing activities of Self-Mutilation Prevention for an adolescent who presents with self-mutilation and emotional instability.

INTERVENTION APPLICATION

Nearly every day, a group of four sophomore girls arrive at the health office during the lunch period. When they visit as a group, much of their conversation focuses on the negative aspects of their lives, who has broken up with whom, and whose parents were fighting or making life difficult. Susan has seemed especially negative and at times says she "doesn't know why she even bothers, it would be easier to be dead." During these conversations, the school nurse listens without expressing too much interest in the negative stories and then focuses her interest when one of the girls describes a situation that includes rational thinking, good problem solving, or good perspective taking. The nurse's open-ended questions often feature thinking ahead. When one of the girls complained about her parent's study rules at home, the nurse asked, "So what's your plan for talking with your parents in a way that will make them seriously consider your point of view?" This statement communicates respect for the adolescent's perspective and plants a suggestion for planning ahead and a constructive approach. When the negativity cannot be refocused, the nurse quickly sends a couple of girls off on an errand or sends the group on its way, claiming to be too busy to chat.

Recently, Susan has come to the nurse frequently for many somatic complaints. One day, she came to the nurse's office alone, complaining of a headache. In the course of discussion, the nurse asked Susan how things had been going and observed three superficial cuts on her wrist. While briefly examining the cuts, other scars were noted on her wrists and forearms. The wounds appeared superficial, so Susan was given materials to clean and dress them herself. After determining the wounds were self-inflicted, the nurse said, "I'm sorry you felt like hurting yourself" in a neutral, nonemotional tone of voice. This was followed by one or two open-ended questions exploring current sources of stress and the final question, "Are any other adults aware of this cutting?" The nurse ascertained that Susan's parents were not aware of the situation and that she was concerned about their reaction. On the basis of observational and assessment data, a nursing diagnosis of Self-Mutilation was made.

The nurse offered to be with Susan while she called her mother or to set up a visit after school so they could talk about it together. Susan chose to have her mother visit after school. During this meeting, the nurse talked with Susan and her mother about choosing a therapist, suggesting ones the nurse had checked out earlier. A release of information was signed allowing the nurse to talk with the therapist. The nurse also suggested referring Susan for the high-risk student group at school and for a humanities class in stress management. In talking with Susan about her favorite classes, she mentioned a favorite teacher. The nurse inquired about Susan being a runner for this teacher during her free period and helping in the office before school. Other volunteer opportunities were explored with Susan and her mother. During problem solving, Susan noted that her group of friends were very negative, and she would work on not spending all her free time with them.

Later, the nurse made it a point to see Susan in different places, greet her warmly, inquire about classes, and reinforce her for keeping in touch with her mentor and for her volunteer work. She did not address the self-mutilation unless Susan mentioned it, in which case she responded with comments that reinforced Susan for any constructive responses. Over time, Susan began to talk more openly about a variety of topics, with only occasional serious negativity that had dominated earlier conversations. Gradually, she seemed slightly more settled and happy and had fewer somatic complaints. The nursing outcome Self-Mutilation Restraint was used to monitor Susan's progress during the school year (Iowa Outcomes Project, 2000).

IMPLICATIONS FOR PRACTICE AND RESEARCH

Nurses in a variety of practice settings confront the challenges posed by adolescents who use self-mutilation or are at risk for self-mutilation. Development of a definition of self-mutilation is central to continued study of the phenomenon and the development of effective interventions. Another challenge is the limited empirical literature. As is the case of many other mental health problems, gathering accurate descriptive data is difficult because of privacy issues. Research is further complicated by the lack of a common understanding and language that is only beginning to be addressed by the work of NANDA, NIC, and NOC in developing standardized language. There are still some who have not differentiated self-mutilation from suicidal behavior in their minds or in their data collection. Because most self-mutilation begins during adolescence, this is an important area for additional research, particularly in outpatient settings in which it is often first seen.

Another challenge is the fact that individuals respond differently to the same intervention. In treating a symptom such as a fever, one can be reasonably sure that treatment with an antipyretic will reduce the temperature, at least temporarily. In treating the symptoms of self-mutilation, the psychological aspects of the situation create wide variation in individual response, making it difficult to develop and evaluate specific practice guidelines.

The nursing activities described in this chapter, including those targeting individuals, those targeting groups, some very basic, and some requiring advanced training, are intended to be used by caring adults in the context of a trusting relationship. This is an essential base on which to develop any nursing plan of care. Therapeutic relationships with adolescents who use self-mutilation are often difficult to establish and maintain. Clinical experience has shown that nurses in a variety of practice settings are often ideally positioned to be significant resource people capable of establishing meaningful relationships that make positive outcomes more likely for adolescents who struggle with self-mutilation.

REFERENCES

American Psychiatric Association. (1994). *Diagnostic and statistical manual of mental disorders* (4th ed.). Washington, DC: Author.

Barstow, D. G. (1995). Self-injury and self-mutilation. *Journal of Psychosocial Nursing, 33*(2), 19-22.

Forman, S. G. (1993). *Coping skills interventions for children and adolescents.* San Francisco: Jossey-Bass.

Haines, J., Williams, C. L., Brain, K. L., & Wilson, G. V. (1997). Coping and problem solving of self-mutilators. *Journal of Clinical Psychology, 53*(2), 177-186.

Iowa Intervention Project. (2000). *Nursing interventions classification (NIC)* (J. C. McCloskey & G. M. Bulechek, Eds.; 3rd ed.). St. Louis, MO: Mosby-Year Book.

Iowa Outcomes Project. (2000). *Nursing outcomes classification (NOC)* (M. Johnson, M. Maas, & S. Moorhead, Eds.; 2nd ed.). St. Louis, MO: Mosby-Year Book.

Lofgren, D. P., Bemporad, J., King, J., Lindem, K., & O'Driscoll, G. (1991). A prospective follow-up study of so-called borderline children. *American Journal of Psychiatry, 148*(11), 1541-1547.

Miller, D. (1994). *Women who hurt themselves: A book of hope and understanding*. New York: Basic Books.

Nichols, P. (1996). *Clear thinking—Clearing dark thought with new words and images: A program for teachers and counseling professionals*. Iowa City, IA: River Lights.

North American Nursing Diagnosis Association. (1999). *Nursing diagnoses: Definitions and classification 1999-2000*. Philadelphia: Author.

Pipher, M. (1994). *Reviving Ophelia: Saving the selves of adolescent girls*. New York: Ballantine.

Rosen, P. M., Walsh, B. W., & Rode, S. A. (1990). Interpersonal loss and self-mutilation. *Suicide and Life-Threatening Behavior, 20*(2), 177-184.

Sebree, R., & Popkess-Vawter, S. (1991). Self-injury concept formation: Nursing diagnosis development. *Perspectives in Psychiatric Care, 27*(2), 27-35.

Stanhope, M., & Lancaster, J. (1996). *Community health nursing: Promoting the health of aggregates, families, and individuals* (4th ed.). St. Louis, MO: C. V. Mosby.

Valente, S. M. (1991). Deliberate self-injury: Management in a psychiatric setting. *Journal of Psychosocial Nursing, 29*(12), 19-25.

Walsh, B. W., & Rosen, P. M. (1988). *Self-mutilation: Theory, research, and treatment*. New York: Guilford.

28

Grief Work Facilitation

Kathleen Ross-Alaolmolki

Marjorie M. Heinzer

Loss, mourning, and grief are universal, timeless experiences for people of all ages and all cultures. Coping with the loss of a parent and the potential death of a child from AIDS may be one of the most overwhelming and catastrophic experiences with grief for family members. Tragically, it is an experience that will be faced by many families today and in the future. We contend that despite the uncertainty and difficulties with regard to the long-term effects of the illness, the surviving parent and siblings can draw on their natural capacity for resilience and emotional healing, which is an integral component of every human being. This chapter discusses an intervention designed to enhance family support and facilitation of grief.

BEREAVEMENT, LOSS, AND THE ROLE OF ATTACHMENT

Death of a mother from AIDS presents many implications for the grieving family. In many instances, the mother may not have had the support of a partner or of a family during her illness. There are multiple losses for the family system that can potentially complicate the grieving process, including (a) the loss of the mother as parent and caregiver, (b) the loss of a spouse for the father, and (c) the threatened loss of a child.

After a parent dies, the children will experience grief and uncertainty. The threatened loss of a sibling with AIDS will further complicate the grieving process. Sibling response to illness in their brother or sister will be influenced by the family response and how the members individually and collectively relate to each other and cope with the circumstances that are encountered. There is no such thing as "generic" grief because each kind of relationship produces a different form of bereavement (Stroebe, Stroebe, & Hansson, 1993).

Bereavement was defined by Worden (1996) as "the adaptation to the loss." *Children's Mourning* was defined as "the process that children go through on their way to adaptation" (p. 11). He used the concept of "grief" to describe the child's personal experience, thoughts, and feelings associated with death. In addition, he suggested that grief counseling is facilitation of uncomplicated or normal grief to a healthy completion of the tasks of grieving within a reasonable time frame. The description of grief as an emotion (Attig, 1996) includes a complex set of responses that are appropriate for children (Averill & Nunley, 1993). Attig (1996) proposed that bereavement is the state or condition of loss through death; to bereave means "to deprive, to dispossess or strip from" (p. 32). He described grieving as the full range of coping responses that a person uses to deal with death. Raphael (1983) defined bereavement as the reaction to the loss of a close relationship. The bereavement process has the potential to be a difficult and uncertain process when an intense and committed relationship is involved (e.g., a parent-child or sibling relationship).

Several reviews and classic studies on the development of children's concepts of death exist in the literature (Anthony, 1971; Gartley & Berasconi, 1967; Koocher, 1981). The conceptualization of death by children is related to age and cognitive developmental level. The literature notes, however, that experience with loss through terminal illness and death can hasten children's understanding of death and its meaning at an even younger age than previously thought (Bluebond-Langner, 1978; Furman, 1986; Worden, 1996). The child's age and cognitive developmental level need to be considered when intervening during the grief process. Cultural and environmental factors are also important in considering children's understanding of serious illness and death.

Loss is considered within the context of attachment theory because the feelings resulting from the perception of loss flow from connections that one human being has for another. If it is the goal of attachment behavior to maintain an affectional bond, situations that endanger this bond give rise to very specific reactions. The greater the potential for loss, the more intense and varied these reactions will be. Change will occur slowly because it will take time for the integration of the reality of the loss and for the development of new cognitive models and schemata to evolve. During this process, the bereaved may exhibit painful emotional responses, such as vulnerability, rage, guilt, and sadness.

Worden (1996) underscores the relevance of attachment theory in understanding the strong emotional reactions that accompany the threat or actual loss of a significant other, whether it be a parent, a caregiver, a child, or other close family member. Attachment is relevant to bereavement following the death of a parent or a sibling because attachment relationships persist. Bowlby's attachment theory provides an approach to conceptualizing the tendency of human beings to make strong affectional bonds with others and to interpret the strong emotional reaction, such as grief, that occurs when these bonds are threatened or broken (Averill & Nunley, 1993; Bowlby, 1979, 1981; Worden, 1996).

BEREAVEMENT AND PARENTAL LOSS

Several authors have identified the importance of family environment on the quality of the relationship and the role of the surviving parent, in particular, both short- and long-term adjustment outcomes (Baker, Sedney, & Gross, 1992; Christ, Siegel, Mesagno, & Langosch, 1991; Furman, 1986; Saler & Skolnick, 1992; Siegel, Mesagno, & Christ, 1990). Silverman, Nickman, and Worden (1992) hypothesized that a helpful family environment would have facilitating effects on mourning in bereaved school-age children. They suggest that the communal or shared representations that each of the family members has of the deceased parent are as important as the bereaved child's own internalized or inner representation (p. 495). Findings from their longitudinal study on 125 bereaved children were consistent with this hypotheses. The bereaved children went through a construction and reconstruction of new connections to the deceased parent. Their ability to reconstruct a relationship enabled them to cope and to make necessary changes in their lives. The authors refer to this process as "accommodation." These authors and Heinzer (1995) found that regardless of age, the children were aware of the meaning of death.

Data from a comparative study on the psychosocial functioning of bereaved school-age children 8 weeks following parental death showed no significant differences between bereaved and nonbereaved children on measures of school behavior, interest in school, peer involvement, enjoyment of peers, and self-esteem. The teachers, using the Child Behavior Checklist (Achenbach, 1991), scored bereaved children as less happy than their nonbereaved counterparts (Fristad, Jedel, Weller, & Weller, 1993).

Empirical data on the long-term effects of parental death are not consistent, and the role of the surviving parent is being examined more closely (Mireault & Bond, 1992; Saler & Skolnick 1992).

Tasks of Mourning

In his classic work on grieving in adults, Lindemann (1944) conceptualized the grief process as including three tasks: (a) emancipation from the bondage of the deceased, (b) readjustment to the environment in which the deceased is missing, and (c) formation of new relationships. The first task can be reformulated as an untying of the invisible threads of loyalty that connect one person to another in families. Parents owe loyalty to their own family of origin in addition to each other and their own children, whereas children owe loyalty to their parents and to each other as siblings (Boszormenyi-Nagy & Spark, 1984).

Worden (1996) modified his original four tasks of mourning to account for the age and developmental level of children. The first task of mourning for people of all ages is to accept the reality of the loss. Adults may experience disbelief and shock when learning about a death. Over time, adults usually are able to accept the loss of significant persons in their lives. Children also must deal with the emotional loss, but to do so they must realize the deceased person will not return. This recognition, however, will be dependent on age and developmental factors related to the child's comprehension of abstractions such as reversibility and finality. It is important that children be given accurate information and their questions, often repetitious, answered consistently so that they do not fill in knowledge gaps with misinformation and fantasy.

Generally, healthy children up to 2 years of age do not understand death, although they fear separation from protective figures who give comfort, nurturance, and protection. Importantly, this age group may be influenced by the grieving of other family members. Children between the ages of 3 and 5 years of age have a vague concept of death, generally believing it is something that happens to someone or something else. Children in this age group are beginning to learn how to tolerate brief periods of separation from their significant caregiver, usually the mother. Children from 6 to 10 years of age are beginning to incorporate ideas about death. It is during these years that children develop the cognitive capacity to understand that death is irreversible, can be personal, is final, and universally happens to everyone at some time, although their thoughts about death tend to remain oriented toward the future. Children 10 or 11 years of age have the intellectual capacity to understand death as universal and permanent, and by adolescence the conception of life and death matures to an adult level of understanding.

The second task of mourning is to experience the pain or emotional aspects of the loss (Worden, 1996). Children, just as adults, must work through the emotions associated with the loss, although they do so in a more gradual way. Worden suggested that children between 5 and 7 years of age may be especially vulnerable due to the intensity of feelings of the loss because of their partial understanding of the permanency of death. Children express feelings such as anger, sadness, guilt, and anxiety in a manner similar to that of adults. It is important, however, that children be able to observe an adult going through the grieving process without being overwhelmed. They will then be better able to process their own pain in dealing with the death of a parent, a particularly painful and bewildering experience.

The third task of mourning is to adjust to an environment in which the deceased is missing (Worden, 1996). Readjustment to an environment without the deceased parent will be experienced differently by the siblings and the surviving parent. The adjustment of children to a parent's death will depend on the roles and relationships that the deceased parent had with the children and the family because the remaining parent will have to shift roles and responsibilities. This shift can be particularly difficult for a father who must assume more caretaking responsibilities on a daily basis. If the deceased is the father, the mother may experience stress related to role changes in the family unit and employment as well as the support needed to undertake the parenting role and responsibilities. Because mothers often take on the emotional caretaker role and that of primary nurturer, the loss of these aspects may be felt acutely by the siblings and the father. Initially, children will also be reminded of the loss of their parent daily. Years after the death, events such as birthdays, holidays, and school events will still be painful.

The fourth task of mourning is to relocate the dead person within one's life and find ways to memorialize the person (Worden, 1996). Rando (1984) suggests that the most critical task in grief work is "untying the ties that bind" the griever to the one who has died (p. 19). To resolve grief and establish new emotional ties and relationships, the relationship to the deceased must be altered. This change in relationship does not mean one forgets or thinks any less of the person who died. The relationship with the person who has died can be thought of in special ways through memories shared with other family members, with friends, or with other parents and children who have experienced a similar loss. In other words, it is necessary for the children and the parent to shift to another meaningful place in how they think and reminisce about the deceased parent. It is impossible for the ties to be completely undone because the memories, both happy and sad, will always remain. Readjustment to an environment previously shared with the deceased person will be experienced differently by both siblings and parent.

GRIEF EXPRESSION WITHIN DIVERSE CULTURES

Mourning is the culturally patterned behavioral response to a death. Feelings of grief as a universal phenomenon are not different among cultural groups, but their form of expression or mourning among groups may vary (Andrews & Boyle, 1995; Raphael, Middleton, Martinek, & Misso, 1993; Rosenblatt, 1993). It is also important to remember that groups within a culture may have different approaches to grieving. For example, the Hispanic culture includes many different cultural groups (Mexican Americans, Puerto Ricans, Cubans, and Hispanic groups from South America or Spain); therefore, sensitivity to the cultural norm for mourning should be considered carefully. For example, it may be inappropriate for the nurse to suggest that it is acceptable for men from the Puerto Rican culture to cry because the male is expected to keep feelings and suffering inside. Furthermore, they may not be receptive to suggestions for counseling. The same consideration must be taken into account with Jewish (Davis, 1991), Arab, Southeast Asian, or Asian families. There may be very different ritual prescriptions and proscriptions specific to each subgroup of the culture.

Bereaved African Americans, particularly those in urban areas and those who come from single-parent households, often rely more heavily on friends, church friends, neighbors, and nonrelatives for support. Their approach to coping with death will be influenced by both their educational and their socioeconomic background (Andrews & Boyle, 1995). The practices of each group reflect the group members' needs. Disregard for their practices may cause disruption in the grief process. Each culture has developed its own approach to ease the suffering of grief by offering the bereaved an explanation for the meaning of the death and a prescription for how to go on living life. For example, the death of a child is viewed as very stressful in certain cultures, but the death of an adult or elderly person may be viewed as very stressful in another culture because emotional attachment to relatives is based on a different concept of kinship (Eisenbruch, 1984a, 1984b; Young & Papadatou, 1997). How a family draws on cultural beliefs and practices will vary greatly with the culture, immigration status, and socioeconomic class, including all the many facets of family circumstances and history (Shapiro, 1994).

NURSING DIAGNOSIS AND
OUTCOME DETERMINATION

Grief is a normal response to loss (Attig, 1996; Bowlby, 1979; Rando, 1988; Stroebe et al., 1993; Worden, 1991, 1996). The terms *grief, griev-*

ing, and *bereavement* are all concepts found in the nursing literature. In their extensive analysis of the evolution of the concept of grief in the nursing and medical literature, Cowles and Rodgers (1991) described grief as a dynamic, pervasive, and highly individualized process with a strong normative component (p. 94). In the nursing diagnosis literature, the term *anticipatory grieving* is used to describe or label ways of dealing with anticipated loss or death. *Dysfunctional grieving* is used to denote that grieving has not taken place. There is no specific diagnosis that addresses the normal processes of grieving. We prefer to use the term *unresolved grief* because it focuses on the potential for resolution, change, and healing through the resilience capabilities characteristic of human beings. Viewing grief as an expression that loss has occurred serves the function of signaling to attachment figures that protection is needed. Protection can be in the form of support and nurturance.

Viewing loss from a family systems perspective provides a broader perspective from which to intervene. The family perspective is stressed because each family member's capacity to grieve is affected by each of the other members, whether they be the children or the parents. In the final analysis, it is the family in interaction that gives permission for its members to grieve. The family members must recognize and validate the feelings of grief that each member is experiencing so that grief can be acknowledged and resolved.

The North American Nursing Diagnosis Association (NANDA, 1999) nursing diagnosis *Anticipatory Grieving* is chosen for this case study. It is defined as "intellectual and emotional responses and behaviors by which individuals work through the process of modifying the self-concept based on the perception of potential loss" (p. 82). In this chapter, we discuss an example in which grieving is in process resulting from the loss of the mother by the two surviving children, one of whom was diagnosed with AIDS within the past 2 months, and the surviving spouse. In addition, anticipatory grieving will occur as a result of the knowledge that the 4-year-old child with AIDS may die soon. Suggested nursing interventions for the outcome of grief resolution that are most appropriate for this case study are Grief Work Facilitation, Family Support, and Sibling Support Intervention (Iowa Intervention Project, 2000).

Assessment of the family system must include a determination of intergenerational losses. This determination should be initiated at the first or second session with the nurse. During the history taking, the nurse should cover at least three generations for losses and conflicts that may have occurred during transitions (Bowen, 1978; Wright & Leahy, 1994). The genogram and ecomap are two structural assessment tools that will be useful for the nurse in family assessment. The genogram will diagram the family constellation, and the ecomap will be a diagram of the family members' connections and relationships with those outside the family. The advantages of using these tools include the discussion that occurs with the nuclear and extended family to complete the tools, the visual nature of the process and outcome, and the family's active involvement in suggesting, planning, and participating in the interventions at their own pace.

An assessment of the grief processes for each family member and factors influencing those processes will be important to determine before the family is given tasks or directives to be completed at home. Questions can be asked and activities performed that elicit the relationship that each of the family members had with the deceased mother to assess the quality of the relationship and each member's feelings regarding his or her loss.

The outcome Grief Resolution would be appropriate to evaluate how individuals and families are progressing through the grief process (Iowa Outcomes Project, 2000). Indicators are that (a) the family will be able to discuss thoughts and feelings related to their loss, (b) they will be able to verbalize their needs for information on an ongoing basis, (c) they will use appropriated resources, and (d) they will maintain constructive interpersonal relationships. Seeking social support and sharing loss with significant others would be important outcome indicators to monitor.

INTERVENTION: GRIEF WORK FACILITATION

Grief Work Facilitation, defined as "assistance with the resolution of a significant loss" (Iowa Intervention Project, 2000, p. 358), is viewed as interactional because relationship issues due to loss are the focus, and the activities are done with the family (Wright & Leahy, 1994). The Iowa Intervention Project suggested activities for grief work facilitation to be used for the intervention (p. 358), although the model used for the discussion of the intervention and specific activities were adapted from previously developed work (Ross-Alaolmolki, 1990; Ross-Alaolmolki, Heinzer, Howard, & Marszal, 1995). Other interventions used are Family Support and Sibling Support, which are critical to the overall grief facilitation intervention.

It is critical that the nurse work with the family over an extended period of time to enable exploration of any other unresolved issues and to maintain open communication among the family members as well as to assign the family tasks to facilitate their grieving. Weekly sessions will be useful during the first few weeks that provide strategies to work on the expression and feelings regarding grief. It is important that the nurse advance at a pace that is comfortable for the family and be very sensitive to their needs.

The mobilization of resources is crucial for every family. Parents can be encouraged to bring supportive family members or friends to the counseling sessions; for example, the grandparents, aunts, or uncles from both sides of the family could be very helpful. If there are older children from a previous marriage or extended family or close and trusted friends in the region, the nurse can encourage the surviving parent to contact them and include them in a supportive linkage for the family and also close and trusted friends. The mobilization of resources can help to empower the surviving parent. The nurse can assist in the identification of family resources and support systems and assist the family to see how these support systems can be mobilized and used. In certain circumstances, the surviving parent may not have performed many of the daily caretaking activities of child care. Therefore, it may be necessary to be very specific about the various activities that need to be included in the daily plan.

Honesty in communication implies trust in family members. Keeping communication lines open is an important skill to foster when the ill child or parent is at home or in the hospital. When dealing with HIV or AIDS, the problem of secrecy and disclosure due to fear about stigma can be a very sensitive issue for both children and parents as well as the extended family (Andrews, Williams, & Neil, 1993; Hughes & Caliandro, 1996; Lipson, 1994). Modification of the expression of emotions by siblings and parents according to their past experiences and the current life situation with which they are confronted can be expected as they struggle with uncertainty and try to maintain a sense of normalcy. Adults have the capacity to shape the emotional climate of family relationships and to be inventive about truth telling. Children in their own way influence other family members and make their choices about concealment and disclosure. Safe topics are learned, and sensitive areas are avoided, often adroitly.

Both parents and children learn over time how to protect each other and the family, but they may need assistance to rehearse new ways of communicating. It is important that the parent be given permission by the nurse to express his or her love and caring openly. The nurse can coach the parent to tell the child in a session how much he or she is loved and valued. The parent can be coached to openly discuss the child's fear of catching AIDS and of dying of the disease. This move will help to change a behavior pattern in the family and open communication. When initiating this strategy, the nurse can have the parent or grandparents speak directly to the child, although this communication can be difficult for them. They may need the nurse to coach them in directly speaking to and looking at the child. This direction can be done very gently. During this process, the emotional integration of the family should be noted (Worden, 1991). Do the family members seem connected to one another? Are the family members able to help each other cope with their loss, or do they need other external sources to assist them, such as referral to a psychologist or other health professional? A family that is not emotionally integrated and is under severe emotional stress may have one or more members develop physical, emotional, or behavioral symptoms.

To explore family relationships, coping, and strengths, a genogram can be a useful as a nonthreatening tool that will assist in opening up communication lines (Wright & Leahy, 1994). Older family members can be a rich resource by sharing family stories and history. In many families, there will be older brothers and sisters that can participate. This work and the sharing of information from the genogram can serve to increase communication between family members so that both good and bad times can be shared and discussed. An effective strategy is to ask the family members to initiate a task between family sessions, such as tracking down information not included in the genogram. This task includes asking extended family members, grandparents, aunts, uncles, or friends about relationships, illnesses, deaths, or other crises that have occurred in the family. This task can be therapeutic because it will facilitate family communication and reinforce the family's extended network. Another strategy is to ask the parent and children to make a list of strengths and bring it to the next session. The parent can be asked to list the strengths of the family of origin. This process will enable the family members, particularly the surviving parent, to realize that the family does have its own strengths as well as strengths received from the family of origin that have enabled them to survive as a family during very trying circumstances.

The sharing of memories in addition to the genogram and the ecomap can serve as vehicles through which feelings can be shared and validated. Questions about what happened since the diagnosis of AIDS in the deceased parent will enable the siblings to talk about relationships within and outside the family system. It is important to talk about whether or not relationships, if temporarily broken, have been reestablished and whether family patterns, such as family activities or sibling activities, are disrupted or ongoing.

In addition to facilitating good sibling-parent interaction with open communication, the nurse can use a variety of other approaches that will enable the siblings and the parents to maintain normal relationships. Appropriate books or films, with attention to the ages and levels of understanding of the siblings, are excellent vehicles to stimulate questions and discussion of feelings. Rehearsal of questions and answers can increase the parents' feelings of confidence in communication. The discussion must be simple, direct, and geared to the age and understanding of the children.

Exploration of family memories, including both parental and sibling relationships, can help open communication lines and release forgotten memories. The sharing of memories about family life and relationships before the diagnosis of HIV or AIDS and the death of the parent can assist the family to reconstruct and reorient to attending to important traditions and special family transitions, such as birthdays, holidays, and events such as the births or adoption of children (Davies, 1987). The genogram and ecomap can be used in a nonthreatening way to provide a family map of members and relationships, reminding members of important family events and rituals, such as how birthdays, christenings or namings, circumcisions, first communions, bar mitzvahs, or bat mitzvahs are celebrated. For example, the following questions can be asked: (a) What part did the parents and the children play in these family events? (b) How were school and extracurricular activities enjoyed, and how did the siblings, including the child diagnosed with HIV or AIDS, participate? and (c) Were these family events? Certificates and prizes won by siblings can be placed in a special book such as a portfolio with a section for each child, or there may be one book for each sibling. These can also be shared with the nurse and health care team as appropriate. This sharing and talking will assist the family to heal and will help the health professionals to understand the family at a more human and caring level.

It may be necessary to plan sessions to assist the family with grieving, the circumstances regarding the illness and death of the parent, the funeral, and the relationship of the siblings and the father with the deceased mother. Questions regarding the death and where each person was on the day of the death inform the nurse of the circumstances regarding the illness and the subsequent death. It is also helpful to ask about the funeral, including who participated in the planning and who participated in the funeral service. A session may be planned to discuss the funeral service. This strategy can be very potent because it gives family members permission to grieve openly and to share special memories of the service. The family can be directed to plan a service at home. In this way, they can bring selected readings or music to share with one another. The family may want to plan a memorial service and invite friends and relatives who were not able to attend the funeral.

Questions about what has happened since the death of a parent in terms of relationships outside the family and the reestablishment of family patterns such as family activities, especially those for the siblings, will give the nurse a chance to examine the family and the support system. Answers to the following questions are important: (a) What other stresses have they experienced since the parent's death? (b) Are the siblings playing with their friends? (c) Are they going to school? (d) Are they having any difficulties with their homework or grades? (e) What is happening at school with friends and other students? (f) Do the children fear questions about their parent's illness and death? and (g) Do their friends understand why and how the death occurred? If the children are experiencing difficulty in school or with friends, the school counselor or teacher can be included in one of the family counseling sessions. Friends who are important to the siblings can be included in selected sessions to enhance their support network.

The nurse is in a position to contact teachers and school nurses to inform them of the family situation and possible effects it may have on the siblings and friends. These contacts may present an opportunity for the nurse to go to the schools to present a workshop to students or teachers or both on HIV or AIDS and include information on grief and grieving and possible interference in sibling-friend relationships. Teachers and nurses can be made aware of behavioral manifestations and plan approaches to assist the siblings, students, and their friends in coping.

A child whose parent has died may harbor guilt over the inevitable disagreements that occurred between the child and the parents. A strategy to absolve some of the guilt might be useful and could be initiated by the nurse. The child could be asked by the nurse to share a story about some mischief or behavior that may have resulted in a reprimand. This strategy can serve to normalize the disagreements that children may have experienced, and humor can be used to reframe the memory into a positive one.

INTERVENTION APPLICATION

Ten-year-old John Barnes had a well child appointment with the nurse in the pediatric primary health care clinic. John was accompanied by his father; his mother had died of AIDS 2 months prior to this visit. Mrs. Barnes was diagnosed with AIDS 2 years ago following the confirmation of the HIV seropositive status of John's 3-year-old sister. Both John and his father tested negative for HIV. For 2 years, the Barnes family dealt with illnesses. John's mother complained of fatigue, weight loss, recurrent yeast infections, and respiratory infections. Her energy in caring for their two children was depleted, and the family's financial status had deteriorated. During this time, John's sister developed gastrointestinal problems with chronic diarrhea, feeding problems, and symptoms of respiratory infections and was diagnosed with AIDS. The family struggled to maintain control of the chronic illness of both the mother and the child. The nursing diagnosis of Anticipatory Grieving was made at that time (NANDA, 1994).

The fact that the HIV infection and consequent AIDS was linked to the mother's unprotected sexual behavior in a previous relationship in her early 20s added complexity to the problem. John's father was angry, and the strain of his parents' relationship was visible to him. John, who was 8 years old when his mother was diagnosed with AIDS, had seen the progressive changes in his mother's health that resulted in her death, and then he saw the changes in his sister's health. He is aware of the diagnosis, has heard the negative meanings associated with HIV and AIDS, and perceives the impending death of his sister. He is fearful that his father will also die, and he will "catch the disease." John has suffered the loss of his mother, perceived the changes in his father's parenting role, and has become withdrawn both at home and at school.

John's father did not talk with him about his mother's illness and death. Now, his sister's health is the primary concern in the home. John's grandparents were stunned by the rapid progression of the disease and death of their daughter and their granddaughter's diagnosis. They were unable to console the father and are having a difficult time with their own grieving.

During the acute illness of his mother, John worried about what would happen to him. He knew the words HIV and AIDS were associated with "bad things" and even dying. He felt uncomfortable when he heard people talk about his mother dying of AIDS. He did not want to go to school and complained he did not feel well. His teachers had contacted John's father because of his lack of interest and participation in class and his increasing sadness. John was alone in his pain and would not talk to anyone about his grief.

In the assessment, the nurse identified the need for increased support for John and his family, and the nursing intervention of Grief Work Facilitation was initiated (Iowa Intervention Project, 1996). Initially, a full health assessment was done for physiological concerns and psychological needs. John's physical examination showed a developmentally appropriate 10-year-old boy. His height was in the 75th percentile and weight was in the 50th percentile, unchanged from his last well child visit for a prekindergarten physical. He was quiet, answered a few questions, offered no comments, tensed his muscles and posture when touched during the examination, and seemed tearful at times. His father was obviously impatient with his lack of response and paced the room. He told the nurse that "John is too quiet at home." He shared the school nurse's comments and the teacher's concerns regarding John's behavioral changes at school.

The father had increased his participation in child care activities prior to his wife's death, and he was still trying to juggle these activities with his work schedule. At that time, he cut back on his work activities. After his wife's death, however, he had resumed a normal working schedule to keep his health benefits. The father was guided in accepting more assistance from his extended family, who planned to take responsibility for car pools, getting the children to day care and school and to and from after-school activities. Both sets of grandparents worked together to assist the father.

Genogram and ecomap work was assigned as a family task, and the extended family members such as grandparents, uncles, and aunts were asked about their experience with relationships, losses, illnesses, deaths, or other crises that occurred in the family. The father was asked to list the strengths that his deceased wife had brought to the family, thus further opening communication and assisting him to acknowledge her strengths to the children. He was coached in speaking to the children about their mother's illness and death, and he was encouraged to tell John about the condition and progress of his sister. The indicators for Grief Resolution began to appear (Iowa Outcomes Project, 1997).

The nurse identified specific concerns for continued work with samily support and the grieving process. The NANDA (1994) diagnosis of Anticipatory Grieving was consistent with John's fear for his sister's death and his behavioral change while still grieving the loss of his mother. Family Support and Grief Work Facilitation With Coping Assistance were the intervention categories (Iowa Intervention Project, 1996) addressed in John's plan of care in the clinic.

RESEARCH AND PRACTICE IMPLICATIONS

There continues to be a paucity of research on the concepts of attachment, loss, and grief and what effect loss and grief in children resulting from a variety of circumstances, such as chronic illness in a parent or impending or actual death in a parent, may have on psychological, physical, and social development. The most extensive approach to systematic knowledge development on grief in siblings was created by Davies (1987, 1988a, 1988b, 1991, 1993), who developed guidelines for investigators conducting studies on bereaved siblings. The responses of children and adolescents to the loss of a family member and their coping strategies over time and within different cultural groups are an important area for nursing research.

When examining a chronic illness, such as parents or children or both who are diagnosed with HIV or AIDS, contemporary investigators suggest that research on loss and grief and its impact on families be examined in terms of positive concepts such as resilience (Cohen, 1994; Hardy, Armstrong, Routh, Albrecht, & Davis, 1994; Sherwen & Boland, 1994) and protective factors such as coping and social support from extended family networks, religious beliefs, and the assistance of older siblings (Lewis, Haiken, & Hoyt, 1994; Mellins & Ehrhardt, 1994; Siegel & Gorey, 1994). A related area of importance is the caregiving aspect and the outcomes for each family member.

Because pediatric HIV or AIDS is a relatively new chronic illness, no systematic longitudinal investigations have examined the effects of loss and grief on the children and their families over time. Importantly, Schumacher and Meleis (1994) suggest that nursing focus on the identification of factors that indicate positive healthy transition outcomes. They identified three indicators of healthy transition that appear to be relevant across all types of transitions: a subjective sense of well-being, mastery of new behaviors, and the well-being of interpersonal relationships. These indicators of healthy transition provide the researcher with a framework for the examination of grief and bereavement in children and their families that identifies strengths and resilience over time and under different conditions.

There are several complicating factors, both theoretical and methodological, that confront the researcher designing a study on children diagnosed with HIV or AIDS and their families. The research on children and families with other chronic illnesses, such as cancer, asthma, and cystic fibrosis, has been conducted on primarily white, middle-class samples (Mellins & Ehrhardt, 1994). The exclusion of minority and ethnic populations from previous studies has resulted in a lack of reliable and valid instrumentation to measure theoretical concepts and models (Sherwen & Boland, 1994). Instruments measuring family dynamics, family functioning, stress, coping, and social support are all normed on majority populations (Cohen, 1994). Furthermore, because of the problems with instrumentation and the exclusion of racial and ethnic minorities who were not ill from differing socioeconomic levels in research, Cohen notes that little is known about family dynamics and family functioning under normal conditions. She extends her critique to include the absence of data-based knowledge that is currently available on racial and ethnic minorities who live in urban versus rural environments and who may or may not have an illness. The methodological problems confronting researchers are enormous in terms of adequate sample size, differing age levels, sensitivity of the topic of HIV and AIDS to families from minority populations, and language barriers between researchers and subjects. Thus, collaborative research across disciplines including multisite research programs would be most efficient.

Tragically, grieving is a universal process experienced by everyone. The process can be facilitated through the intervention presented in this chapter. The facilitation of grief work will promote health and reduce unnecessary health risks related to grief. Thus, this intervention should be central to our nursing practice.

REFERENCES

Achenbach, T. M. (1991). *Child Behavior Checklist.* Storrs: University of Vermont.

Andrews, M. M., & Boyle, J. S. (1995). *Transcultural concepts in nursing care* (2nd ed.). Philadelphia: J. B. Lippincott.

Andrews, S., Williams, A. B., & Neil, K. (1993). The mother-child relationship in the HIV-I positive family. *Image: The Journal of Nursing Scholarship, 25*(3), 193-198.

Anthony, S. (1971). *The discovery of death in childhood and after.* London: Penguin.

Rando, T. A. (1988). *Grieving: How to go on living when someone you love dies.* New York: Macmillan.

Rosenblatt, P. C. (1993). Grief: The social context of private feelings. In M. S. Stroebe, W. Stroebe, & R. O. Hansson (Eds.), *Handbook of bereavement: Theory, research and intervention* (pp. 102-111). New York: Cambridge University Press.

Ross-Alaolmolki, K. (1990). Coping with family loss: The death of a sibling. In M. J. Craft & J. A. Denehy (Eds.), *Nursing interventions for infants and children* (pp. 213-228). Philadelphia: W. B. Saunders.

Ross-Alaolmolki, K., Heinzer, M. M., Howard, R., & Marszal, S. (1995). Impact of childhood cancer on siblings and family: Family strategies for primary health care. *Holistic Nursing Practice, 9*(4), 66-75.

Saler, L., & Skolnick, N. (1992). Childhood parental death and depression in adulthood: Roles of surviving parent and family environment. *American Journal of Orthopsychaitry, 62*(4), 504-516.

Schumacher, K. L., & Meleis, A. I. (1994). Transitions: A concept central to nursing. *Image: The Journal of Nursing Scholarship, 26*(2), 119-127.

Shapiro, E. R. (1994). *Grief as a family process: A developmental approach to family practice.* New York: Guilford.

Sherwen, L. N., & Boland, M. (1994). Overview of psychosocial research concerning pediatric human immunodeficiency virus infection. *Developmental and Behavioral Pediatrics, 15,* S5-S11.

Siegel, K., Mesagno, F. P., & Christ, G. (1990). A prevention program for bereaved children. *American Journal of Orthopsychiatry, 60*(2), 168-175.

Siegel, K. L., & Gorey, E. (1994). Childhood bereavement due to parental death from acquired immunodeficiency syndrome. *Journal of Developmental and Behavioral Pediatrics, 15*(3), S66-S70.

Silverman, P. R., Nickman, S., & Worden, J. W. (1992). Detachment revisited: The child's reconstruction of a dead parent. *American Journal of Orthopsychiatry, 62*(4), 494-503.

Stroebe, M. S., Stroebe, W., & Hansson, R. O. (1993). *Handbook of bereavement: Theory, research and intervention.* New York: Cambridge University Press.

Worden, J. W. (1991). *Grief counseling and grief therapy: A handbook for the mental health practitioner.* New York: Springer.

Worden, J. W. (1996). *Children and grief: When a parent dies.* New York: Guilford.

Wright, L. M., & Leahy, M. (1994). *Nurses and families: A guide to family assessment and intervention.* Philadelphia: F. A. Davis.

Young, B., & Papadatou, D. (1997). Child death and bereavement across cultures. In C. M. Parkes, P. Laungani, & B. Young (Eds.), *Death and bereavement across cultures* (pp. 191-205). New York: Routledge.

PART III

Interventions for Primary Care Health Promotion

As we all work to conserve health care resources, it is imperative that nurses are skilled in health promotion and disease prevention. Pediatric nurses and nurse practitioners have long been providers of anticipatory guidance to parents about children's development and behavior in addition to ensuring that infants and children are properly immunized and reared in safe environments. Interventions appropriate for the ambulatory and community settings include Telephone Consultation, Immunization/Vaccination Administration, and Environmental Management: Automobile Safety.

The importance of school nurses and community health nurses in promoting the health of school-age children and adolescents will become more evident as we seek to ensure that this population develops positive health beliefs and practices that will carry on into adulthood. Although this is a time of relative wellness, many lifestyle behaviors are learned and reinforced during these important years. In addition, many potentially health-altering behaviors are initiated during these years, such as the experimentation with addictive substances, unprotected sexual activity, and risk-taking behavior on bicycles, motorcycles, and motor vehicles. Interventions that address these risk behaviors include Teen Pregnancy: Primary

Prevention, Substance Abuse Prevention, Teaching Sexuality, and Adolescent Suicide Prevention. Examples of interventions designed to encourage health-promoting behaviors are Lifestyle Modification: Nutrition Promotion, Exercise Promotion, and Self-Esteem Enhancement. Finally, Media Management, Teaching Conflict Resolution, and Family Violence Reduction are interventions that can be used with children and families to assist them in understanding and dealing with the contextual factors that influence children and families in today's society. The interventions in Part III are designed for nurses in a wide range of settings and represent the scope of nursing practice characteristic of ambulatory care nurses, nurse practitioners, school nurses, and community health nurses.

29

Telephone Consultation

Julie Osterhaus

Telephone Consultation is an important intervention that nurses and nurse practitioners perform daily in ambulatory settings. For many individuals and families, the telephone is a vehicle for access to the health care system. Nurses perform several services over the telephone, including (a) providing health information and advice about various conditions, (b) providing anticipatory guidance, (c) prescription refills, and (d) making appointments for exams with a health care provider. To assist nurses with this important intervention, many organizations have developed written protocols to ensure that advice and information given are timely, accurate, and consistent.

THEORETICAL FRAMEWORK

Two concepts are important to the framework for telephone consultation. The first is the concept of *helping,* which is essential when dealing with callers who are concerned about themselves or a family member. Egan's (1975) Helping Model (Table 29.1) provides the nurse with a three-

TABLE 29.1   Helping Model

Stage 1	The problem situation is explored and clarified.
Stage 2	Goals based on an action-oriented understanding of the problem situation are met.
Stage 3	Ways of accomplishing goals are devised and implemented.

SOURCE: Egan (1975).

stage process for establishing a helping relationship with the caller to achieve mutual goals.

Nurses can have a profound impact on the way in which individuals and families cope with events in their lives by applying the concept of helping. Proper advice and reassurance over the telephone is one way nurses can have an impact on how families cope with an illness, injury, or concern.

The second concept is *crisis*. Many patients and families view the illness, injury, or concern as a crisis that can significantly cause disruption in their lives. Each person and family views events differently and reacts to crises in different ways. A newborn infant with a fever could be an overwhelming crisis for a tired new mother. Although situational crises occur in unexpected illnesses and injuries, questions about a child's or family member's well-being can reflect a developmental crises. An individual's or family's response to a crisis determines how they will cope with future crises. Although a crisis presents danger, it is also a unique opportunity for growth (Caplan, 1964).

NATURE OF PEDIATRIC PHONE CALLS

The nature of pediatric telephone calls can vary among populations due to age differences and the area of specialty. I found that the most common symptoms and complaints received in a midwestern university-based primary care clinic were fever, cold and upper respiratory infection, ear infection, cough, vomiting and diarrhea, sore throat, conjunctivitis, rash, and chicken pox (Osterhaus, 1995). In another study, the most frequent complaints received in an after-hours program were fever, rash, vomiting, nonpenetrating injuries, and ear complaints (Poole, Schmitt, Caruth, Petersen-Smith, & Slusarski, 1993). Other investigators have studied the nature of phone calls, including the characteristics of callers, the types of calls, and time of day phone calls were received. In one study, 39% of phone calls to a pediatric hotline regarded questions about medical concerns within an 8-hour time period, 39% regarded behavioral concerns, and 22% regarded developmental problems. More than 80% of the calls were from mothers, and approximately 80% pertained to children less than 6 years of age (Troutman, Wright, & Shifrin, 1991). In another setting, 80% of the phone calls received during an 8-hour period were received between 8:00 a.m. and 12:00 p.m., with approximately 50% of the calls received between 8:00 and 9:00 a.m. (Osterhaus, 1995). This information is important for determining how telephone triage and advice lines are staffed.

ROLE OF THE NURSE

Controversy exists in the literature with regard to the appropriate health care personnel to perform telephone consultation. It is evident that nurses perform this function appropriately (Brennan, 1992; Kelly & Mashburn, 1990; Osterhaus, 1995; Poole et al., 1993). Nurses with a strong background in their area of specialty can handle the wide variety of telephone calls that may be received. Several authors cite the roles that nurses of various levels, such as nurse practitioners and registered nurses, must take during telephone consultation. These roles include triaging of telephone calls, facilitating access to the health care system, advising patients and families on how to manage illnesses and injuries at home, anticipatory guidance, counseling, and providing emotional reassurance (Osterhaus, 1997). The goal of the nurse should be to negotiate a mutually satisfactory solution to the problem and to assist parents in making health care decisions about their children (Scott & Packard, 1990).

A problem-solving process must be used when assisting parents on the telephone. Because the nurse does not have the benefit of face-to-face contact and may not have knowledge of the caller's background, he or she must consider several factors. When making decisions regarding the disposition of phone calls, the process centers on the following major considerations (Edwards, 1994): (a) the most likely cause of the presenting problem, (b) the impact of the problem on the caller, (c) the accessibility of alternative sources of health care, (d) the ability of the nurse to control the reactions of the caller, and (e) the nurse's perception of the caller's vulnerability.

USE OF WRITTEN TELEPHONE PROTOCOLS

Several authors advocate the use of written telephone protocols as a means for ensuring that accurate and timely advice is given to callers (Broome, 1986; Brown, 1989; Osterhaus, 1995; Schmitt, 1980; Scott &

Packard, 1990). An important benefit of using telephone protocols is that advice given is accurate and consistent so that patients and families are not faced with differing opinions on how to manage illnesses at home or when to bring the child in for evaluation. Protocols can promote the delivery of consistent advice and prevent the transmission of inappropriate advice. Physicians and other health care providers know what information has been given to patients and families. Appropriate and consistent advice may decrease the number of unnecessary office visits, which can then provide health care professionals more time to see truly ill patients, thus decreasing overall health care costs. Another benefit of telephone protocols is that prompt advice can be given, and nurses do not need to search various references for information. The nurse also has confidence in the accuracy and completeness of the advice when a written, literature-based protocol is used.

Some pediatric centers have developed telephone protocols tailored to their institution and physicians' current practice. At one institution, a committee structure was used to conduct a needs assessment, develop literature- and practice-based written protocols, and evaluate the use of the protocols (Osterhaus, 1995). Protocols were designed to be approximately 1 page in length and were kept in alphabetical order in a three-ring binder at the nurses' station. A system to ensure frequent revisions was also developed so that the protocols reflected recent recommendations. Documentation forms were also refined to ensure all interactions became a permanent part of the patient's medical record.

LEGAL ISSUES

There are inherent risks for a nurse in performing telephone triage because of the lack of a face-to-face encounter with a patient. To minimize the legal risks associated with giving advice over the telephone, nurses should always use specific written protocols or standing orders. Additional ways to minimize legal risks include ensuring patient compliance by being specific about the need to follow the advice given and by keeping a complete permanent record of the telephone encounter (Gobis, 1997). An essential part of telephone consultation that cannot be overlooked is accurate documentation of the interaction. The importance of accurate documentation of phone calls is evident in the literature (Broome, 1986; Brown, 1989; Kelly & Mashburn, 1990; Killila, 1990; Osterhaus, 1995; Scott & Packard, 1990; Tammelleo, 1993). A variety of documentation methods may be used, including preprinted chart forms for single telephone interactions, telephone logs, generic medical record notes, and computerized documents. Logs can provide the nurse with a quick and easy reference to determine what type of calls were taken recently, which calls require follow-up, and which calls were followed up on the next day. Trends can also be noted, especially for parents who make frequent phone calls. This information becomes particularly important when more than one nurse is managing phone calls.

Phone calls in which positive test results are reported while noting when the patient was advised to seek other medical attention or take specific action should be documented. Conversations in which specific medical advice is given should also be recorded, especially when speaking to clients unfamiliar with the clinic (Killila, 1990). Clear, concise, and accurate records can be the best defense against a negligence charge (Tammelleo, 1993). Katz and Wick (1991) report on a case in which a nurse did not document the offer of and the parent's subsequent refusal of an appointment for a child who was later diagnosed with hemophilus influenza Type B meningitis after becoming severely ill. Accurate documentation of the phone conversation may have prevented a lawsuit and judgment against the nurse. Incidents such as this point to the necessity to document all telephone calls. In the future, some may consider tape-recording conversations so that there is a record of the presenting problem and the advice given. If recordings are made, permission from the caller is required prior to taping.

NURSING DIAGNOSIS AND
OUTCOMES DETERMINATION

The North American Nursing Diagnosis Association (NANDA, 1999) nursing diagnosis of Knowledge Deficit is appropriate for many telephone interactions. In the case of a first-time mother or father with a neonate, the knowledge deficit is most often related to inadequate knowledge regarding infant care. The parent may verbalize feelings of inadequacy and make statements such as "I don't know what to do" when calling a nurse for assistance. Knowledge Deficit May also be the result of the parent's inability to retain the information taught in the early postpartum period or the lack of written reference materials at home. The telephone has become a convenient vehicle to educate parents on the care of their children in a less stressful and more convenient setting.

Many parents call with regard to clinical symptoms or complaints. One of the most common parental concerns is a child with a fever. When a parent calls about a child with a fever, the nursing diagnosis Hyperthermia is appropriate (NANDA, 1999). The nurse needs to ascertain what symptoms are present in a child who has a reported fever. The nurse also needs to determine whether other related factors unique to a child with a fever are present. These factors could be illness or trauma, dehydration, or inappropriate clothing.

One of the desired outcomes for parents who seek the advice of a nurse over the telephone is Health-Seeking Behavior, which is listed in the Nursing Outcomes Classification. *Health-Seeking Behavior* is defined as "actions to promote wellness, recovery, and rehabilitation" (Iowa Outcomes Project, 2000, p. 233). Some of the indicators that may apply when a nurse is speaking to a parent of a child with an illness or injury are that the parent completes the health-related tasks suggested by the nurse to relieve the symptoms, the parent asks questions when indicated (i.e., if the advice given is not understood), and the parent contacts health professionals when indicated (i.e., calls the nurse back if the child's condition deteriorates or if additional questions or concerns arise).

A knowledge-related outcome for a concern about a child's illness is Knowledge: Disease Process. This outcome is defined as "the extent of understanding conveyed about a specific disease process" (Iowa Outcomes Project, 2000, p. 262). Appropriate indicators include familiarity with the disease name, description of the disease process, description of the cause and contributing factors, description of the effects of the disease, description of the signs and symptoms, description of the usual course of the disease, description of measures to minimize the disease process, and description of complications and precautions to prevent complications. An example of a telephone interaction with the outcome of knowledge about the disease regards a parent who requests information on how to care for a child with croup. A parent will need to know the clinical course of the disease, the signs and symptoms, and how the symptoms can be managed at home. The education should also include signs and symptoms of worsening respiratory distress and conditions in which the parent should seek additional medical care.

INTERVENTION: TELEPHONE CONSULTATION

Telephone Consultation is an intervention defined in the Nursing Interventions Classification as "exchanging information, providing health education and advice, managing symptoms, or doing triage over the phone" (Iowa Intervention Project, 2000, p. 659). The activities listed as part of the intervention specifically provide the nurse with information on the data to be obtained, how and what information should be provided to the caller, and actions that need to be taken based on the information to be obtained. The activities can be grouped into four phases in the management of telephone calls: information gathering, planning, intervention, and follow-up.

The first phase, information gathering, is perhaps the most important in aiding the nurse to determine what the caller is asking. The nurse gathers information to determine the severity of the concern by asking the right questions. The responsibility of the nurse is to ascertain the caller's needs for additional care rather than to diagnose and treat (Barton, Brown, Curtis, & Lichtenfeld, 1992). There are two key tasks the nurse must keep in mind when gathering information from a parent: developing rapport with the caller and using history-taking skills to gain as much information as possible (Broome, 1986). To develop rapport with a caller, nurses should identify themselves by giving their name and title at the beginning of the conversation and convey a caring and nonjudgmental manner. During the history taking, the nurse must gain as much information as possible. Information collected includes the history of the current illness or concern, allergies, medications, and what home treatment has been given (Broome, 1986). Because telephone contact does not provide the nurse with face-to-face clues, the nurse needs to ask systematic questions that can determine the severity of the illness or concern. The nurse should also rely on the tone of voice of the caller and any emotional statements the caller may make.

The second phase in telephone consultation is careful planning. The nurse should have knowledge of the caller's reliability, resources, and ability to handle the illness or concern (Broome, 1986). The nurse may already be familiar with children and families in smaller primary care settings and therefore will not need to seek this information during the interaction. In larger settings in which individual patients and caretakers are not familiar, the nurses may need to question the parent about financial resources, support systems, and other necessary information.

The intervention phase of telephone consultation is dependent on the information obtained and the planning already performed by the nurse. Generally, three options exist with respect to illness or injury: (a) the patient requires immediate or urgent evaluation by a health care provider, (b) the patient requires same-day evaluation or evaluation within 24 hours by a health care provider, or (c) the illness or injury can be managed at home. It is important that reference materials or in-house protocols precisely state the conditions and symptoms for each disposition. In the case of parents seeking answers to specific questions or concerns, advice and reassurance can be given over the phone. Anticipatory guidance is given by nurses who are well versed in areas such as physical and psychosocial development and parenting concerns. Examples of types of anticipatory guidance that can be given are information related to prenatal care, newborn care, immunizations, growth and development, and behavior management.

The final phase of telephone consultation is evaluation and follow-up. The nurse must determine the caller's understanding of the plan of care. If necessary, the caller should be asked to repeat the information received for verification. The nurse should always ask the caller if there are any unanswered questions and if the caller feels comfortable with the plan. The caller should be instructed to call back if there are any changes in condition and should seek medical advice if he or she is uncomfortable with the situation (Broome, 1986). A follow-up phone call should be offered to increase the caller's comfort if home management advice is given. Another benefit to a follow-up phone call is the conveyance of concern to the family. This can result in parent satisfaction and may influence the family's decision to use that clinic or office for future visits, which is important in a competitive health care environment. During the follow-up phone call, the nurse can determine the outcome of the intervention and also evaluate the effectiveness of the earlier consultation.

INTERVENTION APPLICATION

John is the father of a 2-month-old infant named Benjamin. His wife works the evening shift, and he is the primary caretaker after picking the infant up from day care. He has noticed for the past few weeks that Benjamin is very fussy for a few hours in the evening. He thinks Benjamin may be colicky and decides to call a nurse for suggestions on how to calm the infant. The nurse refers to a telephone protocol on infant crying (Table 29.2) to assist her in counseling and providing information to John. She asks John a standard set of questions to gain basic information about the infant, including age and name of physician or health care practitioner. Next, she asks questions from the protocol to determine the nature of the concern. On the basis of John's answers to these questions, the nurse determines that Benjamin does not have a fever and does not seem to have any symptoms of illness and therefore does not warrant an appointment with a health care provider unless the father is uncomfortable with the situation. A nursing diagnosis of Knowledge Deficit related to managing Benjamin's crying is made based on the assessment data.

John states that he is willing to try something at home first and share the results of his phone call with his wife before setting up an appointment with Benjamin's physician. The nurse gives John suggestions from the protocol on how to care for Benjamin at home. The nurse also informs John of a commercial product called a Sleep Tight (which can be rented or purchased). It is composed of a sound unit that can be attached to the side of a crib that mimics the sound of a car driving and a unit that attaches to the bottom of the crib and gently vibrates the mattress.

The nurse provides John with a great deal of reassurance regarding his ability to handle the situation, which seems to provide John with the

TABLE 29.2   Newborn Crying Telephone Protocol

I. Questions to ask parents or caregiver
   A. Does your child have a fever or other symptoms of an illness?
   B. How long does the crying last?
   C. Is there a pattern to the cryingùthat is, at a certain time of the day, with a feeding, or with a bowel movement or urination?
   D. Is your child inconsolable? What have you done to try to console?
   E. What do you do when you cannot tolerate the crying?
   F. Have you checked the baby from head to toe and noted anything unusual, such as hair or strings tied around a finger or toe, bruises, anal tears, or anything else that could cause the crying?
   G. Has your child had recent immunizations?

II. See immediately
   A. Constant crying lasting more than 2 hours
   B. Persistent crying with fever or cold symptoms
   C. Intermittent crying with abdominal pain (intussusception and currant jelly stools)
   D. Crying so intolerable you fear the caregiver may injure the child

III. See by appointment
   A. Fussiness with pain (otitis media vs. colic)
   B. Change in appetite or stool pattern
   C. Fever with fussiness
   D. Crying with urination or defecation (urinary tract infection or anal fissure)
   E. Suspected formula intolerance

IV. Home management
   A. Burp baby more frequently (hand on abdomen and sit infant upright, knee-chest position, holding upright against caregiver's chest).
   B. Pacifier (overfeeding may cause more crying).
   C. Rock, swing, walk with infant, or swaddle in light blanket.
   D. For colic
      1. Use Sleep-Tight (a system that has a device under the crib mattress that vibrates gently and a sound system that attaches to the side rail that provides a soothing sound).
      2. Ride in car if caregiver not exhausted.
      3. Put baby in care seat and place car seat on top of clothes dryer (parent must be in attendance).
      4. Run vacuum cleaner or hair dryer for noise.
      5. Play soft music.
      6. Lay infant in crib for 10 to 15 minutes and close door (infant may be tired or overstimulated).
      7. Use Mylicon drops for gas (over-the-counter medication).
      8. Reassure caregiver that crying due to colic may disappear by the time the baby is 3 months old.
   E. If caregiver or parent is concerned about formula intolerance, he or she needs to see the family's health care provider.

SOURCES: Hawson, Oberklaid, and Menahem (1987) and Mones and Asnse (1986).

confidence he needs to attempt to try the suggested activities. She also reassures John that crying due to colic typically disappears by approximately 3 months of age. Prior to ending the conversation with John, the nurse validates that John understands what they have talked about and that he is comfortable with the situation at home. She also recites situations in which John should call back for additional advice, including the development of a fever, respiratory distress, and any other deterioration in Benjamin's condition. She ends the conversation by encouraging John to call back if additional advice is needed. She offers a follow-up phone call in a few days to check on the progress of Benjamin. The nurse and John agree that speaking to Benjamin's mother when she is home with Benjamin would be a good idea. The nurse clearly and concisely documents the telephone consultation on her institution's telephone call record sheet, which becomes a permanent part of Benjamin's medical record. She also documents the call in a telephone log and notes when the follow-up phone call should be made. Outcomes appropriate to the Telephone Consultation intervention include Parenting, Knowledge: Disease Process, and other knowledge-related outcomes in the Nursing Outcomes Classification (Iowa Outcomes Project, 2000).

RESEARCH AND PRACTICE IMPLICATIONS

The area of telephone consultation offers many useful and exciting prospects for nursing research for further development of this important nursing intervention. One of the most beneficial areas of research that could validate the importance of this intervention is a cost-benefit analysis. The costs of offering a telephone consultation service and benefits of handling uncomplicated situations over the telephone should be compared, including the actual dollars that could have been saved by keeping patients out of the clinic or office setting. The practice of charging for telephone advice is very controversial and is not widespread. This situation may be due to concern expressed by parents about the uncertainty of health care plans covering this service. One study found that patients were not willing to pay a $10 fee for telephone advice from a nurse but had no consistent opinion for or against paying for a prescription renewal (Ellison & Marr, 1994). Parents may need to be educated on reasons that institutions charge for telephone consultation services and the potential savings they may reap if they contact the telephone counseling service first. In addition, third-party payors need to be convinced that telephone consultation is a cost-effective service that could prevent increased health care costs by identifying and treating problems early, thus resulting in improved health and reduced costs.

Research into patient and family satisfaction with health care providers offering telephone consultation can provide management staff with information to further refine their telephone advice programs. A specific area for additional study in individual settings is the accessibility to advice over the telephone, which should include the parent's perception of whether calls were answered within an acceptable time frame, whether the nurse spent an adequate amount of time addressing the parental concern, and whether appointments for examination could be made within an acceptable time frame. Another area for additional study is the parent's satisfaction with the actual advice received, including whether the parent was comfortable with the recommendations and had the resources necessary to carry out the recommendations.

Staff satisfaction with telephone consultation is another important area of study and has implications for nursing practice. Nurses need to have adequate resources to offer appropriate and consistent advice. These resources may be in the form of written telephone protocols developed specifically for their settings or general telephone advice textbooks. Practicing nurses can also provide valuable feedback on the physical settings in which they are providing advice and whether these settings provide the necessary atmosphere to perform their roles. Nurses need to have a quiet area that is free from interruption, clear and concise protocols, additional reference materials, and access to patient medical records. Aspects of the physical setting include the noise level, potential for distraction, expectations to do a variety of tasks at once, and computer support. The effect of a telephone consultation service on the pediatric practice should also be addressed. Telephone consultation can be a time-consuming activity in an office setting because of the variability in the volume and content of calls. Some settings build telephone advice time into the office schedule or schedule a second nurse at peak times to handle telephone calls (Robinson, Anderson, & Erpenbeck, 1997).

Telephone consultation is an efficient and cost-effective service that families can use as a means to access the health care system, obtain advice about how to manage illnesses and injuries at home, and acquire health promotion and disease prevention information. Early identification and management of common childhood illnesses and injuries can save money in the current environment, in which prudent use of health care dollars is essential. A wealth of information and support is available to families by just merely dialing a telephone to speak to a nurse.

REFERENCES

Barton, E., Brown, J., Curtis, P., & Lichtenfeld, L. (1992). Making phone care good care. *Patient Care, 26*(20), 103-117.

Brennan, M. (1992). Nursing process in telephone advice. *Nursing Management, 23*(5), 62-66.

tion Administration. The need to target parents or caregivers is obvious because these are the persons responsible for bringing them to vaccination services. Immunization/Vaccination Administration is also important for health care providers involved in inpatient or outpatient pediatrics, emergency services, family health care, well child care, or with sick children.

Healthy People 2000 Objectives

The national goal for immunization of this population is based on the *Healthy People 2000* Objective 20.11, which states that 90% of all 2-year-olds should have received the basic immunization series (U.S. Department of Health and Human Services [USDHHS], 1991). The basic immunization series includes the following vaccines: four diphtheria, pertussis, and tetanus (DPT) vaccines; three oral or inactivated polio vaccines (OPV or IPV); one measles, mumps, and rubella (MMR) vaccines; and three haemophilus influenza Type b (HIB) vaccines. Objective 20.11 also includes the goal of Hepatitis B immunization for 90% in the population for infants of surface antigen-positive mothers (USDHHS, 1991). President Clinton's Childhood Immunization Initiative (CII) began in 1993 to increase the immunization rates of 2-year-olds and specified the same goal as Objective 20.11 in addition to a goal to increase Hepatitis B vaccination rates to 70% by 1996 and 90% by 1998 (CDC, 1994a). The midcourse review of *Healthy People 2000* reported the national 2-year-old immunization rate at 67% for the following immunizations: four DPT, three polio, and one MMR (USDHHS, 1995). The National Immunization Survey (NIS) conducted by the CDC in accord with the CII found that 77% of children aged 19 to 35 months had received the basic series during the time period of January to December 1996 (CDC, 1997c). This NIS survey found that 82% of these children also had received three or more hepatitis B vaccines (CDC, 1997c). Individual vaccine data showed DPT, polio, HIB, and measles rates to exceed the national goal of 90%, when not measured as a series (CDC, 1997c). These numbers, the highest recorded, provide encouragement toward meeting the goal of 90% for the series, but the data continue to indicate that many children are not appropriately vaccinated at the ages when they are most susceptible to vaccine-preventable diseases.

LITERATURE REVIEW

Current literature on the immunization status of 2-year-olds can best be described as an ongoing discussion of the changes in policy, schedule, and barriers to adequate vaccination. Vaccination barriers and recommended practice standards to remove or minimize the barriers can be categorized into three areas: (a) administration barriers, (b) parent barriers, and (c) health care provider barriers.

Immunization Policy and Schedule Changes

Direction for practice and policy change was offered by the Ad Hoc Working Group for the Development of Standards for Pediatric Immunization Practices (1993) and CII (CDC, 1994a) with the goal of decreasing the barriers encountered by parents or practitioners that cause inadequate immunization completion for 2-year-olds. The Standards for Pediatric Immunization Practices is an important document that outlines 18 standards for use by health care providers to improve immunization services (Ad Hoc Working Group, 1993). The Childhood Immunization Initiative defines six areas to meet national goals for 2-year-old immunization rates (CDC, 1994a). Included in this initiative is the Vaccine for Children Program, which pays for immunizations for those children who are on Medicaid, have no health insurance, are Native Americans, or whose private insurer will not pay for vaccines administered at government-regulated facilities (CDC, 1994a). In March 1996, the Advisory Committee on Immunization Practices outlined recommendations for inclusion of immunizations tracking and referral associated with Women, Infants, and Children (WIC) programs (CDC, 1996). The National Vaccine Advisory Committee (1999) published recommendations to sustain and further improve immunization delivery.

Another significant change occurred in January 1995 when the CDC introduced a joint childhood immunization schedule endorsed by the Advisory Committee on Immunization Practices, the American Academy of Pediatrics (AAP), the Academy of Family Physicians, and the CDC National Immunization Program (CDC, 1995). Previously, these groups responsible for vaccine schedules had differences in their immunizations requirements. The new, conjoined schedule did not make major revisions in the separate schedules, but it offers a flexible, unified format that is helpful for both parents and health care providers. Since 1990, specific changes to the immunization schedule have been numerous. Staying current for practitioners, let alone parents, has been difficult. Prior to 1989, only one change had been made to the vaccination schedule in 20 years (Hall, 1994). It is easy to understand the challenge of keeping all these modifications straight in everyday health care practice.

Beginning in 1990, the immunizations schedule for 2-year-olds changed with the addition of three haemophilus influenza Type b vaccines; three new Hepatitis B vaccines were added in 1991, and one new varicella virus vaccine was added in 1995. Recommendations for the use of IPV instead of the traditional active OPV for the first two doses of the polio series was instituted in 1997 with the belief that this policy will decrease the eight or nine annual cases of vaccine-associated poliomyelitis in the United States (CDC, 1997a). The change in recommendation for use of acellular pertussis for all the pertussis series versus only the fourth dose was made in March 1997 (CDC, 1997b). Use of acellular vaccines is predicted to lessen the negative side effects of whole-cell pertussis vaccines.

In March 1999, an oral live rotavirus vaccine was added for the purpose of decreasing rotavirus gastroenteritis and sequelae of the disease (CDC, 1999b). In the summer of 1999, the rotavirus vaccine recommendation was suspended because of numerous reported cases of intussusception possibly related to the vaccine (AAP, 1999a).

Finally, in July 1999, a concern was raised regarding thimerosal, a mercury-containing vaccine preservative. Although the risk-to-benefit ratio favored using vaccines with this preservative, recommendations changed to give either thimerosal-free immunizations to 2-month-olds of hepatitis-negative mothers or to initiate the hepatitis B series at 6 months (AAP, 1999b).

Barriers to Vaccination

Administration Barriers

Administration barriers are those that inhibit access to immunizations. These variables are often beyond the control of parents and keep them from following the recommended vaccination schedule. The administration barriers include the cost of vaccines, the lack of health insurance coverage for vaccines, priorities and survival issues for parents, and the inconvenience of the provider system.

Parents view cost as the primary reason why they delay having their children immunized (Salsberry, Nickel, & Mitch, 1993). Often, immunizations are not covered by health insurance plans (Abbotts & Osborn, 1993; Salsberry et al., 1993). In addition, many parents were not aware of vaccination coverage even when offered by their insurance program (Lieu et al., 1994). Lieu et al. also reported that 63% of public clinic users preferred to obtain immunizations for their children from a private provider. Of these parents, 61% had a primary care provider but stated that the cost of the vaccines kept them from seeking them at their private care site. Children without health insurance are at risk of being underimmunized (Abbotts & Osborn, 1993).

Parental priorities play a role in delayed immunization rates. Parents frequently are faced with survival issues, namely, shelter, food, safety, employment, and child care, which may take financial priority over disease prevention. The focus group study of Keane et al. (1993) centered on parental beliefs and perceptions regarding health, illness, and immunizations. This sample of low-income, urban, 19- to 32-year-old parents knew they were involved in the study to discuss health issues. They chose to talk about other life and parenting concerns that they perceived as more important, however, including the exposure of their children to drugs, HIV, and violence. It is understandable that these parents struggle with these conflicts.

Children who are immunized in a public clinic are less likely to be current at 2 years of age than children who receive their immunizations at private clinics (Abbotts & Osborn, 1993; Hueston, Mainous, & Palmer, 1994). This has been related to inconvenient clinic scheduling practices, the need to enroll the child in a well child program, and completion of a physical exam before receiving immunizations. Parents, however, chose public clinic sites as vaccine providers because they were more convenient than private sites. They were relieved when they did not need an appointment at the public facility to have their child immunized. Parents rated a long wait as the third barrier to immunizations after cost and no insurance coverage (Salsberry et al., 1993). Public versus private acquisition of vaccines, however, causes concern regarding the continuity of the child's comprehensive health care. Continuity of care is compromised when the child receives vaccinations at one clinic (public), well child exams at another (private) site, and acute care in potentially another (emergency room) setting.

Parent Barriers

Many studies have involved the identification of parental demographic and socioeconomic risk factors for the underimmunized. Poor, inner-city, and nonwhite parents are most at risk for improper vaccination of their children (CDC, 1991). Single mothers with less that 12 years of education and less than 21 years of age had children who were not up-to-date on their immunizations (Salsberry, Nickel, & Mitch, 1994). Parents who were involved in a government support program, such as Aid to Families With Dependant Children (AFDC) or WIC, and families who relocated in the first 2 years of the child's life were at risk for delayed immunizations (Abbotts & Osborn, 1993). Children who are not current by 3 months of age and children who are second born or later also were more likely to be behind schedule by the age of 2 years (CDC, 1994b).

In addition to demographic variables, parent barriers include a lack understanding about immunizations and the diseases they prevent. Most of the parents of today's generation have no firsthand awareness of the mortality and morbidity of diseases, such as pertussis and polio, because the vaccinations have been effective in nearly eliminating their occurrence. In addition, the greatest misinformation parents have about immunization is that a minor cold or fever is a valid reason to postpone vaccination (Abbotts & Osborn, 1993; Salsberry et al., 1993, 1994). Health beliefs and values of parents have not consistently been found to affect immunization of 2-year-olds. Taylor and Cufley (1996) studied parental health beliefs regarding the benefits, susceptibility, severity, or barriers of vaccine-preventable illness in a private pediatric population and found no difference between parents who immunize their children according to schedule and parents who do not. Another study of poor, urban parents found neither immunization knowledge nor health beliefs to affect the immunization status of their children (Strobino, Keane, Holt, Hughart, & Guyer, 1996). Even with these findings, the Ad Hoc Working Group (1993) supports education of parents as a primary standard. They advise that parents be educated about the importance of immunizations, the diseases they prevent, and the schedule, risks, and contraindications of the vaccines in a culturally appropriate manner.

Health Care Provider Barriers

Health care providers have been criticized for not being aware of appropriate contraindications to vaccination and for failure to assess the immunization status of children. Opportunities to administer vaccinations are missed when vaccines are not given simultaneously or when the child presents for a reason other than immunization. Colds, mild cases of upper respiratory illness, and low fevers are not reasons to delay vaccinations, but studies continue to document children missing shots for these reasons (CDC, 1994b; Fairbrother, Friedman, DuMont, & Lobach, 1996; Hueston et al., 1994; Smith et al., 1999). Ball and Serwint (1996) found that the simple task of failing to review immunization status was the major cause of missed opportunities.

Few providers incorporate an official tracking and reminder system in their practice. A study that examined the Department of Defense clinics, in which immunizations are free and the clinic is accessible, found that failure to immunize and failure to remind parents when immunizations were due kept this ideal situation from reaching the national objective of 90% (Lopreiato & Ottolini, 1996).

In addition, physicians have been described as being poorly informed regarding the correct contraindications and administration and tracking of childhood immunizations (Smith et al., 1999). A nursing study showed that only 7% of hospital nurses had knowledge of proper immunizations for a 2-year-old (Dixon, Keeling, & Kennel, 1994). These nurses understood their role in immunization assessment, but they realized that they were not knowledgeable. Health care providers have a responsibility to maintain a current working knowledge of when and how to administer vaccinations (Ad Hoc Working Group, 1993). This responsibility is especially important considering the frequent changes that have been and continue to be made in the recommended schedule. Providers need to administer vaccines at the same visit according to schedule, decreasing the number of return visits that the patient is required to make. Every contact with the health care system should be an opportunity to assess and update childhood immunization status. Providers should track and audit their patient population to identify patients who are not up-to-date and target interventions toward these preschoolers.

Summary

In summary, many policy and practice changes have occurred in the past decade to improve the immunization delivery system to 2-year-olds. The Standards for Pediatric Immunization Practices offers practice direction. One accepted immunization schedule helps to decrease conflicts of vaccine administration. Numerous new and improved vaccine recommendations have been made to optimize protection of children and minimize side effects. Barriers to properly immunized 2-year-olds are multidimensional, as evidenced by administration, parental, and health care provider factors.

NURSING DIAGNOSIS AND OUTCOME DETERMINATION

The nursing diagnosis appropriate for Immunization/Vaccination Administration is Risk for Infection as indicated by inadequate immunization status (North American Nursing Diagnosis Association [NANDA], 1999). *Risk of Infection* is defined as "the state in which an individual is at increased risk for being invaded by pathogenic organisms" (NANDA, 1999, p. 11). Children without the immunity provided by vaccinations live in a state of increased risk of contracting these diseases. Risk factors to this diagnosis are those that preclude access of this patient population to adequate immunization and include demographic and socioeconomic factors and parent and provider immunization knowledge and practice. Demographic and socioeconomic factors include children who are born to poor, inner-city, and nonwhite parents who receive government assistance, such as AFDC or WIC (Abbotts & Osborn, 1993; CDC, 1991). Children who are second born or later are also at risk (CDC, 1994b). Parent knowledge of the immunization series is truly an indicator of their involvement in the health care of their children. It is the responsibility of the provider to educate and encourage appropriate immunization status. This is difficult to accomplish, however, because many providers are misinformed about the current immunization schedule and standards of practice. Risk for Infection is a relevant clinical judgment for these children. The ultimate goal of Immunization/Vaccination Administration is the prevention of infection due to these childhood diseases. Improper vaccination coverage places the individual and the community at enhanced susceptibility to these vaccine-preventable diseases.

An appropriate evaluation for this nursing diagnosis is the outcome Immunization Behavior from the Nursing Outcomes Classification (NOC; Iowa Outcomes Project, 2000). This outcome is defined as "actions to obtain immunity from a preventable communicable disease" (p. 245). Most of the indicators are applicable for determination of both parent and provider practice associated with the Immunization/Vaccination Administration intervention. Two indicators scored on a Likert-type scale of 1 ("never demonstrated") to "5" ("consistently demonstrated") worth highlighting for parents are "Brings updated vaccination card to each visit" and "Confirms date of next immunization" (p. 245). In addition to knowledge of the disease and the accompanying vaccination, parents should be reminded and consistently demonstrate understanding of the importance of an updated vaccination card and the date of the next immunization in their child's series. It has been shown that when immunization cards are available, the correlation between the card and the child's medical record is high (85%), which is extremely helpful information for providers in maintaining the appropriate immunization status of children (Fierman et al., 1996).

Providers also need to be able to demonstrate knowledge of the vaccine-preventable diseases and the accompanying immunizations. The indicators of this outcome for providers include "Describes contraindications to specific immunization" and "Obtains [or provides] immunizations recommended for age by the [current schedule]" (Iowa Outcomes Project, 2000, p. 245). Providers consistently miss opportunities to update the immunization status of 2-year-olds because of misunderstanding of the current contraindications and schedule.

INTERVENTION: IMMUNIZATION/VACCINATION ADMINISTRATION

The nursing intervention *Immunization/Vaccine Administration* is defined as the "provision of immunizations for prevention of communicable disease" (Iowa Intervention Project, 2000, p. 292-253). Current nursing practice for immunization of 2-year-olds involves the use of a majority of the activities listed for this intervention. Immunization/Vaccination Administration can easily be incorporated into the practice of nurses who care for young children by considering a review of immunization status as another vital sign. Just as temperature, pulse, respiration rate, blood pressure, and height and weight measurements are important, whether the child is well or sick, determination of immunization status can fit into the routine child assessment.

Nursing activities associated with Immunization/Vaccination Administration begin with giving a personal record-keeping card to parents at the time of their child's birth or first well child visit (Iowa Intervention Project, 2000). Parents must be encouraged to bring their child's immunization record to each health care encounter. Education incorporates a written schedule of immunizations, the route of administration, reasons for immunization, benefits, possible adverse reactions, and side effects (p. 392). Vaccine Information Statements (VISs) are required by law to be distributed at the time of immunization administration and are available from the CDC. These statements are 2 pages in length and contain information about the disease(s), vaccine, schedule, risks, and what to do if a serious reaction occurs (USDHHS, 1995). A readability estimate of these statements was determined to be at the seventh-grade level (Fry, 1968). The statements are available in Chinese, French, Spanish, and Vietnamese languages. Information can also include the legal requirements for day care and school enrollment.

In addition to written information and verbal explanation of the vaccines and their potential side effects, special handling of the child such as the use of acetaminophen for comfort and handling of stool with the oral polio vaccine should be provided by the nurse who administers the immunization. Parents should be given an opportunity to ask questions before consent is obtained for each shot given (Iowa Intervention Project, 2000).

It is essential for nurses to have current knowledge of contraindications to immunization administration (Iowa Intervention Project, 2000). True contraindications for all vaccines include "previous anaphylactic reaction to a vaccine and moderate or severe illness, with or without a fever" (Ad Hoc Working Group, 1993, p. 1819). Specific contraindications are identified for DPT, OPV, and MMR vaccines.

Two nursing activities of special note are the recognition "that a delay in series administration does not indicate restarting the schedule" and "help[ing a] family with financial planning to pay for immunizations" (Iowa Intervention Project, 2000, p. 392). Guidelines are specifically written for children who fall behind on the recommended immunization schedule (CDC, 1999a). Financial assistance for vaccinations is provided by programs such as Vaccines for Children and by public health departments, which offer immunizations at reduced costs.

INTERVENTION APPLICATION

Nurses at a tertiary child health clinic became concerned following an audit of their 2-year-old population that showed vaccination rates of 54%. The audit also showed that the main reason for underimmunization in their clinic was missed opportunities to vaccinate children during well child and sick child visits. These data led to a nursing diagnosis of Risk for Infection not only for families served by the clinic but also for the community (NANDA, 1999). An educational intervention was planned and presented to the nursing personnel by the clinic's nurse educator. The education session focused on recent immunizations schedule changes, practice guidelines highlighting true and false contraindications, and the Immunization/Vaccination Administration nursing intervention. Current clinic practice was reviewed, and positive activities were identified, such as the use of the current immunization schedule, use of the VISs for parent education, and appropriate parent anticipatory guidance beginning at the first visit to the clinic and continuing at each immunization encounter. Recommended practice modifications included changing the practice of checking immunization status of children at only well child visits to checking it at every encounter, increasing awareness of true and false contraindications to immunizations, updating immunization cards or replacing cards with each vaccination, follow-up on the underimmunized children, and expanding the educational intervention to include physicians and medical residents who are a part of the clinic staff.

The NOC nursing outcome Immunization Behavior could be used to track immunization status (Iowa Outcomes Project, 2000). A follow-up audit 1 year later showed that the overall rate for all recommended vaccinations improved to 80%. Again, the primary reason for underimmunization was missed opportunities. The clinic nurses saw that progress had been made toward the national immunization goals for their 2-year-old population, but additional intervention was necessary. A separate survey is planned to determine nursing and medical knowledge of the recommended immunization practices and to assess the clinic staff members' individual delivery practices. Appropriate education and continuing audits will track the results of these efforts during the next few years.

NURSING PRACTICE AND
RESEARCH IMPLICATIONS

The problem of underimmunization in 2-year-olds in the United States is multidimensional. Health care providers and parents have had to deal

TABLE 30.1   Immunization Resources and Reference Guide

Resource	*Reference*
Recommended Childhood Immunization Schedule—United States, 1999	*Morbidity and Mortality Weekly Reports, 481*, 12-16
Standards for Pediatric Immunization Practices	*Journal of the American Medical Association, 269*(14), 1817-1822
Every Child by Two	http://www.ecbt.org/
Clinical Assessment Software Application	http://www.cdc.gov/nip/casa
American Academy of Pediatrics	http://www.aap.org
Vaccines for Children	http://www.cdc.gov/nip/vfc

with significant changes in the immunization schedule and practice recommendations during the past decade. Often, providers believe that parents are the cause of the underimmunization problem. Both providers and parents, however, contribute to the problem of inadequate immunization status. Nurses often have the first opportunity to consider every health care encounter as an opportunity to review the immunization status of young children, update as necessary, and educate the parent. Viewing every visit with a child as an immunization opportunity requires a change in mind-set and practice. The Ad Hoc Working Group (1993) noted, "Each encounter with a health care provider, including an emergency department visit or hospitalization, is an opportunity to screen immunization status and, if indicated, administer needed vaccines" (p. 1819). Therefore, it is essential to have not only knowledge of but also adherence to the true contraindications of immunization administration.

In addition, documentation on the patient health care record and on the child's personal immunization card is imperative. Immunization records have been problematic, especially when vaccines are administered at multiple sites, when parents do not carry the card at all times, or when providers simply ask "Are your child's shots up-to-date?" and the parent answers "Yes" without proper knowledge of what vaccines are required for his or her child or official documentation. The personal immunization record should be updated at every visit, or a new replacement card should be completed and issued.

Numerous resources are available to help nurses improve the immunization status in their practice (Table 30.1). The CDC regularly updates the immunization schedule and recommendations of the Advisory Committee in *Morbidity and Mortality Weekly*. Use of tracking devices such as the Clinical Assessment Software Application, which is available at no cost to public and private health care providers, helps to document and improve immunization status (CDC, 1996). Commuter-generated telephone reminders have also been shown to improve immunization rates (Alemi et al., 1996). Strategies to improve immunization rates for 2-year-olds are being developed by the American Nurses Association (ANA) through a partnership with the Every Child by Two, the Carter/ Bumpers Campaign for Early Immunization (Lambert, 1995).

Nursing continues to play a vital research role in the analysis of this timely issue. Long before the concept of disease prevention became fashionable in the health care community, nurses understood the importance of prevention on the health of the nation. Nurses have a responsibility to continue their leadership role in promoting Immunization/Vaccination Administration and improving the immunization status through outcomes research. Future research should focus on testing the proposed intervention and evaluating the implementation of the practice standards, specific methods of tracking immunization status, and the effect of parent and health care provider education on immunization status. Recognizing and acting on this responsibility will protect the 2-year-old population from preventable diseases.

Childhood immunizations are a primary offense for disease prevention. As a nation, the United States continues to make progress toward the goal of immunizing the 2-year-old population at a 90% level. To achieve this goal, continued effort must be directed toward this issue. Improvement in vaccination status can be made if changes in nursing practice are implemented and then evaluated for effectiveness. Through the management of the intervention Immunization/Vaccine Administration, young children throughout the United States can have a healthy start in life.

REFERENCES

Abbotts, B., & Osborn, L. (1993). Immunization status and reasons for immunization delay among children using public health immunization clinics. *American Journal of Diseases in Children, 147*(9), 965-968.

Ad Hoc Working Group for the Development of Standards for Pediatric Immunization Practices. (1993). Development of standards for pediatric immunization practices. *Journal of the American Medical Association, 269*(14), 1817-1822.

Alemi, F., Alemagno, S. A., Goldhagen, J., Ash, L., Finkelstein, B., Lavin, A., Butts, J., & Ghadiri, A. (1996). Computer reminders improve on-time immunization rates. *Medical Care, 34*(10), OS45-OS51.

American Academy of Pediatrics. (1999a). *Possible association of intussusception with rotavirus vaccine* [On-line]. Available: http://www.aap.org/new/ rotapublic. htm.

American Academy of Pediatrics. (1999b). *Thimerosal in vaccines—An interim report to clinicians* [On-line]. Available: http://www.aap.org/new/thimpublic.htm.

Ball, T. M., & Serwint, J. R. (1996). Missed opportunities for vaccination and the delivery of preventive care. *Archives of Pediatric and Adolescent Medicine, 150*(8), 858-861.

Centers for Disease Control. (1991). Measles-United States, 1990. *Morbidity and Mortality Weekly Report, 40*(22), 369-371.

Centers for Disease Control. (1992). Retrospective assessment of vaccine coverage among school-aged children: Selected U.S. cities, 1991. *Morbidity and Mortality Weekly Report, 41*(6), 103-107.

Centers for Disease Control. (1994a). Reported vaccine-preventable diseases—United States, 1993, and the childhood immunization initiative. *Morbidity and Mortality Weekly Report, 43*(4), 57-61.

Centers for Disease Control. (1994b). Vaccination coverage of 2-year-old children: United States, 1992-1993. *Morbidity and Mortality Weekly Report, 43*(15), 282-283.

Centers for Disease Control. (1994c). Rubella and congenital rubella syndrome: United States, January 1, 1991-May 7, 1994. *Morbidity and Mortality Weekly Report, 43*(21), 391-401.

Centers for Disease Control. (1995). Recommended childhood immunization schedule: United States, January 1995. *Morbidity and Mortality Weekly Report, 43* (51/52), 959-960.

Centers for Disease Control. (1996). Recommendations of the advisory committee on immunization practices: Programmatic strategies to increase vaccination coverage by age 2 years—Linkage of vaccination and WIC services. *Morbidity and Mortality Weekly Report, 45*(10), 217-218.

Centers for Disease Control. (1997a). Poliomyelitis prevention in the United States: Introduction of a sequential vaccination schedule of inactivated poliovirus vaccine followed by oral poliovirus vaccine. Recommendations of the advisory committee on immunization practices (ACIP). *Morbidity and Mortality Weekly Report, 46*(RR-3), 1-25.

Centers for Disease Control. (1997b). Pertussis vaccination: Use of acellular pertussis vaccines among infants and young children. Recommendations of the advisory committee on immunization practices (ACIP). *Morbidity and Mortality Weekly Report, 46*(RR-7), 1-25.

Centers for Disease Control. (1997c). Status report on the childhood immunization initiative: National, state, and urban area vaccination coverage levels among children aged 19-35 months: United States, 1996. *Morbidity and Mortality Weekly Report, 46*(29), 657-664.

Centers for Disease Control. (1999a). Recommended childhood immunization schedule: United States, 1999. *Morbidity and Mortality Weekly Report, 48*, 12-16.

Centers for Disease Control. (1999b). Rotavirus vaccine for the prevention of rotavirus gastroenteritis among children. Recommendations of the Advisory Committee on Immunization Practices (ACIP). *Morbidity and Mortality Weekly Report, 48*(RR-2), 1-20.

Dixon, M., Keeling, A. W., & Kennel, S. (1994). What nurses know about immunization. *MCN: American Journal of Maternal Child Nursing, 19*(2), 75-78.

Fairbrother, G., Friedman, S., DuMont, K. A., & Lobach, K. S. (1996). Markers for primary care: Missed opportunities to immunize and screen for lead and tuberculosis by private physicians serving large numbers of inner-city Medicaid-eligible children. *Pediatrics, 97*(6, Pt. 1), 785-790.

Fierman, A. H., Rosen, C. M., Legano, L. A., Lim, S. W., Mendelsohn, A. L., & Dreyer, B. P. (1996). Immunization status as determined by patients' hand-held cards vs. medical records. *Archives of Pediatric and Adolescent Medicine, 150*(8), 863-866.

Fry, E. (1968). A readability formula that saves time. *Journal of Reading, 11*(514), 577.

Hall, C. B. (1994). Childhood immunizations: A strategic maze. *Pediatric Infectious Diseases, 1*(2), 1-4.

Hueston, W. J., Mainous, A. O., & Palmer, C. (1994). Delays in childhood immunizations in public and private settings. *Archives of Pediatric and Adolescent Medicine, 148*(5), 470-473.

Iowa Intervention Project. (2000). *Nursing interventions classification (NIC)* (J. C. McCloskey & G. Bulechek, Eds.; 3rd ed.). St. Louis, MO: Mosby-Year Book.

Iowa Outcomes Project. (1997). *Nursing outcomes classification (NOC)* (M. Johnson, M. Mass, & S. Moorhead, Eds.; 2nd ed.). St. Louis, MO: Mosby-Year Book.

Keane, V., Stanton, B., Horton, L., Aronson, R., Galbraith, J., & Hughart, N. (1993). Perceptions of vaccine efficacy, illness, and health among inner-city parents. *Clinical Pediatrics, 32*, 2-7.

Lambert, J. (1995). Every child by two: A program of the American nurses foundation. *American Nurse, 27*(8), 12.

Lieu, T. A., Smith, M. D., Newacheck, P. W., Langthorn, D., Venkatesh, P., & Herradora, R. (1994). Health insurance and preventive care sources of children at public immunization clinics. *Pediatrics, 93*(3), 373-378.

Lopreiato, J. O., & Ottolini, M. C. (1996). Assessment of immunization compliance among children in the department of defense health care system. *Pediatrics, 97*(3), 308-311.

National Vaccine Advisory Committee. (1999). Strategies to sustain success in childhood immunizations. *Journal of the American Medical Association, 282*(4), 363-370.

North American Nursing Diagnosis Association. (1999). *Nursing diagnoses: Definitions and classification 1999-2000*. Philadelphia: Author.

Salsberry, P. J., Nickel, J. T., & Mitch, R. (1993). Why aren't preschoolers immunized? A comparison of parents' and providers' perceptions of the barriers to immunizations. *Journal of Community Health Nursing, 10*(4), 213-224.

Salsberry, P. J., Nickel, J. T., & Mitch, R. (1994). Inadequate immunization among 2-year-old children: A profile of children at risk. *Journal of Pediatric Nursing, 9*(3), 158-165.

Smith, S. W., Connery, P., Knudsen, K., Scott, K. L., Frintner, M. P., Outlaw, G., & Weingart, S. (1999). Immunization practices and beliefs of physicians in suburban Cook County, Illinois. *Journal of Community Health, 24*, 1-11.

Strobino, D., Keane, V., Holt, E., Hughart, N., & Guyer, B. (1996). Parental attitudes do not explain underimmunization. *Pediatrics, 98*(6), 1076-1083.

Taylor, J. A., & Cufley, D. (1996). The association between parental health beliefs and immunization status among children followed by private pediatricians. *Clinical Pediatrics, 35,* 18-22.

U.S. Department of Health and Human Services. (1991). *Healthy people 2000: National health promotion and disease prevention objectives* (DHHS Publication No. PHS 91-50312). Washington, DC: Government Printing Office.

U.S. Department of Health and Human Services. (1995). *Healthy people 2000 midcourse review and 1995 revisions.* Washington, DC: Government Printing Office.

31

Environmental Management

Automobile Safety

Sara Walsh Arneson

In the past 100 years, many deadly childhood illnesses have been conquered. Despite this progress, children in the United States continue to face many threats to their well-being, especially from unintentional injuries, which remain the leading cause of death in children younger than 14 years of age. Although unintentional injuries occur in a variety of settings and in many circumstances, motor vehicle crashes are the leading cause of death for children of every age from 6 to 18 years (National Highway Traffic Safety Administration [NHTSA], 1998a). *Healthy People 2000* (U.S. Department of Health and Human Services [USDHHS], 1991) challenges the nation to redouble its efforts to reduce unintentional injury deaths to no more than 29.3 per 100,000 people (a 15% decrease) and increase automobile safety restraint use to at least 85% of automobile occupants (a 102% increase). Achievement of these goals will require a concerted effort on the part of health care providers, safety experts, legislators, parents, and law enforcement officers.

LITERATURE REVIEW

Until recently, unintentional injuries were viewed as an unavoidable part of growing up. With the advent of the science of injury prevention, a greater understanding of injuries has emerged that suggests that childhood injuries can be reduced by modifying the associated human and environmental factors.

Sociodemographic Factors

A child's age is one of the most significant factors related to automobile safety practices. In 1994, an estimated 88% of infants younger than 1 year of age were restrained, whereas only 61% of toddlers and preschoolers were observed in safety seats (NHTSA, 1996). Even fewer school-age children have been observed using seat belts correctly. In 1995, 56% of 10- to 14-year-olds involved in fatal automobile collisions were unrestrained (NHTSA, 1996). In addition, studies have demonstrated positive relationships between parents' use of child safety seats and their (a) education levels, (b) personal seat belt use, and (c) attitudes toward seat belt use (Gielen, Erikson, Daltroy, & Rost, 1984; Margolis, Wagenaar, & Molnar, 1992; Webb, Sanson-Fisher, & Bowman, 1988), whereas nonuse of automobile safety restraints tended to increase as parental income decreases (Gielen et al., 1984). Table 31.1 summarizes the results of these studies.]

Environmental Factors

For children younger than 4 years of age, the most effective means of preventing or reducing or both automobile mortality and morbidity is the correct and consistent use of an approved child safety seat. Child safety seats are misused as much as 78% of the time, however (Block, Hanson, & Keane, 1998). *Misuse* is defined as the child being incorrectly harnessed in the safety seat, the seat being improperly anchored, or the seat being positioned incorrectly in the front seat or facing forward when it should be facing the rear or both. Once a child weighs 40 pounds, a child safety seat is no longer recommended. Lap-type and shoulder-lap combination seat belts, however, are designed for adults and frequently cause friction on a young child's neck. The use of a booster seat can minimize this problem, but many parents choose not to purchase one. Use of lap-type seat belts without a shoulder harness have been linked to severe abdominal injuries and lumbar compression fractures in 4- to 9-year-olds (Osberg & DiScala, 1992).

TABLE 31.1 Studies of Relationships Between Parents' Use of Child Safety Seats and Selected Parental Characteristics

Parental Characteristic/Reference	Statistical Test	r or χ^2	Significance
Educational level			
Gielen, Erikson, Daltroy, and Rost (1984)	Pearson correlation coefficient	$r = .12$	$p = .01$
Webb, Sanson-Fisher, and Bowman (1988)	Chi-square	$\chi^2 = 27.77$	$p = <.00$
Parental seat belt use			
Gielen et al. (1984)	Pearson correlation coefficient	$r = .22$	$p = .00$
Margolis, Wagenaar, and Molnar (1992)	Chi-square	$\chi^2 = 111.26$, df = 1	$p < .00$
Webb et al. (1988)	Chi-square	$\chi^2 = 76.61$	$p < .00$
Parental attitudes toward seat belt use and comfort			
Gielen et al. (1984)	Pearson correlation coefficient	$r = .40$	$p = .00$
Margolis et al. (1992)	Chi-square	$\chi^2_2 = 11.55$, df = 1	$p < .00$
Webb et al. (1988)	Chi-square	$\chi^2 = 4.95$	$p < .05$
Income			
Gielen et al. (1984)	Pearson correlation coefficient	$r = .11$	$p = .02$

A significant step in reducing adult mortality and morbidity related to automobile collisions has been the development of air bags. However, from 1996 to 1999, more than 32 children died from injuries sustained when air bags on the passenger side of the front seat deployed ("Update," 1996). In November 1996, the NHTSA (1996) announced a comprehensive plan to minimize air bag danger to children. The plan includes the installation of reduced-power air bags and new air bag testing procedures. A phase-in schedule for reduced-power air bags began in the fall of 1998 (NHTSA, 1998b). While the plan is being implemented, NHTSA recommends that children under 12 years of age sit in the rear seat (NHTSA, 1998a).

NURSING DIAGNOSIS AND OUTCOME DETERMINATION

Assessment

Assessment of automobile safety practices should begin during the prenatal period with questions designed to evaluate prospective parents' knowledge of child automobile safety practices and their plans to acquire a child safety seat. Each well child visit offers an excellent opportunity for ongoing assessment and reinforcement of automobile safety practices. The focus of this assessment shifts as the child progresses through the stages of childhood (Table 31.2).

Toddlers pose a particular challenge with regard to automobile safety practices. Because of their drive for mobility and need to be autonomous, the use of a child safety seat can become a point of significant conflict between the child and parents. As children enter the preschool period, the use of child safety seats becomes a shared responsibility between parent and child. Although primary responsibility continues to rest with parents, preschool children have the capability to not only understand what is expected in regard to automobile safety but also, in many instances, to manage the buckles and harnesses themselves. Children's knowledge of automobile safety practices can be assessed through selected questions, drawings depicting safety seat and seat belt use, or play sessions. School-age children generally take great pride in assuming responsibility for their own behaviors. At the same time, they also come under the increasing influence of peers who may encourage them to disregard automobile safety practices to fit in with the group. As a result, ongoing assessment of automobile safety practices is critical during this developmental period.

Nursing Diagnosis and Outcome Determination

Failure to practice routine and correct child automobile safety practices places children at risk for injury and death and leads to a nursing diagnosis of Risk for Trauma (North American Nursing Diagnosis Association, 1999). The Nursing Outcomes Classification (Iowa Outcomes Project, 2000) outcome Safety Behavior: Personal includes the indicator "use of seat belts or safety seats" (p. 375). More specific indicators to measure the effectiveness of nursing interventions designed to promote automobile safety and prevent trauma, however, include the following:

For infants
    Uses federally approved child automobile safety seat designed for infants
    Positions child safety seat in center of rear seat in rear-facing position
    Anchors child safety seat to automobile according to directions

For toddlers and preschoolers
    Uses child safety seat designed for children weighing up to 40 pounds

TABLE 31.2   Assessment of Automobile Safety Practices by Developmental Level

	Developmental Level				
	Prenatal	*Infant*	*Toddler*	*Preschool*	*School*
Parent					
Knowledge of					
Auto safety	X	X	X	X	X
Types of seats	X	X	X		
Plans to acquire	X	X	X	X	Booster
Barriers to purchase	X	X	X	X	X
Correct installation	X	X	X	X	X
Beliefs about auto safety practices	X	X	X	X	X
Access to adjustable shoulder harness				X	X
Barriers to regular use of seats and seat belts	X	X	X	X	X
Personal use of seats and seat belts	X	X	X	X	X
Positions child in rear seat		X	X	X	X
Positions infant facing rear		X			
Positions toddler or preschooler facing forward			X	X	
Children					
Knowledge of					
Auto safety				X	X
Back seat safety				X	X
Use of seat belt or booster seat				X	X
Personal seat belt practices				X	X
Regular use of seat belts				X	X

   Positions child safety seat in center of rear seat in front-facing po-
      sition
   Anchors child safety seat to automobile according to directions
   Uses booster seat with automobile shoulder-lap combination seat
      belt for children who exceed the height or weight recommen-
      dations for child safety seats
   Positions children using booster seats or shoulder-lap combina-
      tion belts or both in outside position of rear seat
   Adjusts shoulder strap to avoid pressure on child's neck

For school-age children
   Uses shoulder-lap combination seat belts
   Sits in outside position of rear seat

Uses booster seat, if necessary, to avoid neck friction from shoulder strap

INTERVENTION:
ENVIRONMENTAL MANAGEMENT: SAFETY

Activities to encourage the use of child safety seats and seat belts include (a) educational programs for parents and children, (b) distribution of informational material, (c) positive reinforcement and rewards for safety seat or seat belt use, (d) infant safety seat loan programs, (e) community-based educational and enforcement programs, and (f) communitywide incentive programs. The majority of studies designed to test the effectiveness of these activities used quasi-experimental, pretest-posttest designs and included both randomized and convenience samples of varying sizes from statewide populations of children attending selected day care centers and schools (Arneson & Triplett, 1990; Chang, Dillman, Leonard, & English, 1985; Foss, 1989; Roberts & Fanurik, 1986; Robitaille, Legault, Abbey, & Pless, 1990). The activities met with varying success. In most studies, the number of children who were observed using child safety seats or seat belts increased during and shortly following the selected activity. Very few studies conducted long-term follow-up evaluation of ongoing effects.

The Nursing Interventions Classification (Iowa Intervention Project, 2000, p. 311) lists many activities under the nursing intervention Environmental Management: Safety that are relevant to the promotion of automobile safety in childhood.

Education of Parents and Children

The majority of strategies to promote automobile safety practices include a strong educational component. Although child safety seats have been available for many years, adults' knowledge of their correct use continues to be limited. In a 1992 study of 368 adults, both parents and nonparents, only 22% knew that infants should be positioned in the center of the rear seat, whereas 54% knew that infants should be facing the rear (Ruffin & Kantor, 1992). Although information about risks associated with riding in automobiles and the availability of resources for acquiring federally approved child safety seats is important to include in any educational program, emphasizing the direct benefits of using child safety seats is also an essential component. This is especially true when working with parents of toddlers and preschoolers who frequently resist being restrained.

It is important to take into account different learning styles and cognitive abilities when developing educational programs and informational materials. In a study by Ruffin and Kantor (1992), respondents who received their information about child safety seats from prenatal instructors or the manufacturers' written information were significantly more likely to give correct responses on a self-administered questionnaire than those who relied on newspapers and television for their information. Making videotapes, posters, brochures, and sample car seats available in exam and waiting rooms in ambulatory care settings can educate parents while they are waiting to be seen. Videotapes could also be given to parents to take home for viewing at their leisure. Nurses would then review the information with them as part of their health care visit.

When working with high-risk populations, it is important to understand their cultures and communities to provide information in settings that are accepted and frequented by community members. For example, in many cultures the church serves a central focus in family life and may be an ideal location for providing informational sessions on automobile safety practices. This can be especially effective if health care providers collaborate with parish nurses and church leaders in the development and implementation of programs.

Educational programs aimed at preschool and school-age children must be geared to their specific developmental levels and include parents. Some of the most successful programs target both children and parents in group settings, such as day care settings, nursery schools, and elementary schools.

Use of Protective Devices

The correct and consistent use of child safety seats and seat belts and air bags are two of the most effective strategies in reducing automobile injuries and deaths. During the 1980s, many hospitals initiated car seat loan programs. Nurses need to be knowledgeable about the availability of child safety seat loan programs and collaborate with the community organizations that develop and administer these programs. All hospitals with maternity and pediatric services should be urged to adopt and enforce comprehensive automobile safety policies for the discharge of infants and children. To be effective, child safety seats must not only be readily available but also easy to install and use. In February 1997, President Clinton proposed new regulations to standardize child safety seat design to eliminate the difficulties encountered by parents when they try to install safety seats in their cars. According to the new regulations, a universal child safety seat anchorage system will be phased in over a period of 3 years beginning in September 1999. By 2002, all new vehicles will be equipped with the new system (NHTSA, 1999).

Although the majority of infants are currently being transported in child safety seats, older children are not as well protected. Of special concern are children in the 5- to 9-year-old group. The use of a standard shoulder-lap combination seat belt is only 34% effective for 5- to 9-year-old children compared to more than 60% effectiveness of the child safety seat for infants (Johnston, Rivara, & Soderberg, 1994). An approved, crash-tested restraint device for children in this age group is urgently needed. Ideally, such a device should be a built-in component in new automobiles. Nurses can provide automotive designers with data about the perceived barriers and benefits of using various child and adult restraint systems with 5- to 9-year-olds. These data can be gleaned from research studies with sound designs and clinical practice.

Enforcement of Child Restraint Legislation

Legislation can be a powerful adjunct to education in the promotion of automobile safety practices. Nurses are in ideal positions to collaborate with law enforcement officers and other community leaders in the periodic evaluation of compliance with child restraint laws. In addition, information about child restraint laws could be distributed at well baby and prenatal clinic visits. It has been shown that parents who are knowledgeable about child restraint laws are more likely to use child safety seats correctly as measured by direct observation of child safety seat use (Margolis et al., 1992).

Child restraint laws require parents to restrain children younger than specified ages in child safety seats. In theory, mandatory seat belt laws should take over when a child exceeds the maximum age in the child restraint law. In most states, however, there are large gaps in the law that leave many young children at risk. For example, in some states only parents are required to comply with the child restraint law. In other states, the law applies only to drivers who are state residents (Fields & Weinberg, 1994). Amendments to child restraint laws that make all drivers responsible for children younger than 16 years of age would effectively eliminate the majority of current gaps in the law (Fields & Weinberg, 1994). Nurses, as individual citizens and members of their professional organizations, need to be knowledgeable about the law and urge their legislators to close existing gaps.

INTERVENTION APPLICATION

One morning, Dana Jeffries, director of the ABC Day Care Center, received a phone call informing her that 3-year-old Justin had been hospitalized with multiple injuries following an automobile collision. This was the second automobile collision involving a child from the ABC Center in 6 months. In both collisions, the children were unrestrained. Dana wondered how many other children were being transported without the use of optimal child safety restraints. To document the existence of a problem, the center staff systematically observed the arrival of the children for a 2-week period to determine correct use of child safety seats. Data showed that only 54% of the children were correctly restrained.

Dana contacted a faculty member from a nearby university who offers consultation and an educational program on automobile safety as a community service to day care centers and nursery schools. As part of the program, the center staff was encouraged to review their policies related to automobile safety and to convey information about these policies to all parents. In addition, parents were provided information about obtaining child safety seats. The center acquired three child safety seats to loan to families, as needed. Sessions for the children included coloring activities, songs, a video, and opportunities to play with toy cars equipped with seat belts and child safety seats. Informational materials and an educational session were provided for parents at a regularly scheduled parent meeting. Special emphasis was placed on helping parents identify specific strategies for keeping toddlers correctly restrained in their car seats. Reinforcement took place on an ongoing basis through periodic reminders to parents and children and through recognition and rewards for those who practiced correct automobile safety habits.

Six months following completion of the program, the staff again observed the children on arrival at the day care center to determine their use of car seats and seat belts. The average number of children who were properly restrained on arrival at the center increased to 79%.

RESEARCH AND PRACTICE IMPLICATIONS

Studies documenting the effectiveness of various activities to increase automobile safety practices have been conducted for many years. The measures used to determine the success of these activities often relied on parent self-report (questionnaires, phone calls, and interviews) or direct observation of actual child safety seat use or both. Self-report measures are often suspect because there is no way to substantiate the subjects' responses. Similarly, direct observation of safety seat use has many attendant problems that make accuracy questionable. For example, unless the observer is standing directly next to the automobile, it is impossible to determine whether the child is correctly buckled into the safety seat. Researchers of future studies need to consider these issues when designing methodologies and measurement techniques.

Previous studies focused on safety seat and seat belt use among infants, preschool, and school-age children. No studies were found, however, that tested activities to increase compliance with safety seat use among toddlers. This is an especially challenging age because toddlers are striving for autonomy and dislike being restrained. Studies are needed to identify interventions that help parents keep their toddlers safely restrained while riding in the car.

Child restraint laws have been in effect for less than 20 years, with the majority of states passing legislation during the 1980s. Several pertinent questions need to be addressed, including the following: (a) Will consistent and correct use of child safety seats throughout early childhood result in more consistent and proper use of seat belts in later childhood? and (b) Are there differences in seat belt use between adolescents who were raised using child safety seats and seat belts from birth and those who were not required to use any type of restraint?

The 5- to 9-year-old group is at particular risk because child safety seats are designed for younger children and automobile seat belts are designed for adults. Studies need to be conducted to document the effectiveness of booster seats when used with adult shoulder-lap combination-type seat belts. Similarly, some manufacturers have developed adjustable shoulder straps that are intended to accommodate individuals of various sizes. Studies are needed to determine the effectiveness of adjustable straps for 5- to 9-year-olds.

Many nurses and health care providers fail to take advantage of the many opportunities to educate children and parents about the dangers of certain practices and the strategies that they can use to prevent injury. Emphasizing injury prevention through family education in settings in which children and parents congregate, such as day care centers, nursery schools, elementary and secondary schools, hospital emergency departments, community recreational facilities, and churches, will go a long way to decrease the incidence of injuries and deaths associated with automobile collisions. Emphasizing injury prevention should be an integral part of all nursing education curricula and should include didactic content and clinical experiences. The most important thing that can be done to reduce childhood mortality and injury morbidity is to ensure that children are raised in safe, hazard-free environments. This will require commitment on the part of everyone. Nurses in all practice settings are in ideal positions to achieve this goal through education, encouragement, and reinforcement of positive safety practices.

SUMMARY

Automobile collisions continue to be a leading cause of unintentional injury and death in children. Although more children than ever are currently using child safety seats and seat belts when riding in cars, many children, especially those from high-risk, low-income populations and children from 5 to 9 years of age, remain inadequately protected. If injuries are to be prevented, efforts must be doubled to develop and test activities that focus on increasing parental motivation to provide a safe environment for all children when riding in automobiles. Only through such efforts will the goals outlined in *Healthy People 2000* (USDHHS, 1991) be achieved.

REFERENCES

Arneson, S. W., & Triplett, J. L. (1990). Riding with bucklebear: An automobile safety program for preschoolers. *Journal of Pediatric Nursing, 5*(2), 115-122.

Block, D., Hanson, T., & Keane, A. (1998). Child safety seat misuse: Home visiting assessment and intervention. *Public Health Nursing, 15*(4), 250-256.

Chang, A., Dillman, A., Leonard, M., & English, P. (1985). Teaching car passenger safety to preschool children. *Pediatrics, 76*(3), 425-428.

Fields, M., & Weinberg, K. (1994). Coverage gaps in child-restraint and seat-belt laws affecting children. *Accident Analysis and Prevention, 26*(3), 371-376.

Foss, R. D. (1989). Evaluation of a community-wide incentive program to promote safety restraint use. *American Journal of Public Health, 79*(3), 304-306.

Gielen, A. C., Erikson, M. P., Daltroy, L. H., & Rost, K. (1984). Factors associated with use of child restraint devices. *Health Education Quarterly, 11*(2), 195-206.

Iowa Intervention Project. (2000). *Nursing interventions classification (NIC)* (J. C. McCloskey & G. M. Bulechek, Eds.; 3rd ed.). St. Louis, MO: Mosby-Year Book.

Iowa Outcomes Project. (2000). *Nursing outcomes classifications (NOC)* (M. Johnson, M. Maas, & S. Moorhead, Eds.; 2nd ed.). St. Louis, MO: Mosby-Year Book.

Johnston, C., Rivara, F. P., & Soderberg, R. (1994). Children in car crashes: Analysis of data for injury and use of restraints. *Pediatrics, 93*(6), 960-965.

Margolis, L. H., Wagenaar, A. C., & Molnar, L. J. (1992). Use and misuse of automobile child restraint devices. *American Journal of Diseases of Children, 146*(3), 361-366.

National Highway Traffic Safety Administration. (1996). *Traffic safety facts 1995.* Available: http://www.nhtsa.dot.gov.

National Highway Traffic Safety Administration. (1998a). *Overview traffic safety facts 1997.* Available: http://www.nhtsa.dot.gov/people/ncsa/overvu96.html.

National Highway Traffic Safety Administration. (1998b). *Safety fact sheet: Comprehensive air bag plan.* Available: http://www.nhtsa.dot/airbags/factsheets/deact_53.html.

National Highway Traffic Safety Administration. (1999). *Universal care safety seat system.* Available: http://www.nhtsa.dot.gov.

North American Nursing Diagnosis Association. (1999). *Nursing diagnoses: Definitions and classification 1999-2000.* Philadelphia: Author.

Osberg, J. S., & DiScala, C. (1992). Morbidity among pediatric motor vehicle crash victims: The effectiveness of seat belts. *American Journal of Public Health, 82*(3), 422-425.

Roberts, M., & Fanurik, D. (1986). Rewarding elementary schoolchildren for their use of seat belts. *Health Psychology, 5*(3), 185-196.

Robitaille, Y., Legault, J., Abbey, H., & Pless, B. (1990). Evaluation of an infant car seat program in a low-income community. *American Journal of Diseases of Children, 144,* 74-78.

Ruffin, M. T., & Kantor, R. (1992). Adults' knowledge about the use of child restraint devices. *Family Medicine, 24*(5), 382-385.

Update: Fatal air bag-related injuries to children—United States, 1993-1996 (1996, February 13). *Morbidity and Mortality Weekly Report, 45*(49), 1073-1076.

U.S. Department of Health and Human Services. (1991). *Healthy people 2000: National health promotion and disease prevention objectives* (DHHS Publication No. PHS 91-50312). Washington, DC: Government Printing Office.

Webb, G. R., Sanson-Fisher, R. W., & Bowman, J. A. (1988). Psychosocial factors related to parental restraint of pre-school children in motor vehicles. *Accident Analysis and Prevention, 20*(2), 87-94.

32

Sleep Enhancement

Nancy C. Corser

Ann E. Edgil

Sleep is a pattern of increasing and decreasing states of arousal that allow for rest and rejuvenation of the body and mind. Disturbances in this pattern have consequences that affect the child's growth, perceived health pattern, and response to illness and also place strain on the caregiver and family (Mahon, 1995). *Healthy Children 2000* (U.S. Department of Health and Human Services, 1991) recognizes that childhood is a critical time for healthy human development. To support the child through this critical period, consideration must be given to promoting appropriate sleep patterns.

THEORETICAL FRAMEWORK AND LITERATURE REVIEW

Physiological Basis for Sleep

Sleep is two distinct states of central nervous system activity, rapid eye movement (REM) and non–rapid eye movement (NREM) sleep states, that occur in a cyclic pattern. These states are under different neuroendocrine controls, serve different purposes, and have different characteristics. NREM sleep is composed of four stages and is primarily under the control of serotonin, adenosin, and gamma-aminobutyric acid secreted by various neurons (Jones, 1989). NREM sleep is considered to function primarily in physical restoration. After infancy, sleep is initiated into NREM, with progression to Stage 4 within approximately 40 minutes. Each sleep cycle (REM/NREM) is approximately 50 minutes duration in the term infant and increases to the adult duration of 90 minutes during the school-age years.

Stage 1 sleep is a relaxed dreamy state in which the person remains somewhat aware of the surrounding environment. It typically lasts only a few seconds and is characterized by reduced body movement and eye rolling. Eyelids may be closed or slowly blinking. The person is easily awakened. Electroencephalograph (EEG) tracings show low-voltage alpha activity at 4 to 6 cycles per second (Adair & Bauchner, 1993). Stage 2 sleep is a deeper level of sleep in which the person is not aware of the surrounding environment. Respirations vary but tend to become more even. Occasional jerky, muscular contractions may occur in the hands, arms, and legs. In Stage 2 sleep, a person is easily awakened. EEG demonstrates high voltage activity with sleep spindles at 13 to 15 cycles per second and large K complexes (Adair & Bauchner, 1993). In Stage 3 sleep, the person is easily aroused but is in a deeper level of sleep with increasing muscle relaxation and decreasing heart rate, blood pressure, and temperature. EEG recordings show a slow-wave delta pattern at 1 to 4 cycles per second (Adair & Bauchner, 1993). Stage 4 sleep is the deepest sleep. It is the sleep on which people usually judge sleep adequacy. Also, growth hormone secretion occurs during Stage 4 sleep. Pulse and blood pressure are regular, respirations are slow and even, muscles are relaxed, and profuse sweating may occur. If awakened during Stage 4, the person is typically confused. Stage 4 is characterized by a slow-wave delta pattern on EEG (Adair & Bauchner, 1993).

REM sleep is controlled by dopamine neurons in the pons and is important for learning and information processing. It provides for physical restoration while allowing easy coherent arousal if necessary. REM sleep is characterized by complete relaxation of muscle tone, fine twitching movements of face or digits, and irregular respirations, with rapid irregular eye movements under closed eyelids sometimes visible (Adair & Bauchner, 1993). In REM sleep, heart rate, respiratory rate, and blood pressure increase, and temperature regulation is impaired. Although dreams occur in other states, they are not usually recalled. Recall of dreams in REM sleep has contributed to its reputation as the "dreaming" sleep (Adair & Bauchner, 1993).

Sleep as a Developmental Phenomenon

Infants

Newborns sleep approximately 16 hours each day in 2- to 4-hour periods. They enter sleep through REM and transition from one sleep state to another through REM. REM sleep accounts for approximately one third to one half of the total sleep time with REM cycles lasting approximately 50 to 60 minutes. Although accounting for two thirds of every 24 hours, sleep is not distributed in a diurnal pattern. A diurnal sleep concentration is usually first recognized at 2 months of age and stabilizes with the longest sleep period (approximately 7 hours) occurring at night by age 5 months, which remains constant throughout the remainder of the first year of life. At 6 months of age, the ratio of REM to NREM sleep reverses for the first time, and sleep onset through REM is rare. Total sleep time decreases to approximately 13.5 hours each day by the end of the first year of life (Adair & Bauchner, 1993).

Characteristic behaviors and EEG parameters of sleep states are not consistently demonstrated early in infancy. Therefore, infant sleep is generally classified as Quiet (NREM) or Active (REM) sleep on most infant behavioral state systems (Brazelton, 1994). EEG findings that can identify sleep are first demonstrated at approximately 6 weeks of age (Adair & Bauchner, 1993).

Premature infants have shorter sleep cycles than do term neonates, and their cycles are less well defined. Preterm infants and term infants who have experienced anoxia or brain stem stress may demonstrate delays in differentiation of sleep states (Brazelton, 1994). Depending on the severity of the brain injury, these effects may persist into childhood.

Toddlers and Preschoolers

Between the ages of 13 months and 5 years, sleep patterns stabilize. Total sleep time declines, and night sleep lengthens from approximately 7 hours at 12 months to approximately 10 hours at 54 months of age. Night awakenings decrease in number during this time but may persist up to 5 years of age. REM sleep is reduced and shifted to the last third of the night, whereas most Stage 4 sleep occurs in the first third of the night (Adair & Bauchner, 1993; Edgil, Wood, & Smith, 1985).

School-Age Children

During the school-age years, the REM cycle is first established at the adult level of 60 to 90 minutes. REM sleep accounts for approximately

20% of total sleep time. Latency to sleep onset initially increases but then decreases. Total sleep time decreases to approximately 8 or 9 hours a night (Adair & Bauchner, 1993).

Adolescents

REM sleep continues to account for 20% of total sleep time with a cycle of approximately 90 minutes. Total sleep time remains constant or decreases slightly (Adair & Bauchner, 1993). A decrease in daytime alertness at midpuberty with a concurrent delayed phase preference is probably due to a combination of physiological and psychosocial factors (peer pressure, school schedule, and control of own bedtime). The increased need for sleep is recognized by the adolescent, who supplements sleep by daytime napping or sleeping late on weekends rather that going to bed early (Carskadon, Vieira, & Acebo, 1993).

Behavioral Aspects of Sleep Pattern Development

Sleep is a complex process whose development is influenced by individual child temperament, parent-child interactions, cultural expectations, and environmental conditions (Jimmerson, 1991). Feeding patterns during infancy, cultural norms concerning cosleeping, and child-rearing practices can all influence the emerging sleep pattern. Even the onset of age-appropriate separation anxiety creates challenges for parents attempting to foster sleep pattern development. In addition, unrealistic expectations or inconsistent behaviors regarding sleep by parents can alter the normal development of sleep.

Specific Problems Associated With Sleep Loss

Research has demonstrated the physiological consequences of total sleep loss and loss of time in selected sleep stages. Sleep disturbance lowers levels of growth hormones and decreases protein synthesis and immunocompetence (Akerstdt, Palmblad, de la Torre, Mkarana, & Gillberg, 1980; Palmblad, Petrini, Wasserman, & Akerstedt, 1979). Even short periods of sleep disruption can significantly impair an individual's ability to arouse in response to hypercapnia and hypoxia (Phillipson, Bowes, Sullivan, & Woolf, 1980). Loss of REM sleep causes a subsequent recovery of REM sleep that increases cerebral blood flow, cardiac workload, and myocardial irritability (Slota, 1988). In addition, sleep loss causes psychological and cognitive changes that can decrease the child's ability to tolerate difficult situations, develop acceptable behavior patterns, and succeed in

TABLE 32.1 International Classification of Sleep Disorders

Dyssomnias
    Intrinsic sleep disorders
    Extrinsic sleep disorders
    Circadian rhythm sleep disorders
Parasomnias
    Arousal disorders
    Sleep-wake transition disorders
    Parasomnias usually associated with REM sleep
    Other parasomnias
Medical or psychiatric sleep disorders
    Associated with mental disorders
    Associated with neurological disorders
    Associated with other medical disorders
Proposed sleep disorders
    Includes disorders under investigations but not yet classified

SOURCE: Based on data from ASDA (1990).

school (Stores, 1996). Restlessness, disorientation, combativeness, apathy, fatigue, anxiety, irritability, and anorexia are all demonstrated after sleep loss (American Sleep Disorders Association [ASDA], 1990).

NURSING DIAGNOSES AND OUTCOMES DETERMINATION

Sleep Pattern Disturbance

In childhood, normal sleep is restful to the child and not excessively disruptive to others (Adair & Bauchner, 1993). Variations in sleep patterns of a child that do not result in a rested child or that cause disruption in the family routine may be considered sleep pattern disturbances. The North American Nursing Diagnosis Association (NANDA, 1999) developed the nursing diagnosis Sleep Pattern Disturbance, which describes this disruption of sleep time. In addition, the Association of Sleep Disorders Centers established standard diagnostic criteria for sleep disorders that were published as the Diagnostic Classification of Sleep and Arousal Disorders (DCSAD) in 1979 (Adair & Bauchner, 1993). A diagnostic and coding manual of the revised DCSAD was published in 1990 (ASDA, 1990). This revision organized sleep disorders according to known or presumed physiologic causes of the disorders (Table 32.1). Data regarding prevalence, course of the disorder, and polysomnographic features are included with each diagnosis.

According to the DCSAD, sleep problems are classified as dyssomnias, parasomnias, and medical and psychiatric sleep disorders (ASDA, 1990). *Dyssomnias* are defined as disorders of initiating and maintaining sleep. These disorders involve difficulty or resistance to falling asleep or frequent and disruptive night wakening or both. Factors influencing the development of these disorders include neurodevelopmental maturation, temperament, parenting skills, home environment, and life stressors. *Parasomnias* are defined as a group of disorders that have certain discrete and definable clinical features occurring during sleep or sleep-wake transition state. These disorders are characterized by fairly dramatic symptoms, confusion and disorientation of the child, and they are usually treatment resistant. Medical and psychiatric sleep disorders include inappropriate daytime sleepiness, total daily sleep in excess of developmentally appropriate levels, and excessive napping. Etiologies may be obstructive sleep apnea, narcolepsy, medications and toxins, central nervous system lesions, and depression.

Two of the most common sleep problems are classified under dyssomnias. Twenty to 30% of all infants and children experience the problems of resistance to bedtime, difficulty in going to sleep, and night waking (Fox, 1997). These problems typically begin during infancy and decline in early school years. Although these sleep problems are sometimes thought to be transitory, research has shown that they often last for months and sometimes for 1 year or more (Kerr & Jowett, 1994). Other problems are sleep enuresis, early rising, and difficulty in awaking the child in the morning.

Common sleep problems that are classified as parasomnias include nightmares, night terrors, somnambulism (sleepwalking), and somniloquy (sleeptalking) (Clore & Hibel, 1993). Nightmares or bad dreams are extremely common in early childhood, with the peak incidence occurring between 3 and 6 years of age (Leung & Robson, 1993). These dreams occur during the latter period of sleep (REM). There is little motor behavior during the dream. The child is fully awake following the dream, is easily calmed, and usually can recall the content of the dream.

Night terrors are a disorder of arousal that occur during an abrupt transition from Stage 4 NREM sleep to REM sleep (Fox, 1997). This transition time is in the first third of the sleep period. Night terrors have a dramatic, sudden onset. The child may bolt upright from bed, may scream or yell incoherently, or may cry inconsolably. During a night terror episode, the child may have tachycardia, tachypnea, and diaphoresis. The child does not remember the event.

Somnambulism or sleepwalking is a partial arousal disorder of Stage 4 NREM sleep. It peaks in adolescence and declines rapidly by the late teens (Horne, 1992). In a sleepwalking episode, the child may sit up quietly, get out of bed, and move about in a confused and clumsy manner. While sleepwalking, the child is not appropriately responsive to others and may become agitated if attempts are made to interact with him or her. If aroused from the episode, the child may be confused. If informed of his or her behavior the following morning, the child will not remember the event.

Somniloquy or sleeptalking is not specific to either NREM or REM sleep. Sleeptalking can occur during a nightmare. It may be of concern to parents but is of no clinical significance (Adair & Bauchner, 1993). In one study, one half of the sleepwalking children talked in their sleep for 1 year or more before the onset of sleepwalking (Klackenberg, 1987). Sleep disturbance has also been associated with many chronic diseases and conditions. Sleep loss can be a result of early termination of sleep, awakening after sleep onset, or overall decreased quality associated with changes in time spent in various sleep stages. Likely causes of sleep disturbance in chronic illness include performance of treatment and medication regimens, pain, anxiety, fear, symptoms exacerbation, or side effects of medications and treatments. Family reaction to the diagnosis of a chronic condition (parental anxiety, strained family relationships, and overprotectiveness or overpermissiveness) can contribute to poor sleep habits.

Any condition necessitating hospitalization presents many stimuli that can adversely affect sleep, as does the hospitalization. The most frequent sleep disturbances that result from hospitalization are classified as extrinsic sleep disorders, a subclassification of dyssomnias, and include total sleep loss (due to prolonged sleep onset latency, early termination of sleep, and sleep fragmentation) and REM sleep disruption or deprivation. Pain, anxiety, fear, stress, lack of control, separation from parents, an unfamiliar environment, noise, changes in light-dark cycles, disruption of normal routines by staff activities, and use of restraints can contribute to sleep changes (Corser, 1996; Cureton-Lane & Fontaine, 1991; Hagemann, 1981a, 1981b; Slota, 1988). Medications exert differing effects on sleep depending on the action of the medication. Changes in sleep pattern initiated during hospitalization continue after discharge to home (Corser, 1996).

Nurse-Sensitive Outcomes

The goal for nursing is to recognize sleep pattern disturbance and intervene to support the acquisition of sleep to facilitate mental and physical rejuvenation. Accomplishment of this goal is dependent on interventions to enhance sleep and ongoing evaluation of sleep. The Nursing Outcomes Classification's outcome Sleep (Iowa Outcomes Project, 2000) can be used to determine the quality and quantity of sleep and its effects on physical rejuvenation. Outcome indicators most easily evaluated in children are sleep routines, observed hours of uninterrupted sleep, and wakefulness at appropriate times.

INTERVENTION: SLEEP ENHANCEMENT

The Nursing Interventions Classification (NIC) defines *Sleep Enhancement* as "facilitation of regular sleep/wake cycles" (Iowa Intervention Project, 2000, p. 602). Activities to achieve sleep enhancement include determination of the sleep-activity pattern, education, and structuring the environment. Practitioners can work with primary caretakers of the child by setting the stage for normal sleep pattern development at home. It is recommended that discussion of issues of sleep management begin early in the postnatal period (Kerr & Jowett, 1994). A sleep history can determine if a sleep problem exists or if parents simply lack understanding of normal sleep patterns of children (Table 32.2). After parents are taught about normal sleep patterns, they can be given guidance on facilitation of regular sleep-wake cycles and how to manage problems. Facilitation of regular sleep-wake cycles and management of sleep problems is best initiated through prevention.

Anticipatory guidance to parents on facilitation of regular sleep-wake cycles is best addressed for each age group: infants, toddler-preschooler, and school-age child/adolescent. Prevention of sleep disturbance in infants is directed toward infants older than 4 months. In the first 3 or 4 months, diverse sleep patterns are not generally considered sleep problems. For an infant born at term, by 6 months a pattern of night sleeping and day feeding should have developed. Gradual reduction of nighttime feedings can be effective if initiated after approximately 2 weeks (Stores, 1996). Middle-of-the-night feeding after 4 months needs to be discontinued. Parents are encouraged to put the baby to bed drowsy but awake. The baby should not be put to bed with a bottle. If night waking occurs, contacts by the parent need to be reassuring but brief and boring. Parents can avoid stimulation such as changing diapers during the night. Parents should not remove the baby from the crib or bring the baby into the parents' bed in response to night waking. If possible, keeping the crib in the parents' room should be avoided. If living space does not allow separate rooms, the side rails of the crib can be covered with a blanket to minimize environmental stimuli for the infant. Rapid settling and return to sleep after waking are facilitated by previous establishment of comforting conditions. These sleep-onset associations may be objects such as blankets or toys that do not depend on the parents' presence (Stores, 1996). As the infant matures, attention should be given to the number and length of daytime naps. Lengthy daytime naps (more than 2 hours) may need to be shortened or eliminated.

TABLE 32.2   Sleep Behavior Inventory

1. Does (name) have a usual bedtime? If so, what is that bedtime?
2. Who usually puts (name) to bed?
3. In what type of bed does (name) sleep most frequently?
4. Does (name) sleep in a room and bed alone? (If no) Who does (name) sleep with?
5. Has there been a recent change in the room or bed in which (name) sleeps? (If yes) Please describe what has changed.
6. Are there any bedtime routines or rituals that (name) follows? (If yes) Please describe (name)'s bedtime routine.
7. Does (name) sleep with an overhead light, lamp, or night-light on in the room?
8. How long does it usually take for (name) to fall asleep after being put to bed?
9. Does (name) routinely wake up during the night?
   On the nights that he/she wakes up, how many times a night does (name) wake up?
   How long is (name) usually awake when he/she wakes up at night?
   What does (name) act like when he/she wakes up at night?
   What do you have to do to get (name) back to sleep when he/she wakes up at night?
10. Does (name) have a usual time that he/she wakes up in the morning? (If yes) What time does he/she usually wake up?
11. Does (name) still take a nap? (If yes) How many naps a day does (name) take?
    How much time does (name) spend in nap sleep?

Enhancement of sleep or facilitation of regular sleep-wake cycles in children 2 to 5 years old is begun in the infancy period through the establishment of a regular bedtime routine or ritual. Prior to beginning the bedtime routine, which may vary with parental or family values, the child needs a calm-down time. Parents need to create an inviting, comfortable sleep environment. The bedroom should be a place of peace and sleep rather than one for fun and excitement (Horne, 1992). Parents should avoid using the bedroom for time-out. A consistent, firm bedtime should be established. Like the infant, the child should be allowed to self-soothe; the use of comfort or security objects should be encouraged. Parents need to avoid reinforcing bedtime procrastination, such as offering extra drinks or food. Positive reinforcement, such as stickers or stars for staying in bed, may be used. Parents need to be consistent in returning the child to bed gently but firmly. Sympathetic but brief reassurance for nighttime fears should be provided when a child awakens from a nightmare or expresses a fear. Simple explanations of night terrors can be comforting to parents.

Facilitation of regular sleep-wake cycles for older children and adolescents is dependent on keeping regular bed and wake-up times. Like younger children, older children and adolescents need to establish a bedtime routine that includes a quiet time before bed. They should maintain a comfortable sleeping environment with proper temperature, light, and

TABLE 32.3 Sleep Disorders Requiring Referral

Parasomnias

Sleep enuresis: Defined as nocturnal urinary incontinence after 6 years of age. Initial strategies include limiting fluid intake prior to bedtime. Refer to sleep specialist practitioner for evaluation.

Sleep bruxism: Involves clenching, gritting, or grinding of teeth during sleep. Signs include toothwear, misalignment, or c/o temporomandibular joint pain. Stress reduction techniques and referral to a physician or dentist for a tooth guard may be necessary.

Benign neonatal sleep myoclonus: Characterized as asynchronous jerking of limbs and trunk during quiet sleep. An EEG may be required to differentiate it from seizures.

Medical and psychiatric sleep disorders

Obstructive sleep apnea: Repeated 15- to 20-second episodes of apnea terminating in gasps or moans. There is often a history of snoring and mouth breathing during sleep. Complaints of tiredness and daytime fatigue are frequent. It is associated with obesity or enlarged tonsils. Refer to sleep specialist practitioner or sleep center.

Central sleep apnea: Characterized by frequent awakenings with shortness of breath. Repeated 10-second periods of apnea during sleep. It is associated with mild snoring but not obesity or tonsil enlargement. Refer to sleep specialist practitioner or sleep center.

Narcolepsy: Irresistible daytime sleepiness. It may be associated with cataplexy (abrupt loss of muscle tone), hallucinations, or sleep paralysis. It usually manifests in adolescence. Refer to physician or sleep center.

noise level. Watching television, reading, and doing other activities in bed should be avoided. They should get out of bed if they are having difficulty falling asleep. Older children and adolescents having problems getting to sleep also need to avoid daytime naps, caffeine, cigarettes, and heavy meals late at night. They should be encouraged to increase physical exercise, but not just before bedtime (Fox, 1997).

There are several sleep disorders seen in infancy and childhood that may require extensive evaluation and treatment—for example, parasomnias such as sleep enuresis, bruxism, and benign neonatal sleep myclonus and medical sleep disorders, including sleep apnea and narcolepsy. Nursing's role in these situations is the recognition of symptoms and initiation of appropriate referral. Table 32.3 outlines the usual signs and symptoms and indicates the appropriate referral.

Promoting the sleep of children in the hospital setting is a challenging proposition that requires knowledge of normal sleep patterns and habits. It is a process of constantly weighing the sleep needs of the child against the need for nursing intervention to maintain physical integrity. This process must begin with an admission assessment of normal home sleep to determine sleep pattern, sleep rituals, and any preexisting sleep difficulties. The sleep inventory (Table 32.2) provides an initial guide for important data to be acquired. Information gathered should be compared to age-specific norms to identify sleep problems existing prior to hospitalization. These reference norms can be kept in a central location for easy access.

Recognizing that hospitalization is an anxiety-provoking experience, enhancing the sleep of children will be more difficult in the hospital setting and may require additional measures. Sleep-enhancing activities include providing comfort and security measures, manipulating the environment to promote sleep, and organizing nursing care to minimize sleep disruption (Iowa Intervention Project, 2000).

Reinforcement of the child's usual bedtime routines, rituals, or cues will provide security that is lacking in the unfamiliar hospital environment. These rituals usually include activities that can easily be incorporated into the hospital routine. Parental participation in this process can be beneficial for the child and provide parents with a recognized role in their child's care. Bringing familiar objects from home, especially sleep-onset association items, will provide an illusion of consistency. In situations in which parents cannot room-in, they can participate by scheduling visiting times or phone calls to reinforce usual bedtime routines. In other cases, the nurse can serve a key role in perpetuating the bedtime routines. In addition to the usual activities, recorded tapes of stories, massage, affective touch, soft music, and relaxation techniques are of benefit in promoting sleep in more challenging situations (White, Williams, Alexander, Powell-Cope, & Conlon, 1990).

Maintaining an environment to promote sleep in the hospital begins at the point of admission. The child's bed and room should be reserved as a safe area. All painful or anxiety-provoking treatments should be conducted in a treatment room. Observation of these procedures on others (i.e., roommates in semiprivate rooms or other children in open units) is anxiety producing as well. If moving the child is not an option, curtains should be drawn. Content of television viewed at night should also be controlled for younger children. Adjustments in the environment to promote sleep include control of light-dark cycles and noise. The role of day-night cycles in establishing circadian rhythm has been well documented (Ferber, 1987) and can be beneficial in sleep enhancement. A quiet time prior to bed should be arranged. Noise by staff, parents, and others needs to be minimized, and other noise made by telephones, equipment, and televisions should be decreased in volume or eliminated during nighttime hours.

Perhaps the biggest boost to sleep acquisition can be provided by organization of nursing care. Planning should incorporate sleep acquisition as a priority goal. Schedules should be arranged to meet the child's regular sleep-wake cycle. Adjustment of medication administration or procedural schedules may be necessary. If procedures during the nighttime hours cannot be avoided, grouping of care activities while minimizing the number of awakenings and allowing for sleep cycles of at least 90 minutes is recommended. Management of the nurse's work time should account for time needed to assist in sleep rituals for those children whose parents are not present. Anticipate nightmares and frequent awakening and allow time to respond in a comforting, soothing manner.

Ongoing monitoring of the child's sleep in the hospital is required. There are a variety of instruments used to record patient's sleep pattern and number of sleep hours. There are also instruments that solicit patient opinions about the quality of sleep that can be used with older children and adolescents. Signs that indicate loss of sleep (frequent yawning, dark circles under eyes, listlessness, irritability, and disorientation) should be noted in documentation of the nursing assessment and explored. In addition, physical or psychological circumstances or both that interrupt sleep, such as pain, nightmares, anxiety, and need to void or defecate, should be noted. Awakening at night for voiding is associated with intravenous fluid maintenance and the use of certain medication (diuretics), whereas continuous enteral feeds have been associated with awakening due to abdominal discomfort (Holden, Puntis, Charlton, & Booth, 1991). Review the medication history and determine what effects (if any) medications can have on sleep pattern (Nicholson, Bradley, & Pascoe, 1989). Effects of common medications on sleep are listed in Table 32.4. If indicated, encourage the selection of sleep medications such as chloral hydrate that do not contain REM sleep suppressors.

Organization of care should also allow time for daytime sleeping. Approximating the time and routines associated with daytime napping in younger children will facilitate transition into sleep during the day. Daytime sleep in older children and adolescents can help to offset sleep loss but must be controlled to prevent interference with night sleep. Establishing a quiet time when lights are dimmed will promote rest and sleep during these times.

INTERVENTION APPLICATION

Michelle Carter is a 35-month-old white female admitted to the hospital for resection of a spinal tumor. Her past medical history was significant only for periodic episodes of wheezing treated with Ventolin. A sleep history taken on admission to the hospital revealed that Michelle slept 8 hours each night without awakening and took a daily 2-hour nap. The major problem reported by the mother was that despite being put to bed, Michelle would postpone bedtime, resist sleep, and get out of bed repeatedly until she fell asleep approximately 3 hours later. The mother had talked to several friends who told her she would just have to let Michelle "cry it out." Her response was, "I just can't do that! She may really need

TABLE 32.4 Medication Effects on Sleep

Medication	Total Sleep Time	Sleep Onset Latency	REM Sleep	REM Sleep Latency	Subjective Changes	NREM Sleep			
						Stage 1	Stage 2	Stage 3	Stage 4
Antidepressants			↓	↑					
Anticonvulsants									
Ethosuximide			↓			↑		↓	↓
Valproic acid								↑	↑
Phenytoin	↑ᵃ		↓						↑
Analgesics									
Nonopioid							↑	↓	↓
Opioid	↑		↑				↓		
Antiemetics									
Anticholinergics			↓	↑			↑		
Dopamine antagonists					1				
Antihistamines		↓	↓	↑			↑		↓
Barbiturates		↓	↓	↑		↓		↓	↓
Benzodiazepines	↑	↓		↑			↑	↑	↑
H₂ antagonists									
Xanthines	↓				2	↑	↑	↓	↓

NOTE: ↑, increase; ↓, decrease; 1, drowsiness; 2, reduced quality

ᵃ At initiation

533

me like with her wheezing and all. She always seems to have these attacks at night." On the basis of this information, a diagnosis of Sleep Pattern Disturbance would be appropriate.

After surgery, Michelle was admitted to the pediatric intensive care unit (PICU) for a 2-day recovery during which she was treated with antibiotics, steroids, H_2 antagonists, Versed, and morphine. During her stay in the PICU, Michelle averaged 5 hours of sleep each day, with the longest sleep time being 155 minutes. No REM sleep was observed during the PICU stay. She was transferred to the general pediatric unit and then discharged to home after a total hospital stay of 5 days. Upon return home, Michelle maintained the sleep pattern she had established in the hospital, falling asleep shortly after midnight and waking two or three times nightly. She slept more hours by sleeping later in the morning than she had prior to hospitalization. After talking with the nurse at her pediatrician's office, Michelle's mother began to provide calm reassurance during night awakenings, which resolved approximately 1 week after discharge. At the same time, Michelle reverted to her prehospitalization sleep pattern of bedtime resistance. Again, the mother consulted the pediatrician's office, and with guidance and support of the nurse she established bedtime routines and reinforced staying in bed rather than procrastinating behaviors. She started bedtime rituals approximately 15 minutes prior to Michelle's usual bedtime of midnight and gradually moved the bedtime to approximately 9:00 p.m. Despite the setback of a "wheezing" attack that necessitated treatment with Ventolin and antibiotics 10 days after discharge, Ms. Carter continued enforcement of firm limits and positive reinforcement of good sleep patterns. The nursing outcome Sleep could be used to evaluate the effectiveness of interventions used to promote a normal sleep for Michelle (Iowa Outcomes Project, 2000). By 6 weeks after discharge, Michelle had achieved a more age-appropriate sleep pattern.

RESEARCH AND PRACTICE IMPLICATIONS

Assessment of sleep patterns should be an integral part of each well child visit from birth to adolescence. Anticipatory guidance given to parents can prevent poor sleep practices and foster achievement of sleep development milestones. Cultural sleep practices can also mold developing sleep patterns. Although some sleep routines and patterns can be associated with specific cultures (cosleeping and delayed disappearance of daytime sleep), little work has been done to identify the more subtle ways in which culture influences sleep pattern development. Nurse-sensitive outcomes for child development need to be expanded to reflect the achievement of sleep milestones for each age. Continued research in defining sleep problems and testing new measurement techniques for use with children is needed to expand the knowledge available to nurses. Recognition of decreased daytime alertness experienced by adolescents raises questions about the possible role that sleep loss plays in accidental injury in this age group. Injury prevention investigators need to further explore this area.

Sleep disturbance treatments are incorporating behavioral approaches that recognize circadian rhythm. Although many current interventions are theoretically sound, they frequently offer conflicting management strategies. Multidisciplinary research can evaluate the effectiveness of various management strategies. These approaches are not "quick fixes," and parents will need support and reinforcement to progress over time. Knowledge of sleep progression and the stimuli that affect sleep in the hospital should be reflected in unit design, policy development, and care planning. Additional development and testing of interventions to promote sleep in hospital settings needs to occur. Recent confirmation that sleep disturbance continues after hospitalization should dictate education for parents regarding the sleep changes they can anticipate and strategies to facilitate return to a normal sleep pattern for their child. If existing sleep enhancement strategies are not successful, additional study to develop strategies to normalize sleep in chronic illness and after hospitalization should be undertaken.

REFERENCES

Adair, R. H., & Bauchner, H. (1993). Sleep problems in childhood. *Current Problems in Pediatrics, 23*(4), 147-170.

Akerstdt, T., Palmblad, J., de la Torre, B., Mkarana, R., & Gillberg, M. (1980). Adrenocortical and gonadal steroids during sleep deprivation. *Sleep, 3,* 23-30.

American Sleep Disorders Association. (1990). *International classification of sleep disorders: Diagnostic and coding manual.* Lawrence, KS: Allen Press.

Brazelton, T. B. (1994). Behavioral competence. In G. B. Avery, M. A. Fletcher, & M. G. MacDonald (Eds.), *Neonatology: Pathophysiology and management of the newborn* (4th ed., pp. 289-300). Philadelphia: J. B. Lippincott.

Carskadon, M. A., Vieira, C., & Acebo, C. (1993). Association between puberty and delayed phase preference. *Sleep, 16*(3), 258-262.

Clore, E. R., & Hibel, J. (1993). The parasomnias of childhood. *Journal of Pediatric Health Care, 7,* 12-16.

Corser, N. (1996). Sleep of 1- and 2-year-old children in intensive care. *Issues in Comprehensive Pediatric Nursing, 19,* 17-31.

Cureton-Lane, R. A., & Fontaine, D. (1991). *Sleep in the pediatric intensive care unit.* Unpublished master's thesis, University of Maryland, Baltimore.

Edgil, A. E., Wood, K. L., & Smith, D. P. (1985). Sleep problems of older infants and preschool children. *Pediatric Nursing, 11,* 87-89.

33

Lifestyle Modification

Nutrition Promotion

Julie L. Ritland

The prevalence of obesity in children in the United States is escalating despite society's quest for increased health and wellness. Approximately 27% of children and 21% of adolescents are characterized as overweight. This is an increase of 54% and 39%, respectively, from 1970s statistics (Burns, Barber, Brady, & Dunn, 1996). Obesity among children aged 6 to 11 years has shown an increase of 54% when compared with data collected between 1966 and 1970 (Strong et al., 1992). Both physical and psychological risks are associated with obesity. Physical risks include cardiovascular disease, diabetes, hypertension, premature joint destruction, cholecysitis, and premature death (Greydanus & Pratt, 1995). Psychological risks include decreased self-esteem, depression, and impaired social interaction.

Nutrition is a priority area in the objectives set forth in *Healthy People 2000* (U.S. Department of Health and Human Services [USDHHS], 1991). Interventions that would decrease the number of obese children and adolescents could have far-reaching effects and increased health benefits even decades later. There are several goals stated in *Healthy People 2000* pertaining to nutrition. Baseline data from 1976 to 1980 show that the American diet has 36% of its caloric intake derived from fat. It is recommended this be reduced to 30%. Objective 2.7 of the guidelines states the goal to "increase to at least 50% the proportion of overweight people age 12 and older who have adopted sound dietary practices combined with regular physical activity to attain an appropriate body weight" (p. 93). The baseline data collected in 1985 report that 30% of women and 25% of men older than age 18 are overweight. Objective 1.2 identifies the need to "reduce overweight to a prevalence of no more than 20% among people aged 20 and older and no more than 15% among adolescents aged 12 through 19" (p. 91). The nation is clearly moving in the wrong direction because the progress chart indicates an increase of 8% in overweight people. Despite the negative trend shown, the goal still targets a 6% decrease in the baseline (USDHHS, 1995).

LITERATURE REVIEW

The nutritional aspect of weight control for young people needs to be addressed from a different perspective than that of adults. Anticipating a rapid and significant weight loss in a child is unrealistic and could present serious health problems. Careful attention to nutrition is imperative during the rapid growth periods of childhood. Emphasizing dietary moderation rather than restriction is key to ensuring the success of the promotion of healthy eating habits. Food should not be used as a reward or as a comfort measure for adverse situations. In educating young people about portion control, second helpings should be discouraged, as should unhealthy, high-calorie snack foods. Realistic expectations also need to be considered when targeting adolescents. Awareness of body shape and the role played by genetics in general size are important factors (Strong et al., 1992). Adolescents can be guided to more realistic expectations and achievable goals for their body structure when they are taught to consider their inherited characteristics.

A major concern regarding childhood obesity is the severe long-term effects on general health. An adolescent who continues to be overweight will eventually be at increased risk for physical health problems and mortality due to heart disease, stroke, and diabetes (Johnson, 1990). The weight-loss benefits of proper nutrition can be enhanced by an increase in moderate to vigorous physical activity. The Youth Risk Behavior Survey of 1990 validates the importance of physical activity and exercise during childhood as an indicator of exercise patterns in adulthood (Dennison, Straus, Mellits, & Charney, 1988). Childhood is the time when the risk factors associated with cardiovascular disease are known to become established. Physical inactivity in adolescents has also been linked to increased levels of blood lipids and cholesterol, increased blood pressure, and increased anxiety and depression (Strong et al., 1992). A sedentary lifestyle appears to be an independent risk factor for coronary heart disease, nearly doubling a person's risk (Powell, Thompson, Caspersen, & Kendrick, 1987). This information, although not motivating to a child or adolescent, may provide an incentive to parents when considering diet and exercise programs available to their children.

Two major surveys of physical activity behavior in American children have been made since the mid-1980s—the National Children and Youth Fitness Study and the Youth Risk Behavior Survey (Pate, 1993). These studies attempted to examine an array of health behaviors in children between the ages of 10 and 17 years. Normal childhood activities provide the opportunity for most youngsters to maintain a reasonably active lifestyle; there remains a segment of the population, however, that does not engage in an appropriate amount of physical activity on a regular basis. In addition, the correlation between physical activity and adiposity is significant from a statistical perspective (Pate, 1993; see Chapter 34, this volume).

Although parental encouragement and participation are important factors in the involvement of young people in physical activity, this type of support is not reaching enough youth. Parents as role models in establishing healthy nutrition and exercise patterns for children have not been very successful due to the parents' lack of participation in these lifestyle behaviors. It is estimated that 51% of adults are sedentary, and only 15% participate in activities that are strenuous enough to produce any significant health benefits (Bonheur & Young, 1991). Both the individual and the community should be a concern when discussing strategies for health promotion. Risk factor reduction in a set of individuals will in fact result in health benefits. Although the lifestyle changes by individuals are subjective and unique, community health officials should try to make the public aware of the difficulties and misfortunes that can be avoided by healthier lifestyle choices (Greydanus & Pratt, 1995).

The schools and community should be used to support parental guidance in the areas of nutrition and exercise as they relate to the problem of obesity. The community could sponsor health promotion programs, and schools could provide educational curricula that would encourage good nutrition practices. Teaching children about healthy eating habits can be easily incorporated into the existing school curriculum as demonstrated by a study sponsored by the National Heart, Lung, and Blood Institute. Participants in the 3-year project were elementary students from California, Louisiana, Minnesota, and Texas. The children in the study were taught which foods were lower in fat, especially saturated fat, and were encouraged to combine moderate to vigorous exercise with their new eating habits. Teachers and food service personnel needed minimal training to implement the program. A reduction of fat intake to 30.3% from 32.7% was the result of classroom lessons, food games, educating parents about healthy food choices, and offering school lunches that were lower in fat content (Luepker et al., 1996). The use of similar interventions may enhance the possibility that children could acquire the knowledge and the chance to practice healthy lifestyle decision-making skills and help the United States meet its goals.

A supportive social environment is of utmost importance in changing the behaviors that contribute to many of today's leading health threats (USDHHS, 1991). Unfortunately, evidence suggests this supportive environment does not always exist for those suffering from obesity. Obese children, and their adult counterparts, suffer intense discrimination and increased self-consciousness. It is important that families are aware of the psychological ramifications of obesity because it is during the adolescent years that the negative body image that has been slowly developing throughout childhood is internalized (Bandini & Dietz, 1992). Cruel teasing by schoolmates, snide remarks from unthinking adults, and criticism from parents will eventually take their toll on the child's self-esteem.

Several factors may contribute to adiposity, including genetic predisposition and environmental and lifestyle factors. These, however, may be beyond the control of a health care provider. The perception that obesity in children automatically leads to obesity in adulthood suggests that nothing can be done to alter this progression. In theory, this would justify the absence of interventions that help to prevent or to treat the problem of adolescent obesity. Rather than dismiss the problem as an inevitable conclusion to a potentially unhealthy situation, studies suggest that as a nation we should be aware of the subtle trend toward a more overweight and less active youth population. The past two or three decades have provided evidence of an increasing number of overweight children. Fewer children find it necessary to walk to school, and television is often the playmate of choice. Technology has provided an array of computer games that foster more sedentary playtime activities. In addition, physical education classes that once ensured some form of strenuous activity now offer choices for class requirements that, although beneficial, often do not require vigorous physical exertion. Also, fewer physical education classes are being required than in previous years. At some high schools, physical education classes can be eliminated entirely in favor of a full schedule of academic classes.

The need for increased emphasis on childhood physical activity is supported by recent statistics gathered through the National Children and Youth Fitness Survey. In 1984, statistics showed that 61.7% of students participated in vigorous physical activity three or more times per week (Ross, Dotson, & Gilbert, 1985). The statistics from 1990 show a decline to 37% engaging in vigorous activity (Heath, Pratt, Warren, & Kann, 1994). This century has seen many advances in methods of transportation and energy-saving work products and a change in leisure-time activities that have contributed to a decrease in energy output. This decrease in physical activity is a fairly recent phenomenon for most Americans. This generation has also seen a dramatic increase in working mothers. Fast-food meals, which are high in fat, sodium, and calories, have become an occasional necessity in a busy parent's schedule. Television advertisements, a source of information for children concerning food products, primarily promote sugar-filled foods or other salty snacks that are high in fat content and tend to counteract the benefits of regular exercise activities (Perry et al., 1990). The health benefits of a physically active lifestyle of children were evaluated and included weight control, an improved cardiovascular outlook for adulthood, an increased sense of psychological well-being, and a better chance of maintaining a physically active lifestyle into adulthood. Other benefits from participation in sports and physical activity are associated with positive social values, which include interpersonal skills, diffusion of tension, and improved high school performance (Strong et al., 1992).

NURSING DIAGNOSES AND OUTCOME DETERMINATION

Several nursing diagnoses are pertinent to overweight children and adolescents. The primary nursing diagnoses are Altered Nutrition: More Than Body Requirements and Altered Nutrition: Risk for More Than Body Requirements. Pertinent defining characteristics that could be identified in potential candidates for a lifestyle modification program include an accelerated growth pattern that surpasses the normal rate from one growth percentile to the next, a family pattern of obesity that can be observed in one or both parents, evidence of food being used in an inappropriate manner such as a reward or comfort, improper nutritional patterns, associating food with various activities, and the consumption of food in response to improper external and internal cues (North American Nursing Diagnosis Association [NANDA], 1999).

A third nursing diagnosis that may be identified is Body Image Disturbance (NANDA, 1999). Two factors that may be observed to aid in validating this diagnosis are a substantial increase in weight and a change in social activities. The child or adolescent may also verbalize a fear of rejection by others or a negative feeling about appearance, or he or she express a desire to be more like he or she was in the past. These observed or reported behaviors will substantiate the diagnosis.

The fourth diagnosis is Self-Esteem Disturbance. Some of the defining characteristics include self-deprecating behaviors, feeling ashamed, resistance to new activities, the inability to recognize the problem, rationalization of failures, and overreaction to suggestions or criticism from others (NANDA, 1999). A more general nursing diagnosis is Knowledge Deficit. Examples of Knowledge Deficit include nutritional food choices, portion control, fat content, and basic nutrition principles. Ironically, an additional diagnosis that could be a concern is Altered Nutrition: Less Than Body Requirements (NANDA, 1999). Obese children and adolescents may be consuming a large number of calories without fulfilling the proper nutrition needed for growth.

When evaluating the effectiveness of nutrition modification programs, the following nurse-sensitive outcomes should be considered. The first outcome to be observed may be *Health-Seeking Behavior,* defined as "actions to promote optimal wellness, recovery, and rehabilitation" (Iowa Outcomes Project, 2000, p. 233). *Health-Promoting Behavior,* "actions to sustain or increase wellness," is another outcome to be considered (p. 232). These would be demonstrated by the client's concern and involvement in promoting sound nutritional habits based on self-evaluation. The next nurse-sensitive outcome that could be used is *Knowledge: Health Behaviors,* defined as the "extent of understanding conveyed about the promotion and protection of health" (p. 268). Indications of increased knowledge include being able to describe proper nutritional habits and the benefits that result from balancing diet with activity and exercise. The extent of the client's comprehension of sound nutritional practices could be measured with a self-appraisal and physiological measurements.

Three additional outcomes pertaining directly to nutrition have been developed: (a) *Nutritional Status,* which is the "extent to which nutrients are available to meet metabolic needs" (Iowa Outcomes Project, 2000, p. 319); (b) *Nutritional Status: Nutrient Intake,* defined as "adequacy of nutrients taken into the body" (p. 324); and (c) *Nutrition Status: Body Mass,* which is the "congruence of body weight, muscle, and fat to height, frame, and gender" (p. 321). Indicators of the nutritional status outcomes include concrete measurements of intake, body mass, and biochemical measurements. Specific indicators of nutritional status include nutrient intake, energy, and weight. Specific biochemical measures include serum albumin, hematocrit, cholesterol, and glucose. Indicators for body mass include triceps and subscapular skinfold thickness, body fat percentage, and height and weight percentages.

Two psychosocial outcomes have also been developed to assist in the evaluation of the client's self-perception: Body Image and Self-Esteem (Iowa Outcomes Project, 2000). Body image indicators that may be reported by the client include satisfaction with body appearance and a willingness to use the new-found skills to improve body function. A validation of increased self-esteem may be observed through the client's increase in self-acceptance, confidence, and pride. Although significant changes in these areas may not be readily observed, they remain an integral part of the client's successful lifestyle modification.

INTERVENTION:
LIFESTYLE MODIFICATION: NUTRITION PROMOTION

The Nursing Interventions Classification (NIC) (Iowa Intervention Project, 2000) has four interventions related to nutrition, nutrition management, therapy, counseling, and monitoring. These interventions focus more on patients with specific illnesses requiring special diets or patients who are at risk for malnutrition. Nutrition Counseling is most helpful when working with adults. When working with children, however, it is important to tailor activities to their developmental level, personal goals, and family values. It is also important to instill positive values and develop new skills and behaviors early in life as well as involve families in this planning. Therefore, a new intervention, Lifestyle Modification: Nutrition Promotion, was developed to target this unique population. *Lifestyle Modification: Nutrition Promotion* is defined as encouraging the ability to evaluate and improve nutritional choices (Table 33.1). As the benefits of a nutritionally sound lifestyle are assessed, the outlook for substantial health gains for our children and adolescents is evident. The longer children remain overweight, the more likely they are to carry this burden into adulthood. Although prevention of obesity would be ideal, the need for intervention is clearly indicated by the increasing segment of the population that is overweight.Although there is still debate regarding some dietary recommendations, during the 1980s two comprehensive studies on the relationship among dietary factors, health, and disease drew similar conclusions. The Surgeon General's *Report on Nutrition and Health* and the Food and Nutrition Board's report, *Diet and Health,* suggested similar changes in the nation's diet to reduce the risk of coronary heart disease, several cancers, hypertension, chronic liver disease, and obesity. These changes include limiting foods high in fat content, limiting refined sugars and alcohol, and including more fish, poultry, grains, vegetables, and fruits. Recognizing that diet and nutrition are linked to 6 of the 10 leading

TABLE 33.1   Lifestyle Modification: Nutrition Promotion

Definition

Nutrition Promotion is defined as encouraging the ability to evaluate and improve nutritional choices.

Activities

  Assist client in setting realistic short- and long-term goals for nutrition.

  Teach client about Food Pyramid and dietary guidelines.

  Assist client in creating a climate that will optimize success in reaching goals.

  Encourage client to keep food diary to document food consumption to be used for analysis and teaching about nutrition and meal planning.

  Determine non–food-related rewards with client for adhering to nutrition program.

  Encourage limiting foods high in fat, refined sugars, and alcohol.

  Instruct client in reading food labels.

  Promote informed decision making regarding food choices.

  Teach client ideal balance between caloric intake and energy output.

  Instruct on proper portion size using pictures, models, and videotapes.

  Encourage inclusion of more fruits, vegetables, grains, fish, and poultry in diet.

  Provide activities to assist in meal planning.

  Provide experiences that demonstrate newly acquired skills (e.g., grocery shopping and meal planning and preparation).

---

causes of death in the United States has forced consumers to be aware of the labeling of food products and the challenge of implementing the new dietary guidelines for their families (Palmer, 1990).

The process of Lifestyle Modification: Nutrition Promotion can be taught at any age using the following activities as guides to learning (Table 33.1). One of the first activities should include goal setting. Short-term goals that are easily attainable can be an incentive to clients to persevere toward more difficult, long-term goals. The client should be counseled to set realistic goals, and expectations concerning progress should be monitored to reduce discouragement. Rewards for reaching short-term and long-term goals are a motivating part of a nutritional plan. The rewards should be determined by the client and should not be food related. Examples of rewards include movie passes, items of clothing, tickets to plays or sport activities, inexpensive jewelry, compact disks, books, or anything else of value to the client. The value of the reward should be commensurate with the magnitude of the goal attained.

Creating a climate in which clients can succeed will help them to achieve their goals. Although levels of motivation vary, everyone wants to be recognized and successful. Moving from the comfort and security of old behaviors takes drive, energy, and support of family, friends, and peers. An anticipated reward or payoff is a positive reinforcement for accomplishment. Each client may have his or her own perception of success, but nurses can help create a climate in which clients choose to perform at high levels (Lancaster, 1985).

The Food Guide Pyramid is an ideal tool to begin helping children and adolescents make informed food choices. The Food Guide Pyramid, prepared by the United States Department of Agriculture and the United States Department of Health and Human Services, identifies the various food categories and suggests the number of servings needed from each group to achieve a healthy balanced diet. The concepts concerning dietary guidelines are basic and could even be incorporated into a preschool curriculum. The shape of the pyramid suggests the number of servings that should come from each food category and encourages moderate inclusion of fats and sugars in a healthy food plan.

Keeping food diaries is an excellent activity to encourage awareness of current eating habits. The client is asked to record all foods and beverages consumed during a specified time period that could be as brief as 24 hours. Clients are then asked to compare what they have eaten to the suggested items in the Food Guide Pyramid and to analyze the results. Through this analysis of the types of food consumed during the specified period, it becomes clear which categories are being ignored and which are being indulged. Again, this activity could be modified so that it will be appropriate for all age groups, and the length of the diary could be adjusted accordingly.

Appropriate portion sizes are often misunderstood. Advertising leads the public to believe that bigger is often better. Hands-on activities could involve arranging plastic food likenesses on serving plates, holding and measuring a medium-sized apple or orange, measuring out a proper portion of pasta, or pouring a four-ounce serving of orange juice. This helps to reinforce portion control and to eliminate misconceptions about portion size. Actively involving clients in hands-on activities helps them to comprehend and retain new information. Pictures, models, and videotapes will enhance memory and help clients recall correct portions (London, 1995). These types of activities can also be the "fun" part of a nutrition program. Actual food preparation is enjoyable and informative for clients. Meal planning offers the opportunity to put new knowledge into practice. Shopping for the food items can also be a learning tool. Grocery store scavenger hunts in which clients locate specific food items are an interesting activity appropriate for older children and adolescents.

Fast food has become commonplace in today's society; therefore, it is unrealistic to expect adolescents to completely eliminate it from their diets. The private sector has made some effort to comply with dietary guidelines and has responded by producing low-salt, low-fat food and wholegrain cereal products. A trend toward production of leaner meats has also been noted. In addition, many restaurants and fast-food establishments have begun to offer diet menus (Palmer, 1990). Examining the nutrition pamphlets that are available in these establishments can help guide clients to the best food choices. Low-fat items are becoming more readily available at such establishments, and an adolescent can be taught to be selective about food choices while still enjoying the social interaction with peers.

Analyzing the fat content of foods is a helpful exercise in determining which foods are most healthful. Reading food labels to count fat grams and comparing the fat content of various foods, such as vegetables, fruits, meats, and snacks such as potato chips and ice cream, clearly demonstrates to children and adolescents how to make healthy choices. In addition to fat content, it is also important to study the other information provided on food labels. Cholesterol, sodium, carbohydrates, protein, vitamin, and mineral information is routinely provided on the standardized food label and is imperative to sound nutrition. These activities combined with portion control give clients a more realistic idea of the amounts of each type of food they should be selecting.

Developing smart snacking ideas can also be useful given that mid-morning, after-school, and bedtime snacks are popular with children and adolescents. Providing low-fat, healthful alternatives to calorie-laden snacks, such as cookies, chips, and soda, can be helpful in evaluating and improving nutritional choices. Smart snacking would include fruit, low-fat yogurt, pretzels, unbuttered popcorn, or almost any raw vegetable. This also provides an opportunity to introduce new and unusual foods. Learning to prepare healthy snacks ahead of time, making them readily available, will increase the likelihood that a child or adolescent will make the more healthful choice. Knowing which food choices are healthy, however, does not imply that these healthy choices will always be made. Because human beings usually make the easiest choices available to them, it is important for healthful choices to be readily and easily available (Milio, 1976).

An important underlying concept in these activities is the maintenance of a proper energy balance. Children and adolescents need to understand the relationship between caloric intake and expenditure. Knowledge of the importance of exercise can be incorporated into the curriculum while studying energy balance. The different types of exercise, such as aerobic and anaerobic, can be explained. It is useful to compute the calorie expenditure that occurs during normal daily routines, such as walking to school, mowing the lawn, or completing various household chores. It is also effective to compare the expenditure of walking versus running or jogging or to emphasize the time needed to expend the calories from several high-fat snacks. Obesity in an otherwise healthy child is not a reason to omit exercise from his or her daily routine. Being overweight does not automatically indicate abnormal fitness or impaired cardiorespiratory response to exercise. Many obese children have normal fitness for their developmental stage, but care should be taken to identify those who may have more serious cardiac or pulmonary impairment (Cooper, Poage, Barstow, & Springer, 1990).

Exploring the pitfalls of fad dieting may be very beneficial, especially for adolescents. Fad diets often make exaggerated claims for weight loss. They usually limit food choices and may be nutritionally unbalanced. The monotony of this type of diet often leads to an on-again, off-again syndrome in which weight is lost only to be regained. These diets are discouraging to the dieter and most often neglect the good nutrition habits that nutrition modification programs are trying to instill. The unrealistic promises and the health risks involved make fad diets a poor choice for adolescents (Hans & Nelson, 1986). Problems relating to eating disorders, such as anorexia nervosa and bulimia, are also concerns for adolescents. Discussing these problems provides an opportunity to emphasize the link between good health and nutrition.

An effort has to be made to maintain client participation in the ongoing nutritional changes. A supportive relationship with the client's family will be very beneficial. The client may include family members in the learning process by reviewing, organizing, and verbalizing the information to them. This also gives the nurse an opportunity to assess the client's understanding of the nutritional process and identify any needed adjustments that can be made to his or her interpretation of the information (London, 1995). Studies have shown that long-term success in helping overweight children control their weight is more prevalent when parental involvement and family-based intervention are encouraged (Strong et al., 1992). If direct parental involvement is not possible, communication through newsletters or conferences is an appropriate means to facilitate parental commitment. When educating children, it must be remembered that they are not typically responsible for meal preparation or grocery shopping. Parents must help by purchasing and preparing the kinds of food choices that are recommended and by providing long-term support and role modeling.

INTERVENTION APPLICATION

During a routine health screening at a middle school in a midsized, midwestern community, children who had a higher than indicated by the ideal body mass index were identified. These adolescents with a nursing diagnosis of Altered Nutrition: More Than Body Requirements were invited to participate in a free summer nutrition promotion program. Letters were written to parents to notify them of their child's eligibility for the program.

Parents who were interested in having their child participate were required to sign consent forms and received additional information about the program. The participants met two mornings a week for an 8-week summer session. Pretests for dietary habits and physiological measurements were obtained at the initial session, and posttests were conducted at the final session. The program's curriculum consisted of nutrition promotion activities along with exercise and recreation.

Megan, a 12-year-old seventh grader, was a regular participant in the program. Several of the beginning sessions were devoted to the introduction of the food pyramid and its importance in planning daily food intake. Megan kept a dietary diary and compared her meals to the recommendations of the food pyramid. Through simulated meal planning and the use of food modeling, she learned portion control. This was also emphasized by measuring out servings of snacks such as pretzels and grapes. Making fruit kabobs was a time-consuming activity in which the preparation and anticipation of the finished product were as enjoyable for the participants as eating their creations. A session on label reading was beneficial even at the intermediate level. The measures of fat grams, calories, proteins, and vitamins in different foods helped to emphasize the validity of the Food Pyramid. A test tube demonstration comparing the fat content of many fast-food sandwiches was done by filling different test tubes with the appropriate amount of shortening to represent the fat grams. In a session on energy balance, the number of calories burned by various exercise activities was also explored. Any activities that are enjoyed by the child and are considered play rather than exercise are most beneficial. The exercise activities that were used most frequently were walking, bicycling, volleyball, and basketball.

At the beginning of the program, Megan's dietary habits included 2% milk, 7 to 10 regular sodas per week, fried foods more than three times per week, processed meats such as hot dogs and bologna, and unregulated sweet treats such as candy bars and snack cakes. At the culmination of the program, Megan reported in her log that she had switched to 1% milk, was substituting leaner meats for hot dogs and luncheon meat, and had discussed with her family the benefits of using cooking techniques other than frying. These healthy nutritional changes, in addition to an increase in physical activity, resulted in a 6-pound weight loss during the 8-week period. In addition to learning and practicing sound dietary habits, Megan enjoyed the socialization associated with the program. Megan's parents, especially her father, were very pleased with her progress and expressed an interest in the continuation of the program. Megan's reaction to the program was very positive, and she was proud of her newly acquired knowledge and nutritional practices. The Nursing Outcomes Classification outcomes Nutrition Status, Nutrition Status: Body Mass, Knowledge: Health Behaviors, and Health Promoting Behavior all contain indicators that target knowledge and behaviors that would be appropriate to measure as baseline and terminal behaviors of the program described in this case study (Iowa Outcomes Project, 2000).

RESEARCH AND PRACTICE IMPLICATIONS

The link between dietary practices learned at a young age and those carried into adulthood is clearly established. The effort by parents to educate children about nutrition principles and the importance of daily physical activity needs to be reinforced by school and child care center personnel. Good nutrition should be clearly evident in lunch programs provided by schools and day care centers, and appropriate exercise and activities should also be included in the curriculum. Schools play a major role in promoting and maintaining good health in the 48 million children in the United States. Through this education, children will be able to learn about their bodies, the health effects of specific behaviors, and how to choose the appropriate activities to maintain a healthy lifestyle (USDHHS, 1995).

Health promotion is undoubtedly a major focus for nursing intervention. With the incorporation of healthy eating and exercise and recreation promotion into one program, it is anticipated that the participants will exit with increased knowledge and a more positive attitude toward these two health-promoting behaviors. By planning and implementing programs such as this, nurses will eventually be able to fine-tune curriculum into a combination of what clients want and what is needed. Bonheur and Young (1991) noted, "Nurses can help clients choose a more healthy lifestyle by designing strategies to change the client's relative perceptions of barriers to and benefits of exercise" (p. 6). With the development of a solid research base, nursing can provide statistics to support the funding and implementation of various nutritional- and exercise-based programs for America's children and adolescents.

Health care reform and financial restraints have shifted the focus of health care delivery in the United States. High-technology, hospital-based care provided by health professionals who have become increasingly more specialized will be compelled to give way to preventive, community-focused care (Nugent & Lambert, 1996). Health care will become more concerned with prevention of disease rather than high-priced treatment of illnesses. Continuing to educate the public about proper nutrition to ensure early interventions with certain preventable medical problems will prove to be prudent. The emphasis on education and prevention will prove to be very cost-effective when compared to the extreme economic impact associated with treatment of diseases such as hypertension, diabetes, and cardiovascular disease, which are currently associated with poor nutrition. The nursing intervention Nutrition Promotion: Lifestyle Modification is a proactive response to society's increasing health care needs and will help health care providers promote and encourage healthy living.

REFERENCES

Bandini, L. G., & Dietz, W. H. (1992). Myths about childhood obesity. *Pediatric Annals, 21*(10), 647-652.

Bonheur, B., & Young, S. W. (1991). Exercise as a health-promoting lifestyle choice. *Applied Nursing Research, 4*, 2-6.

Burns, C. E., Barber, N., Brady, M. A., & Dunn, A. M. (1996). *Pediatric primary care: A handbook for nurse practitioners.* Philadelphia: W. B. Saunders.

Cooper, D. M., Poage, J., Barstow, T. J., & Springer, C. (1990). Are obese children truly unfit? Minimizing the confounding effect of body size on the exercise response. *Journal of Pediatrics, 116*(2), 223-230.

Dennison, B. A., Straus, J. H., Mellits, E. D., & Charney, E. (1988). Childhood physical fitness tests: Predictor of adult physical activity levels? *Pediatrics, 82*(3), 324-330.

Greydanus, D. E., & Pratt, H. D. (1995). *Adolescence: A continuum from childhood to adulthood* (3rd ed.). Des Moines: Iowa Department of Public Health.

Hans, C., & Nelson, D. (1986). *What you should know about fad diets.* Ames: Iowa State University, Cooperative Extension Service.

Heath, G. W., Pratt, M., Warren, C. W., & Kann, L. (1994). Physical activity patterns in American high school students: Results from the 1990 Youth Risk Behavior Survey. *Archives of Pediatric & Adolescent Medicine, 148*(11), 1131-1136.

Iowa Intervention Project. (2000). *Nursing interventions classification (NIC)* (J. C. McCloskey & G. M. Bulechek, Eds.; 3rd ed.). St. Louis, MO: Mosby-Year Book.

Iowa Outcomes Project. (2000). *Nursing outcomes classification (NOC)* (M. Johnson, S. Moorhead, & M. Maas, Eds.; 2nd ed.). St. Louis, MO: Mosby-Year Book.

Johnson, E. H. (1990). Interrelationships between psychological factors, overweight, and blood pressure in adolescents. *Journal of Adolescent Health Care, 11*(4), 310-318.

Lancaster, J. (1985). Creating a climate for excellence. *Journal of Nursing Administration, 15*, 16-19.

London, F. (1995). Teach your patients faster and better. *Nursing, 25*(8), 68-70.

Luepker, R. V., Perry, C. L., McKinlay, S. M., Nader, P. R., Parcel, G. S., Stone, E. J., Webber, L. S., Elder, J. P., Feldman, H. A., Johnson, C. C., Kelder, S. H., & Wu, M. (1996). Outcomes of a field trial to improve children's dietary patterns and physical activity. *Journal of the American Medical Association, 275*(10), 768-776.

Milio, N. (1976). A framework for prevention: Changing health-damaging to health-generating life patterns. *American Journal of Public Health, 66*(5), 435-439.

Nugent, K. E., & Lambert, V. A. (1996). The advanced practice nurse in collaborative practice. *Nursing Connections, 9,* 5-15.

North American Nursing Diagnosis Association. (1999). *Nursing diagnoses: Definitions and classification 1999-2000.* Philadelphia: Author.

Palmer, S. (1990). Food and nutrition policy: Challenges for the 1990s. *Health Affairs, 9*(2), 94-108.

Pate, R. R. (1993). Physical activity in children and youth: Relationship to obesity. *Contemporary Nutrition, 18*(2), 1-2.

Perry, C. L., Stone, E. J., Parcel, G. S., Ellison, R. C., Nader, P. R., Webber, L. S., & Luepker, R. V. (1990). School-based cardiovascular health promotion: The child and adolescent trial for cardiovascular health (CATCH). *Journal of School Health, 60*(8), 406-413.

Powell, K. E., Thompson, P. D., Caspersen, C. J., & Kendrick, J. S. (1987). Physical activity and the incidence of coronary heart disease. *Annual Review of Public Health, 8,* 253-287.

Ross, J. G., Dotson, C. O., & Gilbert, G. G. (1985). The national children and youth fitness study: Are kids getting appropriate activity? *Journal of Physical Education, Recreation and Dance, 56,* 40-43.

Strong, W. B., Deckelbaum, R. J., Gidding, S. S., Kavey, R. W., Washington, R., Wilmore, J. H., & Perry, C. L. (1992). Integrated cardiovascular health promotion in childhood: A statement for health professionals from the subcommittee on atherosclerosis and hypertension in childhood of the Council on Cardiovascular Disease in the Young, American Heart Association. *Circulation, 85*(4), 1638-1650.

U.S. Department of Health and Human Services. (1991). *Healthy people 2000: National health promotion and disease prevention objectives* (DHHS Publication No. PHS 91-50312). Washington, DC: Government Printing Office.

U.S. Department of Health and Human Services. (1995). *Healthy people 2000: Midcourse review and 1995 revisions.* Washington, DC: Government Printing Office.

34

Exercise Promotion

Cynthia L. Bennett

During the past two decades, American youth have become increasingly inactive and overweight. Young people spend numerous hours engrossed in sedentary pastimes such as watching television, playing video and computer games, and surfing the Internet. These entertainment novelties are gaining popularity as parents seem to tolerate and even condone their use with few restrictions. At the same time, opportunities to be physically active continue to diminish in our schools and neighborhoods. Insufficient and infrequent physical activity is a major contributor to the increasing childhood obesity rate, which is as high as 25% to 30% (Moran, 1999). Growth disturbances, orthopedic problems, respiratory difficulties, abnormal glucose metabolism, hypertension, hyperlipidemia, psychosocial despair, and persistence of obesity into adulthood are the health consequences linked to childhood obesity (Dietz, 1995). The alarming message is that young Americans prefer to spend their free time engrossed in motionless activities rather than engaging in physical activities that will improve their overall health and well-being.

In response to the epidemic of inactivity, high obesity rates, and low physical fitness scores of American children, the U.S. Department of Health and Human Services (USDHHS), the Public Health Service, the Health Resources and Service Administration, and the Maternal and Child Health Bureau joined together to publish *Healthy Children 2000* (USDHHS, 1992). These health promotion and disease prevention objectives included fitness and nutrition goals for children and adolescents. These goals posed a challenge to health care providers, teachers, community leaders, and program directors to find ways to change the health behaviors of our youth. Unfortunately, there have been no significant changes in health behaviors of American children, and the prevalence of childhood obesity continues to increase (Klish, 1998; Moran, 1999).

Promoting physical activity to American youth will not be easy. On a national level, public messages encourage sedentary behavior and portray exercise as recreation for superathletes and bodybuilders. On a community level, schools are reducing the number of physical education classes, activity clubs, and sports teams each year. Neighborhoods may be too dangerous for children and teens to be active outside of their own homes, and community recreation programs are being cut due to lack of public funding. In individual households, working parents are poor role models because they are either absent from the home or are too exhausted after work to participate in physical activities with their children on a regular basis. Nutritious home-cooked meals are given up for easier, quicker microwave meals or fast foods at the end of a long day. The modern American lifestyle is leading to the physical deterioration of young and old alike. American families, schools, and communities must be made aware of the consequences of inactivity and poor nutrition, and efforts should be made to reverse this trend. Increasing the activity level of youth will be the first step to improving the fitness state of all Americans.

Physical activity is often the easiest factor of the energy equation to change. Other components of the energy equation include heredity, which is unchangeable, and family eating habits, which are very difficult to change. An increase in energy output may be achieved by simply stimulating a young person's innate desire to be active. Young people must be exposed early in life to the enjoyment of regular physical activity to bring about a lifelong change in their health-seeking behaviors. This chapter focuses on ways to inspire participation in physical activity during childhood so that the desire to be active will continue throughout adulthood.

THEORETICAL FRAMEWORK AND LITERATURE REVIEW

Theoretical Perspectives

Developmental theorists suggest that children adopt an outside view while projecting themselves into adult roles during play. Arnsten (1990) explains that role playing allows the child to gain insight into new roles, achieve mastery of tasks, learn effective methods of problem solving, and provides an opportunity to express creativity. Parents and family are the most influential role models during school-age years, followed closely by peers and teachers. The development of social skills progresses from general to specific and from simple to complex. Social concepts of moral reasoning, working cooperatively, concern for others, and dealing efficiently with anxiety-producing situations are learned and are reinforced by successful experiences during play and physical activity.

Personal self-esteem and lifelong fitness behaviors are developed by engaging in all types of physical activity. Fox (1988) suggests, from a self-esteem theory perspective, that unless aspects of physical fitness have high social and personal value and provide opportunities to experience feelings of success and competence, they will not be central to the child's self-esteem structures. Arnsten (1990) correlates achievement theory and motivational theory, stating that achievement theory suggests that personal value will be attached to fitness as the child internalizes feelings of success resulting from improved skill, endurance, appearance, and self-acceptance. Similarly, motivation theory suggests that the successes felt as tasks are mastered will inspire the child to willfully participate in activities and seek them out on a regular basis. Children begin learning to be active by exploration, progressing to competency and finally to achievement. This hierarchical concept of motivation contends that children will be motivated toward increasingly complex behaviors by a sense of control that is experienced when less complex challenges are mastered. If failures repeatedly occur with an activity, the child will stop striving for success with that activity. Lifelong fitness behaviors are inspired by an environment that offers appropriate challenges, opportunities for physical success, positive social interactions, and adequate social support (Arnsten, 1990).

Declining Youth Fitness:
A National Concern

Volumes of literature about fitness in children have been written since the 1950s when President Eisenhower first brought attention to the decline in the fitness level of America's children. Fitness testing became popular during that time, and organizations such as the President's Council on Physical Fitness and the American Alliance for Health, Physical Education, Recreation, and Dance were developed to study the problem and prepare recommendations. During the following two decades, the results of fitness testing studies were inconclusive, and the reliability and validity of the testing methods were challenged (Safrit, 1990). Internationally known researchers Bar-Or and Malina (1995) reported difficulty in determining whether children are really less physically fit because there is no universally accepted operational definition of fitness. Pate (1995) contended, however, that the fitness state of America's children is continually declining despite the fitness testing controversy.

Improving the national fitness levels is a prime objective of the U.S. government and many national, public, and private fitness organizations. In 1996, the Surgeon General's *Report on Physical Activity and Health* was released by the President's Council on Physical Fitness; Communicable Disease Center; Office of the Surgeon General; Office of Public Health and Science; National Institutes of Health; American Alliance for Health, Physical Education, Recreation, and Dance; American College of Sports Medicine; and the American Heart Association (President's Council on Physical Fitness and Sports and Centers for Disease Control and Prevention, 1996). The report states that the physical activity patterns for an alarming number of Americans are well below the levels needed to maintain general physical health. Suggestions about appropriate activities and the duration, frequency, and intensity required to improve general health are included in the report. Friends, families, communities, and government agencies are encouraged to cooperatively promote participation in physical fitness activities. The report concludes that the social advantages of regular physical activity are quite clear, and Americans can substantially improve their health and quality of life by including moderate amounts of physical activity in their daily lives.

Promoting Youth Fitness

Researchers have recommended a variety of solutions to combat the decline in the fitness state of America's youth (Barlow & Dietz, 1998; Bar-Or & Malina, 1995; Gidding, Deckelbaum, Strong, & Moller, 1995). Philosophical and strategic approaches to fitness promotion are easily found; methods for teaching healthy fitness behaviors to young people, however, have not been universally agreed on. Corbin (1986) believes lifelong fitness behaviors will be encouraged by the development of each child's intrinsic motivation to be active and by reinforcement of the process of achieving competence and confidence. This philosophy is widely supported by contemporary literature.

In addition to the philosophical approach, Fox (1991) provides recommendations that will strategically guide organized physical fitness instruction. Fox explains that the child's skill level, state of physical fitness, knowledge base, and behavioral level should be considered before choosing activities for a physical fitness program. After careful assessment of these factors, appropriately chosen physical activities will provide feelings of success as the young person masters each task. These positive feelings—intrinsic motivators—will be intensified as the individual experiences skill attainment and personal improvement. While performing activities, competition should be minimized for 5- to 10-year-old children because it may lead to low expectations of success, feelings of powerlessness, and learned helplessness. Fox (1988, 1991) and Whitehead and Corbin (1991) believe that fitness behaviors will be continued longer when competition is avoided and emphasis is placed on enhancing individual intrinsic motivators by offering ample opportunities for mastery of age-appropriate tasks and challenges. Fox (1991) also believes that fitness instruction for children 10 years and younger should focus on "here and now" reality. Children choose to be active to have fun and to feel enjoyment, to attain personal success from physical mastery of tasks, and to obtain whatever social value has been attached to the activity by their role models. Appropriate instruction for this age group should include abundant amounts of fun and enjoyment, suitable challenges that offer opportunities for personal success, positive coach and team interactions, and adequate social support from parents, peers, and teachers. Another approach to increasing the activity level of young people involves increasing the amount of nonorganized recreational activity. Free play and games improve general fitness and develop self-identity and self-confidence in children (Corbin, 1986).

NURSING DIAGNOSIS AND OUTCOME DETERMINATION

The nursing diagnosis that addresses physical inactivity is Activity Intolerance. The nursing diagnoses relating to obesity is Altered Nutrition: More Than Body Requirements, and the desire to achieve a higher level of physical fitness is Health-Seeking Behaviors. These diagnoses deal with the health risks related to physical inactivity and describe how to appraise the desire to change health behaviors and how to prevent illness and seek optimal health.

The fact that America's youth are unable to tolerate the physical activities that will improve their health is most concerning. They lack the opportunity to be active, the social support necessary for an active lifestyle, and the basic knowledge regarding the type, amount, and intensity of activity required to maintain an optimal state of physical fitness and body weight. When children are underconditioned, they tend to avoid physically challenging activities. Activity Intolerance is the nursing diagnosis reflecting the reeducation in physiological capacity to endure activities to the degree desired or required by a normally healthy child or adolescent (North American Nursing Diagnosis Association [NANDA],

1999). Children who show signs of activity intolerance may avoid daily fundamental challenges because they are unable to keep up with their friends. This behavior often leads to social isolation and further deconditioning.

As the young person becomes increasingly deconditioned, the signs of activity intolerance intensify to include respiratory difficulty with exertion and an abnormal response of pulse rate (usually too high) during activity with failure to return to resting rate within 3 minutes of stopping the activity. Blood pressure abnormalities may include failure to change with exertion and an increase more than 15 mm Hg diastolic or an inappropriate decrease. Muscular inflexibility and imbalances may occur, demonstrated by weakness and injury. The extent of the young person's limitations may be assessed by simple physical fitness tests available through organizations such as the American Alliance for Health, Physical Education, Recreation and Dance (1998) and the Cooper Institute for Aerobics Research (IAR, 1987). Although the validity and scoring methods of these tests are controversial (Safrit, 1990), basic information about the young person's state of fitness may be obtained through testing. Vital sign response to the cardiorespiratory endurance testing component should be included because it is not included in most general fitness test batteries.

Activity intolerance is most commonly caused by physical deconditioning as a result of excessive sedentary behavior, an ineffectual exercise regime, low activity level, and poor nutrition. Social and psychological factors often contribute significantly to the severity of the problem. Activity intolerance also occurs with diseases, illnesses, and obesity due to impaired oxygen transport mechanisms and excessive energy demands. The effectiveness of interventions to improve activity tolerance can be measured by the following outcomes described in the Nursing Outcomes Classification (NOC): Knowledge: Health Behaviors, Knowledge: Prescribed Activity, Endurance, and Muscle Function (Iowa Outcomes Project, 2000). Young people should be empowered to continually seek and maintain their optimal level of fitness when the appropriate nursing interventions have been successful.

Underconditioned and activity-intolerant young people are more likely to become obese when energy intake exceeds energy expenditure (Dietz, 1995). Children and teens are consuming excess amounts of fat, sugar, and salt and continue these habits into adulthood. The nursing diagnosis for this problem is *Altered Nutrition: More Than Body Requirements,* defined as "the state in which an individual is experiencing an intake of nutrients which exceeds metabolic needs" (NANDA, 1999, p. 9). The U.S. government has sponsored several large nationally representative surveys beginning in the 1960s called the National Health and Nutrition Examination Studies (NHANES I-III). These surveys show that the incidence of obesity has increased during the past two decades as much as

54% for 6- to 11-year-old children and 39% for 12- to 17-year-old teens (U.S. Department of Commerce, 1989). Related studies report that 40% of obese children become obese adults, and 70% of obese adolescents become obese adults (Must, Jacques, Dallal, Bajema, & Dietz, 1992).

Although the incidence of obesity among children and teens appears to be alarmingly high, controversy exists about the reliability of the commonly used anthropometric methods of measurement. Troiano, Flegal, Kuczmarski, Campbell, and Johnson (1995) state that currently there is no clear consensus on the definition of obesity in children that would precisely detect adiposity and relate to morbidity and mortality outcomes. Skinfold measurements offer the most significant correlation with body fat; weight-for-height comparisons such as body mass index (BMI, kg/m^2), however, are the easiest methods for collecting data for large numbers of children. A child is considered obese when the triceps skinfold measurement is greater than the 85th percentile (Dietz, 1995) or the BMI measurement exceeds the 95th percentile for age (Troiano et al., 1995). As body fat proportion increases above these percentages, skinfold and BMI measurements become less sensitive. Superobesity occurs when a child exceeds a relative median weight for age by 30%. The incidence of superobesity in children has increased 98% in the past two decades along with related health problems, such as hypertension, Type 2 diabetes, impaired glucose metabolism, hyperlipidemia, sleep apnea, activity intolerance, inability to provide self-care, low self-esteem, and social isolation (Moran, 1999).

Many children and teens are predisposed to altered nutritional states because they lack knowledge about basic nutrition and appropriate types of physical activity. Contributing factors include psychological or social dysfunction. Nursing interventions should be aimed at preventing the obesity that is a consequence of overconsumption and physical inactivity. With successful intervention, the child or adolescent will demonstrate improved nutritional status as described in the NOC for Nutritional Status: Body Mass and Nutritional Status: Energy (Iowa Outcomes Project, 2000).

To diminish the health risks related to inactivity and poor nutrition, timely and suitable preventive interventions should be designed and implemented. The nursing diagnosis *Health-Seeking Behaviors* is defined as "a state in which an individual in stable health is actively seeking ways to alter personal health habits and/or the environment in order to move toward a higher level of health" (NANDA, 1999, p. 83). Children or adolescents seeking to improve their current level of fitness will exhibit the desire to search for useful information about physical activity and exercise and then engage in an activity and exercise regime that will improve their body composition, cardiorespiratory endurance, flexibility, and muscle strength.

Barriers to achievement of a higher level of physical fitness may be personal or situational or both. Young persons who cannot identify, manage, and seek out help to maintain or improve their state of health exhibit altered health maintenance. Personal barriers to improving physical fitness include overeating and obesity, frequent musculoskeletal injury and weakness, inability to communicate, lack of education, limited cognitive abilities, poor motivation, or low self-esteem. Situational barriers include the lack of access to health maintenance facilities, improper equipment, insufficient space or finances, and lack of social support. Once the desire to achieve a higher level of fitness has been expressed, the crucial information been gathered, and the barriers reduced, appropriate interventions should be designed that ensure a positive outcome. A positive outcome would include the ability to describe the benefits of activity and exercise, the knowledge of healthy nutritional and physical fitness practices, and improvement in the components of fitness. Improved health-seeking behaviors would be consistent with the NOC outcome Knowledge: Health Behaviors (Iowa Outcomes Project, 2000).

INTERVENTION: EXERCISE PROMOTION

Formulating successful activities for improving physical fitness levels in children and adolescents involves (a) acknowledging and encouraging health-seeking behaviors, (b) promoting exercise as a way of improving activity tolerance, (c) recommending nutritional practices that optimally meet body requirements, and (d) monitoring progress of the activity or exercise routine on a regular basis and modifying as necessary (Iowa Intervention Project, 2000).

Promoting wellness and preventing illness is the most encouraging trend in modern medicine. Maintaining healthy lifelong fitness and nutrition behaviors is becoming a priority with third-party payors and health care providers, and it requires the support of the health care team, families, communities, and government. The moment children or adolescents first express the desire to be more active or to improve one of their fitness components, interventions to encourage lifelong fitness behaviors must begin. The preliminary steps to successful intervention include developing intrinsic motivation to be active; recommending appropriate activity and exercise challenges; limiting sedentary activities such as watching television, playing video games, and using the Internet; locating adequate financial resources; and recruiting sufficient social support.

Interventions to improve activity tolerance require stable self-esteem structures and sufficient intrinsic motivation. Assessment of these factors may identify deficits that should be addressed prior to the start of activity and exercise interventions. Information about the child's general health and level of physical fitness should also be obtained before designing a program to improve activity tolerance. Most children and adolescents can safely participate in routine fitness activities with a basic preparticipation exam (PPE). The PPE includes a medical history, physical exam with vital signs, eye exam, height, weight, Tanner staging, and cardiorespiratory, abdominal, and musculoskeletal exam (American Academy of Family Physicians, 1997). Individuals who have questionable conditions identified on the PPE may require a physical performance assessment, which includes body composition, cardiovascular endurance, muscular strength and endurance, and flexibility measures. The Prudential FITNESSGRAM is an example of a reliable and simple physical fitness test battery (IAR, 1987).

Once the young person's general fitness level is known and physical deficits are identified, an appropriate individual activity and exercise program can be designed. The young person's level of fitness will determine the appropriate training methods to use and the frequency, duration, and initial intensity of the fitness program. Reasonable short- and long-term goals need to be agreed on prior to beginning the program. Short-term goals should be based on the ability of the young person to master age-appropriate skills and his or her potential for improvement. Long-term goals for maintaining fitness should correlate with the recommendations cited in *Healthy People 2000* (USDHHS, 1991). A contract can be established between the young person and the fitness instructor, and social support for the exercise regime should be enlisted. Strategies to enhance the child's intrinsic motivation to be active are continued throughout each training interval by choosing physical activities and exercises that will provide opportunities for success and entertainment. As Exercise Promotion begins, workouts carefully advance the young person from a lower level of fitness to a higher level of fitness. Challenging movements are added to fundamental activities while both intensity and duration are increased as tolerated.

Although individual fitness training is often effective, it is usually costly and lacks the positive influence that may occur in a group program in which the young person has the opportunity to socialize with peers. Children with nearly the same fitness level may benefit from a fitness program designed to meet their collective fitness needs. Group programs are usually more cost-effective and offer the support of peers throughout the instruction. Individual and group programs need to include information to empower the youth to obtain and maintain physical fitness. Physical activity should not be thought of as the equivalent of exercise. Physical activity is movement of the skeletal muscles that results in energy output, and exercise is repetitive body movement to improve physical fitness. Both physical activity and exercise should be incorporated into fitness programs to achieve optimal results. The main objective of the intervention is to expose children at an early age to the enjoyment of routine physical activity and to provide opportunities to be successful so that they will be motivated to continue similar fitness behaviors throughout their lifetimes.

A cardiorespiratory endurance program should begin by introducing a variety of activities meant to entice young people to find enjoyment in being physically active on a daily basis. Demonstrating various activities gives children the opportunity to attempt activities they may not experience on their own and provides opportunities for success with these activities. Simple locomotor skills such as brisk walking around the neighborhood or safe social gathering places such as the mall, playing skill-building games, skipping, jumping rope alone or with teams, rollerblading, running through a homemade obstacle course, circuit running from one exercise station to another to perform skills such as hula hoop or jumping jacks are a few of the fun and worthwhile activities that can be incorporated into a fitness routine. Adding music and encouraging rhythmic expression will enhance fitness training for all ages. Family members and friends should be enlisted as participants and cheerleaders. Regular times to perform activities can be chosen from the menu to ensure that a routine will be established.

The intensity and duration of activities will vary depending on the young person's fitness level and should be increased as tolerated by 10% or less each week. Suitable aerobic activities should be carried out for 20 to 60 minutes, three to five times a week (USDHHS, 1992). Sufficient gratification and support are required to elicit a dedicated effort that will raise and maintain the target heart rate effectively (see Chapter 35, this volume). For children younger than 10 years of age, activities are more effective when varied every few minutes, modified each week, and completely changed every 6 weeks to provide appropriate challenges and to maintain interest. Engaging in the activity with family or friends will also promote enjoyment for young children. Adolescents, however, will chose activities that they enjoy and will discipline themselves to perform them repeatedly. A concern with this behavior is the potential for overtraining. Adolescents should be observed periodically and encouraged to vary their activities when signs of fatigue or failed performance begin to occur. Peers are helpful for social support.

A muscular strength and endurance program includes progressive muscular flexibility, strength, and endurance activities beginning at the appropriate level for each individual. Strength training should occur every other day for the same body regions, three times a week to build strength and endurance and two times a week for maintaining strength (Zwiren, 1993). Before beginning the strength program, age, maturity, developmental level, flexibility, strength, and endurance, in addition to psychological motivators and social support, should be assessed. Instruction should be designed and supervised by a certified youth strength and conditioning or fitness specialist or well-trained fitness professional to provide safe and effective strength training for the preadolescent and the adolescent youth. Proper weight lifting technique is essential, and young persons need to be supervised and follow strict guidelines to bring about maximum benefit without causing serious injury when using these training methods (see Chapter 35, this volume).

Strength training for all ages begins with the development of flexibility. Proper stretching technique will help lengthen and tone the muscles, especially for young people with musculoskeletal imbalances caused by rapid growth. Maintaining or improving flexibility is important through every stage of a cardiovascular and strength program because tight muscles inhibit performance and may lead to injuries. Once flexibility is adequate to move each joint through the full range of motion, the next step in a strengthening program is the development of core (trunk) strength. Core strength involves the muscles of the abdomen, back, trunk, and hips. Typical care strength exercises begin with fundamental steps and progress at a pace dependent on the young person's age and developmental maturity. For example, the basic steps for a curl-up exercise (sit-up) for strengthening the abdomen progress from simply holding the proper position on the floor (beginning with 5- or 6-year-old children) to a pelvic tilt or "dead bug" position as the abdominal muscles are contracted and knees are drawn up, partial curl-ups as the trunk is slightly elevated, and full curl-ups. Other core strength exercises, such as trunk lifts for the back and wall sits for the hips and legs, progress in similar steps. Many challenging and fun modifications of these basic core strengthening exercises can be used to maintain interest and to promote physical success.

When core strength is sufficient to provide balance and stability, weight of the body exercises are introduced. Body weight resistance is the first step of extremity strengthening and includes simple body weight exercises such as push-ups, pull-ups, and tricep dips for the upper body and squats, lunges, and vertical jumps for the lower body. Body weight exercises may be performed in a variety of ways and are the safest and most effective form of extremity strengthening for prepubescent children (IDEA, 1990). The equipment for these exercises is usually found in the house, including walls, stairs, and large balls. Weight lifting with heavy exercise equipment should be avoided until the growth (epiphyseal) plates of the involved appendages are ossified or closed. These growth plates are found on most long bones and close at different times for different areas depending on skeletal maturity. While the growth plates are actively growing and depositing new bone cells, they are vulnerable to injury. For example, the tibial tubercle in Osgood-Schlatter syndrome becomes the site of irritation from contraction of the quadriceps muscle group during jumping and running activities, especially at 12 to 17 years of age. Because the tubercle is the quadriceps tendon attachment site and the growing area of the bone, pain and a bump often occur as a result of repeated trauma. As skeletal maturity occurs at that growth area, the painful symptoms will usually subside. Because of growth-related concerns, weight lifting guidelines for youth are offered by the American Academy of Family Physicians (1997) and IDEA (1990) and are summarized in Chapter 35. A young person's developmental level may not always correspond to chronological age; therefore, individualized strength training programs should be designed and carefully supervised for each participant or group of similar participants.

Other muscular training components that should be included in a comprehensive fitness program are motor skill development drills that enhance speed, agility, quickness, balance, power, and explosive movement (plyometrics). Neuromuscular training methods are most commonly used by elite-level and professional athletes under the guidance of qualified fitness instructors. When broken down into fundamental steps, however, these training methods are very effective in developing motor skills in children of all ages. The steps used to develop proper movement techniques are fun to learn, but to be performed safely they require an acceptable level of fitness. Beginning as young as 5 years of age, a child can participate in games and activities designed to develop basic motor skills used in running, jumping, sprinting, and throwing while simultaneously experiencing success and enjoyment. These techniques may be practiced at home or during sporting activities that include family and friends.

Including the family in activities and ensuring access to space at home and public activity centers will help provide the social support needed for improving physical fitness habits. Attempts are made to encourage each young person to realize the mastery of strength-building tasks, improvement of individual weight lifting skills, and health benefits gained from training are valuable rewards for their efforts. Once social support is enlisted and intrinsic motivation is kindled, the young person is more likely to seek out strength training and other health-promoting activities on a regular basis and for a longer period of time.

When designing strategies to prevent energy excess and reduce obesity, four important areas must be addressed: physical activity, nutrition, eating behaviors, and psychosocial health. Interventions focus on increasing energy expenditure through routine physical activity, providing appropriate nutrition counseling, providing training in behavior management techniques, and providing psychosocial assessment and counseling.

A collaborative effort by the health care team, the family, and the child or adolescent is essential for an optimal outcome. The young person should clearly understand the relationship between activity level and weight. Education and instruction in routine physical activity and exercise must be age appropriate, effective, and fun. A nutrition consult is necessary for identifying eating patterns that contribute to weight gain and to provide education about foods and dieting. Dieting is carefully supervised and avoided whenever possible to prevent omission of vital nutrients essential for growth and development (see Chapter 33, this volume). Psychological counseling is needed to identify problems with self-concept, self-efficacy, and the underlying stressors or barriers to seeking a higher level of fitness. Working with the health care team and supported by family, the young person must be prepared to carry out the suggested weight management interventions and make a commitment to maintaining optimal weight once reached.

Health-promoting activities include eating healthy foods and avoiding tobacco, alcohol, and drugs. Although Altered Nutrition: More Than Body Requirements has been discussed, Altered Nutrition: Less Than Body Requirements may also occur. Lack of vital nutrients during childhood and adolescence may lead to altered growth and development. Maintaining health and physical activity on a regular basis requires proper energy management and special nutritional information for varying intensity levels. Nutritional guidelines for athletes and active people include proper balance of carbohydrates, proteins, and fats needed for the specific type, intensity, and duration of the chosen activity, in addition to information on proper rehydration, vitamin and mineral supplementation, and rest.

The progress of children and adolescents seeking to improve their current level of physical fitness should be monitored periodically. Once the interventions are initiated, the preliminary steps toward fitness should be accomplished within a few weeks. These steps include identifying and stimulating intrinsic motivation, establishing contacts for personal or group training, gaining knowledge about proper nutrition or contacting a dietitian for a personalized nutrition consult, identifying and using the resources that may be available, creating opportunities for social support, and engaging in an appropriate physical activity and exercise regime. The exercise regime then progresses in 6- to 12-week intervals, with evaluation of the components of fitness, the primary motivators, the financial resources, and the social support structures at the end of each interval. The length of training interval depends on the age of the youth, the beginning level of fitness, and the type of training desired. The training program is modified as needed, and barriers to continuing the program are resolved before the next training interval begins. Eventually, young people will be proficient at monitoring their own progress and will be able to increase or maintain their optimal level of fitness as pledged in their long-term goals.

INTERVENTION APPLICATION

In 1996, a physical fitness program was designed for a group of 6- to 9-year-old children. The program included 12 participants and was conducted in a 1,500-square-foot dance studio in an upper-middle-class suburb of Akron, Ohio. The program lasted 6 weeks, and the sessions were 1 hour long. Pretesting included the FITNESSGRAM Sit and Reach flexibility test and two skinfolds measurements (Institute for Aerobics Research, 1987), the results of which remained confidential. The fitness instruction progressed from one week to the next in a sequence specifically designed for this age group by a youth physical fitness specialist/certified personal trainer (CPT), a sports medicine physician, and a pediatric nurse practitioner.

Each session was conducted by the CPT and a certified athletic trainer. The sessions began with simple warm-up activities in a circle, including light muscle warm-up activities and stretching, and then proceeded to station activities with a variety of entertaining skill-building drills and games arranged in a continuous circuit. The skill-building station activities included running, skipping, jumping rope, and using a hoola hoop. Each week these activities became progressively more complex according to the abilities of the group and included quick-feet ladder drills, large ball relays, and bean bag drills. After 20 to 30 minutes of moderate strengthening and endurance circuit activities maintaining the perceived exertion at a level of 6 or 7 out of 10, cool-down activities took place for approximately 10 minutes. At that time, interactive instruction in body systems and nutrition took place to increase the child's self-awareness and knowledge of proper eating habits. Teaching methods included wall drawings, worksheets, flash cards, posters, demonstrations, and open discussion.

At the end of 6 weeks, the results of the posttesting showed an increase in flexibility ranging from 0.5 to 4.0 in. in one or both legs for all but one child. The sum of skinfolds did not show significant change, although theoretically this program was not held frequently enough or long enough to achieve a change in aerobic fitness or body composition. Self-report by the children and observations reported by their parents proved to be the most meaningful measures of change. The children were performing the program activities at home regularly as if they were playing games, they began to watch their intake of high fat and high sugar foods, and they were conscious of their need for adequate sleep and plenty of water each day. Parents were both astounded and inspired by the behavior of their children, and many vowed to continue these newly discovered lifestyle changes as a family. This small pilot program illustrated the fact that children can be motivated to engage in healthy lifestyle activities when fun and innovative training methods are used and family support is enlisted.

RESEARCH AND PRACTICE IMPLICATIONS

Research in the area of Exercise Promotion for children and adolescents currently lacks direction or group effort. Much research comprises isolated studies with specific age groups using measures that lack validity. The physical fitness community must work together to (a) establish a universally agreed on operational definition of fitness, (b) design more reliable and valid instruments for measuring the components of fitness, (c) conduct long-term studies that link childhood activity levels to adult activity levels and health status, and (d) isolate the best methods for motivating a child to maintain healthy lifestyle behaviors throughout adulthood.

In practice, health care providers need to be aware of the state of physical fitness for each child and adolescent in their care. Appropriate referrals should be made or interventions designed so that young people may attain or maintain an acceptable level of physical fitness. Outcomes should be monitored on a regular basis so that progress or backsliding can be recorded and proper follow-up instituted. Young people should be empowered to continually seek and maintain their optimal level of fitness. Increasing the activity level of youth is the first step to improving the fitness level of all Americans.

REFERENCES

American Academy of Family Physicians, American Academy of Pediatrics, American Medical Society for Sports Medicine, American Orthopedic Society for Sports Medicine, American Osteopathic Academy of Sports Medicine. (1997). *Preparticipation physical evaluation (PPE)*. New York: McGraw-Hill.

American Alliance for Health, Physical Education, Recreation and Dance. (1998). *Physical best: The AAHPERD guide to physical fitness, education, and assessment*. Reston, VA: Author.

Arnsten, S. M. (1990). Intrinsic motivation. *American Journal of Occupational Therapy, 44*(5), 462-463.

Barlow, S. E., & Dietz, W. H. (1998). Obesity evaluation and treatment: Expert committee recommendations. *Pediatrics, 102*(3), 29-46.

Bar-Or, O., & Malina, R. M. (1995). Activity, fitness, and health of children and adolescents. In L. W. Cheung & J. B. Richmond (Eds.), *Child health, nutrition and physical activity* (pp. 79-123). Champaign, IL: Human Kinetics.

Corbin, C. B. (1986, May/June). Fitness is for children; Developing lifetime fitness. *Journal of Physical Education, Recreation and Dance*, 82-84.

Dietz, W. H. (1995). Childhood obesity. In L. W. Cheung & J. B. Richmond (Eds.), *Child health, nutrition and physical activity* (pp. 155-169). Champaign, IL: Human Kinetics.

Fox, K. (1988). The self-esteem complex and youth fitness. *Quest, 40*(3), 230-246.

Fox, K. (1991, September). Motivating children for physical activity: Towards a healthier future. *Journal of Physical Education, Recreation and Dance*, 34-38.

Gidding, S. S., Deckelbaum, R. J., Strong, W., & Moller, J. H. (1995). Children's Heart Health Conference. *Journal of School Health, 65*(4), 129-132.

IDEA: The Association for Fitness Professionals. (1990). *Children and teens*. San Diego, CA: Author.

Institute for Aerobics Research. (1987). *FITNESSGRAM user's manual*. Dallas, TX: Author.

Iowa Intervention Project. (2000). *Nursing interventions classification (NIC)* (J. C. McCloskey & G. M. Bulechek, Eds.; 3rd ed.). St. Louis, MO: Mosby-Year Book.

Iowa Outcomes Project. (1997). *Nursing outcomes classification (NOC)* (M. Johnson, M. Maas, & S. Moorhead, Eds.; 2nd ed.). St. Louis, MO: Mosby-Year Book.

Klish, W. J. (1998). Childhood obesity. *Pediatrics in Review, 19*(9), 312-315.

Moran, R. (1999). Evaluation and treatment of childhood obesity. *American Family Physician, 59*(4), 861-868, 871-873.

Must, A., Jacques, P. F., Dallal, G. E., Bajema, C. L., & Dietz, W. H. (1992). Long-term morbidity and mortality of overweight adolescents. *New England Journal of Medicine, 327*(19), 1350-1355.

North American Nursing Diagnosis Association. (1999). *Nursing diagnoses: Definitions and classification 1999-2000*. Philadelphia: Author.

Pate, R. R. (1995). Promoting activity and fitness. In L. W. Cheung & J. B. Richmond (Eds.), *Child health, nutrition and physical activity* (pp. 139-145). Champaign, IL: Human Kinetics.

President's Council on Physical Fitness and Sports and Centers for Disease Control and Prevention. (1996). *Surgeon General's report on physical activity and health*. Washington, DC: Author.

Safrit, M. J. (1990). The validity and reliability of fitness tests for children: A review. *Pediatric Exercise Science, 2*, 9-28.

Troiano, R. P., Flegal, K. M., Kuczmarski, R. J., Campbell, S. M., & Johnson, C. L. (1995). Overweight prevalence and trends for children and adolescents. *Archives of Pediatric and Adolescent Medicine, 149*(10), 1085-1091.

U.S. Department of Commerce, National Technical Information Service. (1989). *National Health and Nutrition Examination Survey (NHANES)*. Springfield, VA: Author.

U.S. Department of Health and Human Services. (1991). *Healthy people 2000: National health promotion and disease prevention objectives* (DHHS Publication No. PHS 91-50312). Washington, DC: Government Printing Office.

U.S. Department of Health and Human Services. (1992). Physical activity and fitness. In *Healthy children 2000* (DHHS Publication No. HRSA-M-CH 91-2). Washington, DC: Jones & Bartlett.

Whitehead, J. R., & Corbin C. B. (1991). Effects of fitness test type, teacher, and gender on exercise intrinsic motivation and physical self worth. *Journal of School Health, 61,* 11-15.

Zwiren, L. D. (1993). Exercise prescription for children. In *The American College of Sports Medicine's resource manual for guidelines for exercise testing and prescription* (pp. 409-417). Philadelphia: Lea & Febiger.

35

Athlete Health Promotion

Cynthia L. Bennett

The number of children and adolescents involved in sports in the United States has increased rapidly in the past decade. According to the National Safe Kids Campaign (1996), more than 25 million children and adolescents between the ages of 6 and 21 years participate in competitive school sports each year, and an estimated 20 million are involved in organized sports outside of school. These estimates do not include the millions of children participating in nonorganized "backyard" sports. Until recently, sports were thought of as recreational activities intended for the entertainment and enjoyment of the participant. Now, however, they are also thought of as big business. With the right blend of genetic potential, appropriate training, and exceptional performance, a young person may be able to finance a college education or become a well-paid professional athlete. These financial opportunities have contributed to the phenomenal increase in the popularity of athletics—a trend that is fervently fed by the media. Because of this trend, children are led into a variety of sports at inappropriate ages and may be encouraged to train with unreasonable methods. Safe training methods and injury prevention guidelines for children have not been thoroughly substantiated by research and are not well-known by the public. Adult training guidelines are inappropriately substituted because of the lack of relevant research relating to the pediatric athlete. Many promising careers have ended prematurely because the young athletes were unable to deal with negative physical or psychological experiences encountered at the hands of poorly informed coaches and parents.

The National Safe Kids Campaign (1996) reported that approximately 20% of all young people involved in sports sustain injuries each year, and 70% of these injuries are incurred by athletes 20 years of age or younger (Backx, 1996). Sports injuries are frequently easy to treat, and full recovery is expected. Approximately one fourth of all sports injuries are serious in nature, however. Many serious injuries could be prevented by complying with conservative and sensible guidelines for performance, age-appropriate training techniques, proper nutrition, adequate hydration, and rest. When these essential safeguards are included in the young athlete's training program and games, the benefits of sports participation will almost certainly outweigh the risks. The ultimate goal of Athlete Health promotion is to prepare youth for the athletic stresses, metabolic demands, and the injury risks that occur with each sport while enhancing psychological well-being and creating positive social interactions (Kibler & Chandler, 1994).

LITERATURE REVIEW

Research related to youth participation in sports is still in the preliminary stage. In the past 10 to 15 years, the popularity of youth participation in organized sports has continued to increase, but comprehensive studies designed to answer important questions about safe participation are still incomplete.

Theoretical models of human development may offer some guidance in assessing readiness for sports, including the theories of Erikson and Piaget (Gallahue & Ozmun, 1989). Erikson's psychosocial theory described success-oriented movement as a means of advancing effectively through developmental crises. Consequently, motor development will not progress if attempts at various movements are not successful. Piaget's theory explained children's behavior on the basis of their level of cognitive development. Cognition is a crucial element in sports training and performance because children are required to learn increasingly complex strategies and apply them to game situations. Gallahue and Ozmun (1989) noted that the growth process is hierarchical in nature, and the formative years of an athlete's life are the most important to reaching optimal performance. Coaches are challenged to combine these theories with common sense and experience to meet the needs of an athlete as a whole person.

Literature combining theory and practice in the training of young athletes is limited. The questions that currently cannot be answered with absolute confidence include the following: (a) When is a child ready to participate in sports? (b) What training methods are appropriate and safe for children and adolescents? and (c) What injuries occur due to youth sports participation and how can they be prevented?

When Is a Child Ready to Participate in Sports?

Researchers have attempted to answer this important question largely from isolated cross-sectional studies, qualifying their assumptions with recently compiled data. Children should be neurodevelopmentally, socially, and cognitively ready for participation in sports (Dyment, 1990). Growth, maturity, and developmental readiness are demonstrated by mastery of motor skills, social competence, emotional control, and cognitive proficient. Performing basic movements necessary for the sport and successfully interacting with the coach are indicators of readiness. If children lag behind in any of these areas, participation in sports can expose them to negative physical, psychological, or social experiences. Petlichkoff (1996) stated that 35% of children and adolescents involved in organized youth sports withdraw each year. Limited studies indicate that young people are often turned off by the following common factors: (a) emphasis on winning, (b) lack of necessary motor skills to be "good enough" to compete successfully, (c) too much pressure from parents or coaches, or (d) too much time required for practicing and competing.

Malina and Beunen (1996) proposed that children be matched developmentally to equalize competition more effectively, enhance chances for success, diminish attrition, and reduce the risk of injuries. They stated that skill, strength, size, and maturity should be determined prior to assigning children to teams. The most objective indicators of readiness are cognitive skills, motor skills, and vision (Nelson & Goldberg, 1991). Each of these developmental components is relatively easy to determine, and when the skills required by the sport are compared with the results of the testing, the child's readiness for that particular sport can be determined. It is important to modify the sport to match the characteristics and needs of children. They suggest that the tasks and rules of performance should be adjusted to accommodate the developmental needs of the young athlete (Malina & Buenen, 1996). Examples that apply for younger athletes are eliminating body checking in ice hockey; making smaller playing areas for football, soccer, and other large-field sports; lowering basketball hoops; and enlarging soccer goals.

What Training Methods Are Appropriate and Safe for Children and Adolescents?

Flexibility, cardiorespiratory endurance, muscle strength and endurance, and body composition are the components of health-related physical fitness that are essential for performing daily motor tasks and an integral prerequisite for all advanced motor skills (Nichols, 1994). Although basic fitness components must be optimized during training for sports, there is also potential for exposure to excessively heavy training and subsequent health consequences (Pate & Ward, 1996). Appropriate guidelines are needed to guide performance-enhancement methods and injury-prevention training techniques.

Flexibility Training

A musculoskeletal flexibility program is usually recommended to accompany all cardiorespiratory, strength, and motor skill training programs, although studies that conclusively prove the beneficial effects are not easily found. Flexibility is a vital part of good posture, sports skill performance, and prevention of injury. The range of motion of each joint varies with genetic endowment, physical condition, body proportion, and the age of each athlete. Consequently, efforts to improve flexibility should be approached differently for each individual. Realistic goals should be established so that less flexible young athletes will not experience disappointment as they compare themselves to athletes with greater flexibility (Nichols, 1994). There is a direct relationship between muscle inflexibility and injury at or near the site of the involved muscle insertion (Smith, 1997). These insertion sites are more vulnerable during adolescence when rapid bone growth applies tension to muscles, bones, and connective tissues. The contours of the epiphyseal (growth) plates found at the ends of long bones and on bony prominence are unlocked and predisposed to injury during growth spurts (Burgess-Milliron & Murphy, 1996). During times of rapid growth, the need for a dedicated stretching routine increases (Smith, 1997). Basic flexibility testing techniques and stretching programs are included in fitness testing batteries through fitness organizations such as the Institute for Aerobics Research (1987), the American Alliance for Health, Physical Education, Recreation, and Dance (1988), and others discussed by Safrit (1995).

Cardiorespiratory Training

The purpose of cardiorespiratory endurance training is to enhance exercise tolerance and ultimately improve performance (Pate & Ward,

1996). Appropriate training methods for improving cardiorespiratory endurance in pediatric athletes, designed to enhance sports performance and prevent injury, have only recently been addressed in the literature (American Academy of Pediatrics [AAP], 1990; Ratliff, 1990; Tanner, 1997). It has been suggested that all young athletes in both aerobic (endurance) and anaerobic (strength and power) sports will benefit from endurance training (Ratliff, 1990). The goals for fitness stated in *Healthy People 2000* (U.S. Department of Health and Human Services, 1991) recommend that all children and adolescents engage in vigorous activity for 20 to 30 minutes a day to promote general health and fitness. General fitness goals are essential prerequisites for higher-level endurance training programs (Pate & Ward, 1996). Sport-specific endurance training is designed to enhance performance by continuing to improve the cardiorespiratory component of fitness beyond the goals required for general fitness. Advanced training should be specific to the sport (specificity); incorporate graduated and progressive increase (overload) in frequency, intensity, and duration (Ratliff, 1990); and allow for recovery, variety, and individuality (Kibler & Chandler, 1994).

Endurance can be defined as the ability to sustain a high rate of aerobic energy expenditure for a prolonged period of time (Pate & Ward, 1996). Maximal aerobic power, lactate threshold, and energy economy are three essential physiological factors that determine tolerance for endurance activities. Maximal aerobic power or maximal oxygen consumption ($\dot{V}O_2$ max) is the product of maximal cardiac output and the maximum arteriovenous oxygen difference. It is the greatest rate at which an individual can use oxygen in the metabolic process. $\dot{V}O_2$ max is a widely accepted index of work capacity that indicates the maximal rate of delivery of oxygen from the inspired air to the skeletal muscles (Smith & Mitchell, 1993). The higher the $\dot{V}O_2$ max, the greater the capacity for energy expenditure. Lactate threshold is the rate of aerobic energy expenditure at which the muscle fatiguing by-product, lactate, begins to build up in the blood. The higher the lactate threshold, the longer the activity can be performed. The third physiological factor, energy economy, is the rate of energy expenditure for a particular pace during an aerobic activity. The greater the energy economy, the less oxygen consumed during an activity at a given pace. Cardiorespiratory endurance training is proposed to improve these three physiological factors.

Although pertinent scientific literature is scarce, the general consensus of well-known fitness and exercise specialists is that prepubescent, pubescent, and postpubescent athletes will benefit to some degree from endurance training if the stimulus is adequate (Pate & Ward, 1996). The measurable benefit in all age groups is, on average, 10%, as demonstrated by an increase in maximal aerobic power and lactate threshold and an overall improvement in the energy economy of the aerobic metabolic system. Careful attention must be paid, however, to the athletes' response to intense, exhaustive training because they may not be able to tolerate the demand for the increased cardiac output and arteriovenous oxygen difference during continuous progressive overload training. Prepubescent children may show less benefit from aerobic training because they usually begin training at a higher level of fitness than do adolescents and adults and therefore have less capacity for improvement (Pate & Ward, 1996). Growth and developmental factors also influence training response, with evidence that $\dot{V}O_2$ max increases regardless of training during pubescence. As the athlete progresses through adolescence, training may increase the $\dot{V}O_2$ max by as much as 29% (similar to the response of an adult), as cardiac stroke volume and output increase and ventilation improves (Smith & Mitchell, 1993). The high-intensity endurance training needed to bring about the greatest increase in $\dot{V}O_2$ max, however, may cause stress injury to vulnerable growing tissues during adolescence (Burgess-Milliron & Murphy, 1996).

Properly designed and supervised endurance training for young athletes improves performance, delays fatigue, and prevents injury (Pate & Ward, 1996). The endurance training techniques are sport specific and are used in combination with a strengthening program. Although training methods are intended to be appropriate and safe, the child's response to training should be carefully monitored for signs of overtraining and boredom (Ratliff, 1990).

Muscular Strength and Endurance Training

Strength is defined as the peak force or torque developed during a maximal voluntary effort and power as the rate or speed at which mechanical work is performed within a given period of time. *Muscle endurance* is the ability to contract the muscle repeatedly or continuously without fatigue (Durnstine et al., 1993). Muscle strength, endurance, and power are important elements when performing activities of daily living and sport skills, and they are developed by training methods that are specific to the desired outcome (Blimkie & Bar-Or, 1996). With strength training during adolescence, significant strength gains and increases in muscle size are observed from all training methods (isometric, dynamic, isotonic, and isokenetic). The amount and type of strength gain in all age groups depend on an optimal combination of training mode, intensity, volume, and duration. Strength training recommendations are found in many sources (Alberta, 1993; Blimkie & Bar-Or, 1996; Cahill, 1988; Harris, 1997; IDEA, 1990; Metcalf & Roberts, 1993).

Neuromuscular Training

Neuromuscular training involves the improvement of the motor skills used during sports. This type of sports-specific movement training occurs after an athlete has achieved reasonable athletic fitness with suitable aerobic and anaerobic endurance (Kibler & Chandler, 1994). Motor skills fundamental to sports movement are described as voluntary, postural, fundamental, transitional, or complex (Nelson & Goldberg, 1991). Voluntary movements are conscious, purposeful, and include hand-eye coordination. Postural movements are automatic responses to changes in position to maintain balance. Fundamental movements are building blocks for subsequent motor activities, and transitional movements are combinations and variations of fundamental skills. Complex movements are the combination of fundamental and transitional skills required in sports competition. Neuromuscular training programs are designed to develop these motor skills in succession (Nelson & Goldberg, 1991). Training sessions should be short, entertaining, and emphasize experimentation and exploration (Johnson, 1988). Competition should be minimized while working on individual motor skills, and challenges should be entertaining and age appropriate. According to Sharkey (1990), motor skill and efficiency are acquired through repetitious movement patterns similar to movements that occur in sports. With proper training in technique of movement patterns, the motions become smoother, coordinated, and consequently require less energy to perform. Practicing sports movement skills results in beneficial neurogenic changes, including muscle fiber recruitment, reduction in inhibition factors, and refined application of power. The training techniques for improving motor skill and efficiency are complex and should be taught and supervised by knowledgeable fitness professionals or coaches. Young athletes should achieve acceptable health-related fitness, then improve on the fitness components demanded by their specific sport, and finally progress to optimizing energy systems and motor skills such as speed, agility, quickness, and balance. Injuries may occur if the objectives of training are not met in sequential fashion (Kibler & Chandler, 1994).

Body Composition

Cardiorespiratory endurance, flexibility, muscle strength and endurance, and motor skills acquisition are influenced by body composition. Body composition, the amount of lean tissue and fat in the body, is dependent on factors such as heredity, metabolism, activity, and nutrition. Improving body composition is a key element to improving general health and athletic performance. Fat and carbohydrates should be optimally available as fuel for sports-related energy systems.

What Injuries Occur Due to Sports Participation and How Can They Be Prevented?

Using available data, it has been estimated that approximately 20% (or 4,379,999) of young people involved in sports and recreation sustain injuries each year (Bijur et al., 1995). Sports injuries account for 36% of all injuries to children and adolescents. Although most sports-related injuries are easy to treat and full recovery is expected, approximately one fourth (or approximately 1,363,000) of these injuries are serious in nature (Bijur et al., 1995). Although rare, permanent disability or death are the most serious consequences of sports participation, usually associated with head and neck injury or sudden death from cardiac abnormalities.

Musculoskeletal injuries, including bruises, inflammation of bones, joints, or muscles, muscle strains, ligament sprain, and minor bone fractures, account for the majority of sports-related injuries. Other systems also at risk but less commonly reported include the cardiovascular, endocrine, integumentary, and immune systems. The severity of sports injury can be defined by the degree of pathology and the number of practice or performance days lost due to injury (Landry, 1992). All sporting activities involve some degree of risk. The older and bigger the athlete and the more contact and collision involved in the sport, however, the greater will be the risk of injury. Baseball has the highest mortality rate and is the leading cause of eye injury with the least amount of mandated safety equipment (Rome, 1995). In baseball, death and serious injury occur from direct impact with the ball to the head or chest. Basketball, soccer, wrestling, and gymnastics are also associated with a high risk of injury. Unfortunately, reliable statistics on the actual number of injuries incurred in each sport, the definition of each type of injury, the severity of injury, the type of treatment given, and response to treatment are not currently available (Rome, 1995). The wide variety of organizational and competition levels, the erratically different frequency and intensity of training methods, and the subjectiveness of injury assessment and reporting make it difficult to collect and analyze meaningful data. Current data on sports-related injury must be interpreted with caution, but these data are often useful in developing preventive interventions.

Physical injuries are not the only type of injury associated with athletic participation. Psychological and emotional injuries commonly occur as children attempt to develop the physical and social skills necessary for participation. The child's body is the instrument of action and communication. Body concept and motivation are developed as physical challenges are attempted (Roberts, 1992). Self-concept is dependent on the perception of self and success with activities. Self-esteem may be lowered when unsuccessful attempts to master physical and social skills occur repeatedly. In one study, children with low motor and social skills valued extrinsic reward more than intrinsic reward, whereas high-skill children related the opposite (Anderson & Pease, 1981). Low-skill children need more positive reinforcement to develop self-esteem than do high-skill children. Many athletes drop out of sports because coaches tell them that they are not good enough to compete (Dulberg, 1995). Common situations include sitting on the bench, making the game-losing error, or being cut from the team. The psychological and emotional scars that occur can be carried for life and affect sports participation in adulthood.

When sports injuries occur, they are usually the result of disregard for proper protection of vulnerable anatomy, growth and developmental needs, or psychological or social sensitivity. Injuries are an unwanted side effect of sports participation that may be reduced by ensuring that sports are age appropriate and the young athlete is responding positively to the training methods and competition (Backx, 1996). Young athletes, parents, coaches, school systems, communities, and trainers should minimize risks by following the recommendations for safe participation (Rome, 1995).

NURSING DIAGNOSIS AND OUTCOME DETERMINATION

The nursing diagnoses that describe concerns of the young athlete are Health-Seeking Behaviors, Knowledge Deficit, and Risk for Injury (North American Nursing Diagnosis Association, 1999). The most relevant outcomes from the Nursing Outcomes Classification are Knowledge: Health Behaviors, Knowledge: Prescribed Activity, Endurance, Muscle Function, Nutritional Status: Body Mass, Nutritional Status: Energy Conservation, and Knowledge: Personal Safety (Iowa Outcomes Project, 2000).

Healthy young athletes are continually striving for better physical and mental condition to enhance their performance. Health-Seeking Behaviors are demonstrated when a young athlete expresses the desire to improve physical attributes or psychological constructs relating to sports participation. Once the young athlete gains the knowledge of how to improve these physical and psychological factors, he or she will be able to describe practices that will promote optimal performance.

The nursing diagnosis Knowledge Deficit can be present when the young athlete exhibits poor training methods, inadequate skills, improper performance techniques, and frequent injuries. These deficits are often the result of lack of knowledge on the part of those involved with teaching

582 PRIMARY CARE HEALTH PROMOTION

or supervising the young athlete. With comprehensive instruction and proper training, the athlete should demonstrate the ability to attain and maintain optimal athletic health.

As the physical, psychological, and social demands on a young athlete increase, so does the risk for injury. Factors related to the athlete's physical, psychological, and social readiness should be determined prior to designing interventions, including level of physical fitness and skill, past patterns of health care, knowledge of proper training methods, intellect, psychological stability, self-esteem, motivation, emotional state, ability to interact socially, and the status of social support systems. As the potential risks are identified, the young athlete needs to be taught to determine factors that may cause injury in the future, how to recognize the early signs of injury and overuse, how to seek proper treatment, and how to participate safely.

INTERVENTION: ATHLETE HEALTH PROMOTION

This intervention is designed to enhance physical skills, to promote growth, development, and psychological well-being, and to create positive social interaction and support. This intervention also should prepare the young person for the anticipated athletic stresses, metabolic demands, and injury risks. Once successful, young athletes should be empowered to maintain and improve their personal level of athletic health throughout their years of participation. Activities that relate to health-seeking behaviors and knowledge deficits will reduce the risk for injury. They should be designed to maintain and improve physical attributes, enhance psychological construct, and encourage positive social interaction and support while preventing physical, psychological, and social injuries. The components of physical fitness that require appropriate training processes to maintain and improve athlete health are flexibility, cardiorespiratory endurance, muscular strength and endurance, and neuromuscular skill.

A musculoskeletal flexibility program accompanies all types of training and is almost always required during the rehabilitation of sports injuries. Realistic goals for improving flexibility should be established for each athlete based on current flexibility. The need to stretch is greater for those with less flexibility. Basic flexibility exercises should be included in both the warm-up and the cool-down phases of each exercise session. Proper form and technique should be required while following the principles for safe stretching (Smith, 1997):

- Warm up muscles prior to stretching.
- Hold each stretch for approximately 30 seconds.

- Perform slow, gradual stretches to end range of motion but not to pain.
- Repeat each stretch three times for maximal benefit.

The beginning cardiorespiratory or aerobic training level depends on the athlete's current level of physical fitness as indicated by preprogram testing. Realistic goals should be established on an individual basis. Durnstine et al. (1993) noted that although prepubescent athletes respond differently to exercise than do adults, the only limitations are low economy of locomotion and poor tolerance for extremes of climate. Endurance training programs for the prepubescent athlete should be goal oriented as demanded by the sport. Increases in the training intensity, duration, and frequency should be no more than 10% per week. Short-term, intermittent sessions with a high recreational component are preferred over long-duration training sessions with high intensity. As long as the child enjoys the activity and is not showing symptoms of overtraining or boredom, participation in the endurance activity should be safe (AAP, 1990). Signs of overtraining include poor appetite, weight loss, poor sleep, increased thirst, mood swings, depressed immune system, amenorrhea in females, increased morning heart rate, positive orthostatic pulse, increased effort with submaximal exercise, poor performance, muscle soreness, and susceptibility to injury (Scott, 1997). Endurance training and competition in extreme heat or cold should be avoided.

Endurance training for enhancing performance and preventing injury should include training that is sport specific and graduated and progressive in frequency, intensity, and duration (Ratliff, 1990). It should also provide time for recovery, variety, and individuality (Kibler & Chandler, 1994). The focus of the training is to develop maximal aerobic power, a higher lactate threshold, and better energy economy. Little is known about the safety of training at these levels for prepubescent children, but experts agree that the principles of adult endurance training are applicable to children. Limits should be placed on volume of training and competition, however. The following are activities for safe aerobic training: (a) obtain medical clearance to participate in aerobic activities; (b) warm-up, cool-down, and stretch appropriately before and after each training session and performance; (c) increase stress gradually—combined changes in intensity, duration, and frequency should be no more than 10% per week; (d) limit mileage for prepubescent runners to 14 to 30 miles per week; (e) match sports performance goals and training procedures; (f) include a high recreational component and positive and enjoyable experiences to the endurance training routine; (g) emphasize proper running form, increasing the efficiency of motion; (h) use cross-training methods (such as swimming, biking, or rollerblading) for at least 20% to 30% of training time when duration and frequency of training are being increased; (i) require proper footwear and suitable running surfaces; and (j) avoid running in extremes of climate.

A well-designed resistance training program will prepare the young athlete physically and mentally for a higher level of sports performance. Significant strength gains occur when methods are individually selected, dependent on preprogram testing results, and they progress in intensity, duration, and frequency. The most important consideration during strength training in the young athlete is the potential for injury to growing tissues.

Recommendations for safe and effective strength training sessions are listed in Table 35.1. These recommendations were formulated from early research results and practical experience to help prevent significant musculoskeletal injury and to provide for safe, effective, and enjoyable strength training sessions.

Neuromuscular training programs are designed to develop motor skills, beginning with fundamental movement skills, incorporating transitional skills, and finally adding and refining complex skills. The training techniques are the most challenging and often the most entertaining of all training methods. Speed, acceleration, quickness, agility, and balance are a few of the skills improved with neuromuscular training. These factors are important when the body has to react quickly during competition. Basic aerobic and anaerobic power and especially the "power zone" located between the chest and the top of the knees (Phelps, 1992) must be developed by adequate cardiorespiratory and strength training prior to beginning neuromuscular training. The initial neuromuscular training level depends on each athlete's motor skill development as determined by preprogram testing. Neuromuscular training techniques are then incorporated into conditioning and technique training days. Strict attention is placed on proper form and execution of the drills. The training methods are entertaining and challenging, including plyometric (power and explosiveness), plyoquicknic (speed and quickness), and combos (combinations of power and speed). Activities include bounding, jumping, hopping, skipping, kicking, and throwing. Neuromuscular training is an effective way to build motor skills beginning as early as 5 or 6 years of age, when programming should incorporate simple postural and fundamental activities that are advanced as children master each skill. Adolescent athletes should also be exposed to neuromuscular training techniques because they are entertaining and challenging, and improvements in performance are quickly realized.

The optimal training for many sports includes a combination of cardiorespiratory endurance, muscular strength and endurance, and neuromuscular training methods designed to improve each fitness component at the appropriate time. Fitness intervals begin at the athlete's current level of fitness and advance to competition level in a predetermined

TABLE 35.1   Recommendations for Strength Training for Children and Adolescents

1. Preparticipation evaluation should be performed by physician or nurse practitioner knowledgeable in sports medicine. Preclude physical and medical conditions from participation as necessary.

2. Choose good quality, durable, stable, and safe equipment suitable to the size, age, and maturity of the athletes.

3. Appropriate warm-up before and cool-down period after the strength training with appropriate stretching exercises should be performed.

4. Select sports-specific exercises appropriate to the level of physical and emotional maturity of the participant.

5. Attention to instruction and supervision of proper technique should be provided by a well-trained adult. Lift with slow, controlled, smooth technique through full range of motion to allow for maximum muscle development and maintenance of flexibility. Exhale while lifting to avoid Valsalva maneuver and control breathing pattern to avoid hyperventilation. Avoid back hyperextension and excessive muscle fatigue.

6. Avoid maximal and near maximal lifts (e.g., clean and jerk, squat lift, and dead lift) until skeletal maturity is reached (Tanner Stage 5).

7. Train all major muscle groups and both flexors and extensors. Place emphasis on dynamic concentric contractions, and avoid eccentric overload exercises until skeletal maturity. Balance routine with upper and lower body exercises and pushing and pulling maneuvers. Place emphasis on sets of high repetitions with low resistance for prepubescent youth.

8. Sample program for *prepubertal child:* The child may perform 15 to 20 repetitions, one or two sets, for two 20-minute sessions per week. Increase weights in 1- to 3-pound increments. Sample program for *postpubertal youth:* The child may perform 8 to 10 repetitions, three sets, in three or four sessions per week lasting 30 to 60 minutes.

9. Individualize the training program. Balance routine with upper and lower body exercises and pushing and pulling maneuvers. Vary the training modalities (e.g., free weights, machines, resistance bands or cords, balls, and springs).

10. Competition, in addition to weight lifting, power lifting, and bodybuilding, should be prohibited until skeletal maturity is reached. Discourage intraindividual competition.

SOURCE: Summary of recommendations by Harris (1997), Blimkie and Bar-Or (1996), Alberta (1993), Metcalf and Roberts (1993), IDEA (1990), and Cahill (1988).

amount of time, usually in 12 to 16 weeks. Tables 35.2 and 35.3 are examples of a general fitness interval and an athletic fitness interval designed by Deanna Langford, CPT (personal communication, October 1, 1997) for a prepubescent female soccer player. Daily training activities include flexibility, cardiorespiratory, strength, and motor development arranged in a sequence that is age appropriate and follows the principles of periodization. Periodization is a training plan based on the manipulation of intensity, volume, and duration of workload in which an athlete engages during various periods of the athletic season—that is, preseason, during the season, and off-season (Kibler & Chandler, 1994). When athletes are involved in sports year-round, periodization training will be the most suc-

TABLE 35.2   General Physical Fitness Interval (Foundation)

Goal	To increase general fitness, develop a greater work capacity, and prepare the body for sport-specific training interval
Frequency	3 to 5 days per week, 20 to 45 minutes per session
Rest	48 to 72 hours between sessions, depending on intensity of training; aerobic workout requires active rest from regular activities; cross-training used
Intensity	Progressive increase in energy expenditure, 5% to 10% per week; minimal concern for exercise intensity; increase volume and duration; use circuit training

	Monday	*Tuesday*	*Wednesday*	*Thursday*	*Friday*
Weeks 1 and 2	Run/walk	Swim	Run/walk	Cycle	Run/walk
	1 mile	30 minutes	1 mile	3/5 mile	1 mile
	Core[a]	Body weight[b]		Core	Body weight
Weeks 3 and 4	Run	Run/walk	Tennis/B-ball	Run	Run/walk
	½ mile	1½ mile		½ mile	1½ mile
	Core	Body weight		Core	Body weight
Weeks 5 and 6	Run	Roller blade	Run	Aerobics	Run
	1 mile		1 mile		1 mile
	Core	Body weight	Core	Body weight	Core
Weeks 7 and 8	Run	Run	Swim/baseball	Run	Cycle
	½ mile	1 mile		½ mile	

NOTE: A 10- to 15-minute warm-up and cool-down period should be incorporated into each flexibility drill.

a. Trunk strengthening exercises that include abdominal crunches, reverse crunches, lunges, step-ups, trunk twists, wall squats, and ball squats; 4 or 5 exercises are chosen for each session to work a variety of muscles. The number of repetitions depends on the ability to perform the exercise with good form. Increasing the volume will improve work capacity.

b. Extremity strengthening exercises using the weight of the body as resistance, including push-ups, chin-ups, triceps dips, ball squats, and toe raises.

cessful way to enhance performance and prevent injuries. Proper nutrition, adequate rest, and ample fluids are vital elements in all athletic fitness training programs.

Activities that enhance performance and prevent injury should provide a positive and enjoyable experience and include the following: (a) offer positive reinforcement for skill attainment, hard work, and team play; (b) minimize competition when working on skills and for children 6 to 10 years of age; (c) ensure that all tasks and challenges are age appropriate and provide opportunity for success whenever possible; (d) allow ample participation for all members of the team; (e) promote healthy social interaction; (f) restrict antisocial, overly aggressive, and demeaning behavior; and (g) enthusiastically recruit the support of family and friends.

Throughout the Athlete Health Promotion intervention, recommendations for prevention of sports-related injury are emphasized. Even when all the proper preventive measures are taken, however, injuries still occur. Early detection and proper treatment can lessen the severity and disability of injuries. Early signs of significant injury that require assessment and treatment include pain with activity that is present the next day,

TABLE 35.3   Sports Fitness Training Interval

Goal	To develop sport-specific energy systems, cardiorespiratory endurance, strength, speed, ability, quickness, proper technique, and execution of sports movement
Frequency	3 to 5 days per week, 20 to 45 minutes per session
Rest	24 to 48 hours of rest between exercises and workout sessions; sports-specific nutrition and fluid intake required; incorporate light free exercise, relaxation, stretching, walking, and games
Intensity	Combination of general and specific training; aerobic/speed, strength/power, stability/agility; intensity will increase as work capacity demand increases

	Monday	*Tuesday*	*Wednesday*	*Thursday*	*Friday*
Weeks 1 and 2	Interval running[a] 1 mile	Cross-training	Running ½ mile	Interval running 1 Mile	Cross-training
	Core body weight	Balance stability[b]	Core body weight	Balance stability	Core body weight
Weeks 3 and 4	Continuous running	Cross-training	Speed training	Interval running	Cross-training
	Sports movement training[c]		Strength circuit	Sports movement training	Strength circuit
	Speed training		Pattern running		
Weeks 5 through 8	Interval sports movement training	Speed strength circuit	Cross-training	Speed sports movement	Internal strength circuit

NOTE: All workouts start with a 10- to 20-minute warm-up period. General and sports-specific flexibility exercises are included in every session. Examples of sports-specific flexibility exercises are hip flexion/extension swing, straight leg flexion/extension swing, straight leg abduction/abduction swing, torso twist with ankle pivot, and shoulder swing crossing the midline. Sports movements are slowly performed, gradually increasing the intensity during the remainder of the warm-up.

a. Distance running is combined with sprinting, 3 minutes running—40-m sprint, 3 minutes running—60-m sprint, 3 minutes running—100-m sprint.

b. For example, a series of drills on a line or tape while concentrating on balance and control. Perform single leg stand, one leg squat, and hold for 5 seconds.

limping, inability to complete the training plan, symptoms of overtraining, and the need for pain medication on a regular basis or to get through a competition. Prompt assessment by a physician or nurse practitioner knowledgeable in sport medicine is warranted for these signs.

The first phase of treatment will usually follow the principals of RICE (rest, ice, compression, and elevation) so that pain will be decreased and the inflammatory response will be limited (Arnheim & Prentice, 1993). The second phase of treatment involves stretching to improve range of motion (ROM), progressing to strengthening when ROM is full and pain free. The third phase of treatment involves attempting sport-specific movements in a functional progression (gradually increasing in difficulty) to carefully prepare the athlete for return to play. Once the athlete returns to play, the area must be protected by bracing or taping until strength and stability are 100% or normal. Return to play is not recommended if strength and stability are less than 85%, if limping occurs, or if the young athlete cannot perform the functional progression skills without pain. Volume is often limited for the first few days or weeks after returning to play. Parents should be made aware of the early signs of injury and where to seek appropriate treatment for sports-related injuries.

Outcomes

Monitoring the outcomes of the physical training and psychosocial activities should occur every 3 or 4 months or at the end of each training interval. Assessment methods used prior to the program should be used again and differences noted. Desired outcomes should be identified and deficiencies resolved before the next training interval begins. Training activities should be reviewed with athletes and their families, and modifications should be made that will encourage continuation of the performance-enhancing activities.

INTERVENTION APPLICATION

In the 1994 and 1995 school year, a winter conditioning program was designed for adolescent student athletes at a private secondary academy. The program was designed by a CPT, a youth fitness specialist, a pediatric sports medicine physician, and a pediatric nurse practitioner. The program instruction was provided by a CPT and a certified athletic trainer or a strength and conditioning assistant for 5 days a week, 2 hours per day, for a period of 12 weeks. Forty-nine students voluntarily participated in the performance enhancement program as one of many selections offered on campus for winter conditioning.

Preprogram assessment included physical fitness testing and preprogram student questionnaire. Physical fitness testing was labor intensive and not very popular with the students; the results were valuable, however. Results of the preprogram testing showed that 93.3% of the students were in the healthy fitness zone for cardiorespiratory endurance at the beginning of the program. This result reflected favorable on the physical fitness curriculum of the academy and allowed performance-enhancement training to begin immediately. In addition, 94% of the students tested scored in the healthy fitness zone for percentage body fat, and 97% scored in the healthy fitness zone for abdominal strength. Any student who did not score in the healthy fitness zone was considered to be At Risk for Injury. Significant weaknesses were also detected: 43% had lower body flexibility scores below the healthy fitness zone, and 43.7% scored below the healthy fitness zone for upper body strength. This reflected the underde-

velopment of balance among abdominal, trunk, and upper body muscula-
ture. A confidential questionnaire served to determine fitness goals, current fitness habits, and interest areas for each student.

After pretesting was completed, the coeducational program to enhance athletic performance and maintain general fitness began. Training
methods included generalized and advanced flexibility techniques, neuromuscular facilitation, and sports movement techniques such as proprio-
ception (balance), speed, agility, and quickness. These techniques were
taught using drills and team competitions with equipment such as agility
ladders, cones, minihurdles, various types and sizes of balls, and bean
bags. Obstacle courses, station activities, and line activities were well received by the participants.

Strength training was included in the program. Trunk (core) strength
was emphasized throughout the program because it is fundamental to all
athletic movement and performance and aids in the prevention of back injuries. Extremity strengthening began once core strength was sufficient,
and many hours were spent in the weight room focusing on proper lifting
technique and form with minimal weight resistance. Weights were gradually increased on an individual basis under careful supervision. All the
training techniques were modified to meet the various fitness levels of students.

Although the program went well, some of the situational barriers
were significant and were difficult to overcome. The school had only one
small weight room, one set of free weights, and one circuit of nautilus
equipment. Students had to wait to use the equipment instead of continuously moving through their workout. Aerobic endurance training was
also limited by the lack of space, and many of the speed agility and quickness drills had to be performed and practiced one at a time instead of simultaneously. This led to boredom and provided less individual training
time. The school agreed to improve these factors prior to the next program session.

At the end of the 12-week program, students were retested using the
same fitness testing battery and a postprogram questionnaire. Remark-
ably, 62% of the students showed improvement in lower body flexibility,
and 40% showed improvement in abdominal and upper extremity
strength. A perceived overall improvement in these fitness components
was verbalized by the students and was reflected on the postprogram
questionnaire. The students expressed marked improvement in their own
athletic performance and self-confidence. Teachers and coaches also offered positive comments and a genuine interest in continuing the program. This program served as a model for future athlete health promotion
programs designed to enhance performance and prevent injuries.

RESEARCH AND PRACTICE IMPLICATIONS

Longitudinal research studies involving pediatric athletes need to be conducted to examine the effects of childhood participation in athletes. The objective of research would be to discover the best methods to prepare the youth for athletic stresses, metabolic demands, and injury risks that occur with each sport while promoting growth and development, enhancing psychological well-being, and creating positive social interactions. Efforts can be made to define and test the training methods and injury prevention methods to determine those that are most effective. The resulting data need to be shared with coaches, parents, and health care professionals. Conservative and sensible guidelines for performance, age-appropriate training techniques, proper nutrition, adequate hydration, and rest must be established and included in all youth training programs.

Uniform methods of reporting and treating sports-related injuries will provide the data necessary to establish a more reliable indicator of the risk of sports participation. Health care professionals, especially office and school nurses, need to be more knowledgeable about safe sports participation and be prepared to offer advice to young athletes and their parents about the most effective methods to enhance performance and prevent injuries. The large number of athletes who are injured every year can be reduced. Nurses must play a major role in that reduction.

REFERENCES

Alberta, F. G. (1993). Strength training vs. "pumping iron." *Contemporary Pediatrics, 18,* 36-52.

American Academy of Pediatrics. (1990). Risks in distance running for children. *Pediatrics, 86*(5), 799-800.

American Alliance for Health, Physical Education, Recreation, and Dance. (1988). *The AAHPERD physical best program.* Reston, VA: Author.

Anderson, D. F., & Pease, D. F. (1981). Children's motor and social skills and attitudes toward sport team involvement. *Journal of Sport Behavior, 4*(3), 128-136.

Arnheim, D. D., & Prentice, W. E. (1993). *Principals of athletic training* (8th ed.). St. Louis, MO: Mosby-Year Book.

Backx, F. J. (1996). Epidemiology of pediatric sports-related injuries. In O. Bar-Or (Ed.), *The child and adolescent athlete* (pp. 163-172). Champaign, IL: Human Kinetics.

Bijur, P. E., Trumble, A., Harel, Y., Overpeck, M. D., Jones, D., & Scheidt, P. C. (1995). Sports and recreation injuries in U.S. children and adolescents. *Archives of Adolescent Medicine, 149*(9), 1009-1016.

Blimkie, C. J., & Bar-Or, O. (1996). Trainableness of muscle strength, power and endurance during childhood. In O. Bar-Or (Ed.), *The child and adolescent athlete* (pp. 113-129). Champaign, IL: Human Kinetics.

Burgess-Milliron, M. J., & Murphy, S. B. (1996). Biomechanical considerations of youth sports injuries. In O. Bar-Or (Ed.), *The child and adolescent athlete* (pp. 173-188). Champaign, IL: Human Kinetics.

Cahill, B. R. (Ed.). (1988). *Proceedings of the conference on strength training and the prepubescent*. Chicago: American Orthopedic Society for Sports Medicine.

Dulberg, H. (1995). Emotional injuries in youth sports. *Sidelines, 4*(2), 1-4.

Durnstine, J. L., King, A. C., Painter, P. L., Roitman, J. L., Swiren, L. D., & Kenney, W. D. (Eds.). (1993). *American College of Sports Medicines: Resource manual for guidelines for exercise testing and prescription* (2nd ed.). Philadelphia: Lea & Febiger.

Dyment, P. G. (1990). Neurodevelopmental milestone: When is a child ready for sports participation? In J. A. Sullivan & W. A. Grana (Eds.), *The pediatric athlete* (pp. 27-29). Park Ridge, IL: American Academy of Orthopedic Surgeons.

Gallahue, D. L., & Ozmun, J. C. (1989). *Understanding motor development* (3rd ed.). Madison, WI: Brown & Benchmark.

Harris, S. S. (1997). Strength training for children and adolescents. In R. E. Sallis & F. Massimino (Eds.), *Essentials of sports medicine* (pp. 504-508). St. Louis, MO: C. V. Mosby.

IDEA: The Association for Fitness Professionals. (1990). *Children and teens*. San Diego, CA: Author.

Institute for Aerobics Research. (1987). *FITNESSGRAM user's manual*. Dallas, TX: Author.

Iowa Outcomes Project. (2000). *Nursing outcomes classification (NOC)* (M. Johnson, M. Maas, & S. Moorhead, Eds.; 2nd ed.). St. Louis, MO: Mosby-Year Book.

Johnson, C. (1988). Are we really going in the right direction? *Athletic Coach, 22,* 17-20.

Kibler, W. B., & Chandler, T. J. (1994). Sport-specific conditioning. *American Journal of Sports Medicine, 22*(3), 424-432.

Landry, G. L. (1992). Sports injuries in childhood. *Pediatric Annals, 21*(3), 165-168.

Malina, R. M., & Beunen, G. (1996). Matching opponents in youth sports. In O. Bar-Or (Ed.), *The child and adolescent athlete* (pp. 202-213). Champaign, IL: Human Kinetics.

Metcalf, J. A., & Roberts, S. O. (1993). Strength training and the immature athlete: An overview. *Pediatric Nursing, 19*(4), 325-332.

National Safe Kids Campaign. (1996). *Fact sheet-promoting sports safety. A program of Children's National Medical Center.* Washington, DC: Author.

Nelson, M. A., & Goldberg, B. (1991). Developmental skills and children's sports. *The Physician and Sports Medicine, 19*(2), 67-79.

Nichols, B. (1994). *Moving and learning: The elementary school physical education experience* (3rd ed.). St. Louis, MO: C. V. Mosby.

North American Nursing Diagnosis Association. (1999). *Nursing diagnoses: Definitions and classification 1999-2000*. Philadelphia: Author.

Pate, R. R., & Ward, D. S. (1996). Endurance trainableness of children and youths. In O. Bar-Or (Ed.), *The child and adolescent athlete* (pp. 130-137). Champaign, IL: Human Kinetics.

Petlichkoff, C. M. (1996). The drop-out dilemma in youth sports. In O. Bar-Or (Ed.), *The child and adolescent athlete* (pp. 418-430). Champaign, IL: Human Kinetics.

Phelps, S. M. (1992). *Plyometrics and the high school athlete. A training guide to developing an explosive high school program.* North Valley: Author.

Ratliff, R. A. (1990). Endurance training of the pediatric athlete. In J. A. Sullivan & W. A. Grana (Eds.), *The pediatric athlete* (pp. 7-15). Park Ridge, IL: American Academy of Orthopedic Surgeons.

Roberts, G. C. (Ed.). (1992). *Motivation in sport and exercise.* Champaign, IL: Human Kinetics.

Rome, E. S. (1995). Sports-related injuries among adolescents: When do they occur, and how can we prevent them? *Pediatrics in Review, 16*(5), 184-187.

Safrit, M. J. (1995). *Complete guide to youth fitness testing.* Champaign, IL: Human Kinetics.

Scott, W. A. (1997). Overuse injuries. In R. E. Sallis & F. Massimino (Eds.), *Essentials of sports medicine* (pp. 517-527). St. Louis, MO: C. V. Mosby.

Sharkey, B. J. (1990). Neuromuscular training. In J. A. Sullivan & W. A. Grana (Eds.), *The pediatric athlete* (pp. 21-26). Park Ridge, IL: American Academy of Orthopedic Surgeons.

Smith, A. D. (1997). Musculoskeletal injuries unique to growing children and adolescents. In R. E. Sallis & F. Massimino (Eds.), *Essentials of sports medicine* (pp. 495-498). St. Louis, MO: C. V. Mosby.

Smith, M. L., & Mitchell, J. H. (1993). Cardiorespiratory adaptation to exercise training. In J. L. Durnstein, A. C. King, P. L. Painter, J. L. Roitman, L. D. Swiren, & W. D. Kenney (Eds.), *American College of Sports Medicines: Resource manual for guidelines for exercise testing and prescription* (2nd ed., pp. 75-81). Philadelphia: Lea & Febiger.

Tanner, S. M. (1997). Growth and developmental concerns for prepubescent and adolescent athletes. In R. E. Sallis & F. Massimino (Eds.), *Essentials of sports medicine* (pp. 218-225). St. Louis, MO: C. V. Mosby.

U.S. Department of Health and Human Services. (1991). *Healthy people 2000: National health promotion and disease prevention objectives* (DHHS Publication No. PHS 91-50312). Washington, DC: Government Printing Office.

36

Self-Esteem Enhancement

Shelley-Rae Pehler

Self-esteem can be defined as perceived self-worth. It is the evaluative dimension of self-concept. Self-esteem evolves through lifelong experiences as a learned phenomenon (Sieving & Zirbel-Donisch, 1990). Self-esteem is an integral part of health (Overbay & Purath, 1997; Pastore, Fisher, & Friedman, 1996; Torres & Fernandez, 1995). A lowered self-esteem has been associated with increased risk for the major health concerns of depression, drug abuse, teenage pregnancy, and tobacco use (Amos, Gray, Currie, & Elton, 1997; Lesser & Escoto-Lloyd, 1999; Wasson & Anderson, 1995). These health concerns are targeted in the *Healthy People 2000* objectives (U.S. Department of Health and Human Services, 1991). The three leading causes of death in the adolescent age group are unintentional injuries (motor vehicle accidents account for three fourths of the injuries in this category), homicide, and suicide. Alcohol and drug use has been linked as a contributing factor in many accidents and homicides (p. 17). A positive self-esteem has been shown to increase school performance, protect against gang involvement, and improve job productivity (Filozof et al., 1998; Willoughby, Polatajko, & Wilson, 1995). As Youngs (1991) noted, children's actions stem from what they believe about themselves and influence how they treat themselves and other people through-out their lives.

THEORETICAL FRAMEWORK

William James (1890/1981), a nineteenth-century psychologist, discussed three possible influences of self-esteem development. The first influence was whether or not individuals meet their personal goals. Individuals who were able to achieve their dreams held high self-esteem. Individuals who are unable to reach their goals are more likely to have low self-esteem. James called his second influence the "social self." An individual's social self weighs self-worth against one's perception of others. By nature, humans constantly compare themselves with others. When making a comparison of oneself to others, judgment of self-worth is based on perceived successes or failures. James's third influence on self-esteem is the "extended self." The extended self is concerned with outer images, such as body, clothes, house, job, bank accounts, or significant others. Self-esteem is higher if matters that concern the extended self are close to personal expectations.

Mead (1962) extended James's definition of social self to describe how self-esteem develops. Children internalize the criteria of those around them as their gauge of self-worth. Children use these criteria to judge themselves as they grow, using them to determine their own self-worth. If children have parents who treat them with respect and concern, they will grow into adults who have respect and concern for themselves and others. If children are continually told they are no good or second-rate, they will develop a low self-esteem that will show itself in their treatment of others. The significance of Mead's theory is that an individual's self-esteem is influenced by the treatment of significant others.

Sullivan (1953) also emphasized the importance of the social origins of self-esteem. He believed that experiences that a child has with parents and siblings lay the foundation of a child's self-worth. Sullivan also introduced the concept of defense mechanisms. Defense mechanisms are used by individuals to avoid loss of self-esteem. The development of defense mechanisms lies in a child's early experiences in the family. Mayberry's (1990) study of children with disabilities supported Sullivan's concept of defense mechanisms. Mayberry found that children became defensive when rating their self-esteem, especially in their areas of disability.

Alfred Adler (Ansbacher & Ansbacher, 1956) examined the social self and took James's theory one step further in describing how low self-esteem is developed. Adler placed importance on the actual weaknesses of the child. He found that children's feelings of inadequacy and insufficiency are related to children's actual impairments, such as being smaller in size than their peers, not as athletic, or not as intelligent. These actual impairments, or "organ inferiorities" as Adler called them, have a significant effect on children because these are things that cannot be changed by the children. The support of parents, siblings, and friends, however, can make a difference concerning whether or not a child will have low or high self-esteem. Adler warns, however, that overindulgence of this support can cause a child to have an unrealistic, inflated value of his or her worth. Such a child will likely be self-centered, demanding, and have a difficult time with social relationships.

Coopersmith (1967) did an extensive study regarding the antecedents of self-esteem. In this study, he examined how self-esteem is affected by social background, parental characteristics, and parent-child relationships. He also took into consideration the individual's own characteristics, early history, and experiences. Coopersmith found that parents who provided clear and consistent rules, appropriate punishments, and accepted children for their unique strengths were more likely to raise children with high self-esteem than were parents who were more open and permissive. He also found that family environments with structure provide boundaries that children need to determine whether or not they have reached a goal. These children then learned to trust their judgment and interpretations of events and consequences.

In addition, Coopersmith (1967) found that parental respect and self-esteem were antecedents that influenced a child's self-esteem. Coopersmith believed that these two antecedents were important because parents modeled these behaviors to their children. Parents with high self-esteem are more likely to treat their children with respect and show acceptance. These parents are decisive and lead active personal lives. Such parental characteristics and behaviors were influential in developing similar characteristics, resulting in high self-esteem for their children. Bowles and Fallon's (1996) replication study confirmed their previous study that showed a relationship between family functioning and self-concept. The study compared 35 male and 28 female adolescents who sought help for school or family problems with those adolescents who did not seek help. Higher levels of intimacy and a democratic parenting style were associated with higher scores on self-concept dimensions and correlated with those adolescents seeking help. In families with higher levels of conflict, the adolescents' self-concept scores were lower, and they were less likely to seek assistance. Coopersmith also integrated the defense mechanisms proposed by Sullivan. When an individual's self-esteem is threatened, that person becomes uncertain of the ability to handle the threat. This creates anxiety and raises doubts concerning his or her capabilities. Conversely, people with high self-esteem feel more confident, powerful, and able to handle the threat.

The first three antecedents are success, power, and the value that the child places on his or her goals. An individual must feel accomplishments in tasks that the individual values, and the individual must believe that he or she has the capability and capacity to achieve goals. Nurses must identify a child's personal goals and the value placed on these goals. Sometimes, a child's goals are unrealistic; in these cases, nurses can influence a child's self-esteem by lowering these goals to a more realistic and achievable level. By agreeing on incremental goals, the self-esteem of the child can improve through the success in accomplishing each of the smaller goals. Nurses can give rewards and realistic praise as a child achieves the goals, further reinforcing the child's ability to be successful.

Nurses can provide experiences that increase a child's autonomy and feelings of success. This is especially true for children who are physical by nature. It is important to help children maintain their physical mobility and autonomy in basic activities of daily living. This can be accomplished by using the least restrictive devices for maintaining an intravenous site or ensuring that the intravenous pole has wheels. Nurses in a community setting can assist parents to adapt the physical layout of the home to accommodate wheelchairs, walkers, and crutches. Simple rearrangement of furniture for easier mobility can go a long way in helping a child feel more independent.

In a health promotion setting, nurses can influence the self-esteem of a developing child in the areas of goal accomplishments and power. Teaching parents about the child's ever-increasing need for independence and autonomy and how they can encourage this growth becomes an important tool for the nurse to indirectly influence the child's self-esteem. Working with parents to create an environment that provides structure, realistic expectations for each developmental level, and realistic praise and encouragement affects a child's lifelong feelings of self-worth.

Sometimes, parents have unrealistic expectations for their child. These situations cause the child to believe that parental expectations can never be met. These children have lower self-esteem because success cannot be achieved. In these situations, the parents may withhold love and affection or belittle the child because the child was not able to do what the parents expected. Teaching the parents about normal growth and development can give the parents a more realistic expectation of their children's achievements. In situations in which a child has an educational or physical handicap, parents may need to redefine their expectations for the child based on the child's abilities, despite the handicap. Helping the parents and the child identify other strengths, such as the child's inherent friendliness, warm smile, or compassion toward others, begins the process of redefining successes and the value placed on these successes. Parents, teachers, and health care professionals must refrain from negatively criticizing or teasing children. When these people convey confidence to a child that realistic goals can be accomplished, the child will receive the message that he or she is valued. Increased confidence affects goal achievement, thereby increasing self-esteem.

Showing interest in and supporting things that are important to the child also increases the child's self-esteem and feelings of self-worth. When Nintendo was first introduced, it was used as a diversional activity in the hospital unit. Most nurses did not know anything about the machine or how to play the games. Nurses would ask the children to explain the games and their strategies for winning. This attention gave the children the message that the nurses were interested in them. These simple strategies took less than 5 minutes of time but allowed the children to feel valued. It was also an opportunity for the children to share their talents and accomplishments.

Positive, supportive relationships are the third antecedent necessary for the development of positive self-esteem. Nurses become instrumental in helping parents recognize parenting styles that are supportive but that set firm and fair limits for their children (Killeen, 1993). Coopersmith's (1967) research showed that children with well-defined limits had higher self-esteem than children who had parents who were more lenient. Children must feel love and acceptance from others before they can love and accept themselves (Filozof et al., 1998; Sweeting & West, 1995). Love and acceptance are conveyed when parents and significant others spend time with the child. Taking time to read a book, play a game, or go for a walk all convey the message that the child is worthy. Physical contact is also important for children. As children grow older and avoid touching, parents should still place a hand on their shoulder, give a pat on their back, or give them a wink. These forms of communication convey to children that their parents feel they are worthy and loved.

Children need reliable significant others. Meisenhelder (1985) defined *significant others* as "those with high-contact, intimate, long-term relationships" (p. 131). Nurses, both in the hospital and in the community setting, can be significant others for children and affect their self-esteem (Miller, 1987). School and parish nurses have ongoing relationships with the children they see and can influence the development of self-esteem. Meisenhelder defined three ways that nurses as significant others can influence self-esteem. First, the nurse must establish a trusting, credible relationship with a child. Behaviors basic to self-esteem enhancement include genuine warmth, acceptance of the child, and respect for the child's uniqueness and rights (Norris, 1992). Within this relationship, the nurse can then provide verbal feedback on tasks that the child strives to accomplish. A child who needs to learn skills in self-care or specific skills necessary to manage an illness will benefit from verbal feedback. Such responses provide positive appraisals to increase self-esteem.

The second way in which Meisenhelder (1985) identified that significant others are helpful is that they help the person identify positive aspects of himself or herself that may go unrecognized. Providing and encouraging positive appraisals of the child's cognitive, emotional, and spiritual aspects can help the child understand that physical limitations are only a small part of his or her's identity.

Meisenhelder's (1985) third activity is the use of nonverbal reflected appraisals that are very powerful in influencing self-esteem. Facial expressions, body language, and voice tone reflect the nurse's attitude toward the child's worth and value. Taking the time to listen to children's concerns and acknowledging their feelings as legitimate and valid reinforces to children their self-worth.

Meisenhelder (1985) suggested strategies for nurses in acute care settings who only see a child for a short period of time. Reinforcing the attention that the child may be receiving from family and friends indicates to the child that he or she has worth within the circle of significant others. Encouraging parents, siblings, and friends to visit or stay with the child overnight or making them feel welcomed by providing extra chairs and a drink not only reinforces the relationship between the child and significant others but also is important for the child's self-esteem (Miller, 1987).

The final theoretical contribution to self-esteem is the development of defense mechanisms that children use to protect themselves from lowered self-esteem. This is important because those with low self-esteem often present themselves as overconfident and controlling. They show interest in self only and attempt to escape a threatening situation or deal with it by picking fights (Adler as cited in Ansbacher & Ansbacher, 1956). Individuals use these defensive mechanisms to protect themselves from the fear of failure and resultant lowered self-esteem. An erroneous initial assessment might indicate a positive self-esteem rather than a lowered self-esteem. Nurses frequently see these behaviors in acute care and community settings and must be aware of the underlying lowered self-esteem to be effective in working with the child. Interventions must support the child in accepting new challenges, praise and reward progress toward reaching goals, and support the child in accepting dependence on others as appropriate.

INTERVENTION APPLICATION

Adam is a 9-year-old boy in the third grade. He was recently diagnosed with an attention-deficit hyperactivity disorder with an associated learning disability. He took Ritalin twice a day and started a behavior management program for his frequent outbursts and inability to get along with other children. Adam was approximately 20 pounds overweight based on height and was disheveled in appearance. His shoes were untied, his shirt was half tucked into his pants, and his hair was uncombed. He lived at home with both parents and was the elder of two children.

The school nurse was involved with the assessment phase of Adam's academic testing. When the nurse talked with Adam, he made no eye contact and constantly squirmed in his chair. He revealed that no one liked him in school, and the other children teased him because of his weight. He said that he wished he could "cut out his brain because it was so dumb." He was aggressive within groups to try to gain acceptance and would often start fights with children who teased him.

In talking with the parents, the school nurse identified that the mother was overprotective of Adam. She used food as a way to calm Adam when he was upset, and she discouraged any contact with peers because of her fear that Adam would be ridiculed. The father rarely interacted with Adam because he was frustrated by Adam's behavior and disappointed in his academic performance.

The school nurse made the nursing diagnosis of Chronic Low Self-Esteem (NANDA, 1999). Adam exhibited an interruption in the development of the three theoretical antecedents necessary for positive self-esteem. Adam's feelings of success and power were low. He recognized that he had a more difficult time with academic subjects, and he felt powerless to change. He also has not felt successful at any physical activities, due in part to his weight. Unlike most children his age, he did not dream of what he wanted to be as he grew up, and therefore he did not value any achievements.

At home, Adam received conflicting messages. His mother's overprotectedness undermined his confidence in himself and his ability to make decisions and choices. His father's withdrawal undermined Adam's feelings of value and worth. Adam learned that by doing mischievous things he could get his father's attention. The father then attempted to manage this behavior with the use of ridicule and statements such as "I wish you were like your sister." This style of discipline further diminished Adam's feelings of self-worth and ability to control himself. Because of his low self-esteem, Adam developed the defense mechanisms of fighting with others, avoiding new situations, and trying to control others.

Direct nursing intervention with Self-Esteem Enhancement was begun with Adam. Through daily contact with Adam, the nurse worked on developing a supportive environment that enhanced his self-esteem. Rewards and praise were given to Adam for remembering achievable goals, such as coming to the nurse's office for his medication without reminders. The nurse also helped Adam set realistic goals and provided encouragement and confidence in Adam's ability to achieve his goals.

Ansbacher, H. L., & Ansbacher, R. R. (Eds.). (1956). *The individual psychology of Alfred Adler.* New York: Basic Books.

Bowles, T. V. P., & Fallon, B. J. (1996). Self-concept, family functioning and problem type: A replication and extension of a study of clinic and non-clinic adolescents. *Journal of Adolescent Health, 19,* 62-67.

Coopersmith, S. (1967). *The antecedents of self-esteem.* New York: Freeman.

Erikson, E. (1963). *Childhood and society* (2nd ed.). New York: Norton.

Filozof, E. M., Albertin, H. K., Jones, C. R., Steme, S. S., Myers, L., & McDermott, R. J. (1998). Relationship of adolescent self-esteem to selected academic variables. *Journal of School Health, 68*(2), 68-72.

Harter, S. (1983). The development of the self-system. In M. Hetherington (Ed.), *Carmichael's Manual of Child Psychology: Social and personality development* (pp. 275-385). New York: John Wiley.

Iowa Intervention Project. (2000). *Nursing interventions classification (NIC)* (J. C. McCloskey & G. M. Bulechek, Eds.; 3rd ed.). St. Louis, MO: Mosby-Year Book.

Iowa Outcomes Project. (1997). *Nursing outcomes classification (NOC)* (M. Johnson, M. Maas, & S. Moorhead, Eds.; 2nd ed.). St. Louis, MO: Mosby-Year Book.

James, W. (1981). *The principles of psychology.* Cambridge, MA: Harvard University Press. (Original work published 1890)

Killeen, M. R. (1993). Parent influences on children's self esteem in economically disadvantaged families. *Issues in Mental Health Nursing, 14*(4), 323-336.

Lesser, J., & Escoto-Lloyd, S. (1999). Health-related problems in a vulnerable population: Pregnant teens and adolescent mothers. *Nursing Clinics of North America, 34*(2), 289-312.

Mayberry, L. (1990). Self-esteem in children: Considerations for measurement and intervention. *American Journal of Occupational Therapy, 44*(8), 729-734.

Mead, G. H. (1962). *Mind, self, and society: From the standpoint of a social behaviorist.* Chicago: University of Chicago Press.

Meisenhelder, J. B. (1985). Self-esteem: A closer look at clinical interventions. *International Journal of Nursing Studies, 22*(2), 127-135.

Miller, S. A. (1987). Promoting self-esteem in the hospitalized adolescent: Clinical interventions. *Issues in Comprehensive Pediatric Nursing, 10,* 187-194.

Norris, J. (1992). Nursing intervention for self-esteem disturbances. *Nursing Diagnosis, 3*(2), 48-53.

North American Nursing Diagnosis Association. (1999). *Nursing diagnoses: Definitions and classification 1999-2000.* Philadelphia: Author.

Overbay, J. D., & Purath, J. (1997). Self-concept and health status in elementary school aged children. *Issues in Comprehensive Pediatric Nursing, 20*(2), 89-101.

Pastore, D. R., Fisher, M., & Friedman, S. B. (1996). Fellowship forum. Abnormalities in weight status, eating attitudes, and eating behaviors among urban high school students: Correlations with self-esteem and anxiety. *Journal of Adolescent Health, 18*(5), 312-319.

Rickert, V. I., Hassed, S. J., Hendon, A. E., & Curriff, C. (1996). The effects of peer ridicule on depression and self-image among adolescent females with Turner syndrome. *Journal of Adolescent Health, 19,* 34-38.

Sieving, R. W., & Zirbel-Donisch, S. T. (1990). Development and enhancement of self-esteem in children. *Journal of Pediatric Health Care, 4*(6), 290-296.

Stanwyck, D. J. (1983). Self-esteem through the life span. *Family and Community Health, 6*(2), 11-28.

Sullivan, H. S. (1953). *The interpersonal theory of psychiatry.* New York: Norton.

Sweeting, H., & West, P. (1995). Family life and health in adolescence: A role for culture in the health inequalities debate? *Social Science & Medicine, 40*(2), 163-175.

Torres, R., & Fernandez, F. (1995). Self-esteem and value of health as determinants of adolescent health behavior. *Journal of Adolescent Health, 16,* 60-63.

U.S. Department of Health and Human Services. (1991). *Healthy people 2000: National health promotion and disease prevention objectives* (DHHS Publication No. PHS 91-50213). Washington, DC: Government Printing Office.

Wasson, D., & Anderson, M. A. (1995). Chemical dependency and adolescent self-esteem. *Clinical Nursing Research, 4*(3), 274-289.

Willoughby, C., Polatajko, H., & Wilson, B. (1995). The self-esteem and motor performance of young learning disabled children. *Physical and Occupational Therapy in Pediatrics, 14*(3/4), 1-30.

Wolman, C., & Basco, D. E. (1994). Factors influencing self-esteem and self-consciousness in adolescents with spina bifida. *Journal of Adolescent Health, 15*(7), 543-548.

Youngs, B. B. (1991). *The 6 vital ingredients of self-esteem and how to develop them in your child.* New York: Rason Associates.

37

Media Management

Janice Denehy

Television (TV) is a major source of information and entertainment for people of all ages. Since the advent of this medium, there has been optimism about its potential to disseminate information and enrich the lives of viewers. This optimism, however, has been tempered by voices of concern about the potential adverse effects of TV viewing on children who are developing values and beliefs about the world in which they live. Health care professions are echoing this concern because studies have demonstrated negative effects of TV on the developing health beliefs and behaviors of children and adolescents. Currently, parents are concerned not only about TV but also about other media, such as video games, movies, and the Internet, which are accessible in many homes. This chapter focuses on television, but it also considers other media, such as movies and computer games, in its discussion and recommendations for children and families.

In 1990, *The Journal of Adolescent Health Care* published reports on the effects of TV on the health beliefs and behaviors of children and adolescents. Each article critically reviewed and synthesized the literature on TV viewing in a specific area, and a study group report with recommendations for additional research, programming, public education, and policy implications was provided. These reports have provided valuable data for health professionals as they seek to monitor the health effects of TV on children and to educate families about the selection of programs appropriate for children at different age levels. The American Academy of Pediatrics (1997) has taken the following stand on TV viewing to guide health professionals and parents in understanding its effects on children:

> Parents need to monitor what their children see in the media. TV advertising and programming can adversely affect learning and behavior of children and adolescents and detract from time spent reading or using other active learning skills. TV viewing also has been associated with obesity. The Academy therefore recommends that TV viewing by children be limited to 1 to 2 hours per day.
>
> The Academy also supports legislative and regulatory efforts, such as the Children's Television Act of 1990, to improve children's programming content and promote more constructive viewing.
>
> *Commercial TV:* The primary goal of commercial children's TV is to sell products to children. Young children cannot distinguish between programs and commercials, and often don't understand that commercials are designed to sell products. TV also conveys unrealistic messages regarding drugs, alcohol, tobacco, and sexuality.
>
> *Media violence:* Children are exposed to violence in TV, movies, video games, and music. Media glamorize the use of guns and wrongly teach youngsters that it is alright to use violence to resolve problems. Children need to know that violence on TV and in the movies is not real. By watching TV with their children, and discussing the content, parents can address objectionable content and use the medium as a springboard for family discussion.
>
> *Media literacy:* Parents and schools should also teach children to become more "media literate." This involves learning about how the media work, the intent of commercials and programming, and whether media messages are appropriate. Children who are "media literate" are more likely to withstand potentially harmful effects.

It is estimated that children spend 3 or 4 hours per day watching television, and each year they will view 1,000 murders, rapes, robberies, and assaults. The Children's Defense Fund (1997) noted, "In 1992, children's shows featured 32 acts of violence an hour" (p. 68). By high school graduation, it is estimated that children will have spent more time in front of the TV than in the classroom. In addition, they will have viewed more than 20,000 commercials each year. Indeed, TV is pervasive and a major socializing agent of today's children. Its values are imprinted on the minds of passive and intrigued viewers with little thought about the long-term effects on health or values. By the time they reach their 70th birthday, today's adolescents will have spent 7 years of their lives watching TV (Comstock & Strasburger, 1990).

There is a TV in approximately 99% of all American homes, and two thirds of homes have more than one set (Comstock & Strasburger, 1990). Approximately two thirds of adolescents report having their own TV set (Brown, Childers, & Waszak, 1990), a phenomenon not uncommon among younger children as well. Many homes also have cable TV and videotape recorders that can bring a wide variety of movies and other entertainment into the home. In addition, today's family homes often are equipped with personal computers that can be used for a variety of activities, including computer games and access to the Internet. In addition to concerns about TV and movies, currently there is much discussion about violence in computer and video games and sexually explicit content on the Internet. The development of the "V" chip to screen out violent TV shows and that is required on all new TV sets sold beginning in 1998 and software to prohibit access by children and teens to sexually explicit material on the Internet are two methods to assist parents in preventing inappropriate viewing. The responsibility of monitoring media, however, belongs to parents, who find it increasingly difficult to monitor all the activities of their developing children. In addition, parents often do not have sufficient knowledge or advance information to make informed decisions about what to watch and what to avoid. Therefore, rating systems developed in 1996 and 1997 for TV shows and developed in 1995 for computer games are an attempt to give viewers and parents more information about the content of media. In August 1999, the American Academy of Pediatrics urged parents to avoid TV viewing for children younger than 2 years of age because infants and toddlers have a critical need for interaction with parents and other caregivers to promote the development of social, emotional, and cognitive skills. They also suggest a media-free environment in children's rooms and avoiding the use of TV as an electronic baby-sitter (American Academy of Pediatrics, 1999).

Many objectives for the health of the nation stated in *Healthy People 2000* (U.S. Department of Health and Human Services, 1991) are relevant to the concerns being articulated by health professions, educators, and parents related to the effects of media on the health of children and adolescents. Objectives related to physical activity and fitness relate not only to fitness but also to the reduction of overweight and obese children and adolescents. Nutrition objectives call for a reduction of weight among those overweight and a reduction of dietary fat and an increase in consumption of complex carbohydrates, as well as fruits and vegetables, for Americans of all ages. Objectives related to substance use indicate the need for a reduction in the number of children who initiate smoking and become regular smokers to no more than 15% by age 20 (the current baseline is 30%). Similar goals are stated for alcohol and illegal drugs.

Finally, there are many objectives that propose a decrease in violence as indicated by lower rates of suicide, homicide, domestic violence, and rape. A protective strategy to reduce violence is to increase to at least 50% the number of schools teaching nonviolent conflict resolution skills, preferably as part of comprehensive health education programs.

THEORETICAL FRAMEWORK AND LITERATURE REVIEW

Social learning theory is relevant when examining and predicting the impact of TV on the behavior of children and when developing programs to promote healthy behaviors (Hanrahan, Campbell, & Ulrich, 1993). Social learning theory explains "human behavior in terms of a continuous interaction among cognitive, behavior, and environmental determinants" (Parcel & Baranowski, 1981, p. 14). It expands on the principles of operant conditioning by predicting that behavior can be learned and imitated vicariously by having the participant observe a behavior in the absence of obvious reinforcement. This process is known as social modeling. Observation of a behavior prepares the child for performance of the behavior. Models for behavior can be found in the family, society, and media (Bandura, 1973). Of particular concern is the relationship between violence modeled in the media and aggression in children. This is especially potent if the learner identifies with the person performing the violent behavior; the violent behavior is reinforced or viewed as justified or shows good triumphing over evil through violence. Children who witness violence in the home or experience violence in the form of physical punishment or abuse are more likely to use violence as a method of conflict resolution (Kalmuss, 1984). Although it is unlikely that most viewers would actually imitate violence portrayed in the media, recent reports of shootings in schools by students imitating violence from a specific movie illustrate the potential for such action on the part of some individuals. Social learning experience, however, is frequently used as the theoretical basis for health education programs. For example, after viewing a health-promoting behavior modeled in a class skit, film, or videotape, students are given an opportunity to practice the desired behavior, such as resisting drugs and sexual activity or selecting low-fat snack foods.

Sexuality and the Media

At a time when American society has become more tolerant of sexual activity among teens, unmarried parenthood, abortion, and divorce and teens are engaging in sexual activity at younger ages, one has to question the role of media in promoting these attitudes and behaviors (Bearinger, 1990). Studies of sexual references in TV programming found that their frequency has increased and become increasingly explicit (Brown et al., 1990). Studies have also showed that teens who watched numerous shows in which sexual behavior was a major theme believed premarital and extramarital intercourse with multiple partners was acceptable; they were unlikely to learn about the need for protection against disease or pregnancy, however. Sex in TV and movies is often portrayed as glamorous and risk free. Contraceptives are rarely mentioned or used, and TV characters rarely get pregnant or infected with sexually transmitted diseases (STDs). Unfortunately, information about sexuality from other sources, such as parents, schools, and churches, is often minimal or absent and pales in comparison to the repeated messages delivered to viewers via mass media (Brown et al., 1990).

Sexual appeal is also used in advertisements to draw attention to products and entice viewers to purchase products. Models and actors in commercials may set unrealistic and unattainable standards for physical attractiveness and weight among adolescents. Emphasis on beauty and gender stereotypes influence views that adolescents have about their developing bodies and may contribute to poor self-esteem, eating disorders, and depression. Such images also promote a $4 billion cosmetic industry among teens and a growing industry in plastic surgery and body alterations requested by adolescents (Brown et al., 1990).

In action-adventure TV shows and movies, sexual behavior is often associated with violence or a display of power—not in a caring, long-term relationship or as an expression of mutual affection. In fact, sexuality in the context of marriage is rarely portrayed, nor are contraceptives discussed or used during sexual intercourse (Brown et al., 1990). Despite pleas for social responsibility, there is evidence that sexual content on TV is increasing, especially during soap operas and prime-time situation comedies—shows popular with adolescents. The same concerns are being expressed with regard to sexuality in movies. A frequent theme is having intercourse on the first meeting with a person of the opposite sex, even among characters who are portraying roles as scientists or physicians. A recent concern is the easy access to explicit sexual materials, including pornographic pictures and chat rooms, on the Internet.

Nutrition and the Media

Because there is currently concern about the increasing numbers of children and adolescents who are obese, the poor diet of American teens, and eating disorders, there is interest in the effects of TV programs and advertisements on the nutritional health of youth. Although there is little research regarding these effects on adolescents, many studies have been done on young children with regard to the effects of Saturday morning programs and commercials on attitudes and food preferences. Program monitoring has shown that a "television diet" consists primarily of foods with little nutritional value—mostly high-sugar and high-fat snack foods (Story, 1990). Young children who watch advertisements attempt to influence their parents' food purchases based on what they have seen on TV. Constant promotion of foods low in nutritional value is of concern because dietary preferences and patterns established during childhood and adolescence persist throughout life.

The relationship between inactivity and obesity in children is not clear, however. Dietz (1990) stated that perhaps as much as 25% of the recent increase in obesity in youth is attributable to increased TV viewing. Data gathered between 1965 and 1980 indicate that the incidence of obesity, defined as triceps skinfold measurements in excess of the 85th percentile, has increased by 39% and the incidence of superobesity, defined as triceps skinfold measurements in excess of the 95th percentile, has increased by 64%. These data suggest that 3.5 million adolescents in the United States are obese, one third of whom can be considered superobese (Dietz, 1990). Controlling for prior obesity and socioeconomic class, the author found that the amount of TV viewed by nonobese children was the most powerful predictor of future obesity. Additional analysis found that obesity increased approximately 2% with each additional hour per day of TV viewing. No other leisure-time activity was significantly associated with the development of obesity.

In addition to lack of activity during TV viewing, children are more likely to snack on high-calorie food while watching TV, particularly programs in which there are food advertisements. Small amounts of excess energy intake or reduced energy expenditure over time can probably account for increased obesity among heavy TV viewers. Klesges, Shelton, and Klesges (1993) reported in a study of 31 females aged 8 to 12 years that metabolic rate during TV viewing was significantly lower than during rest. They concluded that "children who watch an excessive amount of television are more at risk for becoming obese because their resting energy expenditures are lower than if they were doing nothing at all" (p. 284). Although this study had a small sample and a passive nonviolent viewing segment, interesting questions were raised about the effects of action-packed programs or interactive computer games on metabolic rates on both normal-weight and obese children of both sexes in nonlaboratory settings. Finally, in summarizing a study of the relationship between obesity and the consumption of high-fat foods and low physical activity, Muecke, Simons-Morton, Huang, and Parcel (1992) reported that neither were independent risk factors for obesity, but there appeared be a synergistic effect when both were present in the same child. Although the mechanisms of obesity in childhood are complex and poorly understood, treatment of the problem is equally challenging and long-term results are not encouraging. Decreased activity through lengthy periods of sitting seems to contribute to the problem of obesity of children and adolescents.

The relationship between eating disorders and media has also been discussed, particularly the contradictory messages portrayed in both programming and advertisements in which consumption of nonnutritious high-calorie foods is promoted while visual images of individuals in these programs or advertisements are lean and fit. In this context, Dietz (1990) states that bulimia can be viewed as an adaptive response because bulimics can remain thin while eating everything they wish. There is also a preoccupation with eating and weight among today's preadolescents and teens, with one study reporting that 80% of 10-year-old girls stated that they were currently dieting to lose weight (Mellin, Scully, & Irwin, 1986).

Substance Use and the Media

Although there has been considerable study of substance use, it is clear that factors influencing substance use are complex, interactive, and difficult to isolate (Resnick, 1990). Television, however, provides a continuous learning environment in which messages to youthful viewers encourage the use of alcohol. Such messages may communicate that alcohol is a constant, integral part of everyday life in today's society. Every year, teens encounter more than 1,000 beer and wine commercials and several thousand fictional drinking episodes in TV and movies (Atkin, 1990). Particular concern has been expressed about commercials that promote alcohol consumption as necessary to have a good time, as a reward after a hard day's work, to promote sociability and romance, and as a method to attract females. These commercials also convey messages about new situations in which drinking is socially desirable. Most of these settings, however, are away from the home and without any recognition of how those drinking will achieve safe transportation home. Such commercial messages are especially plentiful during major sporting events, such as the Super Bowl and the World Series. Rarely shown are the negative effects of drinking on behavior, such as getting drunk, hangovers, violence, and acting foolishly or irresponsibility. A critical review of research indicates that alcohol commercials contribute to a modest effect on teen consumption and a slight impact on alcohol misuse and drunk driving (Atkin, 1990).

Another concern relates to the use of cartoon characters used in the advertising of tobacco and alcohol products after studies showed that these characters were more familiar to young children than Mickey Mouse and other child-oriented cartoon characters. These characters were "retired" in the fall of 1997 in favor of more adult themes in advertising. On a more positive note, one brewery has produced numerous commercial messages promoting responsible alcohol use, the use of designated drivers, and the fact that drinking is for adults. It also offers free information and a videotape for parents about how to talk to their children about alcohol and using it responsibly when they become of legal age to drink.

Although tobacco advertisements have been banned from TV for decades, the brand names of many cigarettes are prominently displayed on the stands during sporting events, on race cars sponsored by tobacco companies, and in the titles of sporting events sponsored by the tobacco industry that give their product name visibility, such as the Virginia Slims Tennis Tournament. A phenomena noted in the second half of the 1990s was the marked increase in the number of actors smoking in movies, especially actors popular with teen and young adult viewers of both sexes. When questioned about the social responsibility of this trend, film producers stated the need for freedom of artistic expression and for new and creative situations for characters. Another interesting trend is the popularity of cigar smoking among adolescents and young adults, which is promoted by many celebrities through the media.

Violence and the Media

There is a considerable body of literature describing the relationship among viewing TV violence and aggressive and antisocial behavior in children. In 1972, the surgeon general commissioned several studies on TV violence, including content analyses of programming and a study of the effects of viewing violence on child behavior. Since that time, numerous studies have been done on TV violence. Meta-analyses on approximately 300 articles involving more than 130,000 subjects give support to the hypothesis that exposure to TV violence increases the likelihood of aggressive behavior (Comstock & Strasburger, 1990). An additional hypothesis considered was that children who display more aggressive behavior prefer and choose to watch violent programming. This hypothesis, however, was not supported by subsequent analysis.

Another concern with violent programs is that they can evoke a generalized arousal that affects subsequent behavior. The frenzied fast pace of children's programming, particularly cartoons, with rapid sequences, loud music, and frequent commercials, is linked to aggressive behavior and restlessness in preschoolers who are heavy TV viewers (Comstock & Strasburger, 1990). Observing justified violence in which the good guy triumphs over the villain is likely to promote aggression in the viewer and is a persistent theme of cartoons designed for young children. Even a brief exposure to violent programming can make a child more tolerant of violence in others. Children are also more likely to view violence as a necessary and desirable way to solve problems (Hoberman, 1990). The desensitization of violence and a lack of understanding of the consequences of violence to the victim or his or her family and friends is another concern. Computer and video games are another example of media violence in which players are actual participants in inflicting violence on game characters, and the fast-paced action and sound effects amplify the violent encounters.

Finally, amidst the increasing violence in American society, the depiction of guns in the media no doubt affects what young people know about guns and their use. A study by Price, Merrill, and Clause (1992) provided considerable data about how guns were portrayed in prime-time network programs. Guns were displayed or used in an average of 2.5 scenes per hour. The users were more likely to be male (88%), white (79%), and middle-aged (60%). Most often, the person with the gun was a legal authority, such as a police officer (34%); citizens used guns (23%) nearly as frequently as criminals (25%), however. Victims of gun violence were more likely to be killed, but only 33% of programs demonstrated the pain experienced by the victim and only 7% showed the suffering of the victim's family. Guns used for defense were commonly portrayed, giving the impression that guns are necessary to protect oneself or one's property. Television programming, however, did not depict how guns should be properly stored. Finally, there were frequent displays of unpunished acts of gun violence that may increase the perception that gun use without retribution is characteristic in society (Price et al., 1992).

Network programming that is not designed for children should not be broadcast during the early hours of the evening, times when children represent a significant viewership. Gun violence increases later in the evening (Price et al., 1992). With the widespread availability of videotapes, however, it is difficult to control what children, particularly adolescents, view and when. Although there is considerable pressure on networks and producers to be more socially responsible in the development of programs and movies that children and teens are likely to view, there is little evidence to indicate the trends of increasing media violence and sexually explicit scenes will be reversed. Gannett News Service ("Research," 1997) reported that the percentage of programs with violence increased from 58% in 1995 to 61% in 1996.

In summary, TV and other media are a pervasive part of today's society. Although TV holds great potential for education and information dissemination, there is evidence that what is learned through this powerful medium is not always prosocial and may not promote healthy attitudes and behaviors in children and adolescents. Because there is no evidence that programming will change in the near future, parents need to take greater responsibility in understanding the possible effects of TV and other media, both positive and negative, on their developing children and manage the amount and content viewed by children in their homes.

NURSING DIAGNOSIS AND OUTCOME DETERMINATION

Nursing diagnoses that would be appropriate when considering the effects of media on children include Altered Nutrition: Potential for More Than Body Requirements, Body Image Disturbance, Risk for Infection (STDs), and Risk for Violence (North American Nursing Diagnosis Association, 1999). Outcomes developed for the Nursing Outcomes Classification (Iowa Outcomes Project, 2000) would be appropriate to monitor the effects of media on children. Particularly relevant are the outcomes Health Beliefs, Growth, Body Image, Risk Control, and Aggression Control. The indicators provide a method not only to evaluate behavior but also to gather baseline data prior to health education programs. This information may be valuable in monitoring the effects of media over time in specific groups of children or in children with differing viewing habits or at multiple data points. Especially needed is information on the effects of media on children's attitudes and behavior relating to lifestyle behaviors that influence health.

INTERVENTION: MEDIA MANAGEMENT

Media Management is a nursing intervention designed to educate parents and children about the effects of media, about how to carefully select appropriate programming, and to provide ideas about alternate activities. Nurses who work with children and families in all settings have an opportunity to educate parents about the effects of media, both positive and negative, on children. It is particularly important that nurses who see children in ambulatory clinics for child health maintenance visits make information about Media Management a part of anticipatory guidance given to parents at regular intervals (Denehy, 1990). This is particularly true during the toddler and preschool years, when parents are most receptive to health promotion for their families and TV viewing begins. It is also critical, however, during the school-age and adolescent years when children exercise more autonomy in selecting programs and there are many programs easily available that are not appropriate for these age groups. Nurses can discuss the rating systems for TV programs, computer games, and movies with parents and help them understand how these can be used in making judgments about appropriate programs for their child. They can also encourage parents to join with other parents to form groups or organizations that monitor TV programs and give feedback to local stations, networks, and advertisers about content that is not appropriate for children or does not reflect family or community values. Parents also need information about where to get reports from parent watch groups so that they can benefit from the efforts of others.

Media Management for parents of preschoolers includes knowledge of how programming designed for this age group can stimulate the imagination and assist children in learning concepts, colors, shapes, and words. It essential, however, to emphasize the importance of limiting TV viewing to 1 or 2 hours per day. A good practice for families to develop is to establish a weekly schedule of TV viewing based on selection from a TV-programming guide and then to stick to the programs selected. Parents should also be encouraged to watch TV programs and movies with their children to determine the appropriateness of the content, to determine the child's reaction to the programs viewed, and to be able to discuss what was seen with the family. This also gives parents an opportunity to evaluate not only the programming but also the commercials shown during the programs selected. When selecting videotapes and computer programs, ones that have been made for the preschool age group and that are educational as well as entertaining should be chosen.

If preschoolers start having difficulty sleeping, concentrating, or are modeling violent or silly behaviors seen on TV, particularly prominent in cartoon programs, parents may want to more carefully select programming or decrease viewing time. Parents of preschoolers can assist their young children in distinguishing between fantasy and reality seen in programming, particularly as it relates to unrealistic physical feats and killing of characters in cartoons. In addition, parents must help children understand the rationale for not buying every product, food, or toy being promoted in commercials. Parents of preschoolers also need to monitor what their children are exposed to in day care centers or in the homes of babysitters because TV is often used as a method to keep children occupied.

Families of school-age children need to follow the same guidelines for limiting TV viewing time, selecting programs ahead of time, and viewing programs with children. At this age, children should be involved in the decision-making process and understand criteria used by the family to make decisions about what programs are appropriate. This is a good time to explain the TV and movie rating system to children and how it can be used to guide program selection. Additional ratings now warn of sexual content, violence, or language and dialogue unsuitable for childhood viewing. Parents need to limit programs with sexual and violent content as well as programs that promote stereotypes based on gender or race. Parents can take the opportunity to discuss values portrayed in the programs selected and how they fit with the values the family holds. There are many programs that are family oriented and educational in nature, and parents can encourage and show genuine interest in such programs. These programs can serve as springboards for more reading about a topic of interest or an exploration of maps to locate where a particular program originated. Parents should be more vigilant in surveillance of their children's viewing habits because many children view TV in the homes of friends, while parents are at work or out of the home, or on TV sets located in their bedrooms, away from the watchful eyes of parents. This is also true of computer games and use of the Internet. Parents can stipulate the amount of time spent in alternative activities to provide balance in their children's lives—for example, for every hour of TV, children need to spend equal time in physical activity or homework as appropriate.

Teenagers often watch hours of TV after a busy day at school to relax or as an escape from the many demands placed on them. Limiting the amount and type of programs teens watch becomes more challenging. Teens, who are striving to become independent, often resent parents imposing restrictions on TV viewing. Also, parents often put a lower value on monitoring TV and videotapes, activities that frequently occur in the home, than on monitoring dating, driving, drinking, and drugs (Bearinger, 1990). Therefore, it is essential to establish communication and values for media use prior to the adolescent years. Watching TV with teens gives parents an opportunity to discuss the themes of the programs or movies teens choose, such as risky behavior, sexual content, and violence. They can also discuss alternative scenarios for problems solving and risky behaviors shown in programs. Parents can promote the viewing of news and prosocial programs that illustrate contributions made by teens and other citizens to society. Discussing local, national, and world events seen on TV can be used in meeting assignments for school and can also widen the perspectives of teens with regard to the world around them. Teens can also learn about occupations and careers from TV programs. Teens need to be cautioned, however, about the images portrayed in the media and how these affect their developing body images. Also, the impact of commercials that use sexual messages to promote products should be pointed out to teen viewers. Many high schools offer classes in media awareness, how to evaluate programs and commercials, and the effects of media on behavior, buying habits, and American life in general. Such classes can emphasize the motives of the entertainment industry and the sponsors that support their programming and can assist teens in becoming intelligent and selective viewers.

Parents should communicate with other parents about what their family values are and how these influence what is appropriate media for their child when in the homes of others. Adults can serve as good role models for limiting and carefully selecting media. In today's busy families, in which there is little opportunity for time together, children often have greater access to TV than to working parents (Bearinger, 1990). It is important to emphasize a time during which families can meet together and communicate about their day, their plans for the future, and their values. This is often accomplished during the dinner hour, a time that competes with the ubiquitous TV set in many homes. Nurses can encourage parents to restore the family mealtime as a time that will remain TV free. Parents also need to be supported in their decision to say no to unacceptable programs or to turn off the TV if a program is not acceptable. Too often, parents feel they have no control over what their children watch; they can be empowered to take control of the media entertainment that is ushered into their homes, however.

An important part of Media Management is giving parents and children ideas of alternative activities that can be done by children or by the family unit that are fun, creative, and encourage family togetherness and communication. Regarding younger children, reading stories to the child not only meets these goals but also promotes cognitive development, increases the child's vocabulary, and creates a lifelong interest in reading and books. Having children participate in arts and crafts encourages creativity and a sense of accomplishment. Children also enjoy hobbies, starting collections, or corresponding with relatives or friends in other parts of the country or world. Also important are activities that stimulate physical activity, such as playing outside, going to a park, recreational area, or zoo, or participating in organized activities for children. School-age children need to be encouraged to engage in alternative activities, physical activities such as sports or dance, hobbies or music lessons, or scouting or other organizations for children. Many churches and community organizations offer programs and activities for children that provide opportunities for children to engage in interesting activities and to make new friends. All these activities encourage involvement with others and the development of new interests and skills that can provide an alternative to hours spent in front of the TV or computer.

INTERVENTION APPLICATION

Gail is a recent graduate of a Master's of Nursing Science–Pediatric Nurse Practitioner program. During her graduate education, she worked in an ambulatory clinic and identified the need to provide information to parents on TV viewing. As a class project, she developed a pamphlet to distribute to parents with guidelines for TV viewing for children at different developmental stages. Particularly helpful were suggestions of alternative activities for children and families that would be fun and provide enjoyment and learning away from the TV set. Pamphlets were distributed to families at regular well child visits, at which time Gail took the opportunity to talk to parents about the effects of TV on children. She also gathered information about viewing patterns and favorite programs. For her master's project, she designed a study to determine parents' attitudes about TV because from her earlier work with parents she believed they were tuned in to what their children were watching. She received permission to conduct the study in a large pediatric clinic in a city serving both urban and rural families. Responses from parents of 50 families indicated that parents had a good awareness of the negative effects of TV on children, and they practiced positive viewing habits. Parents indicated a need for more positive programs that portrayed positive role models and a rating system that would assist them in choosing appropriate programs. Parents were quite negative about commercials and their influence on their child's requests for purchasing products. One finding of concern was that the programs listed as favorites by children 9 to 12 years of age were not suitable for this age group because of inappropriate sexual content and the adult nature of the programs (Baughman, 1997).

After graduation, Gail took a job as a nurse practitioner in a pediatric clinic in a large city. Her work with children and families has given her additional insights into parent's attitudes about TV and what types of programs children prefer. She continues to use this information to provide anticipatory guidance about Media Management to parents and children and to provide information about alternative activities for families that provide entertainment and fun away from TV. She also assists parents in carefully selecting TV programs and movies for children because these are an important part of children's lives in today's society.

IMPLICATIONS FOR PRACTICE AND RESEARCH

Television has great potential for disseminating information to large segments of the population. Although there is great concern about the negative effects of TV on children, it may be time to focus on planning positive content. The wide availability and acceptability of this medium needs further exploration as a vehicle to transmit information regarding health. The potential impact is great in terms of shear numbers of people who can be reached, particularly the poor, the poorly educated, and minorities— groups that have had the least exposure to and are the least responsive to traditional health education strategies (Warner, 1987). Innovative strategies need to be developed and tested on different target audiences and age groups to determine what methods produce the desired outcomes. One of the biggest obstacles to using this medium for health education is the cost because commercial program costs are prohibitive for strictly educational programming. Health educators are often loathe to couple health messages with commercial products, believing this cheapens and commercializes the message. There is evidence, however, that this strategy often results in a greater public awareness of health information about nutritional content of specific foods or groups of foods (Warner, 1987). The strategies used by advertisement agencies in successfully planning slick, engaging commercials that sell target products need to be applied to media-based health education. Public service announcements are another method of transmitting health information to a wide segment of the public. Such messages can balance negative images portrayed in the media. These public service messages, however, need to be broadcast at a time when the target audience is likely to be viewing, not after midnight when children are least likely to be watching TV.

Nurses who work in hospitals should be selective about what programs hospitalized children are allowed to watch based on the family's values and the age of the children. Too often, the TV is on all day as a diversion, even when programming is not appropriate for children. Nurses can take this opportunity to educate parents about the effects of TV viewing on children and how to choose programs based on the child's developmental level, the type of program, and the goals of the family. A recent trend is for pediatric units to have a library of videotapes or computer games for children to provide them with more child-centered activities; caution needs to be taken, however, with regard to the amount of time children spend using media in the hospital. This is particularly important for children with serious illnesses or chronic diseases that may limit other options for activities. Too often, nurses are busy or believe that it is none of their business what children or parents select to watch during hospitalization (Adrian, 1993). These same nurses, however, would not consider serving food inappropriate for age or nonnutritious snacks at all hours of the day to children just because it makes them happy or keeps them occupied or quiet. If parents desire to watch adult programs, it might be possible to have a TV in a parents' waiting room that could be used for such programs.

Another concern is TVs in waiting rooms that are continuously on to entertain or distract children and families while they are waiting for appointments. For families who are selective about their TV viewing, such placement of TVs may be offensive or overstimulating at a time when their child is ill or waiting for a well child visit. Parents' attention might better be averted by bulletin boards or health education information carefully placed in the waiting room. Children's books provide parents an opportunity to read to their children while they are waiting. If TVs are to be located in waiting rooms, they might be used for parent education on topics of concern to parents, such as car safety or nutrition, that are short and portray a positive image for the clinic. Parents should be encouraged to speak up if they believe that TV is being used inappropriately in any health care setting. Nurses should not assume that TV is given in all environments; they, too, can speak out for wise and judicious use of media in all settings in which children receive care.

In addition to providing information to children and families about Media Management as part of anticipatory guidance offered to all families, nurses need to become advocates for children's health in their communities and professional organizations. To accomplish this goal, nurses must be aware of the health effects of media, both positive and negative, and be knowledgeable of current research and how it can be used in practice. Nurses are well positioned to conduct research on TV viewing patterns of children in their community, in hospital units, and in other clinical areas. In addition, they can survey parents about the type of information they would find helpful in managing the media, TV, videotapes, and computers that are in their homes. Nurses should also be aware of what programs children are currently watching to be able to communicate intelligently with children and families about which programs are or are not good choices. They can also encourage children to be TV sleuths, recording the types of images portrayed in the programs and commercials they commonly watch and discussing these with family and peers. These activities will assist the next generation to be thoughtful consumers of media that are and will continue to be a pervasive part of our technologically oriented society.

REFERENCES

Adrian, E. (1993). *Television viewing and the chronically ill hospitalized child*. Unpublished master's thesis, University of Iowa, Iowa City.

American Academy of Pediatrics. (1997). *Where we stand* [On-line]. Available: http://www.aap.org/advocacy/wwestand.htm.

American Academy of Pediatrics. (1999). *AAP discourages television for the very young child* [On-line]. Available: http://www.aap.org.advocacy.releases/augdis.htm.

Atkin, C. K. (1990). Effects of televised alcohol messages on teenage drinking patterns. *Journal of Adolescent Health Care, 11,* 10-24.

Bandura, A. (1973). *Aggression: A social learning analysis*. Englewood Cliffs, NJ: Prentice Hall.

Baughman, G. (1997). *Television and children: Parents' perspectives*. Unpublished master's thesis, University of Iowa, Iowa City.

Bearinger, L. H. (1990). Study group report on the impact of television on adolescent views of sexuality. *Journal of Adolescent Health Care, 11,* 71-75.

Brown, J. D., Childers, K. W., & Waszak, C. S. (1990). Television and adolescent sexuality. *Journal of Adolescent Health Care, 11,* 62-70.

Children's Defense Fund. (1997). *The state of America's children—Yearbook 1997.* Washington, DC: Author.

Comstock, G., & Strasburger, V. C. (1990). Deceptive appearances: Television violence and aggressive behavior. *Journal of Adolescent Health Care, 11,* 31-44.

Denehy, J. A. (1990). Anticipatory guidance. In M. J. Craft & J. A. Denehy (Eds.), *Nursing interventions for infants and children* (pp. 53-67). Philadelphia: W. B. Saunders.

Dietz, W. H. (1990). You are what you eat—what you eat is what you are. *Journal of Adolescent Health Care, 11,* 76-81.

Hanrahan, P., Campbell, J., & Ulrich, Y. (1993). Theories of violence. In J. Campbell & J. Humphries (Eds.), *Nursing care of survivors of family violence* (pp. 3-35). St. Louis, MO: C. V. Mosby.

Hoberman, H. M. (1990). Study group report on the impact of television violence on adolescents. *Journal of Adolescent Health Care, 11,* 45-49.

Iowa Outcomes Project. (2000). *Nursing outcomes classification (NOC)* (M. Johnson, M. Maas, & S. Moorhead, Eds.; 2nd ed.). St. Louis, MO: Mosby-Year Book.

Kalmuss, D. (1984). The intergenerational transmission of marital aggression. *Journal of Marriage and the Family, 46,* 11-19.

Klesges, R. C., Shelton, M. L., & Klesges, L. M. (1993). Effect of television on metabolic rate: Potential implications for childhood obesity. *Pediatrics, 91*(2), 281-286.

Mellin, L. M., Scully, S. M., & Irwin, C. E. (1986). Disordered eating characteristics in preadolescent females. *American Dietetic Association Abstracts, 79.*

Muecke, L., Simons-Morton, B., Huang, I. W., & Parcel, G. (1992). Is childhood obesity associated with high-fat foods and low physical activity? *Journal of School Health, 62,* 19-23.

North American Nursing Diagnosis Association. (1999). *Nursing diagnoses: Definitions and classification 1999-2000.* Philadelphia: Author.

Parcel, G. S., & Baranowski, T. (1981). Social learning theory and health education. *Health Education, 12*(3), 14-18.

Price, J. H., Merrill, E. A., & Clause, M. E. (1992). The depiction of guns on prime time television. *Journal of School Health, 62,* 15-18.

Research: TV violence rampant, enticing kids. (1997, March 26). *Iowa City Press Citizen.*

Resnick, M. D. (1990). Study group report on the impact of televised drinking and alcohol advertising on youth. *Journal of Adolescent Health Care, 11,* 25-30.

Story, M. (1990). Study group report on the impact of television on adolescent nutritional status. *Journal of Adolescent Health Care, 11,* 82-85.

U.S. Department of Health and Human Services. (1991). *Healthy people 2000: National health promotion and disease prevention objectives* (DHHS Publication No. PHS 91-50312). Washington, DC: Government Printing Office.

Warner, K. E. (1987). Television and health education: Stay tuned [Editorial]. *American Journal of Public Health, 77*(2), 140-142.

38

Substance Abuse Prevention

Sandra Rae Powell

Harmful substances have been abused throughout human history. Treatments for substance abuse and substance dependence have also existed for a long time, as evidenced by national efforts to create treatment programs, enact laws to contain addiction, and even take part in wars, such as opium wars and the current war on drugs (Eells, 1991). The use of alcohol, tobacco, and other drugs (ATOD) among children and adolescents continues to be a concern. *Healthy People 2000* has approximately 19 goals specifically related to ATOD for children and adolescents (U.S. Department of Health and Human Services, 1991). These goals speak to the societal importance of ATOD prevention. Prevention helps to increase knowledge, decrease the suffering of individuals and families, and decrease health care costs. The earliest prevention programs for substance abuse used information and even scare tactics, such as showing people going "mad" as a result of smoking marijuana, to frighten potential users in attempts to influence behavioral change. Research has shown, however, that information alone is not enough to bring about behavioral changes, and other interventions are needed (Allen, 1996). This chapter describes an intervention that is a more comprehensive approach to prevention and can be used for individuals, families, groups, and communities.

LITERATURE REVIEW

The Alcohol, Drug Abuse, and Mental Health Administration's Office for Substance Abuse Prevention (OSAP) was established to initiate programs to provide prevention and early intervention services for young people, especially high-risk youth. The starting point for OSAP was the identification of theories and models to provide a background body of knowledge. The goal has been to use these theories and models to develop strategies that can prevent or reverse adolescent alcohol use (Johnson, Amatetti, Funkhouser, & Johnson, 1988).

The public health model has emerged from this work as a useful conceptual framework for developing alcohol and drug prevention strategies. It provides the opportunity to use a synthesis of multiple theories. This model of prevention planning requires knowledge of the host (individual adolescent), the agent (ATOD), and the environment (social milieu). Furthermore, knowledge of the interaction among these factors is necessary (Johnson et al., 1988).

Risk Factors for Drug Abuse

Primary prevention for ATOD use and abuse includes identifying risk and protective factors (Belcher & Shinitzky, 1998). A *risk factor* can be defined as an attitude, belief, behavior, situation, action, or all these that may put a person, a group, an organization, or a community at risk for experiencing drug use, abuse, addiction, and its effects (Allen, 1996). Family risk factors include "(a) lack of clear behavioral expectations, (b) lack of monitoring/supervision, (c) lack of caring, (d) inconsistent or excessively severe discipline, (e) history of alcohol and other drug abuse, (f) positive parental attitudes toward alcohol and other drug abuse, and (g) low expectations for children's success" (Allen, 1996, p. 95).

Protective Factors
Against Drug Abuse

Protective factors mediate or moderate the effects of risk. A *protective factor* can be defined as an attitude, belief, situation, action, or all three that protects an individual, group, organization, or community from the effects of drug use (Allen, 1996). Many protective factors have been found to be effective in preventing ATOD use (Belcher & Shinitzky, 1998). For instance, relationships with caring adult role models, who support the ability to cope with life and realistic expectations about their abilities, and a positive outlook help to deter ATOD use. Healthy individuals who are effective in work, play, and relationships are more likely to have positive self-esteem and an internal locus of control, characteristics that provide protection from ATOD abuse (Allen, 1996). Certain attributes, such as self-discipline, problem-solving and critical thinking skills, a sense of humor, and strong identification with ethnic or cultural groups, also provide some protection from ATOD use (Allen, 1996).

Concepts of vulnerability and resiliency have been advanced to identify the extent of individual susceptibility to risk. *Vulnerability* denotes intensified susceptibility to risk; *resiliency* is the ability to withstand or surmount risk. Rutter (1985) suggests that resilient children display a repertoire of social problem-solving skills and a belief in their own self-efficacy. Protection involves enhancing resilient responses to risk exposure. For the concept of protective factors to be useful, it must apply to differences in outcomes among individuals exposed to the same risks.

Brook, Brook, Gordon, Whiteman, and Cohen (1990) identified two mechanisms by which protective factors reduce risk for adolescent drug use. The first is a "risk/protective" mechanism through which exposure to risk factors is moderated by the presence of protective factors. They reported that the risk posed by drug-using peers was moderated by a strong attachment or bond between parent and adolescent and by parent connectionality. The second is a "protective/protective" mechanism through which one protective factor potentates another protective factor, strengthening its effect. They found that a strong attachment between the adolescent and the father enhanced the effects of other protective factors, such as adolescent connectionality, positive maternal characteristics, and marital harmony in preventing drug use. Approaches targeting these risk factors provide a relatively quick reduction of ATOD use if they are effective.

One way to reduce the prevalence of substance abuse is to target measures to reduce the availability of drugs. If reduction in the prevalence of drug abuse is the goal, the evidence does not support those who advocate the legalization of currently illegal drugs such as marijuana and cocaine, although this approach is currently being tried with heroin in Switzerland (Hawkins, Catalano, & Miller, 1992). Since the repeal of prohibition in 1933, the supply of alcohol has been manipulated in several ways, including taxation, age restrictions on consumption, and restrictions on hours of purchase and on liquor-by-the-drink sales. Of these strategies, data indicate that restricting of availability and increasing the price of alcohol by increasing taxes on the purchase price can reduce rates of cirrhosis of the liver and alcohol-related traffic fatalities (Hawkins et al., 1992).

The availability of drugs is a risk factor that has been manipulated in many ways. Reducing availability of drugs through interdiction and arrests of drug dealers does not have a similar effect on reducing rates of drug addiction. Neither doubling of interdiction nor increased arrests of drug dealers seems to affect the retail process or availability of illegal drugs (Polich, Ellickson, Reuter, & Kahan, 1984). A second approach is changing social norms about drug- and alcohol-influenced behaviors. This approach includes "Just Say No!" activities, community coalitions against drugs, media campaigns, and certain policy changes, such as policies for drug abuse prevention and intervention in the schools.

One of the strongest correlates of teenage drug-using behavior is the association with others who use drugs. The most heavily researched strategy for addressing social influence to drug use is classroom-based skills training for adolescents in Grades 5 through 10, especially Grades 6 and 7. The training teaches students through instruction, modeling, and role play to identify and resist influences to use drugs (Hawkins et al., 1992, p. 89). In some cases, this training also prepares students for associated difficulties and stresses anticipated in the process of resisting such influences (Botvin, 1986). Grounded in social learning theory (Bandura, 1977), social influence resistance strategies view drug use as a socially acquired behavior, initiated and reinforced by drug-using peers and family members (Bukoski, 1986).

Social influence resistance approaches have also been combined with training in problem-solving and decision-making skills, skills to increase self-control and self-efficacy, adaptive coping strategies for relieving stress and anxiety, interpersonal skills, and general assertive skills (Botvin, 1986; Flay, 1985). Botvin's skill training program combined elements of both social influence resistance training and social competence skills training (Botvin & Wills, 1985). Students who participated in the peer-led social influence resistance training intervention achieved greater reductions in drug use compared with students in interventions led by teachers (Botvin, Baker, Renick, Filazzola, & Botvin, 1984).

One of the obvious interventions for prevention of substance abuse is education about specific substances and ways to make choices regarding them at age-appropriate levels. Jones, Corbin, Sheehy, and Bruce (1995) studied 34 third graders randomly assigned to treatment groups in a lower-middle-class neighborhood located in a small rural community in Virginia. Subjects showed significant improvement regarding drug knowledge on a posttest. The group that received information and rehearsal showed the most improvement in behavioral skills such as drug refusal.

Gropper, Livaz, Portowicz, and Schindler (1995) studied 700 fifth and sixth graders in a poverty-stricken urban community in Jaffa, Israel. The subjects included high-risk preadolescent Jewish and Arab children 11 and 12 years old. This age is identified as the optimal time to implement drug prevention education to lessen later adolescent peer pressure associated with drug experimentation and use. A computer program with a positive cartoon role model and role playing were used. Three components were included: (a) increasing knowledge; (b) changing beliefs, attitudes, feelings, and values; and (c) teaching drug-resistance, decision-making, and coping skills. The program has been widely accepted by the children, parents, teachers, and school principals who have participated. Research will need to be conducted to evaluate the program's effectiveness and impact in preventing future drug use among the program participants.

Hahn (1995) studied 317 primary caregivers in two counties in Indiana. Beginning Alcohol and Addictions Basic Education Studies (BABES) was targeted at caregivers and children ages 4 to 8 years. Puppets were used to introduce young children to concepts of self-image, feelings, decision making, peer pressure, coping skills, alcoholism, getting help, and sexual abuse. Six instruments were used to assess parental attitudes. Parents were asked to estimate the risk that their children would use ATOD in the future and its severity if it occurred. Parents were taught how to improve family management practices. More than one fourth (29%) of caregivers attended BABES three to seven times. Less than half (43%) did not attend BABES lessons at all. Classroom involvement had the strongest association with parent attendance. Race was the only demographic variable associated with parent attendance, with parents who were Caucasian more likely to attend than African-American parents.

Peer support is a method identified to postpone or decrease ATOD use. Nelson-Simley and Erickson (1995) studied 4,000 youths, Grades 7 to 12, in the state of Nebraska. The program for youths included a complex residential training retreat of 3 or 4 days, with an average-size group of 130. Initial training consisted of the following components: (a) education sessions on the reasons to be alcohol and drug free, (b) team-building commitment to organize drug-free youth groups, (c) adult-sponsored training sessions, (d) drug-free social activities, and (e) a contract for alcohol abstinence until 21 years of age and to be free of tobacco and illegal drugs for a lifetime—a pledge to be renewed annually. In addition, follow-up support and on-site consultation two times per year, training for sponsors, winter reunion, and a newsletter were provided. Results showed that the program appeared to assist in delaying onset of alcohol, tobacco, and other drug use for youths in the program and to assist in decreasing or eliminating use of alcohol and tobacco by adolescents who used before participating (Nelson-Simley & Erickson, 1995, p. 49). Average membership in the group lasted 22.7 months. Adult support was related to long-term group maintenance.

Several studies have included suggestions to enhance children's coping skills (Gropper et al., 1995; Jones et al., 1995). Kalnins et al. (1994) studied 24 children, ages 9 or 10, in Grade 4 in Toronto, Canada, who attended 90-minute weekly sessions conducted by a program facilitator and classroom assistant during the school year. The general focus was on local community health problems that the children considered important. The children's major concern was drugs and drug dealers across the street from their school. Specific community health activities were devised weekly in response to decisions made by the children. The children were able to successfully progress through identifying common problems, mobilizing resources, and implementing strategies to address goals they had set.

An overall view of the empirical work shows that one intervention used in all the studies was education about drugs. In addition, most studies also included support of others, either peers or adults. Currently, a more comprehensive, multisystem approach is recommended to prevent substance abuse. An example of a primary prevention model was developed by Allen (1996) (Table 38.1). The strength of this model is that it covers the life span and targets a range from individuals to communities. The model includes many prevention programs, which serves to build a supportive environment that enhances protective and resiliency factors. These programs must be culturally sensitive and specific. In addition, they should focus across the life span, from prenatal to senior years. The programs must continue for a long period of time if they are to be effective, as opposed to a short, one-time intervention.

No single approach has been identified as effective for prevention. Different factors in separate programs appear to be effective in certain communities or with certain age groups. Therefore, a multifaceted approach to prevention is necessary. For maximum effectiveness, a prevention strategy needs to address parental and peer influences, teachers, and community leaders. Furthermore, norms, marketing and availability of alcoholic beverages, and alcohol-related laws, regulation, and policies need to be addressed.

Hawkins et al. (1992) reviewed many research reports to identify risk and protective factors for ATOD in adolescent and early adulthood with implications for substance abuse prevention. They found that the most promising route to effective strategies for the prevention of adolescent ATOD is a risk-focused approach. The authors reviewed risk and protective factors for drug abuse, evaluated many approaches for drug abuse prevention potential with high-risk groups, and made recommendations for research and practice.

Hawkins et al.'s (1992) conclusion was that it is difficult to ascertain, for instance, which risk factors or combination of risk factors are most virulent, which are modifiable, and which are specific to drug abuse rather than generic contributors to adolescent problem behaviors (p. 65). They also noted that when two or more risk factors exist, the likelihood of problem behavior with harmful substances multiples rapidly with each added risk. A risk-focused prevention approach does not require that risk factors be manipulated directly. It may be impossible to reduce or change certain risk factors directly through preventive intervention. In these instances, the goal of prevention efforts will be to mediate or moderate the

TABLE 38.1   A Comprehensive Model of Primary Prevention

Methods	*Target Groups*				
	Individual (across the life span)	Family	Peers	School/Work	Community (culture specific)
Education/ information	Posters	Programs	Seminars	Teacher/ supervisor training	Brochure distribution
Personal development	Skill building	Parenting training	Work teams	Supportive environment	Wellness programs
Alternative	After-school programs	Family night	Mentors	Company teams	Park facilities
Norms/ standards	ATOD use principles, beliefs, and behaviors	Health care coverage for treatment	Peer-support programs	SAP/EAP	Money to agencies
Community mobilization	Cleanup projects	Family support	Alcohol-free events	Coalition building	Media campaign

SOURCE: Reproduced with permission from Allen (1996).

NOTE: ATOD, alcohol, tobacco, and other drugs; SAP, student assistance programs; EAP, employee assistance programs.

effects of the identified but nonmanipulable risk factors. A family history of alcoholism cannot be changed. It may, however, be possible to moderate the effects of family history by intervening with children who are at risk. When drug-abusing parents were provided with parenting skills and they developed effective discipline methods, children had a decreased intention to smoke or use alcohol. One task of risk-focused prevention research is to determine which risk factors can be manipulated, which risk factors cannot be changed but can be mediated or moderated, and which risk factors cannot be affected at all. The apparent failure of early prevention interventions, such as drug information programs that did not address known risk factors for drug abuse, supports this approach.

Many of the risk factors for adolescent drug abuse also predict other adolescent problem behaviors (Table 38.2). There is evidence that adolescent drug abuse is related to delinquency, teenage pregnancy, school misbehavior, and school drop out. Comprehensive risk-focused efforts can probably prevent or reduce other adolescent problem behaviors in addition to drug abuse.

A comprehensive risk-focused program needs to be developed that targets high-risk youth groups and high-risk communities and schools while avoiding individual and community labeling. It is necessary to intervene early, before negative behaviors can stabilize.

NURSING DIAGNOSES AND
OUTCOMES DETERMINATION

The North American Diagnosis Association (NANDA, 1994) diagnosis of Health-Seeking Behaviors is an appropriate focus for prevention of substance use. Data support the contention that the more healthy coping behaviors children or adolescents have, the more prepared they are to resist using ATODs.

Health-Promoting Behavior from the Nursing Outcomes Classification (NOC; Iowa Outcomes Project, 1997) is a suitable outcome measure for this NANDA diagnosis. The following health-promoting behaviors are all important in preventing substance abuse: the use of risk avoidance behaviors; seeking balance among exercise, work, leisure, rest, and nutrition; using effective stress reduction behaviors; and maintaining satisfactory social relationships (Iowa Outcomes Project, 2000, p. 232).

INTERVENTION:
SUBSTANCE USE PREVENTION

General prevention activities suggested by the Center for Substance Abuse Prevention (CSAP, 1994) are information dissemination, development of life coping skills, provision of alternatives, community development, advocacy for a healthy environment, and problem identification. To make a prevention program as effective as possible, CSAP and Hawkins et al. (1992) suggest the use of multiple systems, such as youth, families, schools, workplace, community organization, and media.

Information dissemination provides awareness and knowledge of the nature and extent of ATOD use and abuse. Knowledge about addiction and its effect on persons, families, and communities needs to be presented to increase the perception of risk. In addition, data about healthy lifestyles should be presented. Information dissemination needs to provide knowledge and awareness of prevention policies, provide information on program services, help set positive societal norms, and reinforce positive societal norms.

Development of life coping skills is an activity performed to influence critical life and social skills (Allen, 1996), including (a) decision-making skills, (b) referral skills, (c) critical analysis systematic and judgmental abilities, (d) communication techniques, (e) goal-setting skills, (f) values clarification skills, (g) problem-solving techniques, (h) self-responsibility (self-care) skills, (i) responsible attitude toward alcohol and drugs, and (j) stress management techniques (Allen, 1996).

TABLE 38.2   Risk Factors Contributing to Adolescent Drug Abuse

Societal	*Individual*	*Interpersonal*

1. Laws and norms favorable toward behavior
  A. Taxation (alcohol consumption is affected by price; specifically tax on purchase price)
  B. Laws stating to whom it can be sold
  C. Laws regarding how alcohol is to be sold
2. Availability: alcohol/drugs
3. Extreme economic deprivation
4. Neighborhood disorganization
	1. Physiological
	  A. Sensation seeking MAO (monoamine oxidase)
	  B. ALDH (aldehyde dehydrogenase)
	  C. Slow-wave electroencephalograph activity
	  D. Genetic factors (predisposition)
	2. Early and persistent problem behaviors
	  A. Academic failure
	  B. Low degree of commitment to school
	  C. Alienation and rebelliousness
	  D. Attitude favorable to drug use
		Family alcohol and drug behavior and attitudes (modeling)
		Poor and inconsistent family management practices
		Family conflict
		Low bonding to family
		Peer rejection in elementary grades

SOURCE: From Hawkins, J. D., Catalano, R. F., and Miller, J. Y. (1992). Risk and protective factors for alcohol and other drug problems in adolescent and early adulthood; Implications for substance abuse prevention. *Psychological Bulletin, 112,* 64-105. Copyright © 1992 by the American Psychological Association. Reprinted with permission.

Attractive alternative activities need to be planned for children and adolescents that exclude the use of ATOD (Allen, 1996). Goals of the alternative prevention strategies include a positive self-image, development of satisfaction and self-esteem, growth in personal skills, development of respect for self and others, provision of positive role models, creation of opportunity for positive interaction with others, and alleviation of boredom, unrest, and apathy (Allen, 1996).

Community development attempts to increase the ability of the community to provide prevention and treatment services related to ATOD use disorders and includes activities such as (a) organizing, (b) planning, (c) enhancing efficiency and effectiveness of services, (d) implementation, (e) interagency collaboration, (f) coalition building, (g) and networking. These activities increase ownership and participation of the community in problem solving. Nurses may facilitate the prevention process or participate as members of a task force, in a forum, or in community-based activities.

Advocating for a healthy environment will change written or unwritten community standards, codes, and attitudes that influence incidence and prevalence of ATOD use in the general population. Included are laws to restrict availability and access, price increases, and communitywide action. There are many prevention activities a nurse could choose to do to become an advocate for a healthy environment, including (a) becoming involved in efforts to change policies, laws, and community norms; (b) lobbying decision makers; (c) supporting measures to limit the availability of ATOD; (d) increasing access to health care and social agency assistance; (e) developing activities to reduce discrimination; (f) participating in organizations with influence; and (g) running for election to political office or becoming a member of boards (Allen, 1996).

It is essential that substance abuse prevention be multifaceted. The more areas of risk and protection that can be addressed, the more likely there way be a reduction in ATOD use. The general prevention strategies suggested by CSAP (1994) training systems and the activities listed in Nursing Interventions Classification (NIC) for the intervention Substance Use Prevention (Iowa Intervention Project, 2000) are very similar. NIC activities for preventing alcohol or drug use lifestyle can be categorized in three areas: legal, educational, and coping (Table 38.3).

INTERVENTION APPLICATION

Eric, 13 years of age, is the third of six children. His mother is a health care professional, and his father is a stay-at-home dad. Eric's whole family is active in the Mormon Church. No one in the immediate family uses drugs, cigarettes, alcohol, or caffeine. Eric's biochemical history is positive for substance abuse. His maternal grandfather was in all probability an alcoholic. His father has a "half-uncle" who was an alcoholic. His father has a past drug history: He used drugs at age 14. He smoked, drank alcohol, and used marijuana, speed, and hash, but he quit using everything at age 22. Eric's father occasionally talks to the children about his drug use. Eric has taken part in Drug Abuse Resistance Education (DARE) for 2 years.

A nursing diagnosis of Health-Seeking Behaviors (NANDA, 1999) would be appropriate for Eric. An assessment of Eric's risks and protective factors shows that, in terms of risk, he has a family history of substance abuse on both his paternal and maternal sides. In terms of protection, both schools Eric has attended had an alcohol and drug prevention program. Eric's immediate family is free of alcohol, tobacco, caffeine, and drug use. His family lived in a mid-sized midwestern city and then moved to a very small town. In the first city, the school system placed DARE in the fifth grade. In the small town to which his family moved, DARE was placed in the sixth grade curriculum. Eric said DARE was very helpful to him in learning what drugs can do to one's body. He also said that in DARE "they don't try to push you into anything. They just tell you this drug does this to your body." He said you make "friends" with the police. Eric also stated that drugs "mess up your thinking, coordination, and

TABLE 38.3 Nursing Interventions Classification Substance Use Prevention Activities

Legal	Educational	Coping
Support measures to regulate the sale and distribution of alcohol to minors and also lobby for increased drinking age.	Recommend changes in the alcohol and drug curricula.	Assist patient (individual) to tolerate increased level of stress, as appropriate.
	Conduct programs in schools on the avoidance of drugs and alcohol as recreational activities.	Prepare patient (individual) for difficult or painful events.
	Recommend media campaign on substance use issues.	Reduce irritating or frustrating environmental stress.
	Instruct parents in the importance of example in substance use.	Reduce social isolation, as appropriate.
	Instruct parents and teachers in the identification of signs and symptoms of addiction.	Encourage responsible decision making about lifestyle choices.
	Support or organize community groups to reduce injuries associated with alcohol.	Assist in the organization of postactivities for teenagers for functions such as prom and homecoming.
	Survey students in grades 1 to 12 on the use of alcohol and drugs.	
	Instruct parents to support school policy that prohibits drug and alcohol consumption at extracurricular activities.	
	Facilitate coordination of efforts between various community groups concerned with substance use.	

SOURCE: Iowa Intervention Project (2000, p. 615).

muscles." He added that he knew a kid in his fourth-grade class (age 10) who brought a suitcase-sized box to school with marijuana and tattoo stickers that could be licked (for acid). He was arrested and suspended from school for a year or two. Eric has peers who have used drugs, like most adolescents. Currently, however, Eric has not been involved in drug use. A useful NOC outcome would be Health-Promoting Behaviors (Iowa Outcomes Project, 2000). Only time will tell whether Eric's protective factors are sufficient to prevent his experimentation with ATOD. Some indicators of Health-Promoting Behaviors for Eric are performing health habits correctly, maintaining satisfactory social relationships, and social support to promote health. The family is using Covey's material on families to write a family mission statement (Covey, 1997, 1998). Eric attended Covey's presentation with his mother. Thus far, the Substance Use Prevention intervention seems to be working for Eric.

IMPLICATIONS FOR NURSING PRACTICE AND RESEARCH

Nurses must first examine their own ATOD use and make a decision about whether or not it is consistent with personal and professional responsibility. Individual nurses should also examine their knowledge, ideas, beliefs, and attitudes regarding substance use and abuse and then learn what they can do to contribute to ATOD prevention in general. Initially, a nurse can give information about the use and abuse of ATOD along with information on consequences of abuse and addiction to all clients.

Nurses can also work with the health care delivery system to institute primary ATOD prevention for clients. First, the nurse needs to become familiar with available resources that can be used for referral. Another necessary activity is to inform clients and families about the effects of combining alcohol and other drugs and drug-drug interactions when prescribing or discussing medication (Allen, 1996). Preventive interventions targeted at clients may include (a) information and education programs (lectures, videos, and pamphlets); (b) awareness events and seminars (lifestyle and early warning signs); (c) general health risk appraisals, screenings, and follow-up for persons identified as potentially having an ATOD problem; (d) early intervention and counseling related to health risk behaviors and workshops for lifestyle management (smoking cessation and parenting); and (e) counteradvertising (CSAP, 1994).

Strategies targeting the community and social policy that can be used by nurses include (a) school health education, (b) educating local and state legislation on topics such as limiting access to ATOD and creating tax incentives to reduce consumption, (c) counteradvertising, (d) seminars and materials targeting the corporate community, (e) employee assistance programs, (f) student assistance programs, (g) participation in posttraumatic event debriefings, and (h) collaboration with community-sponsored events that increase prevention capacity. With health care increasingly moving into the community, nurses will find more opportunities to use prevention strategies and to work with children, adolescents, and families.

In designing interventions to reduce the negative effects of identified risk factors, it is important to focus attention on the potential effects of protective factors. The available evidence suggests that to be viable, a prevention strategy requires attention to risk and protective factors related to individual vulnerability, poor child rearing, school achievement, social influences, social skills, and broad social norms, all of which are implicated in the development of adolescent drug abuse. Because risks are present in several social domains and cumulate in predicting drug abuse, multicomponent prevention strategies focused on reducing multiple risks and enhancing multiple protective factors hold promise. Such interventions would be designed to build up protection while reducing risk.

Each risk factor targeted should be addressed during the developmental period during which it begins to stabilize as a predictor of subsequent drug abuse. If the prevalence of drug abuse is to be reduced significantly through prevention efforts, interventions must also target populations at greatest risk, such as groups and individuals that are exposed to many risk factors.

More research is needed to determine effective interventions. The following are considered to be essential components of effective interventions:

- Communicating a clear, nonuse message for youth through all community channels, policies, and practice
- Role modeling of moderate, low-risk use of ATOD by adults of legal age
- Promoting bonding and attachments to family, peer, school, and religion and belief in general social norms, values, and expectations
- Increasing the perceived benefits of health-enhancing behaviors and decreasing the perceived benefits of health-compromising behaviors
- Providing referral, counseling, or treatment services for children or families in need of help

Many questions remain unanswered because prevention of substance abuse is a complex area to study and existing research is weak. Some of the research problems are related to inadequate sample size, nonrandom samples, and methodology.

Risk-focused prevention studies require research designs that address threats to validity posed by mixed units of analysis, differential attrition, and differential implementation as well as the interpretive challenge presented by heterogeneous effects across risk groups and along the developmental life course. Careful theoretical specification and multiple and varied statistical analysis techniques can be used to meet these challenges (Hawkins et al., 1992). Studies that address several areas of concern and are longitudinal would also be helpful.

SUMMARY

Past efforts for the prevention of substance abuse have focused on education. New paradigms are broadening the intervention focus to address the complexity of variables influencing substance abuse. Continued effort in the testing of interventions is needed to determine which interventions are effective to improve quality of life for individuals and their families and to reduce the cost of substance abuse to individuals, families, and society in lost human potential and productivity.

REFERENCES

Allen, K. M. (1996). Prevention. In K. M. Allen (Ed.), *Nursing care of the addicted client* (pp. 91-99). Philadelphia: J. B. Lippincott.

Bandura, A. (1977). Self-efficacy: Toward a unifying theory of behavioral change. *Psychological Review, 84*(2), 191-215.

Belcher, H. M. E., & Shinitzky, H. E. (1998). Substance abuse in children: Prediction, protection, and prevention. *Archives of Pediatric & Adolescent Medicine, 152*(10), 952-960.

Botvin, G. J. (1986). Substance abuse prevention research: Recent developments and future directions. *Journal of School Health, 56*(9), 369-374.

Botvin, G. J., Baker, E., Renick, N. L., Filazzola, A. D., & Botvin, E. M. (1984). A cognitive-behavioral approach to substance abuse prevention. *Addictive Behaviors, 9*(2), 137-147.

Botvin, G. J., & Wills, T. A. (1985). Personal and social skills training: Cognitive-behavioral approaches to substance abuse prevention. In C. Bell & R. J. Battjes (Eds.), *Prevention research: Deterring drug abuse among children and adolescents 8-49* (NIDA Research Monograph No. 63). Washington, DC: Government Printing Office.

Brook, J. S., Brook, D. W., Gordon, A. S., Whiteman, M., & Cohen, P. (1990). The psychosocial etiology of adolescent drug use: A family interactional approach. *Genetic, Social, and General Psychology Monographs, 116*(2).

Bukoski, W. J. (1986). School-based substance abuse prevention: A review of program research. In S. Griswold-Ezekoye, K. L. Kumpfer, & W. J. Bukoski (Eds.), *Childhood and chemical abuse* (pp. 95-115). New York: Haworth.

Center for Substance Abuse Prevention. (1994). *Invest in prevention: Prevention works in health care delivery systems.* Rockville, MD: U.S. Department of Health and Human Services, Substance Abuse and Mental Health Services Administration.

Covey, S. R. (1997). *The 7 habits of highly effective families: Building a beautiful family culture in a turbulent world.* New York: Golden Books.

Covey, S. R. (1998, November 16). *Strengthening families.* Family Dialogue Workshops, Des Moines, IA.

Eells, M. A. (1991). Strategies for promotion of avoiding harmful substance. *Nursing Clinics of North America, 26*(4), 915-927.

Flay, B. R. (1985). Psychosocial approaches to smoking prevention: A review of findings. *Health Psychology, 4*(5), 449-488.

Gropper, M., Livaz, Z., Portowicz, D., & Schindler, M. (1995). Computer integrated drug prevention: A new approach to teach lower socioeconomic 5th and 6th grade Israeli children to say no to drugs. *Social Work in Health Care, 22*(2), 87-103.

Hahn, E. J. (1995). Predicting head start parent involvement in an alcohol and other drug prevention program. *Nursing Research, 44,* 45-51.

Hawkins, J. D., Catalano, R. F., & Miller, J. Y. (1992). Risk and protective factors for alcohol and other drug problems in adolescent and early adulthood: Implications for substance abuse prevention. *Psychological Bulletin, 112,* 64-105.

Iowa Intervention Project. (2000). *Nursing interventions classification (NIC)* (J. C. McCloskey & G. M. Bulechek, Eds.; 3rd ed.). St. Louis, MO: Mosby-Year Book.

Iowa Outcomes Project. (2000). *Nursing outcomes classification (NOC)* (M. Johnson, M. Maas, & S. Moorhead, (Eds.; 2nd ed.). St. Louis, MO: Mosby-Year Book.

Johnson, E. M., Amatetti, S., Funkhouser, J. E., & Johnson, S. (1988). Theories and models supporting prevention approaches to alcohol problems among youth. *Public Health Reports, 103*(6), 578-586.

Jones, R. T., Corbin, S. K. T., Sheehy, L., & Bruce, S. (1995). Substance refusal: More than "just say no." *Journal of Child and Adolescent Substance Abuse, 4*(2), 1-25.

Kalnins, I. V., Hart, C., Ballantyne, P., Quartaro, G., Love, R., Sturis, G., & Pollack, P. (1994). School-based community development as a health promotion strategy for children. *Health Promotion International, 9*(4), 269-279.

Nelson-Simley, K., & Erickson, L. (1995). The Nebraska "network of drug-free youth" program. *Journal of School Health, 65*(2), 49-53.

North American Nursing Diagnosis Association. (1999). *Nursing diagnoses: Definitions and classification 1999-2000.* Philadelphia: Author.

Polich, J. M., Ellickson, P. L., Reuter, P., & Kahan, J. P. (1984). *Strategies for controlling adolescent drug use.* Santa Monica, CA: RAND.

Rutter, M. (1985). Resilience in the face of adversity: Protective factors and resistance to psychiatric disorder. *British Journal of Psychiatry, 147,* 598-611.

U.S. Department of Health and Human Services. (1991). *Healthy people 2000: National health promotion and disease prevention objectives* (DHHS Publication No. PHS 91-50312). Washington, DC: Government Printing Office.

39

Teaching Sexuality

Barbara Neitzel-Schneider

Adolescent sexual activity has been a concern of parents, clergy, teachers, communities, health care providers, and the government. The percentage of adolescent females 15 to 19 years of age who have had sexual intercourse has steadily increased during the past two decades. In 1970, 29% of adolescent females in this age group had had intercourse: This percentage increased to 36% in 1975, 47% in 1982, 53% in 1988, and 55% in 1990. In 1995, a promising trend showed that the percentage of female adolescents 15 to 19 years of age who have ever had intercourse declined to 50% (Abma, Chandra, Mosher, Peterson, & Piccinino, 1997). There was also a decline from 60% in 1988 to 55% in 1995 for adolescent males 15 to 19 years of age who have ever had intercourse (Children's Defense Fund, 1997). The number of teens who are sexually active remains high, however, putting them at risk for pregnancy, sexually transmitted diseases (STDs), and the psychological sequelae of early initiation of sexual activity.

There is no definite reason for the decline in adolescent sexual activity and birth rate. Experts in the field of adolescent sexuality presume that programs that provide adolescents with information about abstinence, birth control methods, and safer sex to prevent HIV and STDs, as well as comprehensive youth development programs that encourage adolescents to choose healthy lifestyles and work toward productive futures, are contributing to this decline. Despite the promising trends of adolescent sexual activity, the adolescent birth rate in the United States is the highest of any industrialized nation and nearly twice as high as that of the United Kingdom, which has the second highest adolescent birth rate (Robin Hood Foundation, 1996). The purpose of this chapter is to review the literature on research-based multifaceted sexuality education curriculums and identify nursing activities and outcomes for teaching sexuality.

SCOPE OF THE PROBLEM

Many diseases can be transmitted through sexual activity and may cause serious health problems, such as HIV, cancer, and infertility. Three million adolescents acquire STDs every year, and adolescents account for 25% of the 12 million new sexually transmitted infections that occur annually in the United States (Alan Guttmacher Institute, 1994). The number of reported AIDS cases among adolescents is small, but 20% of AIDS cases are diagnosed in people in their 20s and these people are thought to have contracted the virus during adolescence (Alan Guttmacher Institute, 1994).

The adolescent birth rate in the United States had decreased for decades until 1986: The birth rate per 1,000 adolescents 15 to 19 years of age increased from 50.2 in 1986 to 62.1 in 1991. Since 1991, there has been a reversal in adolescent childbearing, with the rate of childbearing per 1,000 adolescents 15 to 19 years of age declining to 56.9 in 1995 (Children's Defense Fund, 1997). This decline in adolescent childbearing is thought to be due to the decline in the number of adolescents engaging in sexual intercourse and the increased use of contraception. Two thirds of adolescents use some method of birth control the first time they have sexual intercourse, and between 72% and 84% of adolescents continue to use a birth control method with sexual intercourse, primarily the condom or the birth control pill (Alan Guttmacher Institute, 1994). Condom use in adolescents at first intercourse tripled between the 1970s and 1990s. In the 1970s, 18% of adolescents having their first intercourse used a condom compared to 36% in the 1980s and 54% in the 1990s (Abma et al., 1997). The use of birth control pills increases with age, as does the likelihood for an adolescent to make an appointment at a family planning clinic. There are differences in birth control use depending on race. White adolescents are more likely than African American and Hispanic adolescents to use some method of birth control; African Americans, however, are more likely than whites to use the birth control pill (Alan Guttmacher Institute, 1994).

While there has been an increase in adolescent use of birth control methods, there has been a decrease in the number of adolescent pregnancies resulting in abortion. Adolescent abortion rates increased in the years prior to the legalization of abortion in 1973 and then became stable in the late 1980s. Abortion rates among sexually active adolescents have declined steadily and account for approximately one fourth of all abortions performed annually (Alan Guttmacher Institute, 1994). Adolescents who are from a higher socioeconomic status and have high academic achievement and aspirations are less likely to become pregnant but are more likely to have an abortion if they do have an unintended pregnancy (Children's Defense Fund, 1997).

Two trends make these declines in adolescent sexual activity and births even more compelling. During the past century, the onset of puberty has been steadily declining, and on average female sexual maturity is now reached between 12 and 12½ years of age. Full-time employment, economic independence, and marriage have been traditional indicators of adulthood. Young adults have been delaying marriage into their 20s, with the average age of marriage now 24 years of age for women and 26 years for men. This is 3 or 4 years later than the average age of marriage in the 1950s (Children's Defense Fund, 1997).

Developmental Perspective

Society is in agreement that adolescent pregnancy is an unfortunate reality, but there is disagreement on how to prevent this multidimensional problem. It may take multiple interventions to address the concern of unintended adolescent pregnancy. To effectively implement interventions, it is important to understand the cognitive and psychosocial development of adolescence. According to Piaget's theory of cognitive development, the adolescent is beginning to develop operational or abstract thinking (Wadsworth, 1971). This is necessary for planning the future but is not fully developed in the young adolescent. Adolescence has also been characterized as a period of cognitive egocentricism, labeled the "personal fable." These are beliefs that adolescents have about their lives that have a theme of invulnerability. The adolescent's immature cognitive development may explain why many are unable to perceive preventive behavior or comprehend the consequences of their behavior. In Erikson's (1963) psychosocial developmental theory, adolescents are in the stage of identity versus role confusion. They are trying to find their identity in an adult world. The adolescent is observing the adult roles in society and attempting to incorporate those roles that fit with his or her personal identity to form a new adult identity. This gives adolescents a sense of individuality, control, and power over their lives. Adolescents experiment with and explore behavior as they strive to establish this adult identity. Experimentation often includes sexual exploration to test new sexual feelings and capabilities, but adolescents are not yet capable of comprehending the consequences of such behavior.

Epidemiological Perspective

There are many long-term consequences for adolescent parents and their children. Many adolescents who become parents are disadvantaged socially, economically, and educationally before they have children, which is often sustained throughout their lives. Approximately 60% of adolescents who become pregnant are living in poverty at the time they give birth (Alan Guttmacher Institute, 1994). Seven of 10 adolescent mothers will drop out of high school, with 70% finishing high school by the time they are 35 to 39 years of age. Adolescent mothers earn an average of $5,600 annually, less than half the poverty level, during the first 13 years of parenthood. These wages are not adequate for the adolescent to be self-sufficient; therefore, more than 70% of adolescent mothers will be welfare recipients, with 40% continuing to be welfare recipients for 5 or more years during the decade after their first birth (Robin Hood Foundation, 1996).

Adolescent mothers are more likely then their peers to have grown up in a single-parent household and spend nearly five times more of their young adult years as single parents than women who delay childbearing until 20 or 21 years of age. Of those adolescents who choose to marry, nearly one third will be divorced within 5 years. In fact, even second marriages of females who have became mothers before age 20 are at risk for marital instability (Alan Guttmacher Institute, 1994; Robin Hood Foundation, 1996).

Almost half of adolescent mothers will give birth to their second child within 2 years. Births that are closely spaced early in an adolescent's life inhibit educational attainment and employment security and thus increase welfare dependency. Additional children, welfare dependency, and the delays in educational attainment and employment add more stress to the life of the adolescent and her children. Children of adolescents are prone to high rates of health problems and often start life as low-birth-weight infants (Robin Hood Foundation, 1996). Adolescent mothers are not inclined to spontaneously play with their infants and tend to use non-verbal forms of interaction (Ruff, 1990). They become easily frustrated with their children's misbehavior and are likely to discipline using physical punishment (Reis, 1988; Reis & Herz, 1987). The children of adolescent mothers consistently score lower than children of later childbearers on measures of cognitive development, and they are 50% more likely to repeat a grade and drop out of high school (Alan Guttmacher Institute, 1994; Robin Hood Foundation, 1996). The cycle of adolescent parenting continues: Daughters of adolescent mothers are 83% more likely than their peers to become mothers before their 18th birthday. The sons of adolescent mothers are 2.7 times more likely to spend time in prison than the sons of mothers who delayed childbearing until their early 20s (Robin Hood Foundation, 1996).

Objective 5.1 in *Healthy People 2000* (U.S. Department of Health and Human Services [USDHHS], 1991) is to reduce adolescent pregnancies to no more than 50 per 1,000 girls aged 17 and younger. Sexuality education is a primary prevention strategy to reduce adolescent pregnancy. Sexuality education provides children with the knowledge needed to understand sexuality so that they can make responsible, healthy choices in their lives. According to Roseman (1991), information leads to informed decision making and awareness of the power over one's life. There is controversy, however, regarding what information should be included in sexuality education programs, who should provide this information, at what age education should begin, and even whether this education influences the decisions that adolescents make about their sexual behavior. Nurses can be instrumental in providing families, schools, and communities with research-based educational strategies, sexuality information, and support to provide children with the information and skills needed to make healthy lifestyle choices. Sexuality education begins at birth, and parents can be provided with anticipatory guidance to enable them to be the primary sexuality educators for their children. Unfortunately, some children do not receive this education at home, and it becomes imperative that schools provide sexuality information and skills to children.

LITERATURE REVIEW

Sexuality education begins at birth and continues as a lifelong process, with parents as the primary sexuality educators. Parents may need help in this important role that can be provided by health and education professionals, religious leaders, extended family members, and community leaders (Finan, 1997; Sexuality Information and Education Council of the United States [SIECUS], 1995). SIECUS acknowledges that "sexuality is a natural and healthy part of living, and encompasses the sexual knowledge, beliefs, attitudes, values, and behaviors of individuals" (p. 1). SIECUS further recognizes and supports comprehensive school-based education beginning with kindergarten and continuing through 12th grade that is appropriate to students' age, developmental level, and cultural background.

There are a wide variety of approaches and curriculums for sexuality education. Kirby, Barth, Leland, and Fetro (1991) grouped sexuality education into four generations. The first generation emphasized the risk and consequences of pregnancy by focusing on increasing students' knowledge about sexuality. The second generation also included increasing students' knowledge of sexuality but added the dimension of value clarification, decision making, and communication skills. It was believed that obtaining these skills would make it more likely that students would avoid risk-taking behavior and effectively communicate their values and decisions to their partners. Most of the research on sexuality education has evaluated first- and second-generation curriculums and indicates that these programs increased the students' knowledge (Kirby, 1992; Kirby et al., 1991; Marsiglio & Mott, 1986; Parcel & Coreil, 1985; Thomas et al., 1985). Research also indicates, however, that increased knowledge had little if any effect on sexual activity, contraception, and adolescent pregnancy (Kirby, 1985, 1992; Kirby et al., 1991; Marsigilio & Mott, 1986; Stout & Rivara, 1989).

Third-generation sex education curriculums focused on teaching abstinence. These programs emphasized that adolescents should postpone sexual intercourse until marriage and did not discuss contraception to avoid communicating a double message. Evaluation of abstinence-only programs showed that they did not delay the onset of sexual intercourse (Roosa & Christopher, 1990). The fourth-generation sexuality education curriculums represent a combination of the three previous generations. This generation emphasized delaying sexual intercourse until adolescents achieve adult maturity and discussed the importance of safer sex practices, including contraception, for teens who chose to engage in sexual activity. These curriculums have shown effectiveness in promoting responsible sexual behavior in adolescents.

The School/Community Program for Sexual Risk Reduction Among Teens is an example of a fourth-generation sexuality education program that has decreased the occurrence of pregnancies in adolescents younger than 18 years of age (Vincent, Clearie, & Schluchter, 1987). This is a public health education model that targeted the intervention messages to parents, teachers, community leaders, ministers, and children, kindergarten through 12th grade, in the western portion of a South Carolina county public school system. The goal for including adults in educational opportunities was to develop their skills as positive role models for children in the community. The primary behavioral objective is "to postpone initial voluntary sexual intercourse among never-married teens and preteens" (p. 3383). The secondary behavioral objective is "to promote among never-married teens and preteens who choose to become sexually active and who do not desire a pregnancy to occur, the consistent use of effective contraceptive" (p. 3383). The educational objective is "to promote the postponement of initial voluntary intercourse as a positive, preferred sexual and health decision" (p. 3383). This educational objective has five subcomponents—to "increase decision-making skills, improve interpersonal communication skills, enhance self-esteem, align personal values with the families, church, and community, and to increase knowledge of human reproductive anatomy, physiology, and contraception" (p. 3383).

The program Helping Teenagers Postpone Sexual Involvement is another example of a successful sexuality education curriculum (Howard & McCabe, 1990). This program was added to an existing school curriculum that gave 8th-grade students information about reproduction, family planning, and STDs. The presenters were trained students from 11th or 12th grade. The program emphasized the effectiveness of peer education and counseling in an interactive process of role playing. The program students postponed sexual involvement and were more likely to continue postponing sexual intercourse into the 9th grade. Students who did engage in sexual intercourse after completing the program were more likely to use effective contraceptives. Those students who were sexually active before beginning the program, however, were neither more likely to use contraceptive nor to reduce sexual intercourse than students who had not been involved with the program.

Reducing the Risk is another fourth-generation curriculum that emphasized avoiding unprotected intercourse by abstinence or using effective contraception. Components of the program include identifying social pressures to have sex; developing and practicing effective strategies to resist pressure; activities to personalize information about sexuality, reproduction, and contraception; and training in decision making, assertive communication skills, and applying these skills in personal situations (Kirby et al., 1991). The curriculum provided factual information to 9th- through 12th-grade students and gave students opportunities to practice the skills they learned in decision making and communication by role playing common situations they face concerning their sexuality. The curriculum also encouraged teens to ask their parents about abstinence and birth control. This program significantly increased the students' knowledge about abstinence and contraception. Communication concerning abstinence and birth control was increased between program students and their parents. The curriculum also reduced the incidence of sexual intercourse among program students up to 18 months after the program, although the curriculum did not significantly increase the use of contraception with those students who chose to be sexually active after participating in the program. The program also did not affect the frequency of sexual intercourse or use of contraception among those adolescents who were already sexually active.

Safer Choices is a multicomponent program with the primary purpose of reducing the number of 14- to 18-year-old students engaging in unprotected intercourse by reducing the number who begin having intercourse in high school and to increase the condom use among those who engage in sexual intercourse (Coyle et al., 1996). The primary components of Safer Choices are school organization, curriculum, and staff development, peer resources and school environment, parent education, and school-community linkages (Coyle et al., 1996). A School Health Promotion Council is established at each program school to serve as the organizational mechanism to ensure the intervention becomes schoolwide and is part of the school culture. The council consists of parents, teachers, administrators, staff, students, and local community agency staff (Coyle et al., 1996). The curriculum consists of a 10-lesson series for 9th- and 10th-grade students and is based on the successful curriculum, Reducing the Risk: Building to Prevent Pregnancy. The lessons address attitudes and beliefs, social skills, functional knowledge, social and media influences, peer norms, and parent-child communication. Peer modeling is an important component of this curriculum, and trained students are facilitators for activities such as skill development. Safer Choices Peer Teams and adult peer coordinators plan and host events to saturate the school environment with activities, information, and services to create an environment that supports HIV, STD, and pregnancy prevention. The parent education component is designed to provide parents with information through newsletters and student homework assignments about HIV, STD, and pregnancy and about how to communicate with teenagers regarding these issues. School-community linkages are achieved through the development of resource guides of youth service agencies for families, students, and school personnel. Also through homework assignments, students are expected to gather information about local support and services outside of the school system (Coyle et al., 1996). Safer Choices is currently being evaluated in 20 schools.

It appears from the results of these effective sexuality education curriculums that it is important to implement educational programs before adolescents become sexually active. Because the statistics report that 30% of adolescents have engaged in sexual intercourse by age 15 (SIECUS, 1994), curriculums must be implemented in grade school and junior high school.

NURSING DIAGNOSIS AND OUTCOME DETERMINATION

The nursing diagnoses that apply to the nursing intervention Teaching: Sexuality include Knowledge Deficit, Decisional Conflict, Risk for Infection (STDs) (North American Nursing Diagnosis Association [NANDA], 1999), and At Risk for Unintended Pregnancy: Adolescents (Merry, 1995). Several outcomes from the Nursing Outcomes Classification are applicable, including Knowledge: Health Behaviors, Decision-Making, Risk Control: Sexually Transmitted Diseases (STDs), and Risk Control: Unintended Pregnancy (Iowa Outcomes Project, 2000).

Knowledge Deficit is defined as an "absence or deficiency of cognitive information related to a specific topic" (NANDA, 1999, p. 118). Adolescents who choose inappropriate, risky behavior may not have an adequate knowledge base to identify or provide protection from the potential consequences of sexual activity, which include pregnancy and contracting HIV or other STDs. *Knowledge: Health Behaviors* is a nursing-sensitive outcome defined as the "extent of understanding conveyed about the promotion and protection of health" (Iowa Outcomes Project, 2000, p. 268). Adolescents who have achieved a level of understanding of health behaviors will be able to describe methods of family planning and measures to prevent transmission of infectious disease.

Decisional Conflict is defined as "the state of uncertainty about course of action to be taken when choice among competing actions involves risk, loss, or challenge to personal life values" (NANDA, 1999, p. 82). Many factors are involved in making decisions, such as identifying personal beliefs or values, acquisition of relevant information to make informed decision, identifying consequences of alternative choices, and experience in decision making. Adolescents need guidance and skills in decision making to make healthy lifestyle choices. The outcome *Decision-Making* is defined as the "ability to choose between two or more alternatives" (Iowa Outcomes Project, 2000, p. 194). Decision making involves identifying relevant information and the alternatives and potential consequences of each alternative.

Risk for Infection (STDs) is defined by NANDA (1999) as "the state in which an individual is at increased risk for being invaded by pathogenic organisms" (p. 14). Adolescents who do not practice safer sex are at increased exposure to STDs and HIV. In many cases, adolescents may not have sufficient knowledge to avoid exposure to these potentially deadly viruses. "Actions to eliminate or reduce behaviors associated with STDs" is the definition of the nursing-sensitive outcomes *Risk Control: Sexually Transmitted Disease (STD)* (Iowa Outcomes Project, 2000, p. 362). Adolescents who have achieved risk control will acknowledge individual risk for STDs and the personal consequences associated with STDs and use methods to control STD transmission.

At Risk for Unintended Pregnancy: Adolescents is defined as "any unanticipated pregnancy during a female's adolescent developmental stage, which is 11 to 19 years old, in which there was a failure to utilize abstinence, contraception, counseling, or contraception failure" (Merry, 1995, p. 20). Adolescents with minimal or no adult supervision, low self-esteem, who are vulnerable to peer pressure, and who have not achieved cognitive maturity are at risk for adolescent pregnancy. The nursing outcome *Risk Control: Unintended Pregnancy* is defined as "actions to reduce the possibility of unintended pregnancy" (Iowa Outcomes Project, 2000, p. 366). Indicators of a successful outcome include the acknowledgment of risk for unintended pregnancy, understanding the physiological processes of conception, and the development of effective pregnancy prevention strategies that may include the identification of appropriate birth control methods.

INTERVENTION: TEACHING: SEXUALITY

The definition of *Teaching: Sexuality* is "assisting individuals to understand the physical and psychosocial dimensions of sexual growth and development" (Iowa Intervention Project, 1996, p. 558). The development of healthy sexuality begins at birth and is a developmental process much like feeding, sleeping, elimination, and motor development. Sexuality not only involves sexual feelings and reproduction but also involves the capacity for intimacy, security, affiliation, communication, mutual respect, and responsibility (Haka-Ikse & Mian, 1993). Erikson's (1963) developmental theory can guide nurses in assisting children and supporting parents as primary educators in the development of healthy sexuality. At each health maintenance examination, time can be spent with parents and children to address their developing sexuality and explore the meaning of sexual roles. Nurses serve as role models for parents and children. An accepting, nonjudgmental atmosphere should be established during the newborn period and maintained through childhood and adolescence. Sexuality education is a continuum, and nurses can educate parents on sexual growth and development through the life span beginning at their first encounter and continuing at each visit. During the newborn exam, parents should be informed of the normal enlargement of the sex organs in the first few weeks of life, and the correct name for body parts should be encouraged. Infants learn basic trust when their needs for food, elimination, sleep, and physical stimulation are met in a comforting manner. This allows infants to trust people and begin to understand their relationship with others. Parents should be informed that cuddling, massage, kissing, and singing to their infants is vital for development. Infants also begin to learn to trust themselves as control over body movements begins to develop. Parents should receive anticipatory guidance on safety and their role in protecting infants while they learn to control body movements.

The toddler enters the stage of autonomy versus shame and doubt (Erikson, 1963). In this developmental stage, the toddler continues to gain independent control over his or her body. Opportunities for physical activities are necessary the toddler to experience his or her body's strengths and limitations. Through parenting, the toddler begins to learn social and family norms while separating self from parents. Rules about sharing, communication, assertiveness, and negotiation will help toddlers experience pleasant and supportive relationships. Toddlers become intensely curious about their bodies and frequently touch all body parts. Parents should be encouraged to use the correct terminology for body parts and not shame toddlers for exploring their bodies.

Preschoolers begin to exercise their own initiative in activities and thought. This stage gives rise to fantasy and modeling of parental behavior. The preschooler's imitating behavior strengthens the role of male versus female. Nurses can support parents in their explanations of anatomical differences and questions about where babies come from. Nurses can provide parents with a bibliography of age-appropriate sexuality education materials to use in answering the preschoolers' questions. Television and other media begin to become major influences during this period. Parents need support in setting limits on the content and amounts of time children view television and other media sources. Parents also need to promote values and explain and model what they are, how they are obtained, and their effect on choices in life.

In middle childhood, feelings of competency in intellectual and physical skills develop in the stage of industry versus inferiority (Erikson, 1963). The child usually focuses on what is happening in his or her environment and begins to learn about the world. Nurses should encourage parents to be good role models of family values and discuss with their children the effects of values on choices in life. When puberty approaches, nurses should spend time with the child and parents to explain human anatomy and physiology of the male and female body, physical and emotional development, and the anatomy and physiology of human reproduction. Sufficient time should be spent discussing peer and social pressures regarding sexual activities and the meaning of sexual roles. This is also an important time to discuss STDs, HIV, and pregnancy prevention. Parents should be encouraged and supported in an open discussion with their children on sexual behavior and appropriate expressions of feelings. The nurse should encourage abstinence with a concrete discussion on the benefits of postponing sexual activity and negative consequences of early childbearing. Nurses should develop or provide or both parents and children with age-appropriate sexuality reading materials to further educate and facilitate conversation of sexuality at home.

Adolescence is a time of identity versus role confusion (Erikson, 1963). During this stage, adolescents are establishing an adult identity and experiment with ideas, behaviors, and relationships with others. Adolescence is a time of discovering one's place in the world. The adolescent should be given the opportunity to be alone with the health care provider during the health maintenance examination. Information and guidance provided in previous office visits should be reinforced, and the responsibility of actions of the adolescent when developing his or her personal identity should also be discussed. Nurses must create an accepting, nonjudgmental, and confidential atmosphere so that adolescents may express their sexual concerns and behaviors. A discussion of the benefits of abstinence and responsibility for sexual behavior should occur. The nurse should use appropriate questions to assist the adolescent to reflect on what is important personally. Sexually active adolescents should be provided with information about safer sex, contraceptive options, and accessibility. Assistance should be provided to the sexually active adolescent in choosing an appropriate contraceptive. The adolescent and parent should be seen together at some point during the health maintenance visit. This provides the nurse with the opportunity to observe and facilitate communication between adolescent and parent.

Nurses can provide information and support to parent groups and schoolteachers and administrators as they develop and implement research-based sexuality education curriculums. Nurses may be viewed by children as sympathetic, trained professionals in the discussion of sexuality issues. Therefore, they are in an ideal position to provide sexuality education in school settings. They can also be instrumental in training students as peer group facilitators as they role play assertiveness and communication skills to resist peer and social pressures of sexual activity. Self-esteem is enhanced through peer role modeling and role playing.

The nurse can use other nursing interventions from the Nursing Interventions Classification (Iowa Intervention Project, 2000) to complement the activities for Teaching: Sexuality, including Self-Esteem Promotion, Decision-Making Support, Teaching: Safe Sex, Family Planning: Contraception, and AIDS Prevention.

INTERVENTION APPLICATION

Brook is a 13-year-old, seventh-grade student. She lives with her parents and two brothers in a small midwestern community and attends the local middle school. Brook has received her health care from a local family practice clinic that has a family practice physician and a pediatric nurse practitioner (PNP) available for health maintenance examinations (HMEs) and treatment of acute illnesses. Brook feels particularly comfortable with the PNP and has seen the PNP for all of her health care needs. During scheduled HMEs, the PNP has provided Brook and her parents with age-appropriate discussions about sexual growth and development, the meaning of sexual roles, and about emotional development during childhood. The PNP supports the parental role as the primary sexuality educator and has resources available to assist parents in promoting healthy sexuality in their children. A bibliography is also made available to parents for sexuality education materials at the local library.

The PNP has been instrumental in developing a local multicomponent school-based pregnancy, STD, and HIV prevention program with teachers, school administrators, parents, clergy, and local small business owners in the community. The program is designed to provide sexuality education and STD and HIV prevention information to teachers, students, parents, and the community; it also encourages the school and community to support healthy lifestyle choices. There are four sections to this program that involve education and year-round activities for students from kindergarten to 12th grade. Section 1 focuses on the anatomy and physiology of the male and female body and human reproduction. Section 2 explores values, sexual roles and responsible behaviors, and the media, peer, and societal influences on values and sexual roles. Section 3 concentrates on the benefits of postponing sexual activity and provides education on STDs, HIV, and adolescent pregnancy. The last section informs students about contraceptives and their proper use, effectiveness, and accessibility. In each section, there is an assignment that facilitates communication between student and parents. Parents are sent a quarterly newsletter that provides them with a schedule of school activities as well as information on STDs, HIV, and adolescent pregnancy. The newsletter also provides parents with tips on talking with their children and adolescents about sexuality. Parents are also invited to parent meetings at the school that provide them with education, support, and time to establish networks with other parents.

Brook has been involved in this program since kindergarten and is training to be a peer role model and facilitator who, along with other students and adults, plans and implements schoolwide activities. Currently, Brook is working on a schoolwide contest that creatively displays messages on abstinence, the consequences of sexual activity, and overcoming the peer and societal pressures to become sexually active. The displays will be used on bulletin boards, monthly calendars, and T-shirts. Brook's brother, Adam, belongs to the high school drama team, which periodically performs skits at schoolwide assemblies that entertain and provide students with information on STD, HIV, and pregnancy prevention. In classrooms, students form small groups and role play preventive behavior. The school has a student newspaper that has a section composed of anonymous stories written by peers about abstinence and personal experiences in choosing not to have sex.

The PNP has created a caring, accepting, and nonjudgmental rapport with the students through the involvement at the school level and accessibility at the family practice clinic. The family planning clinic and local businesses have used contest displays to reinforce the message about STD, HIV, and pregnancy prevention. The PNP and teachers evaluated the program using outcomes from the Nursing Outcomes Classification (2000) and found that the program has been successful in increasing student knowledge, preventive behavior, self-esteem, decision making, and assertiveness skills.

RESEARCH AND PRACTICE IMPLICATIONS

Information is the tool nurses can provide for adolescents to make responsible decisions about sexual activity. There is controversy regarding what should be taught in sexuality programs, at what age children should be educated, and who should be the educators. There are many sexuality education curriculums, but only a few have been evaluated using research methods or have been evaluated for their long-term effects. Additional research should evaluate existing sexuality education curriculums not only for their effectiveness in increasing knowledge but also for the effect that they have on behavior. Longitudinal studies are needed to determine the long-term effects in reducing sexual activity and unintended pregnancy, STDs, and AIDS. Existing curriculums should be revised to include components of successful programs.

The current climate of health care and government-funded programs is focusing on prevention services and research-based programs. Nurses are employed in a variety of settings with diverse populations in the community, school-based clinics, family planning clinics, primary care clinics, and hospitals in which research-based primary prevention programs can be developed. Nurses should educate the community about the multifaceted issue of adolescent pregnancy. They can be instrumental in organizing and supporting community adolescent pregnancy prevention coalitions and programs in which multiple strategies can be developed that involve parents, teachers, community leaders, and clergy in delaying sexual activity and preventing STDs, HIV, and unintended adolescent pregnancy. They are also in the unique position to counsel, educate, support, and facilitate parents as the primary educators about sexuality. This can be accomplished during each health maintenance visit and should be a continuum much like education of other development during life. Many nurses may feel uncomfortable discussing sexuality issues with children, adolescents, and parents. Experienced practitioners should publish teaching strategies that diminish the discomforts encountered when teaching sexuality. Role playing may be a strategy for the nurse to overcome the uneasiness in teaching sexuality. Nurses may want to start an Internet discussion group with other practitioners to share the most current information on the most effective ways of teaching about sexuality. Research should be conducted on the support and guidance that parents perceive they need in communicating with their children about sexuality and incorporated into practice. To reach the goal of *Healthy People 2000* Objective 5.1 (USDHHS, 1991), nurses must implement the intervention Teaching: Sexuality in schools, the community, and primary health care settings and continue to evaluate the effectiveness of these programs on adolescent knowledge and behavior.

REFERENCES

Abma, J. C., Chandra, A., Mosher, W. D., Peterson, L., & Piccinino, L. (1997). Fertility, family planning, and women's health: New data from the 1995 National Survey of Family Growth, National Center for Health Statistics. *Vital Health Statistics, 23*(19).

Alan Guttmacher Institute. (1994). *Sex and America's teenagers.* New York: Author.

Children's Defense Fund. (1997). *The state of America's children.* Washington, DC: Author.

Coyle, K., Kirby, D., Parcel, G., Basen-Engquist, K., Banspach, S., Rugg, D., & Weil, M. (1996). Safer choices: A multicomponent school-based HIV/STD and pregnancy prevention program for adolescents. *Journal of School Health, 66*(3), 89-94.

Erikson, E. H. (1963). *Childhood and society* (2nd ed.). New York: Norton.

Finan, S. (1997). Promoting healthy sexuality: Guidelines for the school-age child and adolescent. *Nurse Practitioner, 22*(11), 62-72.

Haka-Ikse, K., & Mian, M. (1993). Sexuality in children. *Pediatrics in Review, 14*(10), 401-407.

Howard, M., & McCabe, J. B. (1990). Helping teenagers postpone sexual involvement. *Family Planning Perspectives, 22,* 21-26.

Iowa Intervention Project. (2000). *Nursing interventions classification (NIC)* (J. C. McCloskey & G. M. Bulechek, Eds.; 3rd ed.). St. Louis, MO: Mosby-Year Book.

Iowa Outcomes Project. (2000). *Nursing outcomes classification (NOC)* (M. Johnson, M. Maas, & S. Moorhead, Eds.; 2nd ed.). St. Louis, MO: Mosby-Year Book.

Kirby, D. (1985). Sexuality education: A more realistic view of its effects. *Journal of School Health, 50*(10), 421-424.

Kirby, D. (1992). School based programs to reduce sexual risk-taking behaviors. *Journal of School Health, 62*(7), 280-287.

Kirby, D., Barth, R., Leland, N., & Fetro, J. (1991). Reducing the risk: Impact of a new curriculum on sexual risk-taking. *Family Planning Perspectives, 23*(6), 253-263.

Marsiglio, W., & Mott, F. (1986). The impact of sex education on sexual activity, contraceptive use and premarital pregnancy among American teenagers. *Family Planning Perspectives, 23*(6), 253-263.

Merry, K. (1995). *High risk for unplanned pregnancy: Adolescents.* Unpublished master's thesis, University of Iowa, College of Nursing, Iowa City.

North American Nursing Diagnosis Association. (1999). *Nursing diagnoses: Definitions and classification 1999-2000.* Philadelphia: Author.

Parcel, G., & Coreil, J. (1985). Parental evaluations of a sex education course for young adults. *Journal of School Health, 55,* 9-12.

Reis, J. (1988). A comparison of young teenage, older teenage, and adult mothers on determinants of parenting. *Journal of Psychology, 123*(2), 141-151.

Reis, J., & Herz, E. (1987). Correlates of adolescent parenting. *Adolescence, 22*(87), 599-609.

Robin Hood Foundation. (1996). *Kids having kids: A Robin Hood Foundation special report on the costs of adolescent childbearing* (R. Maynard, Ed.). New York: Author.

Roosa, M., & Christopher, F. (1990). Evaluation of an abstinence-only adolescent pregnancy prevention program. *Family Relations, 39*(10), 363-367.

Roseman, L. (Writer). (1991). *If you can talk to your kids about sex, you can talk to them about anything* [Videocassette]. East-West Media Productions.

Ruff, C. (1990). Adolescent mothering: Assessing their parenting capabilities and their health education needs. *Journal of the National Black Nurses Association, 4,* 55-62.

Sexuality Information and Education Council of the United States, National Guidelines Task Force. (1994). *Guidelines for comprehensive sexuality education: Kindergarten-12th grade.* New York: Author.

Sexuality Information and Education Council of the United States, National Guidelines Task Force. (1995). *Position statement on sexuality issues.* New York: Author.

Stout, J. W., & Rivara, F. P. (1989). Schools and sex education: Does it work? *Pediatrics, 83*(3), 375-379.

Thomas, L. L., Long, S. E., Whitten, K., Hamilton, B., Fraser, J., & Askins, R. V. (1985). High school students' long-term retention of sex education information. *Journal of School Health, 55*(7), 274-278.

U.S. Department of Health and Human Services. (1991). *Healthy people 2000: National health promotion and disease prevention objectives* (DHHS Publication No. PHS 91-50312). Washington, DC: Government Printing Office.

Vincent, M. L., Clearie, A. F., & Schluchter, M. D. (1987). Reducing adolescent pregnancy through school and community-based education program. *Journal of the American Medical Association, 257*(24), 3382-3385.

Wadsworth, B. J. (1971). *Piaget's theory of cognitive development.* New York: David McKay.

40

Teen Pregnancy

Primary Prevention

Mary Lober Aquilino

The teen pregnancy rate in the United States is higher than that of all other developed nations, with approximately 11% of females ages 13 to 19 years becoming pregnant each year. Although the figure for males is much more difficult to track, it is estimated that up to 7% of teen males become fathers annually. The majority of teen parents are unmarried (Maynard, 1996; Moore, Driscoll, & Lindberg, 1998). In addition, more than half of all adolescents report having had sexual intercourse by the age of 19 years, and age at first intercourse continues to decline (Office of Technology Assessment [OTA], 1991b). In fact, 17% of students in grades 7 and 8 report having had sexual intercourse (Blum & Rinehart, 1997). Although the number of pregnancies for all teens has declined slightly, there has been an increase in the pregnancy rate for teens younger than 16 years of age. The problem of adolescent pregnancy is not limited to any geographic area, social class, or ethnic group, and the annual public cost of teen pregnancy is estimated to be more than $7 billion (Holmes, 1996; Quint, 1996).

Teen pregnancy affects not only the teen parent(s) but also the off-spring, relatives, friends, taxpayers, and related professionals. Social, economic, and health consequences of teen pregnancy include truncated education, lower paying jobs, increased unemployment, increased likelihood of poverty, larger family size, a closer spacing of children, increased likelihood of marital disruption, and increased likelihood of future out-of-wedlock childbearing. Children of teen parents are more likely to have low birth weight and slower development, and they tend to do less well academically than other children (Card, 1999; Kirby, 1999; Maynard, 1996).

Because teen pregnancy affects and is affected by the teen's community, intervention for the primary prevention of this problem needs to be a communitywide effort. Parents, teachers, counselors, youth group leaders, health care providers, community leaders, legislators, law enforcement personnel, and other adults responsible for teen welfare need to be involved in the intervention. It must be recognized that factors that contribute to and prevent teen pregnancy are not all within the control of the individual or even the family.

Family planning is a priority area identified by *Healthy People 2000* (U.S. Department of Health and Human Services [USDHHS], 1991). National objectives specifically related to adolescents are to reduce pregnancies among girls, especially African Americans and Hispanics, aged 15 to 17 years; to reduce the proportion of adolescents who have engaged in sexual intercourse; to increase to at least 40% the proportion of ever-sexually active adolescents aged 17 years and younger who have abstained from sexual activity for the previous 3 months; to increase to at least 90% the proportion of sexually active, unmarried people aged 19 years and younger who use contraception; to increase to at least 85% the proportion of people aged 10 to 18 years who have discussed human sexuality, including values regarding sexuality, with their parents or have received information through another parentally endorsed source or both; and to increase to at least 60% the proportion of primary care providers who provide age-appropriate preconception care and counseling.

Midcourse reviews indicate mixed results in achieving the *Healthy People 2000* objectives that have been tracked (USDHHS, 1995). On the negative side, pregnancies among adolescent females 15 to 17 years of age and the number of 15- to 17-year-old adolescent males and females who have ever had sexual intercourse have increased. On the positive side, the proportion of teens who are choosing abstinence has increased slightly, and contraceptive use has increased between 40% and 50%.

THEORETICAL FRAMEWORK
AND LITERATURE REVIEW

The Interactive and Organizational Model of Community as Client provides a useful framework for discussing the complexity of preventing adolescent pregnancy (Kuehnert, 1995). This model suggests that nursing intervention be directed toward three distinct but related units: the individual and family, the aggregate, and the community. For each unit, the goal is health improvement or preservation. The primary function of the nurse in this model is the provision of direct service or advocacy (Figure 40.1).

The literature concerning teen pregnancy is extensive, often conflicting, and therefore difficult to summarize. Certain risk and protective factors, however, have been consistently associated with either the initiation of sexual activity or the use of contraception. These include (a) individual characteristics such as age at puberty, race, religiosity, personal aspirations, and personality traits; (b) family factors such as structure, relationships, and communication; (c) peer influence, including group norms; and (d) community characteristics such as norms and economic conditions.

Community and Aggregate Risk
and Protective Factors

Community factors that influence the sexual behavior of young people include the prevailing attitudes about sexuality and sexual behavior, norms and expectations for youth, and communication about sexually related matters. These may be generally accepted or culturally and ethnically defined. For example, the general norm in an industrialized society is to delay childbearing until education is completed, but certain subgroups within a society may exhibit different norms. For some first-generation Hispanic families, adolescent childbearing is not considered deviant but acceptable. Similarly, African American teens are more likely to give birth than whites, Native Americans, or Hispanics (Centers for Disease Control and Prevention, 1994).

A sense of connection to school and future promise seem to be the most influential factors in the prevention of teen pregnancy. Teens who participate in school activities and feel a part of their school are less likely to become sexually active at an early age. Likewise, teens growing up in an environment in which there is "more to life" after high school, who experience academic success, and who see a potential future in the marketplace are more likely to delay childbearing. Teens who have only a mini-

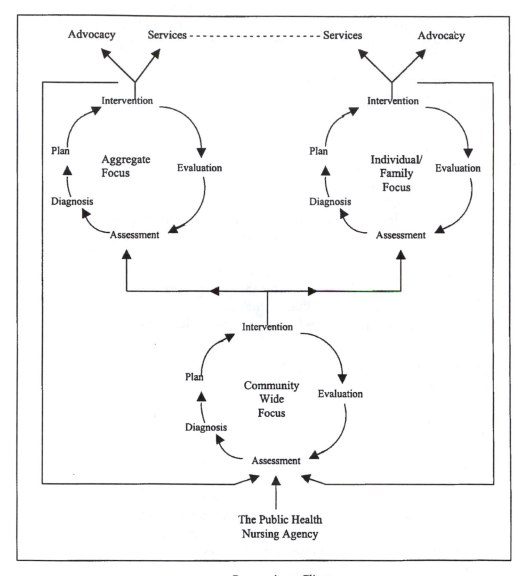

Community as Client

Figure 40.1. The Interactive and Organizational Model of Community as Client (From Community Health Nursing and the AIDS Pandemic: Case Report of One Community's Response, by P. L. Kuehnert, 1991, *Journal of Community Health Nursing*, Summer, pp. 137-146. Copyright © 1991 by Lawrence Erlbaum Associates. Reprinted with permission.)

mum-wage job with no potential for advancement to look forward to, however, are less likely to be concerned about the timing of childbearing.

Community involvement in youth development, community expectations for adolescents, values exhibited in the community, accessibility of health care and related services to adolescents, and the general economic welfare of the community all affect both the timing of initiation of sexual activity and the use of contraception.

Individual and Family Risk and Protective Factors

Within the family structure, family values and expectations, communication patterns, and family involvement seem to have the greatest influence on teen sexual behavior. Factors associated with early initiation of sexual activity include sexual behavior and fertility patterns of the teen's mother, family intactness, history of sexual abuse in the family, family composition, mother's age at marriage, the mother-daughter relationship, and household communication about sex and contraception.

Personal expectations, knowledge, decision-making ability, and sense of future are individual characteristics that influence sexual activity. Individual factors strongly associated with early initiation of sexual activity include perception that peers are sexually active, early pubertal development, African American ethnicity, limited religious affiliation, low intellectual ability, poor academic achievement, lack of educational goals, and early dating behavior. Protective factors associated with contraceptive use include a stable relationship with a sexual partner, knowledge of reproduction and contraception, acceptance of one's own sexuality, academic aspirations, selected developmental characteristics such as self-esteem and low risk-taking behavior, parental support for contraception use, and open communication with mothers.

Adolescent Pregnancy Programs

In addition to research concerning risk and protective factors for teen pregnancy, the literature presents discussions of the various interventions that have been implemented. Although many initiatives are discussed, few have been systematically evaluated. Programs addressing early pregnancy began in the late 1950s and early 1960s. Initially, interventions included "homes" for unwed mothers and federal aid for teen parents through federal programs such as Women, Infants, and Children, Aid to Families With Dependent Children, and Head Start. In the 1970s, health care and educational assistance programs were instituted to support teen moms in the prenatal and postpartal periods. Teens were encouraged to stay in school. Prevention of pregnancy was not an intervention focus until the 1980s. At that time, sex education in the schools that was first introduced in the early 1900s was revisited. The "Just Say No" campaign was launched as a theme for youth to avoid risk behaviors, including sexual activity and drug use. Counseling programs emphasized self-esteem building and hope for the future. Since the late 1980s, the fear of HIV and AIDS has predominated. Contraceptives have become more available to youth; condoms are openly displayed in stores and restrooms and distributed through some school health programs. Television media campaigns are encouraging good decision making in engaging in sexual activity and condom use (Kirby, 1997; Miller, Card, Paikoff, & Peterson, 1992; OTA, 1991b).

NURSING DIAGNOSIS AND OUTCOME DETERMINATION

Assessment and Nursing Diagnosis

The nurse who works with teens must be aware of the characteristics that place a teen at risk for pregnancy. This requires that the nurse do the following:

1. Assess the socioeconomic status of both the community and the family. Adolescents with social and economic disadvantage from poor, isolated, or racially segregated neighborhoods in which early pregnancy is the norm are far more likely to bear children during the teen years than their more affluent and socially integrated peers.
2. Identify teens living in households with family disruption, poor parent-child communication, limited parental supervision, or only one parent.
3. Identify teens with poor academic status who often drop out of school, thus limiting future potential.
4. Assess teens for signs and symptoms of drug use. Drug use is frequently associated with early initiation of sexual activity and subsequent pregnancy.
5. Ask teens about current partner relationships, dating behavior, and sexual activity.
6. Assess physical development at each visit.
7. Assess knowledge about biology and contraception.
8. Assess teens for desire to have a child. Although the number of teens who desire to be pregnant is relatively low, these teens are very likely to become pregnant.

Currently, there is no diagnosis that specifically addresses unintended adolescent pregnancy, but there are several diagnoses related to recognized antecedents of this problem, including Knowledge Deficit (Family Planning), Decisional Conflict, Altered Family Processes, Health-Seeking

Behaviors (Family Planning), Hopelessness, Powerlessness, Self-Esteem Disturbance, and Potential for Community Coping (North American Nursing Diagnosis Association, 1999). Not all diagnoses will be appropriate in all cases of adolescent pregnancy.

Nurse-Sensitive Outcome

Risk Control: Unintended Pregnancy, the desired outcome of pregnancy prevention, is defined as "actions to reduce the possibility of unintended pregnancy" (Iowa Outcomes Project, 2000, p. 366). There are 15 indicators for this outcome, including acknowledges risk for unintended pregnancy, understands physiological processes of conception, develops effective pregnancy prevention strategies, and uses community resources for information and service.

It has been suggested that an additional or perhaps more desirable outcome for pregnancy prevention is "sexual competence." Rather than focusing on adolescent sexual activity as a "risk behavior," possibly focusing on it as a normal aspect of human development will enhance the scope and direction of intervention. Programs that address adolescent sexual behavior need to take into account the fact that sexual feelings and behaviors are a normal part of development from early childhood on, and the unintended consequences of a narrow focus on fear and disease may lead to increased rates of sexual dysfunction (Ehrhardt, 1996).

INTERVENTION: PREGNANCY PREVENTION: ADOLESCENT

No single intervention in the Nursing Interventions Classification (Iowa Intervention Project, 2000) specifically addresses the primary prevention of teen pregnancy. There are several related interventions, including Health Education, Teaching: Safe Sex, Teaching: Sexuality, Family Planning: Contraception, Family Integrity Promotion, Family Mobilization, Assertiveness Training, Behavior Modification: Social Skills, Behavior Management: Sexual, Self-Responsibility Facilitation, Self-Esteem Enhancement, and Health Policy Monitoring. As evidenced by the preceding discussion, however, prevention of pregnancy in adolescents requires a complex, multidisciplinary approach. Therefore, a proposed intervention called Pregnancy Prevention: Adolescent, which will be submitted to the Iowa Intervention team for consideration, is presented in this chapter (Table 40.1). As reflected in the proposed intervention, responsibility for the prevention of teen pregnancy rests not only with the teen or the couple but also with the family, the community, and the greater society. Using

TABLE 40.1   Proposed Intervention: Pregnancy Prevention: Adolescent

Definition

The Pregnancy Prevention: Adolescent intervention provides sexuality education, counseling, support, and reproductive health services to individuals, families, and communities.

Activities

Create an environment in which adolescents feel comfortable seeking help for sexually related concerns.

Address sexual development and behavior at every health maintenance visit.

Provide accurate information about sexual knowledge, beliefs, attitudes, and behaviors.

Support teens who are dealing with issues related to sexual development and behavior.

Guide teens in exploring and affirming personal values and readiness for mature sexual relationships.

Enhance teen skills in decision making and negotiating with peers.

Reinforce the benefits of abstinence and the decision to delay sexual activity.

Promote consistent and effective use of contraceptives for sexually active adolescents.

Support efforts to make contraceptives readily available to sexually active adolescents.

Support efforts to educate teens regarding effective use of contraceptives.

Provide contraceptives as needed.

Facilitate family communication regarding sexual development and behavior.

Target individuals, families, and communities at risk for teen pregnancy.

Educate adults who work with teens regarding teen sexual development and behavior.

Educate the community about the benefits of comprehensive sexuality education.

Initiate measures to remove environmental barriers to abstinence or effective contraceptive use.

Initiate and participate in the development of teen pregnancy prevention programs.

Participate on community boards or task forces concerned with adolescent sexual development and behavior.

Support media messages that encourage abstinence or encourage contraceptive use for sexually active teens.

Denounce sexual exploitation.

Educate lawmakers regarding legislation related to sexual development and behavior (e.g., sex education in schools, parental notification, right to privacy, abortion, and statutory rape).

Monitor legislation related to sexual development and behavior.

Support improved access to affordable, sensitive, and confidential reproductive health care services.

Support funding for continuation and evaluation of pregnancy prevention programs.

Support federal and state data collection and research on adolescent sexual activity, pregnancy, and birth outcomes.

Support community development efforts that improve the economic and social structure and the provision of youth-related activities, facilities, and services.

Kuehnert's (1995) model, each of these units will be discussed, followed by the nurse's role in involving teens, families, and communities in this endeavor.

Most children develop within the context of family. Intervention for teen pregnancy prevention in this unit begins at birth. Families need to be supported in their efforts to minimize household disruption and to foster the developmental enhancement of children. Because communication patterns are established early, parents need to recognize the importance of how they react to their child's sexuality and talk about sexual topics in the home. In addition to being provided with age-appropriate sex information, children need to develop a sense of power and control over there own lives, strong self-esteem, and a sense of hope for the future. The family is the primary influence on these individual characteristics. The nurse has the responsibility to recognize the needs of teens and their families with regard to sexual development and to provide education, counseling, and referral when needed.

From the perspective of the aggregate, tracking and communicating support for or opposition to legislation and health policy are critical interventions. To prevent teen pregnancy, nurses need to support legislation directed toward improving economic opportunity, support media messages that encourage abstinence but educate on the potential consequences of unprotected sex, support sex education, and support improved access to related health services and contraceptives (OTA, 1991a). Federal and state governments need input from nurses on the importance of funding for continuation and evaluation of pregnancy prevention programs. Nurses can also be influential in educating lawmakers on the importance of parental consent and right to privacy legislation. These laws need to be written to protect not only the rights of parents but also the rights of teens.

Within communities, efforts must be made to improve the economic and social structure in a way that promotes a feeling of optimism and a sense of future opportunity. There needs to be an expressed concern for the welfare of youth and a demonstrated commitment to improving the health of teens through provision of youth-related activities, facilities, and services. Nurses can be instrumental in community enhancement by participation on community boards or task forces concerned with these issues.

Community Programs

Although it is apparent that many preventive interventions can be implemented at the individual and family unit level, it is the community that sustains the development of youth and can potentially enhance the lives of youth that come from disadvantaged backgrounds. Thus, community programs addressing teen pregnancy have evolved. When planning a pregnancy prevention program, goals should be specific and well defined. Goals might include imparting knowledge, influencing attitudes, improving access to contraceptives, encouraging contraceptive use, delaying or decreasing sexual activity, enhancing life options and future orientation, or some combination of these. The target of intervention should likewise be well defined to answer the following questions: (a) Will the intervention be targeted at male teens, female teens, all teens, parents, younger children, educators, health care providers, law enforcement, teachers, coaches, clergy, or counselors? and (b) Should the intervention be designed for delivery to individuals, families, groups, or communities? Evaluation should be based on the stated goals and designed during program planning. Decisions need to be made regarding what to evaluate (knowledge, attitude, behavior, or all three), when to evaluate (before, during, or after the program and at what intervals), and how to evaluate (methods and source of data) (Dignan & Carr, 1992).

There are certain philosophical concerns that planners need to address before agreement on a particular approach can be reached. How one views teen sexuality and the rights of teens will impact the decisions to be made. The following assertions could be used to stimulate discussion:

1. Teens are sexual beings influenced by biology, socialization, and personal development.
2. There is often a conflict between biological need and societal values.
3. Society delivers mixed messages about sexual behavior and intimacy.
4. Access to information, services, opportunity, education, and other resources is unequal.
5. Although there are limitations in what role adults can play in teen pregnancy prevention, they have a responsibility to intervene.
6. Adult perspectives may be limited; therefore, adults must make an effort to understand the social, cultural, and moral values of teens, particularly those of teens of different socioeconomic or ethnic backgrounds.

Within each unit of Kuehnert's (1995) model, the nurse has a role in the prevention of adolescent pregnancy. At the societal level, the nurse needs to be cognizant of the prevailing political climate regarding sex education in the school; regulation of the media with regard to sexual messages in advertising and programming; abortion regulation, fornication, and statutory rape laws; and the need for parental consent for health care services. Through monitoring legislation and personal contact with local, state, and federal representatives, the nurse can support initiatives related to adolescent health.

Within the community, the nurse can assume the role of group leader or participant. The community health nurse, nurse practitioner, school nurse, or clinic nurse can identify the need for teen pregnancy prevention and initiate the development of a task force to study the problem and propose solutions. The nurse can educate members of the community about the benefits of sex education programs, dispelling the myth that such programs increase sexual activity. The nurse might also be a participant in a program planning group. In addition, nurses can educate adults working with teens on how to provide open environments, facilitate adult and youth communication, and talk about sexuality and sexual behavior with youth and their parents.

When working with adolescents and their families, the nurse can facilitate family communication about sexually related topics from birth on and help parents and teens understand the normal biological and psychological development of children and adolescents as it relates to sexual behavior. In this regard, the nurse must be comfortable addressing the topic of sexual development and behavior at every encounter with families. In addition, the nurse can educate the family regarding the need for teens to feel a part of the family and to sense parental concern for their welfare. A teen's perception of connection to the family has been shown to decrease the likelihood of early initiation of sexual activity (Blum & Rinehart, 1997).

The nurse should also be an educator and advocate of preteens and teens as they struggle with sexual development. Adolescents not only need accurate and specific information about sexual development, sexual behavior, and contraception but also need a knowledgeable adult to confide in and depend on for support. Several studies have suggested that the presence of a nurse who is accessible and perceived by the teens as an advocate is a crucial element of any program addressing teen pregnancy prevention. Nurses can educate teens and their families during scheduled office visits or through school or community sex education programs.

Nurses can provide contraceptive counseling and, in some cases, gynecological examination, provision of contraceptives, and pregnancy testing. Although such services are sometimes met with resistance from parents and other community members, particularly when they are school based, research indicates that these services have been successful in reducing the incidence of teen pregnancy (Card, 1999; Kirby, 1999; OTA, 1991b).

In summary, intervention for adolescent pregnancy prevention requires a multigenerational approach with intervention at the individual and family, aggregate, and community levels. Interventions should be directed at enhancing the life options of disadvantaged youth, delaying the initiation of sexual activity, and increasing contraceptive use among teens who are sexually active. The unique needs of at-risk populations need to be identified, including the needs of male adolescents. Both health education and health service components are essential to success. Intervention must be interactive, not merely didactic, and it must include both individual and group strategies. Educational and service components must be coordinated and sustainable. Services are needed year-round within walking distance of the youth that they serve. They are more attractive when they are cost free and sensitive and provided at times when youth can attend. The environment should be comfortable, confidential, and private for both males and females.

INTERVENTION APPLICATION

The School/Community Program for Sexual Risk Reduction Among Teens was a communitywide pregnancy prevention effort in rural South Carolina. The goal was primarily to reduce the number of teen pregnancies by delaying initiation of sexual activity and secondarily to promote consistent contraceptive use among the already sexually active. This program involved adolescents, teachers, school administrators, professionals in the community, church officials, peer counselors, parents, the local media, and a school nurse. Adults were provided with sexuality education training, and sex education was taught at all grade levels in the schools. Peer counselors were trained, and the local newspaper and radio station promoted the program. The nurse in the target school provided condoms, took female students to a local clinic for contraceptives, and provided information and counseling. Although not part of the original program, a school-linked health center opened and was staffed by the school nurse and other family planning personnel.

Although it was difficult to design a rigorous evaluation of this intervention, a comparison study of the county that was the home of this community with three similar South Carolina counties found that the pregnancy rate for adolescents ages 14 to 17 years in the target community declined from 61.7 per 1,000 adolescents to 25 per 1,000, whereas those in the three comparison counties increased an average of 8.5 per 1,000 in the first year following implementation of the program. In the second year, the pregnancy rate remained the same in the target community, whereas it increased by an average of 4.5 pregnancies per 1,000 in the three comparison counties. Subsequent research found that the pregnancy rate decline persisted for only 3 years following the program implementation, and by the fourth year the target community pregnancy rate had returned to the level at which it was before the program began. Suggested reasons for this were that the education program lost momentum, the state of South Carolina banned contraceptive distribution in school-based clinics, and the school nurse resigned.

Unfortunately, specific aspects of the program that may have been responsible for the reduction in pregnancy rates were not identified. Success has been attributed to adequate funding and time for training, implementation and follow-up, a receptive target population, and inclusion of an entire small, cohesive target community in the intervention process. In their 1990 reevaluation of the program, Koo, Dunteman, George, Green, and Vincent (1994) concluded that the provision of contraceptives by the school nurse was probably a key factor in the program's success. The nurse seemed to develop trusting relationships with the adolescents and provided sexual counseling and contraceptive services in a school system that supported her effort. In addition, specially trained teachers undoubtedly supported the school nurse.

This case study suggests that a well-designed comprehensive program, including the provision of sexuality counseling and contraceptive services by a trusted school nurse working within and supported by the school system, can reduce adolescent pregnancy (OTA, 1991b).

RESEARCH AND PRACTICE APPLICATIONS

It is difficult to determine the success of many pregnancy prevention programs because evaluation is not always planned for or executed (OTA, 1991a). Sometimes, the explicit goals of programs in relation to teen pregnancy prevention are not defined. It can be assumed that reduction in teen pregnancy was the ultimate goal, but it is unclear whether or not most programs intended to encourage the delay of sexual activity, decrease the frequency of sexual intercourse, increase contraceptive use, or some combination of the these. Programs that have been identified as successful are frequently resource intensive, making them difficult to implement in some settings and difficult to sustain over extended time periods. There are no reports indicating teen participation in program development.

There is an urgent need for program effectiveness research using rigorous methods with implications for health policy. Despite innumerable programs directed at pregnancy prevention being offered nationwide, few have been systematically evaluated. Because measuring change in pregnancy rate and attributing causal relationships to a specific program require rigorous methods, longitudinal study with collection of data regarding other plausible factors for rate change is critical. Because pregnancy rates are not always available, these statistics must often be inferred from birth and abortion data, which may not be available in states that do not report abortion statistics. In this case, the identification and monitoring of intermediate intervention outcomes as well as pregnancy rates becomes important.

Meta-analysis of existing programs, including comparative cost-benefit analyses, would appear to be useful. For this to occur, however, more programs need to be designed and evaluated using sound methodology so that valid comparisons can be made. Similarly, common components of successful programs could be identified using comparison methods.

There is a paucity of research on adolescent males. Only recently have studies begun to address the needs of males with regard to teen sexual behavior and parenting, and there is often a punitive flavor to discussions of male involvement in teen pregnancy. This view is reflected in recent efforts on the part of several states to revive fornication and statutory rape laws as a way to discourage teen sexual activity, and it is due in part to the perception that male impregnators are usually not teens and should therefore be held more responsible. Although it is generally the case that males are older than their female partners, at least 30% of fathers of teen pregnancies are teens, and most are younger than the age of 25 years.

There is a need for continued research on contraceptives, including development of new technologies and determination of teen preferences. One reason why teens are poor contraceptive users could be due to the types of contraceptives readily available to them. Real and perceived side effects as well as ease of acquisition and use seem to be critical factors that need to be examined.

A better understanding of the risk of and protective factors for initiating sexual activity and using contraception would be useful in developing interventions. Although this is probably the most researched area, evidence is still controversial. It is unclear if there are certain factors that are more relevant than others (OTA, 1991a).

Teen Pregnancy Prevention and the Health Care System

Current trends in health care suggest a shift to a multidisciplinary, community-based, aggregate-focused model of care. This shift will necessitate the identification of at-risk aggregates in the community. In addition to teen aggregates with known ethnic or socioeconomic risk factors, identification of groups at risk for teen pregnancy should include negative pregnancy testers and siblings of pregnant adolescents. Program development is a primary intervention strategy for addressing the health care needs of at-risk groups. In addition, there has been a shift in the focus of health care to prevention. Pregnancy Prevention: Adolescent not only involves primary prevention in the form of education, counseling, and health services for abstinence and contraception but also involves secondary prevention for pregnant teens and tertiary prevention for the teen parents and child. Finally, because many of the risk factors for teen pregnancy relate to socioeconomic status, universal access to care is a critical component of any program that attempts to alleviate this problem.

REFERENCES

Blum, R., & Rinehart, P. (1997). *Reducing the risk: Connections that make a difference in the lives of youth.* Minneapolis: University of Minnesota.

Card, J. (1999). Teen pregnancy prevention: Do any programs work? *Annual Review of Public Health, 20,* 257-285.

Centers for Disease Control and Prevention. (1994). *Pregnancy, sexually transmitted diseases, and related risk behaviors among U.S. adolescents* (Adolescent Health: State of Nation Monograph Series No. 2, CDC Publication No. 099-4630). Atlanta, GA: Author.

Dignan, M., & Carr, P. (1992). *Program planning for health education and promotion* (2nd ed.). Philadelphia: Lea & Febiger.

Ehrhardt, A. (1996). Editorial: Our view of adolescent sexuality—A focus on risk behavior without the developmental context. *American Journal of Public Health, 86*(11), 1523-1525.

Holmes, S. (1996, July 13). Public cost of teen-age pregnancy is put at $7 billion this year. *The New York Times,* p. A19.

Iowa Intervention Project. (2000). *Nursing interventions classification (NIC)* (J. C. McCloskey & G. M. Bulecheck, Eds.; 3rd ed.). St. Louis, MO: Mosby-Year Book.

Iowa Outcomes Project. (2000). *Nursing outcomes classification (NOC)* (M. Johnson, M. Maas, & S. Moorhead, Eds.; 2nd ed.). St. Louis, MO: Mosby-Year Book.

Kirby, D. (1997). *No easy answers: Research findings on programs to reduce teen pregnancy.* Washington, DC: National Campaign to Prevent Teen Pregnancy.

Kirby, D. (1999). Reflections on two decades of research on teen sexual behavior and pregnancy. *Journal of School Health, 69*(3), 89-94.

Koo, H., Dunteman, G., George, C., Green, Y., & Vincent, M. (1994). Reducing adolescent pregnancy through a school- and community-based intervention: Denmark, South Carolina, revisited. *Family Planning Perspectives, 26*(5), 206-211.

Kuehnert, P. L. (1991, Summer). Community health nursing and the AIDS pandemic: Case report of one community's response. *Journal of Community Health Nursing,* 137-146.

Kuehnert, P. L. (1995). The interactive and organizational model of community as client: A model for public health nursing. *Public Health Nursing, 12,* 9-17.

Maynard, R. (Ed.). (1996). *Kids having kids* [Special report]. New York: Robin Hood Foundation.

Miller, B., Card, J., Paikoff, R., & Peterson, J. (Eds.). (1992). *Preventing adolescent pregnancy.* Newbury Park, CA: Sage.

Moore, K., Driscoll, A., & Lindberg, L. (1998). *A statistical portrait of adolescent sex, contraception and childbearing.* Washington, DC: National Campaign to Prevent Teen Pregnancy.

North American Nursing Diagnosis Association. (1999). *Nursing diagnoses: Definition and classification 1999-2000.* Philadelphia: Author.

Office of Technology Assessment. (1991a). *Adolescent health: Vol. 1. Summary and policy options* (Publication No. OTA-H-468). Washington, DC: Government Printing Office.

Office of Technology Assessment. (1991b). *Adolescent health: Vol. 2. Background and the effectiveness of selected prevention and treatment services* (Publication No. OTA-H-466). Washington, DC: Government Printing Office.

Quint, E. (1996). Adolescent pregnancy: An update. *Female Patient, 21*(12), 13-18.

U.S. Department of Health and Human Services. (1991). *Healthy people 2000: National health promotion and disease prevention objectives* (DHHS Publication No. PHS 91-50012). Washington, DC: Government Printing Office.

U.S. Department of Health and Human Services. (1995). *Healthy people 2000: Midcourse review and 1995 revisions.* Washington, DC: Government Printing Office.

41

Adolescent Suicide Prevention

Leonie Pallikkathayil

Tammie L. Willis

Suicidal behavior in the adolescent population is a major public health concern.

—*Pearce and Martin (1994, p. 324)*

Adolescent suicide, a phenomenon that has reached epidemic proportions in the United States (Mauk, Gibson, & Rodgers, 1994), is the second leading cause of death for 15- to 19-year-olds (Berman & Jobes, 1995). Recognizing the need for planned intervention, *Healthy People 2000* (U.S. Department of Health and Human Services [USDHHS], 1991) targets adolescents in its key health status objectives, stating "the dominant preventable health problems of adolescents and young adults fall into two major categories: injuries and violence that kill and disable many before they reach the age of 25 and emerging lifestyles that affect their health many years later" (p. 16). The goal of Objective 6.1a is to "reduce suicides among youth aged 15 to 19 to no more than 8.2 per 100,000" (p. 99). Attempted suicide is a morbid, potentially lethal event, a risk factor for future completed suicides, a potential indicator of other health problems, or all three. The target goal of *Healthy People 2000* Objective 6.2 is to "reduce by 15% the incidence of injurious suicide attempts among adolescents aged 14 to 17" (p. 99). Before the tragic nature of suicide in teens can be discussed, terminology used must be clarified. Suicide is the intentional and voluntary cessation of one's life. Suicidal behaviors and self-destructive acts have the potential to end one's life. Suicidal ideation, however, is the thought of causing harm to one's self. The dramatic and frightening rates of adolescent suicide point to the need for prevention and intervention programs to reduce this tragic waste of both human life and potential. The purpose of this chapter is to present the intervention Adolescent Suicide Prevention, which has been created to reverse the increasing number of teen suicides and suicide attempts.

INCIDENCE AND DEMOGRAPHY

The act of adolescent suicide devastates a home, a school, and a community. It removes from the world individuals who no longer have the opportunity to grow, love, and share lessons learned. Annually, 5,000 adolescents between the ages of 15 and 19 years commit suicide. This averages approximately 14 lives per day (Henry, Stephenson, Hanson, & Hargett, 1994). The largest increase in the rate of suicide has been accounted for by young white males (Henry et al., 1994). White males from ages 15 to 19 years reportedly are approximately five times more likely to commit suicide than white females in the same age group (Ladely & Puskar, 1994). Although white males are more successful in their attempts, white females attempt suicide two or three times more often than their male counterparts (Ladely & Puskar, 1994). Nonwhite rates of suicidal behavior for both males and females tend to be lower. The white to African American ratio of suicidal behavior in 1990 was 2.3:1, and for nonwhite males and females the suicide rates were 13.0 and 2.5, respectively (Berman & Jobes, 1995). In viewing behaviors prior to the event of suicide, females were found to be four times more likely than males to speak about the act on the day of death, and males were more likely to leave a suicide note. The majority of adolescents who die from their own hand lived with their parents at the time of the suicide (Ladely & Puskar, 1994).

THEORIES

There are multiple theories that attempt to explain suicide in adolescents. A basic understanding of these theories can be helpful in explaining what may be occurring and how to prevent it. The biological foundation for suicidal behavior in adolescents centers around the genetic transmission of suicidality and psychiatric disorders, such as affective disorders. Biochemical changes during puberty make adolescents more vulnerable to affective disorders (Henry et al., 1994). Although the contribution of heredity is unclear, researchers focusing on the incidence of suicidal behavior in families found that half of the persons with a family history of suicide attempt suicide themselves. In addition, more than half of all individuals with a family history of suicide had a primary diagnosis of affective disorder (Blumenthal, 1990). When considering the general population, it was discovered that 6 of 100 suicide completers had a parent who committed suicide, providing a strong basis for genetic factors in both the transmission of affective disorders and suicide potential (Blumenthal, 1990).

The intrapsychic theory of suicide follows the psychoanalytic viewpoint. Internally, suicide is viewed as an attempt to deal with rejection and deprivation that results in the loss of love and support (Henry et al., 1994). Thus, the core component of the "suicidal personality" in adolescents is the perception of loss of love (Holinger & Offer, 1981). This loss of love during a crucial period of development (puberty) places adolescents at great risk with respect to self-destructive drives (Henry et al., 1994). It is believed that these tendencies emerge as the product of an unconscious death wish resulting from anger turned inward (Henry et al., 1994).

From a developmental perspective, suicide in adolescents is viewed as an inability to cope with developmental changes. Adolescents often lack the ability to solve problems effectively. This situation can cause confusion, doubt, and fear in the adolescent who lacks past experiences to draw from, making solutions to problems appear hopeless. Without the hope that circumstances will change, suicidal behavior is a quick escape from problems to which there appear no answers.

Interpersonal theories of suicidal behavior focus on interpersonal conflicts that the adolescent may have with friends, family, and other social affiliations. The adolescent is unable to resolve conflicts, and the result is a suicide attempt. Similar to this theory is the family systems theory of suicidal behavior. From this perspective, the suicidal behavior is not the result of an individual problem but rather a result of family dysfunction, such as maladaptive family communication and coping. In some cases, adolescents view the suicidal act as freeing the family of painful issues and family conflict (Henry et al., 1994).

The sociological perspective focuses on the individual's degree of integration into social institutions. When there is a mismatch between social norms and adolescent expectations or beliefs, suicidal behavior results. Social learning theory dictates that adolescents learn suicidal behavior by what they view around them. If a parent or friend attempted suicide, then suicide is seen as an acceptable means of problem solving. Here, adolescents learn a pathological rather than an adaptive coping strategy (Henry et al., 1994).

Easy access theory accounts for the increase in availability of lethal means of self-destructive behaviors. More than ever before, firearms are easily accessible to American youth. The availability of firearms to suicidal youths is thought to be a key factor in differentiating suicide attempters from suicide completers (Ladely & Puskar, 1994). Over-the-counter prescription medications are also prominent, making their usage a common method of suicidal behavior. In addition, alcohol is more readily available to adolescents struggling in the midst of confusion for an easy way to escape.

Systems theory identifies multiple factors working in combination that push the adolescent toward suicidal behaviors. No one factor acts independently of another. Family stressors, the inability to cope with personal issues, and a lag in cognitive developmental levels are all essential in determining suicidal risk and potential. Much like the systems theory, the ecological theory provides a multidisciplinary approach to understanding adolescent suicide. This theory incorporates individual, environmental, and social system factors that may be related to suicidal behaviors (Henry et al., 1994). It brings together the interplay of biological, psychological, social, and cultural forces.

NURSING DIAGNOSIS AND RISK FACTORS

To prevent suicidal behaviors in adolescents, attention must be given to who is at risk and what propels an adolescent to such extremes (Gex, Ferron, & Michand, 1998). Identification of risk factors helps nurses and other professionals as well as families, schools, and communities to intervene prior to a tragic event. There are multiple factors to consider in determining who is at risk for suicidal behaviors. In an attempt to clarify physical symptomatolgy, verbal and nonverbal cues, Smith et al. (1997) discussed

36 operational definitions of indicators that can assist in identifying adolescents at risk. Indicators presented by these researchers include hopelessness, anger, feelings of worthlessness, and recent loss. There is no North American Nursing Diagnosis Association (1999) diagnosis applicable for the focus of primary prevention of suicide. Therefore, At Risk for Suicide is being proposed as a working diagnosis in the identification of risk factors.

Affective disorders are generally acknowledged to be a key risk factor for suicide in adolescents (Berman & Jobes, 1995). Depression is a relatively common psychiatric disorder and is associated with many completed suicides (Forster, 1994). A relatively new area of study in relation to suicidal behavior is the neurobiology of suicide and alterations found in the brains of suicide victims. The serotonergic phenomenon implicated in depression represents the most compelling evidence to date for a biological correlation to suicidal behavior (Blumenthal, 1990). Studies have found a common biochemical association among aggression, impulsivity, and reduced serotonergic function (Blumenthal, 1990). In addition, chronic alcohol usage is associated with depletion in serotonin function, which is frequently linked to an increased risk of suicidal behavior (Pfeffer, 1989). These findings in adults may be promising for studying the relationship of the significantly increased rate of suicidal behaviors among adolescent males who demonstrate an increase in alcohol use and aggressive behaviors.

Research studies of adolescents who commit suicide point to specific personality traits, including the tendency to be withdrawn, perfectionistic, explosive, hypersensitive, impulsive, and aloof. These adolescents also have more interpersonal difficulties, lower self-esteem, and are less trusting than nonsuicidal adolescents (Blumenthal, 1990; Ryland & Kruesi, 1992).

In addition to certain personality traits, specific behaviors are frequently observed in adolescents who commit suicide, including sexual promiscuity, serious delinquent behavior, impaired communication, academic decline, and signs of impaired judgment. Adolescents with suicidal behaviors have been found to display increased levels of anger and poor anger control (Ladely & Puskar, 1994). Substance abuse has been diagnosed in more than one third of adolescent suicide victims. Research literature suggests that at least 70% of adolescent victims suffered from alcohol or substance abuse problems (Blumenthal, 1990).

Perceptions of self and significant others has been shown to influence adolescent suicidal behaviors (Rubenstein, Halton, Kasten, Rubin, & Stechler, 1998). Adolescents who believe they have no one to talk to or who perceive themselves to be in poor health were more likely to attempt suicide (Blumenthal, 1990). These negative perceptions are believed to lead to low self-esteem, anger, and a belief that it is impossible to cope effectively. Adolescents who attempt suicide tend to experience significantly more life-change events than do nonsuicidal adolescents. Examples of life-change events are the death of a parent, separation or divorce of parents, or the diagnosis of a debilitating physical illness in the adolescent. Without adequate support, these events exceed adolescents' ability to cope effectively and further diminish their self-esteem (Ladely & Puskar, 1994). The adolescent's failure to believe in his or her own self-efficacy and ability to cope deprive the teen of the "cognitive buffer" that prevents suicidal behaviors (Cole, 1989).

Psychosocial, environmental, and specific life events are important in understanding suicidal behavior in adolescents. Recent bereavement, separation, early loss, and poor social support are all potentially important factors that can affect the lethality of an adolescent's suicide attempt (Blumenthal, 1990). Adolescents who come from homes with marital discord that results in divorce or separation often feel torn between their parents. They frequently believe they are the cause of disruption and try desperately to fix the situation (Blumenthal, 1990). For many, it may be the first time experiencing loss or grief. The process of grieving can evoke extreme feelings of separation, anxiety, and hopelessness with which the adolescent is unfamiliar. Due to developmental immaturity and inability to cope effectively, suicide becomes the option of choice to end the painful nature of what is being experienced.

Other precipitants of suicidal behavior in adolescents include humiliating life events, such as impending disciplinary crisis or threat of incarceration. Situational factors, such as a being the victim of physical or sexual abuse, increase the likelihood of suicidal acts if the adolescent is not removed from these stressors (Blumenthal, 1990). Failing grades and high expectations by parents, learning disabilities, being taunted and teased by peers, not fitting into the "in crowd," or simply feeling ostracized by peers in all relationships can lead to acts of self-violence. There is evidence that knowing someone who committed or attempted suicide or exposure to suicide through the media may render some adolescents more vulnerable to imitation of suicidal behaviors. Research has demonstrated that the reporting of a suicide on the front page of newspapers and on multiple television channels increases the rate of suicide for a 7-day period. Furthermore, adolescent suicide victims are more likely to have known a relative or friend who exhibited suicidal behavior (Blumenthal, 1990).

The lack of social supports is an important risk factor for adolescents. It has been well documented that the strength and quality of social supports are important in the etiology of psychiatric problems, compliance with treatment, and response to treatment regimens (Blumenthal, 1990). Another important determinant of suicidal behavior in adolescents is the degree of hopelessness. Hope serves a protective mechanism against suicidal behavior (Blumenthal, 1990).

Access to lethal means is a powerful risk factor (Kruesi et al., 1999). Greater availability of firearms in the American home is one of the most often cited findings related to both the observed increased incidence of adolescent suicide and the increased use of firearms (Ladely & Puskar, 1994). Brent et al. (1991) concluded that guns were twice as likely to be found in the homes of suicide victims as in the homes of attempters or psychiatric controls. Suicide with firearms is identified as the most common method for both males and females aged 15 to 19 (Ladely & Puskar, 1994).

Although there are many documented risk factors for suicide, no one is immune to this self-destructive act. The possession of a healthy sense of self and satisfactory interpersonal social relationships are good protectors from self-destructive acts. More immediate behavioral warning signs of adolescent suicide include sudden changes in behavior, dramatic brightening of mood after a period of despondency, excessive risk taking, having multiple "accidents," changes in appetite, sleep disturbances, persistent feelings of guilt, acting-out behaviors, self-reproach and hopelessness, loss of interest in usual activities such as work, school, or sports, decreased concentration, suicide "talk," and the giving away of prized possessions (Blumenthal, 1990).

The Nursing Outcomes Classification (NOC) outcome Suicide Self-Restraint can be used to measure the effectiveness of Adolescent Suicide Prevention. Specific indicators are highlighted in Tables 41.1 through 41.3. (Iowa Outcomes Project, 2000)

INTERVENTION:
ADOLESCENT SUICIDE PREVENTION

All prevention programs essentially focus on three levels: primary, secondary, and tertiary. The most effective way to prevent a problem is to intervene at the primary stage, before the problem actually occurs. The proposed intervention focuses exclusively on primary prevention. The essence of primary prevention for adolescent suicide is realizing that a national problem does exist and accepting that there is reason to be concerned. Despite the media attention given to adolescent suicide since the 1970s, suicide is generally still not widely regarded as a major public health issue by many (Berman & Jobes, 1995). It continues to receive less media attention than homicide, even though it tends to be a more frequent cause of death (Berman & Jobes, 1995). Prevention with a resulting decrease in the overall suicide rate to meet the goals established in *Healthy People 2000* (USDHHS, 1991) cannot become a reality if all are not involved in the prevention efforts. Suicidal behavior in adolescents is an individual, school, community, and national issue. Responsibility for its reso-lution must be accepted by all at all points of contact with the adolescent.

Promoting age-specific developmental task accomplishments is a ma-jor focus of primary prevention. Enhancing individual strength and wellness is the foundation for preventing at-risk behaviors. Also, primary prevention involves what is known about who is at risk for suicidal be-haviors. Attention must be given to what has already been noted about who is at risk. To negate this important issue completely destroys the con-cept of primary prevention. Known risk factors, precipitating events, and life circumstances must be accounted for and perceived as important. Be-fore they reach adolescence, children should be taught that life is not with-out problems. Furthermore, adolescents need to learn that it is illogical to approach a temporary problem, such as boy-girl relationship difficulties, with a permanent solution—suicide. Adolescents should be assisted to de-velop healthy thoughts, feelings, interpersonal communication patterns, and spiritual practices. Assisting individuals to develop healthy coping is the key to primary suicide prevention. Role modeling is the best way to teach children healthy behaviors. Adolescents should be taught and helped to seek assistance in coping with stress from family, school, and community resources when needed.

Attention must also be given to strengthening family life in the com-munity (McKeown et al., 1998). Kerfoot, Harrington, and Dyer (1995) stress the importance of a family's acknowledgment and acceptance that suicidal behavior could be a likely result of crisis experiences within the home, school, and community. They believe that improved family com-munication is the cornerstone in identifying suicidal behavior. Another highlight of this approach is the development of problem-solving skills. Family members can be taught the necessary skills to be sensitive in han-dling the distress of others (Kerfoot et al., 1995). Adolescents are vulner-able members of society. The period of adolescence is filled with uncer-tainty, change, and experiences that are difficult to comprehend. Commu-nity resources for families are needed for this turbulent time to intervene for safety.

Primary prevention can be carried out in the school and other com-munity settings in which adolescents are involved. Teachers, counselors, and school nurses have critical roles as agents of suicide prevention within the school setting. If permitted, teachers and school nurses can identify primary referral sources for students and families and assist in developing an effective network for suicidal peers (Shaffer & Craft, 1999). Shneidman (1985) describes several commonalities of suicidal behavior, including that the purpose of suicide is to seek a solution. With the in-volvement of school professionals and community and civic leaders, help can be given before the situation gains momentum.

Primary prevention involves three levels of intervention: the individual, the family, and the community. Table 41.1 presents activities to be implemented by professionals and outcome indicators for the individual. Tables 41.2 and 41.3 present activities and outcome indicators on the family and community levels. The Iowa Intervention Project (2000), Smith et al., (1997), and Stolte (1996) present various interventions and outcome indicators to guide and assist the care provider in developing an action plan. We have created activities and outcome indicators that bring together the works of these authors and present new ideas from a primary prevention focus for decreasing the incidence of suicidal behaviors at all three levels.

INTERVENTION APPLICATION

Cindy, a 16-year-old high school student, had been a very outgoing young woman up until a few months ago. She was a member of the student council, head cheerleader, and active in the French club. She had a grade point average of 3.5 and was in the running for prom queen. The school nurse was asked to see Cindy by her homeroom teacher because she had noticed an erratic change in Cindy's behavior. The teacher reported that Cindy was becoming increasing irritable, inconsistent with turning in assignments, and had begun isolating herself from her peers. When the teacher approached Cindy about these issues, she simply stated, "Everything is OK." The nurse met with Cindy twice; on the second visit, Cindy began to open up. She voiced that her parents had been divorced for 1 year, and now her father, with whom she had a good relationship, was relocating because of his job. Cindy stated that her mother was continuing to deal with depressive and anxiety symptoms that began prior to the divorce, and her mother's condition was worsening. She voiced that she felt responsible for the breakup of her parent's marriage and her mother's condition by not being the "best daughter." Cindy believed she could not try any harder to be the "perfect" daughter to bring her mother out of the pain and suffering she was experiencing. She also stated that she had seen her boyfriend with another girl and believed that her situation would only get worse, and she was tired of all the pain.

The school nurse recognized that Cindy was At Risk for Suicide and immediate action was required. Attention had to be given to the entire family in addition to the individual and her surrounding environment. Cindy's problem is not unusual. Parental divorce, illness, and boy-girl relationship issues are all frequent teenage problems in today's society. What will equip Cindy to deal with her hopelessness and pain are her ability to seek and accept help and her ability to problem solve. From what is

TABLE 41.1   Interventions and Outcomes for Adolescents at Risk for Suicide

Intervention	*Activities*	*Outcome*	*Indicators*
Personal Identity Promotion[a]	Assist the adolescent in identifying The need for developing personal identity[a] Personal values[a] Personal values compared with those of peer group[a]	Positive Self-Identity[a]	Verbalization of Acceptance of self and personal values[b] Support in peer group[a] Personal expression of self with and among peer group[a]
Cognitive Development Promotion[a]	Problem-solving skills and conflict-resolution skills[a] Consequences of behavior[a] Decision-making ability[a]	Problem-Solving Ability[a]	Ability to logically outline a problem and arrive at a solution[a] Ability to defend personal position[a] Ability to predict future as well as present events[a] Ability to analyze and synthesize material[a]
Occupational Goals Promotion[a]	Exploring occupational interests[a] Resources for particular occupations[a] Development of personal goals[a]	Occupational Interests[a]	Strengths and weakness, which can lead to interest in particular occupations[a] Resources available to learn more about occupations[a] Personal goals[a]
Self-Awareness Enhancement[c]	That he or she is unique[c] Usual feelings about self[c] Negative self-statements[c] Positive self-attributes[c] Self-destructive behaviors[c]	Self-Esteem[b]	Self-acceptance[b] Open communication[b] Confidence level[b] Description of pride in self[b]
Anger Control Assistance[c]	Feeling of anger[c] Appropriate expression of anger[c] Destructive aspects of anger[c]	Aggression Control[b]	Appropriate outlets[c] Decrease in harmful behaviors to self[c]

TABLE 41.1   *Continued*

Intervention	Activities	Outcome	Indicators
Impulse Control Training[c]	Problems or situations that require thoughtful action[c] Personal strengths Restraint[c]	Impulse Control[b]	Harmful behaviors[b] Feelings leading to impulse actions[b] Consequences of impulsive actions[b] Risk in environment[b] Control of impulses[b]
Coping Enhancement[c]	An objective appraisal of situation/events[c] Specific life values[c]	Coping[b]	Effective coping[b] Ineffective coping[b] Sense of control[b] Decreased stress[b] Adaptation to developmental changes[b]
Support System Enhancement[c]	Existing social networks[c] Degree of family support[c] Barriers to using support systems[c]	Social Support[b]	Emotional assistance provided by others[b] Persons who can help[b] Willingness to call on others for help[b] Adequate social networks and contacts[b]
Hope Instillation[c]	Expanding repertoire of coping mechanisms[c] Hopelessness[c] Hope[c]	Hope[b]	A positive future[b] Faith[b] A reason to live[b] Meaning in life[b] Belief in self and others[b] Inner peace[b] Zest for life[b]

a. From Stolte (1996).
b. From Iowa Outcomes Project (2000).
c. From Iowa Intervention Project (2000).

known about Cindy, she is a healthy teenager with much strength who is experiencing a great deal of stress and pain. It is appropriate that her concerned teacher referred her to the school nurse.

The nurse was able to locate an after-school counselor for Cindy free of charge through a local community crisis center who would work with Cindy on her normal individual and family developmental crises. With Cindy's approval, the nurse contacted both of Cindy's parents to discuss

TABLE 41.2   Interventions and Outcomes for Families With Individuals at Risk for Suicide

Intervention	Activities	Outcomes	Indicators
Parent Education: Childrearing Family[a]	**Identification of:**	Parenting[b]	**Verbalization of**
	Developmental tasks[a]		Provides for the child's needs[b]
	Teaching normal physiological, emotional, and cognitive characteristics[a]		Stimulates cognitive development[b]
			Stimulates emotional growth[b]
	Power/control issues[a]		Demonstrates a loving relationship with child[b]
			Avoids power struggles[b]
			Realistic parental roles[b]
			Demonstrates empathy for child[b]
Family Support[a]	Family disruptions, changes, and roles[a]	Family Adjustment[c]	Increased external relationships
	Access to support networks[a]		Verbalization of feeling to each other
			Mutual support

a. From Iowa Intervention Project (2000).
b. From Iowa Outcomes Project (2000).
c. From Stolte (1996).

the issues at hand. The nurse assessed the home environment for access to lethal means of harm and asked if someone within the family would be willing to increase time spent with Cindy to get her through her crisis period. The nurse was able to involve both parents in family therapy and assisted the mother in receiving treatment for her depressive symptoms. Mobilizing family and community resources assisted Cindy in dealing with her normative crisis.

Within a few months, Cindy was doing much better. The nurse observed that Cindy was once again involved in her usual social activities. Although her father had moved, family therapy continued via telephone conference. Her mother was beginning to show improvement, and she and Cindy were talking about issues. These behaviors could be monitored by those working with Cindy and her family using the NOC outcome Suicide Self-Restraint (Iowa Outcomes Project, 2000). Cindy never made that trip to the hospital emergency department because someone was alert to risk factors of suicide and intervened at the individual, family, and community levels.

TABLE 41.3 Interventions and Outcomes for Communities With Individuals and Families at Risk for Suicide

Intervention	Activities	Outcome	Indicators
Gun Safety Training[a]	**Identification of:** Access to firearms[a] Federal firearms laws and protections[a]	Decreased Firearm Availability[a]	**Results** Decreased death by firearms[a] Increased community awareness and support for prevention and use of firearms[a]
Suicide Prevention[b]	Those at risk[b] Individual, family, and community resources Plan and means to harm[b] Safety needs[b] Removal of hazards[b]	Suicide Self-Restraint[c]	Help seeking when feeling self-destructive[c] Control of impulses[c] An informed community[c] Discloses a suicidal plan[c] Does not attempt suicide[c] Support from multiple systems[c]

a. From Brent et al. (1991).
b. From Iowa Intervention Project (2000).
c. From Iowa Outcomes Project (2000).

IMPLICATIONS FOR PRACTICE AND RESEARCH

Prevention of suicidal behaviors requires timely recognition of the problem. Therefore, the main emphasis for practice is placed on education so that the at-risk individual can be identified and resources in the home, schools, and community provided. Once education has been done, prevention focuses on proper assessment of at-risk individuals and intervening to provide family and individual support. Nurses are in a unique position to promote adolescent development and reduce the incidence of suicidal behaviors for several reasons. They possess strong communication skills that enable them to facilitate education, and they are located in strategic health promotion leadership roles in a variety of settings within the community. Nurse practitioners in particular are in an ideal setting to do screenings and physical examinations with the adolescent and the family. When properly assessed and identified, referral to appropriate community resources can be made.

Research in the area of prevention for adolescents at risk for suicidal behavior has increased dramatically during the past three decades (Berman & Jobes, 1995). From a research standpoint, the question of whether there will ever be sufficient monies available to fund psychosocial and public health prevention research remains. Past empirical research has provided important and useful data on which to build future prevention efforts (Berman & Jobes, 1995). Research of the past two decades has provided a clearer understanding of who is at risk for completing suicide and has also suggested significant biological and psychosocial directions for additional study (Berman & Jobes, 1995).

Legislative concerns have not translated into suicide prevention dollars, despite the compelling need to prevent adolescent suicide (Berman & Jobes, 1995). Federal spending cutbacks have limited the research monies available for additional basic and applied investigation. In the ever-changing field of health care and managed care organizations, uncertainty does exist. If the survival of our youth is a priority, mental health resources that produce the most cost-effective results must be identified. Despite the success of recent national legislation limiting access to firearms, more needs to be done on the local level to promote education about safe storage of firearms in homes with children and adolescents.

Our nation's youth are our future. What is done for them today influences tomorrow. Primary prevention in the home, school, and community can reduce the incidence of self-destructive behavior before it has the opportunity to take a young life.

REFERENCES

Berman, A. L., & Jobes, D. A. (1995). Suicide prevention in adolescents (age 12-18). *Suicide and Life-Threatening Behavior, 25,* 143-154.

Blumenthal, S. J. (1990). Youth suicide: Risk factors, assessment and treatment of the adolescent and young adult suicide patient. *Psychiatric Clinics of North America, 13*(3), 510-550.

Brent, D. A., Perper, J. A., Allman, C. J., Monitz, G. M., Wartella, M. I., & Zelenak, J. P. (1991). The presence and accessibility of firearms in the homes of adolescents suicides. A case control study. *Journal of the American Medical Association, 266*(21), 2989-2995.

Cole, D. (1989). Psychopathology of adolescent suicide: Hopelessness, coping beliefs, and depression. *Journal of Abnormal Psychology, 98*(3), 248-255.

Forster, P. (1994). Accurate assessment of short-term suicide risk in a crisis. *Psychiatric Annals, 24*(11), 571-578.

Gex, R. C., Ferron, F. N. C., & Michand, P. A. (1998). Suicide attempts among adolescents in Switzerland: Prevalence, associated factors and co-morbidity. *Acta Psychiatrica Scandanavica, 98,* 28-33.

Henry, C. S., Stephenson, A. L., Hanson, M. F., & Hargett, W. (1994). Adolescent suicide and families: An ecological approach. *Family Therapy, 21,* 63-80.

Holinger, P. C., & Offer, D. (1981). Perspectives on suicide in adolescence. *Research in Community and Mental Health, 2,* 139-157.

Iowa Intervention Project. (2000). *Nursing interventions classification (NIC)* (J. C. McCloskey & G. M. Bulechek, Eds.; 3rd ed.). St. Louis, MO: Mosby-Year Book.

Iowa Outcomes Project. (2000). *Nursing outcomes classification (NOC)* (M. Johnson, M. Maas, & S. Moorhead, Eds.; 2nd ed.). St. Louis, MO: Mosby-Year Book.

Kerfoot, M., Harrington, R., & Dyer, E. (1995). Brief home-based intervention with young suicide attempters and their families. *Journal of Adolescence, 18*(5), 557-568.

Kruesi, M. J. P., Grossman, J., Pennington, J. M., Woodward, P. J., Duda, D., & Hirsch, J. G. (1999). Suicide and violence prevention: Parent education in the emergency department. *Journal of American Academy of Child Adolescent Psychiatry, 38*(3), 250-255.

Ladely, S. J., & Puskar, K. R. (1994). Adolescent suicide: Behaviors, risk factors and psychiatric nursing interventions. *Issues in Mental Health Nursing, 15*(5), 497-504.

Mauk, G. W., Gibson, D. G., & Rodgers, P. L. (1994). Suicide postvention with adolescents: School consultation practices and issues. *Education and Treatment of Children, 17*(3), 469-483.

McKeown, R. E., Garrison, C. Z., Cuffe, S. P., Walker, J. L., Jackson, K. L., & Addy, C. L. (1998). Incidence and predictors of suicidal behaviors in a longitudinal sample of young adolescents. *Journal of American Academy of Child Adolescent Psychiatry, 37*(6), 612-675.

North American Nursing Diagnosis Association. (1999). *Nursing diagnoses: Definition and classification 1999-2000.* Philadelphia: J. B. Lippincott.

Pearce, C. M., & Martin, G. (1994). Predicting suicide attempts among adolescents. *Acta Psychiatrica Scandinavica, 90*(5), 324-328.

Pfeffer, C. R. (1989). Assessment of suicidal children and adolescents. *Psychiatric Clinics of North America, 12*(4), 861-872.

Rubenstein, J. L., Halton, A., Kasten, L., Rubin, C., & Stechler, G. (1998). Suicidal behavior in adolescents: Stress and protection in different family contexts. *American Journal of Orthopsychiatry, 68*(2), 274-284.

Ryland, D. H., & Kruesi, M. J. P. (1992). Suicide among adolescents. *International Review of Psychiatry, 4*(2), 185-195.

Shaffer, D., & Craft, L. (1999). Methods of adolescent suicide prevention. *Journal of Clinical Psychiatry, 60*(2), 70-74.

Shneidman, E. S. (1985). *Definition of suicide.* New York: John Wiley.

Smith, J. E., Early, J. A., Green, P. T., Lauck, D. L., Oblaczynski, C., Smochek, M., & Wright, G. (1997). Risk for suicide and risk for violence: A case for separating the current violence diagnoses. *Nursing Diagnosis, 8*(2), 67-78.

Stolte, K. M. (1996). Wellness nursing diagnoses for adolescents. In K. M. Stolte (Ed.), *Wellness nursing diagnosis for health promotion* (pp. 134-143). Philadelphia: Lippincott-Raven.

U.S. Department of Health and Human Services. (1991). *Healthy people 2000: National health promotion and disease prevention objectives* (DHHS Publication No. PHS 91-50212). Washington, DC: Government Printing Office.

42

Teaching Conflict Resolution

Kathleen Ross-Alaolmolki

Violence and its consequences are having devastating effects on children and adolescents. This chapter addresses opportunities for children and adolescents to learn alternative dispute resolution skills and conflict resolution that can enhance self-regulatory behavior and social competence that prevent violence. *Healthy People 2000* (U.S. Department of Health and Human Services [USDHHS], 1991) addresses goals to reduce violence through the introduction of conflict resolution programs in schools. Goal 7.16 is to "increase to at least 50% the proportion of elementary and secondary schools that teach nonviolent conflict resolution skills, preferably as a part of quality school health education" (p. 101). Efforts to achieve this goal can be spearheaded by nurses who are an integral part of the communities in which children and adolescents live and attend school. Programs that focus on violence prevention and teach children and adolescents to resolve conflicts nonviolently are being evaluated positively (Beauchesne, Kelley, Lawrence, & Farquharson, 1997; Farrell & Meyer, 1997; Hausman, Prothrow-Stith, & Spivak, 1995; Hausman, Spivak, & Prothrow-Stith, 1995; Johnson, Johnson, Dudley, & Burnett, 1992). More such intervention programs are needed. The purpose of this chapter is to discuss one such intervention, Teaching Conflict Resolution.

Incidence of Conflict and Violence

There has been a shift in the leading causes of death for youth from natural to violent etiologies, including unintentional injuries, homicide, and suicide (Sells & Blum, 1996). Most violent events occur because of conflict among families, friends, and acquaintances, with 90% of the perpetrators and victims being young and of the same race (Prothrow-Stith, 1995).

Violence is an expression of alienation and can be turned inward or outward. According to the Children's Defense Fund (1997), more than 1.6 million children ranging in age from 12 to 17 reported that they had been the victims of violent crime, other than murder, in 1994. Sadly, most of the victimization of these children was committed by adults, and four of every five juveniles murdered in 1994 were killed by adults. This statistic does not include child abuse, another form of violence perpetrated by parents and caretakers. Between 1983 and 1993, guns were associated with the doubling of the number of children younger than 20 years who died from violent causes. In 1993, one child was killed every hour and a half, which equates to a classroom full of children being killed every 2 days. African American children have been found to be at the greatest risk. African American males aged 15 to 19 disproportionately suffer the greatest toll, and they are five times more likely than their white male counterparts to die from gunfire. Violence has crossed all socioeconomic and racial and ethnic groups, however, as the availability of handguns and other weapons has increased (Brady, 1994). Socially and culturally sanctioned violence is suspected to play a major role in affecting the psychological and physical health of children and their parents (Nelms, 1997; Wolfe & Korsche, 1994).

CONFLICT RISK FACTORS

Poverty

Both racism and poverty are associated with inequalities. They are viewed by many as forms of social violence that deter access to health, education, and criminal justice. Importantly, they contribute to expressions of individual and group violence (Stiffman, Earls, Dorr, Cunningham, & Farbers, 1996). Other factors that increase children's risk for fatal violence include being male, being a resident in an environment in which there is a high rate of violence, and being a victim of violence during early childhood (Prothrow-Stith, 1995). Children and youth at high risk for engagement in violent behaviors are likely to come from environments that predispose them to vulnerability, such as those with few social resources, high levels of stress, and a lack of institutional support. Importantly, the proportion of adolescents from socioeconomically disadvantaged groups is increasing, and they are at higher risk for engaging in risk behaviors at increasingly younger ages (DiClemente, Hansen, & Ponton, 1996). In 1992, there were more than 35 million youth aged 10 through 19, representing 14% of the population (Hollman, 1993). By 2020, it is estimated that the youth population will increase to approximately 43 million, with the majority being youth of differing racial and ethnic minorities.

Racial and Ethnic Minorities

In 1995, there were 14.7 million children (21% of all American children) younger than 18 years of age living in poverty, an increase of 2.1 million since 1989 (Children's Defense Fund, 1997). Specifically, 16% of white children, 41.3% of African American children, 39.5% of Hispanic children, 41.4% of Native American children, and 19.2% of Asian American children were living below the poverty level in 1996. Moreover, 56.9% of African American children, 36.5% of Native American children, and 28.6% of Hispanic children were living with one of their parents—their mother. The Children's Defense Fund estimates that current child poverty levels will cost the nation $36 billion in lost future productivity due to lack of education and ineffective work habits of adults. Thus, communities and neighborhoods that are experiencing a higher level of underemployment, unemployment, availability of illicit drugs, the presence of gangs, and availability of sophisticated weapons have increased violence (Stiffman et al., 1996).

Media Influences

In his review of the behavioral science and medical literature, Barry (1993) noted that studies point to media violence consistently as a causative factor in the crime rate. This evidence is largely ignored. Children 2 to 11 years of age watch an average of 28 hours of television per week. Prime-time programming contains an average of 5 violent acts per hour, equal to 100 acts of violence per week and 5000 per year. Furthermore, cartoons that are watched by many young children contain more violent acts than do adult programming, with 25 acts of violence per hour—six times higher than the rate of violence for television drama. Interestingly, toy commercials ranked with cartoons in violent content. By the seventh grade, the average child has watched 8000 screen murders and more than 100,000 acts of violence (see Chapter 37). These figures double by the end of adolescence (p. 8). Without question, vulnerable children and adolescents are given the message that power and force resolve conflict and disagreements.

Experience with violence begins early and may continue to influence how children and youth behave as they develop through adolescence. The Metropolitan Life Survey (1994) concluded that children and young adults who have experienced violence are more likely than their peers to have negative experiences in their school lives such as failure to achieve academically, the belief that their schools offer a lesser quality of education, and attending schools in which there are serious problems with vandals. Children who had been victims of violence reported their parents had less frequent communication with their schools than others students' parents, such as individual meetings with teachers, parents, or group meetings, or visits to the schools. These children also believed that they ran the risk of becoming victims of violence and were more likely than their peers to be critical of their schools and their relations with teachers and other students. They were also more likely to approach their personal relationships with underlying assumptions that enhanced their vulnerability to confrontations or violence episodes and to distrust and be disrespectful of their peers. Therefore, violence and use of violent acts to solve conflict may influence children and adolescents from any socioeconomic or racial or ethnic group.

COGNITIVE DEVELOPMENT AND INTERNALIZATION OF RULES

The process of attachment is a key component of the development of trust and empathy toward others. Inborn, basic motives are activated that lead to exploration, learning, and internalized shared meaning from early infancy (Emde, 1993). This developmental progression includes the internalization and organization of moral motives and continues within the context of caregiving. Internalization includes the "do's" and "don'ts" of experiences (p. 120). From infancy through adolescence, rules become a shared experience between the child and the caregiver. These rules usually include experiences of conflict and pleasure. They are learned or internalized through the child's natural tendency to initiate, maintain, and terminate social interactions and through the expectation that the caregiver relationship experiences will continue. Thus, children learn very early the rules that govern reciprocity in face-to-face and turn-taking interactions as well as other forms of communication. The concepts of turn taking in communication and social interaction also may be connected to the development of empathy (Emde, Biringen, Clyman, & Oppenheim, 1991).

Toward the end of the second year, the tendency for "getting it right," another aspect of basic morality, is differentiated (Emde, 1993). Anxiety or distress may be experienced when internal standards or expectations are violated, such as experiences of violence or being a witness to violence. Children as young as 16 months are reported to have memories of stressful events (Taylor, Zuckerman, Harik, & Groves, 1994). In 1987, the *Diagnostic and Statistical Manual of Mental Disorders* (American Psychiatric Association, 1987) recognized posttraumatic stress disorder (PTSD) as a condition that occurs in children and adults. The diagnostic criteria for PTSD was further refined by Pynoos (1993) for children 3 years of age and older. The criteria include experiencing an event that would be distressing for anyone, reexperiencing the trauma in various ways, avoidance, psychological numbing of responsiveness, and increased or decreased arousal. Several reports document that children exposed to the chronic stress of living in actual war zones and in urban war zones exhibit PTSD symptoms (Dubrow & Garbarino, 1989; Garbarino, Dubrow, Kostelny, & Pardo, 1992; Garbarino, Kostelny, & Dubrow, 1991; Osofsky, 1995). The extent to which PTSD influences conflict in children and adolescents is unknown but deserves further study.

Adolescence has been known historically as a time of experimentation and risk-taking behavior, with an increase in levels of independence and autonomy that prepares the adolescent for the shift to adult status. In the United States and Canada, many adolescents work through their role identities by being involved in work and recreational activities as they progress on the path to development of values, goals, and careers (Marcia, 1987). A second hallmark of adolescent development is the concern with the self-concept. During childhood, self-concept is integrated with concrete experiences, such as school, name, sports, or games. During adolescence, the self-concept is associated more with abstract psychological and emotional concerns, such as feelings and thoughts (Harter, 1990).

RISK-TAKING BEHAVIOR

Risk-taking behavior is a concept used to link conceptually several health behaviors that can be destructive, including substance use, precocious or risky sexual behavior, reckless vehicle use, homicidal and suicidal behavior, eating disorders, and delinquency (Igra & Irwin, 1996). Because risk-taking involves the possibility that a decision is made at some level, engagement in risk behaviors connotes volition, with some consideration given to alternative courses of action. These behaviors usually share similar physiological, environmental, biological, or all three antecedents. Reviews of the theories of risk-taking behavior can be found in the literature (Igra & Irwin, 1996; Millstein & Igra, 1993).

The biopsychosocial model (Igra & Irwin, 1996) includes social environmental factors from the ecological model and factors from the biological, developmental, and problem behavior model. Developmental considerations include psychosocial and cognitive changes characteristic of the adolescent period, such as independence, autonomy from family, peer affiliation and its significance, sexual awareness, identity formation, and physiological and cognitive maturation. The premise of problem behavior theory (Jessor, 1982, 1991) is that problem behaviors are a part of normal adolescent development and are important factors in the transition to adulthood. Smoking, drinking, illicit substance use, risky driving, and early sexual activity are viewed as purposeful, meaningful, goal-oriented, and functional ways to gain respect and acceptance from peers and as the means to establish autonomy from parents by negating conventional norms and values. Engagement in risk behaviors can help adolescents to learn to cope with anxiety and frustration and to anticipate failure. Thus, Igra and Irwin suggest that risk-taking behaviors must be viewed from a developmental context.

It is important that engagement in risk-taking behaviors be considered along with other cofactors such as changes in the social environment, which includes culture and individual differences. The biopsychosocial model allows a broader perspective from which to view risk-taking behavior and is a useful framework for nurses using holistic approaches to assessment and intervention. This approach is embedded in conflict resolution programs because consideration is given to the age, cognitive, and developmental level of the children and adolescents, cultural differences such as racial, ethnic, and cultural considerations.

Nurses have the knowledge and skill to develop intervention programs that provide appropriate information for children and adolescents on both biological and psychosocial influences on their health and well-being. A creatively developed psychoeducational approach is useful for intervention programs targeted at children, adolescents, and their families. The community approach to violence prevention is a good example in nursing (Beauchesne et al., 1997), as is violence prevention incorporated into anticipatory guidance during well child visits (McCarthy & Hobbie, 1997).

NURSING DIAGNOSIS AND
OUTCOME DETERMINATION

Conflict is a normal part of the everyday response to disagreement or ambivalence about a situation. Violence, however, is a learned response to perceived sources of environmental stressors. Children or adolescents may or may not have the necessary knowledge to work through conflict, and the outcome may be anxiety provoking or distressful and may escalate to violence. The North American Nursing Diagnosis Association (NANDA,

1999) diagnosis of *Ineffective Individual Coping* is defined as "impairment of adequate adaptive behaviors and problem-solving abilities of a person in meeting life's demands and roles" (p. 70). This choice of diagnosis is based on the difficulty children or adolescents may have in dealing constructively with conflict. Ineffective coping can be viewed in terms of one or more individuals, as in the case of children or adolescents, involved in conflict. Another alternative diagnosis is Knowledge Deficit, although this diagnosis is defined in terms of illness and currently does not apply to healthy persons in normal everyday communication problems. It could be adapted for use in conflict situations to deal with children or adolescents who have the requisite knowledge and skills to handle conflict situations.

Assessment of the ways in which children and adolescents resolve or do not resolve conflict is important. It is essential for the nurse to establish the meaning of conflict, discomfort, and distress with verbal or nonverbal encounters. Prior to beginning conflict resolution training, it is important to engage students in ice-breaking strategies, games, and other activities to assess their knowledge about feelings such as anger, love, hatred, fear, distrust, trust, and anxiety.

An expected outcome related to the nursing diagnosis of Ineffective Coping is that children and adolescents would exhibit more effective ways of coping. The Nursing Outcomes Classification (NOC) outcome Coping has many indicators that measure coping effectiveness, including identifying effective coping patterns, verbalizing acceptance of the situation, avoids unduly stressful situations, and verbalizing need for assistance (Iowa Outcomes Project, 2000, p. 192). Other outcome indicators include the ability to use listening and verbal skills to engage constructively in the resolution of conflict. It is expected that children and adolescents will be able to acknowledge, reflect, paraphrase, question, and, importantly, credit others. Many of these outcome indicators are captured in the NOC (Iowa Outcomes Project, 2000) outcome Aggression Control. Finally, it is important that the children and adolescents learn to use resources such as family, friends, teachers, health professionals, mentors, or mediators in their school environments to resolve their potential, impending, or actual conflicts before they escalate.

INTERVENTION: CONFLICT RESOLUTION

Conflict is a universal phenomenon that can have beneficial effects or harmful consequences ranging from emotional hurt to severe physical disabilities or psychological trauma for all concerned or both. The importance of skills to mediate conflict is becoming of increasing concern to nursing (Beauchesne et al., 1997; Johnson & Rudy, 1990) and related disciplines as both teaching (Johnson et al., 1992) and health disciplines (Farrell & Meyer, 1997; Hausman, Prothrow-Stith, et al., 1995) encounter children, adolescents, and their families who are embroiled in a variety of conflicts or see the consequences of conflict that led to violence in trauma units, emergency rooms, and later in the hospital and community. School nurses witness the effects of unresolved conflict in their daily encounters as they often deal with the aftermath of serious conflict between students in classrooms, the gym, the playground, or the health clinic.

Conflicts arise as the result of the common tendency of human beings to enter into them. Many children and adolescents do not know that there are nonviolent alternatives to resolve conflict. An important component of conflict resolution training is teaching children and adolescents how to become aware of and recognize feelings. Exercises that increase awareness of feelings of anger, fear, and humiliation, as well as positive feelings of happiness, joy, and love, are critical to the successful integration of conflict resolution skills. Many children are not aware of their feelings and do not know the words to use to describe them. Children and adolescents, through the acquisition of conflict resolution skills, can handle their own feelings of anger and frustration in a constructive manner and settle conflicts peacefully. They can be taught to problem solve by using active listening skills and recognizing feelings. Children and adolescents can be taught to recognize a problem, such as name calling, pushing, shoving, teasing, psychological intimidation, unprovoked meanness, or impending violent acts, and stop their escalation. They are also encouraged to acknowledge their own feelings and the feelings of others and to communicate to others their own feelings without putting others down. The goal of conflict resolution or mediation programs is to increase students' sense of self-responsibility and self-regulatory behavior. Through participation in the conflict management/mediation process students develop valuable social and problem-solving skills.

It is customary to label school-age children trained in conflict resolution as conflict managers and the process as conflict resolution. Adolescents are referred to as mediators and the process as mediation. Conflict situations or disputes can be referred for conflict resolution in different ways. Children and adolescents may request their conflicts or disputes be brought to a conflict resolution session or teachers, parents, support staff, administrators, or counselors may refer them. The children and adolescents must agree and not be forced to enter into mediation.

The conflict resolution process has four ground rules that must be adhered to throughout the training: (a) do not interrupt, (b) no put-downs, (c) no name calling or gossip, and (d) respect each other. There are five phases to the conflict resolution intervention. The first phase is seeing the problem, during which children and adolescents are taught how to identify a problem as it arises or to recognize one that already has developed.

The second phase is acting on the problem, during which children and adolescents are introduced to the ground rules "do not interrupt" and "no put-downs" so that they can see the problem and begin to act on it. The important factor underlying these ground rules is the need to practice active listening. It is important that the ground rules are adhered to throughout the conflict resolution process. The third phase is listening to both sides of the story. Each participant in the problem must be able to present his or her side of the story. This phase is a critical step. The children are taught to use words that describe their feelings and what the problems mean to them. They are also taught how to actively listen with exercises to reinforce listening skills. The fourth phase is thinking of solutions and coming to an agreement. Both participants must think of alternative approaches to solving their problem. They are taught to be creative and derive as many solutions as possible so that parties can negotiate a solution agreeable to all concerned. Finally, departure is a friendly and respectful termination to the conflict resolution session.

Children and adolescents are trained in active listening skills that include acknowledging, reflecting, paraphrasing, questioning with an emphasis on differentiating open- and closed-ended questions, and giving credit to the other party in the dispute. Nonverbal listening and observation skills train them to use positive body language, which includes how a person looks, speaks, sits, stands, and uses facial expressions in interaction with another person. Role modeling, games, and discussion can be used to demonstrate the many aspects of conflict resolution. The use of positive words of encouragement is taught and modeled. Both children and adolescents are informed of their civil rights and given the Children's Bill of Rights. Resources listed in Table 42.1 are very helpful to nurses who want to implement conflict resolution programs in schools or the community.

INTERVENTION APPLICATION

A commonly occurring boyfriend-girlfriend dispute among adolescents is chosen for this study. Monica, age 16, and Paul, age 17, dated for 2 years before Monica ended their relationship at the beginning of the school year. Recently, Monica started dating Eric, age 17, a student in the same high school. At a recent rock concert on a Saturday evening, Paul saw Monica and Eric together and was furious, the first indication that he was coping ineffectively (NANDA, 1999). On Monday morning, between classes he angrily confronted Monica and Eric in the hallway. He accused her of dating Eric before their breakup and accused Eric of being the cause of his and Monica's breakup. Paul had talked a lot about his anger to his friends and

TABLE 42.1   Resources

The Center for Nonviolent Communication
P.O. Box 2662
Sherman, TX 75091-2662
Phone: (903) 893-3886

The Community Board Program
1540 Market Street, Suite 490
San Francisco, CA 94102
Phone: (415) 552-1250

The Iowa Peace Institute
917 Tenth Avenue
P.O. Box 480
Grinnell, IA 50112
Phone: (515) 236-4880

National Association for Mediation in Education (NAME)
205 Hampshire House, Box 33635
University of Massachusetts
Amherst, MA 01003-3635
Phone: (413) 545-2462

Peacebuilders, Heartsprings, Inc.
P.O. Box 12158
Tucson, AZ 85732
  Phone: (520) 322-9977

had told them he was going to make Eric stop seeing Monica even if he had to beat him up. He made several calls to Monica during the weekend, but her sister and brothers fielded the calls, which further infuriated Paul.

Paul's friends were worried about his behavior. One friend, who was a student mediator in the mediation program, suggested to Paul that it might be a good idea for Paul to convince Monica and Eric attend a mediation session with him to settle this escalating dispute. Paul agrees to participate in mediation because he believes the conflict will be resolved in his favor, but he refuses to directly request the participation of Monica and Eric. He says he will attend if his friend arranges the mediation with Monica and Eric. They agree to the request, and at lunchtime they meet in the mediation room.

The mediator asks Paul to give his side of the story, and he calls Eric a jerk and tells him Monica belongs to him and that she really wants to be with him but is afraid of Eric. He also wants Eric to stop seeing Monica and Monica to start dating him again. Monica reveals that she had not been seeing Eric before the breakup and she had decided last year to stop seeing Paul because he was interfering with her studies and was becoming too serious. Eric wants Paul to stop pestering Monica; he also wants to continue his relationship with Monica. In addition, Eric requests that Paul apologize to him for trying to start a fight in the school hallway and for embarrassing him in front of teachers and other students.

Monica wants Paul to stop bothering her and to stop asking her for dates because she does not want to go out with him. She tells Paul she did not date Eric while they were seeing each other. She is also becoming frustrated with Eric, who she believes might be fueling Paul's anger through some of his friends. Eric told Paul's friends that Monica had decided to work at the same summer camp at which he was planning to work. Monica tells Paul and Eric she has not decided to work at the summer camp, and she wants Eric to stop spreading rumors.

The participants reach an agreement. Paul states that he will not contact Monica anymore, although he does not apologize to Eric. He states that he will not confront Eric or start fights with regard to Monica. Monica decides that she does not want to continue dating Eric because she believes they are all friends, and she does not want to have a serious relationship with either of them. She informs Eric and Paul that she wants to see several friends and not be tied to any one person. Rather, she wants to have fun and concentrate on her schoolwork to prepare for college. Through the Conflict Resolution intervention, all parties were able to neutralize their dispute. The desired outcome indicators for aggression control were reached, and the parties were able to depart peacefully.

RESEARCH AND PRACTICE IMPLICATIONS

Abdullah and Levine (1994) reiterated the need for research on violence and the development of field models for intervention with vulnerable and high-risk populations such as children. Furthermore, the development and testing of interventions focused on conflict resolution are needed. Nurses could both initiate the development and implementation of conflict resolution programs and test different approaches to implementing these interventions. Funding, however, must be allocated to this important component of violence prevention for children and adolescents and their families.

Risk behavior is tied to both a developmental sequence and a pattern of etiology (DiClemente, Ponton, & Hansen, 1996). Use of violence and delinquency follow a trajectory of increasing prevalence and intensity during adolescence that make evaluation of interventions difficult. Therefore, it is important to target multiple risk behaviors simultaneously. Interventions must not only be done with the individual but also be extended to the family and community and to the peer group (Stiffman et al., 1996). Furthermore, the development and evaluation of intervention programs aimed at health promotion and prevention of engagement in risk behaviors would be best achieved with an interdisciplinary focus.

A related area important to research on adolescents is the identification of protective factors associated with engagement in risk-taking behaviors and the consequent morbidity, mortality, or development of disease. Qualitative approaches that facilitate greater understanding of the complexity underlying risk factors in children and adolescents are needed. Quantitative approaches could use secondary data analysis of existing large national data sets that might facilitate identification of protective factors such as resilience, coping behaviors, and social and/or cultural factors that predispose youth to engage or not engage in risk-taking behavior.

Health promotion activities must occur at the family, community, and societal levels (USDHHS, 1993). Meleis (1990) suggests that strategies for fostering health include the primary health care concepts of community participation, consciousness raising, appropriate local resources, access, options, and empowerment. All these health care concepts need to be used in developing the climate for and implementing conflict resolution intervention programs. Nurses in academic nursing centers, school-based clinics, ambulatory clinic settings, and other traditional or nontraditional community environments are in a position to engage in collaborative efforts with community members who serve as resources who can address problems stemming from poverty and violence. A collaborative approach to the development of conflict resolution interventions for children and youth at risk that uses the strengths and knowledge of multiple discipline is essential.

Certain risk behaviors could be targeted as a group in the development of interventions and their evaluation. Intervention programs that foster skill development and empowerment would teach youth alternative options for solving disagreements and disputes among their peers and their families. Adults, such as grandparents or mentors (Schirm, Ross-Alaolmolki, & Conrad, 1995), could be instrumental in the development and maintenance of conflict management programs in schools and in the community. A natural extension of these types of programs could be offered to parents and other adults in the community.

Findings from the evaluation of Conflict Resolution intervention programs could be used to influence public policy initiatives at the state and national levels and to justify the allocation of increased funding to target risk-reduction factors as advocated in *Healthy People 2000* (USDHHS, 1991). Finally, the importance of the role of advocacy by nurses cannot be underestimated. There are many associations and organizations in the community concerned with youth in which nurses can participate. Nurses see and deal with the consequences of poverty and violence in many areas of their practice, both in the hospital and in the community. Therefore, they are in prime positions to be spokespersons to advocate against violence and to teach conflict resolution to parents and teachers as well as children and youth. There is no intervention with more potential to save lives and protect public health.

REFERENCES

Abdullah, F. G., & Levine, E. (1994). *Preparing nursing research for the 21st century: Evolution, methodologies, challenges.* New York: Springer.

American Psychiatric Association. (1987). *Diagnostic and statistical manual of mental disorders* (3rd ed.). Washington, DC: Author

Barry, D. S. (1993). Growing up violent: Decades of research link screen mayhem with increase in aggressive behavior. *Media & Values, 62,* 8-11.

Beauchesne, M. A., Kelley, B. R., Lawrence, P. R., & Farquharson, P. E. (1997). Violence prevention: A community approach. *Journal of Pediatric Health Care, 11*(4), 155-164.

Brady, M. (1994). Educating youths and their parents about the prevention of firearm injury. *Journal of Pediatric Health Care, 8*(3), 127-129.

Children's Defense Fund. (1997). *The state of America's children: Yearbook.* Washington, DC: Author.

DiClemente, R. J., Hansen, W. B., & Ponton, L. E. (1996). Adolescents at risk: A generation in jeopardy. In R. J. DiClemente, W. B. Hansen, & L. E. Ponton (Eds.), *Handbook of adolescent health risk behavior* (pp. 1-4). New York: Plenum.

DiClemente, R. J., Ponton, L. E., & Hansen, W. B. (1996). New directions for adolescent risk prevention and health promotion research and interventions. In R. J. DiClemente, W. B. Hansen, & L. E. Ponton (Eds.), *Handbook of adolescent health risk behavior* (pp. 413-420). New York: Plenum.

Dubrow, N. F., & Garbarino, J. (1989). Living in the war zone: Mothers and young children in a public housing development. *Child Welfare League of America, 67,* 4-20.

Emde, R. N. (1993). The horror! The horror! Reflections on our culture of violence and its implications for early development and morality. *Psychiatry, 56,* 119-123.

Emde, R. N., Biringen, Z., Clyman, R. B., & Oppenheim, D. (1991). The moral self of infancy: Affective core and procedural knowledge. *Developmental Review, 11,* 251-270.

Farrell, A. D., & Meyer, A. L. (1997). The effectiveness of a school-based curriculum for reducing violence among urban sixth-grade students. *American Journal of Public Health, 87*(6), 979-984.

Garbarino, J., Dubrow, N., Kostelny, K., & Pardo, C. (1992). *Children in danger: Coping with the consequences of community violence.* San Francisco: Jossey-Bass.

Gabarino, J., Kostelny, K., & Dubrow, N. (1991). What children can tell us about living in danger. *American Psychologist, 46*(4), 376-383.

Harter, S. (1990). Self and identity development. In S. S. Feldman & G. R. Elliott (Eds.), *At the threshold: The developing adolescent* (pp. 352-387). Cambridge, MA: Harvard University Press.

Hausman, A. J., Prothrow-Stith, D., & Spivak, H. (1995). Implementation of violence prevention education in clinical settings. *Patient Education and Counseling, 25*(2), 205-210.

Hausman, A. J., Spivak, H., & Prothrow-Stith, D. (1995). Evaluation of a community-based youth violence prevention project. *Society for Adolescent Medicine, 17*(6), 353-359.

Hollman, F. W. (1993). *U.S. population estimates, by age, sex, race and Hispanic origin: 1990-1992.* Washington, DC: U.S. Bureau of the Census, Population Division, Population Projections Branch.

Igra, V., & Irwin, C. E. (1996). Theories of adolescent risk-taking behavior. In R. J. DiClemente, W. B. Hansen, & L. E. Ponton (Eds.), *Handbook of adolescent health risk behavior* (pp. 35-52). New York: Plenum.

Iowa Outcomes Project. (2000). *Nursing outcomes classification (NOC)* (M. Johnson, M. Maas, & S. Moorhead, Eds.; 2nd ed.). St. Louis, MO: Mosby-Year Book.

Jessor, R. (1982, May). Problem behavior and developmental transition in adolescence. *Journal of School Health,* 295-300.

Jessor, R. (1991). Risk behavior in adolescence: A psychosocial framework for understanding and action. *Journal of Adolescent Health Care, 12,* 597-605.

Johnson, D. W., Johnson, R. T., Dudley, B., & Burnett, R. (1992, September). Teaching students to be peer mediators. *Educational Leadership,* 10-13.

Johnson, M. L., & Rudy, C. A. (1990). Teaching children to resolve conflicts cooperatively. *Journal of Pediatric Health Care, 4*(5), 237-243.

Marcia, J. (1987). The identity status approach to the study of ego development. In T. Honess & K. Yardley (Eds.), *Self and identity: Perspectives across the lifespan.* London: Routledge Kegan Paul.

McCarthy, V., & Hobbie, C. (1997). Incorporating violence prevention into anticipatory guidance for well child visits. *Journal of Pediatric Health Care, 11*(5), 222-226.

Meleis, A. I. (1990). Being and becoming healthy: The core of nursing knowledge. *Nursing Science Quarterly, 3,* 107-114.

The Metropolitan Life Survey of the American Teacher 1994. (1994). *Violence in American public schools: The family perspective.* New York: Harris & Associates.

Millstein, S. G., & Igra, V. (1993). Theoretical models of adolescent risk-taking behavior. In J. L. Wallender & L. J. Siegel (Eds.), *Adolescent health problems: Behavioral perspectives* (pp. 52-71). New York: Guilford.

Nelms, B. C. (1997). Helping the victims and the bullies. *Journal of Pediatric Health Care, 11*(5), 205-206.

North American Nursing Diagnosis Association. (1994). *Nursing diagnoses: Definitions and classification 1995-1996.* Philadelphia: Author.

Osofsky, J. D. (1995). The effects of exposure to violence on young children. *American Psychologist, 50*(9), 782-788.

Prothrow-Stith, D. B. (1995). The epidemic of youth violence in America: Using public health prevention strategies to prevent violence. *Journal of Health Care for the Poor and Underserved, 6*(2), 95-101.

Pynoos, R. S. (1993). Traumatic stress and developmental psychopathology in children and adolescents. In J. M. Oldham, M. B. Riba, & A. Tasman (Eds.), *American Psychiatric Press review of psychiatry* (Vol. 12). Washington, DC: American Psychiatric Press.

Schirm, V., Ross-Alaolmolki, K., & Conrad, M. (1995). Collaborative education through a foster grandparent program: Enhancing intergenerational relations. *Gerontology & Geriatric Education, 15*(3), 85-94.

Sells, C. W., & Blum, R. W. (1996). Current trends in adolescent health. In R. J. DiClemente, W. B. Hansen, & L. E. Ponton (Eds.), *Handbook of adolescent health risk behavior* (pp. 5-34). New York: Plenum.

Stiffman, A. R., Earls, F., Dorr, P., Cunningham, R., & Farbers, S. (1996). Adolescent violence. In R. J. DiClemente, W. B. Hansen, & L. E. Ponton (Eds.), *Handbook of adolescent health risk behavior* (pp. 289-312). New York: Plenum.

Taylor, L., Zuckerman, B., Harik, V., & Groves, B. M. (1994). Witnessing violence by young children and their mothers. *Journal of Developmental & Behavioral Pediatrics, 15*(2), 120-123.

U.S. Department of Health and Human Services. (1991). *Healthy people 2000: National health promotion and disease prevention objectives* (DHHS Publication No. PHS 91-50312). Washington, DC: Government Printing Office.

U.S. Department of Health and Human Services. (1993). *A report of the NINR priority expert panel on health promotion: Health promotion for older children and adolescents* (NIH Publication No. 93-2420). Bethesda, MD: National Institutes of Health.

Wolfe, D., & Korsche, B. (1994). Witnessing domestic violence during childhood and adolescence: Implication for pediatric practice. *Pediatrics, 94*(4, Pt. 2), 594-599.

Index

About the Editors

Martha Craft-Rosenberg, PhD, RN, FAAN, is Chairperson for the Parent, Child, and Family Area of Study. She is a professor at The University of Iowa College of Nursing and has conducted research on siblings of ill children for 20 years and on families of critically ill patients for 10 years. In addition, she has been an investigator on the Nursing Interventions Classification research team for 10 years. During the past 5 years, she has been the principal investigator for the Nursing Diagnosis Extension and Classification research team on a collaborative project with the North American Nursing Diagnosis Association (NANDA) to refine and extend the nursing diagnosis nomenclature. She is a member of the NANDA taxonomy committee and reviews grant proposals regularly for Sigma Theta Tau and the American Nurses Foundation. She has received awards from the American Association for Critical Care Nursing and the Midwest Nursing Research Society for her research on children and families. In addition, she is editor of the first book on *Nursing Interventions for Infants and Children,* which received the American Journal of Nursing Award and the Pediatric Nursing Book of the Year Award. This book is a modification and enlargement of that book.

Janice Denehy, PhD, RN, is Associate Professor at The University of Iowa College of Nursing. She is involved in the graduate program, teaching child health nursing, nursing education, concepts and theories in nursing, and health promotion. Her research interest is school-age children's knowledge of their bodies, health, and illness. She is also an investigator on the Iowa Intervention Project and has developed interventions related to children and families for the Nursing Interventions Classification. In addition, she is coprincipal investigator of the Nursing Diagnosis Extension and Classification research team, serving as the Parents/Infant/Child Diagnosis Work Group Chair. She is a frequent speaker on the importance of using standardized language in nursing education and school nursing. She is executive editor of *The Journal of School Nursing*.

About the Contributors

Arnette Marie Anderson, PhD, RN, is Associate Professor of the Faculty of Nursing, University of Alberta, Edmonton. Research interests include the development of the mother-twin relationship, during the infant's first year of life, the father-infant relationship, and the father-twin relationship.

Mary Lober Aquilino, PhD, RN, FNP, at the time of this writing was Assistant Professor in The University of Iowa College of Nursing. She conducts research in the area of teen pregnancy prevention. As a member of the University of Iowa Nursing-Sensitive Outcomes Classification Research Team, she is involved in developing and measuring standardized nursing outcomes. Her academic interests include community health and primary care. She is a member of the board of directors of the Family Planning Council of Iowa.

Sara Walsh Arneson, PhD, RN, is Associate Professor in the School of Nursing at the University of Virginia. Her area of specialization is child health with a special emphasis on health promotion responsibilities. She also serves as a health consultant to the Monticello Area Community Action Agency's Head Start Program. In addition, she writes a bimonthly column that is distributed to ambulatory health care settings. Her research interests focus on health promotion and injury prevention strategies among young children.

Deborah K. Bahe, MSN, RN, PNP, has been a member of the Oelwein School Health program in Oelwein, Iowa, for the past 10 years.

Cynthia L. Bennett, MSN, RN, CPNP, is a nurse practitioner at the Sports Medicine Center of the Children's Hospital Medical Center of Akron, Ohio. She has been involved in research projects to improve the validity of youth fitness tests, to develop a performance enhancement curriculum for physical education classes, and to determine the most effective way to deliver an antismoking campaign to school-age children. An athlete all her life, she is dedicated to preparing children to meet their optimal potential for physical, mental, and spiritual health.

Kathryn Moore Breitbach, MA, ARNP, CPNP, RNC, is a pediatric nurse practitioner in the high-risk infant follow-up program at The University of Iowa Hospitals and Clinics. She is a member of the Iowa Association of Nurse Practitioners and Sigma Theta Tau, Iota Tau Chapter.

Marion E. Broome, PhD, RN, FAAN, is Professor and Associate Dean for Research at the University of Alabama at Birmingham. Her area of expertise is the reduction of child distress during pain using relaxation, distraction, and simple imagery. She is a member of the Nursing Science Study Section at the National Institute of Nursing Research and serves on several professional organization governing boards, including the Midwest Nursing Research Society and the Association for Care of Children's Health. She is editor of the journal *Child and Family Nursing* (Lippincott, Williams, & Wilkins).

Stephanie Clatworthy, EdD, RN, is Professor of Nursing at Kent State University. Her research on the impact of hospitalization on school-age children began in 1978 and progressed and was extended to include not only the state of Ohio but also the state of Michigan. The support of many graduate students and external funding made it possible to collect information on the impact of hospitalization on school-age children.

Nancy C. Corser, DSN, RN, RNC, is Dean of the Health Division at Wallace State Community College in Hanceville, Alabama. Her research and publications have focused on sleep of infants and children.

Judith A. Coucouvanis, MA, CS, RN, NP, is a clinical nurse specialist and nurse practitioner in the Department of Child and Adolescent Psychiatry at the University of Michigan Medical Center. She works with families to design behavior modification plans to change or decrease troublesome behaviors. In addition, she lectures and provides workshops and consultation services to schools, parent groups, and other service agencies. She has published articles and lectured extensively in the areas of behavior management, autism, and social skills training.

Jo Ellen Crowe, MSN, RN, ARNP, CPNP, is a staff nurse on the Inpatient Child and Adolescent Psychiatry Unit at The University of Iowa Hospitals and Clinics. Her experience has focused on the mental health of school-age and adolescent children.

Janet A. Deatrick, PhD, RN, FAAN, is Associate Professor at the University of Pennsylvania School of Nursing. Her interests are the day-to-day management by families who have children with chronic conditions and the contribution of qualitative research to understanding that phenomenon. She was elected a member of the American Academy of Nursing in 1992 and received the Christian and Mary Lindback Award for Distinguished Teaching at the University of Pennsylvania in 1995. She won the 1998 Distinguished Nurse Alumnus Award of the University of Illinois College of Nursing.

Christine L. Doyle, MSN, RN, CPNP, works in a family practice rural health clinic and also for the Maternal-Child Health Program for several counties in the state of Iowa. Her master's project was the premise for her chapter. She has worked in neonatal intensive care units, obstetrical nursing, and wellness pediatrics.

Ann E. Edgil, DSN, RN, CPNP, recently retired as Professor at the University of Alabama School of Nursing, where she chaired the Pediatric Nurse Practitioner Option in the master's program. She has published in the areas of family functioning, high-risk behaviors of adolescents, and sleep of children. She has numerous nonresearch publications in the areas of pediatric nursing and nursing education.

Lynn Eidahl, MA, RN, is the Early Childhood Tracking Coordinator of the Minnesota Children With Special Health Needs Section of the Minnesota Department of Health. She has worked as a genetics clinical nurse specialist. Genetic counseling and preconception counseling were the focus of her graduate studies.

Susan M. Elek, PhD, RN, CPNP, is Associate Professor in the College of Nursing at the University of Nebraska Medical Center. Currently, she is researching fatigue during the transition to parenthood. She has developed and taught two nursing courses via the Internet.

Michele J. Eliason, PhD, RN, is Associate Professor of Nursing at The University of Iowa College of Nursing. She is also coprincipal investigator on the Prairieland Addiction Technology Transfer Center, a research-based center for the collection and dissemination of information about substance abuse. Her research interests are in the areas of substance abuse and sexuality studies.

Sandra Jane Hahn, MSN, RNC, is In Vitro Fertilization Coordinator, Advanced Practice Nurse in Children's and Women's Services, Department of Nursing, The University of Iowa Hospitals and Clinics. Her areas of research interests are decision making related to multifetal reduction and disclosure of birth origins to children.

Kirsten Sueppel Hanrahan, MA, RN, CPNP, is an Advanced Registered Nurse Practioner in the Special Care Nurseries at the University of Iowa Hospitals and Clinics. Her clinical and research interests include parenting, child neglect and abuse, and invasive lines in children.

Marjorie M. Heinzer, PhD, RN, CS, CRNP, is Assistant Professor at La Salle University and Associate Director of Nursing for Research at the Albert Einstein Medical Center. Her area of expertise is child and adolescent health nursing. Research interests include resilience and coping of adolescents who have lost a parent and chronic illness issues related to children and their families.

Pamela D. Hill, PhD, RN, is Associate Professor at the University of Illinois at Chicago, College of Nursing, Quad Cities Regional Program. She has been involved with lactation research for the past 12 years and has published in numerous journals. Her particular research area of interest is insufficient milk supply among mothers of term, low-birth-weight, and preterm infants.

Cynthia S. Hockman, MSN, RN, CPNP, works for the Blank Developmental Screening Program at Blank Children's Hospital. Blank Developmental Screening is a neurodevelopmental screening program that provides ongoing follow-up and case management to infants who have been hospitalized in the neonatal intensive care unit (NICU) at Blank Children's Hospital. She developed the follow-up program in 1980 and continues to be the clinical coordinator and pediatric nurse practitioner of the program. She is a certified NIDCAP observer and participates in the family-centered and development caregiving in the NICU.

Myra Martz Huth, MSN, RN, is a doctoral candidate at the Frances Payne Bolton School of Nursing, Case Western Reserve University. She is conducting research to reduce postoperative pain in children using an imagery intervention. She is on the editorial board and writes a bimonthly instrument section for the *Journal of Child and Family Nursing*. Past publications include topics on a theory of acute pain management, children's spirituality, the Gastronomy Feeding Button, and hospital tours.

Adrienne Kirby, PhD, RN, is Vice President of Operational Improvement at the Christiana Care Health Services and also Adjunct Associate Professor at the University of Delaware College of Nursing. She has research interests in and has published on topics such as taxonomic classification of nursing interventions, the impact of nursing care on patient satisfaction, and performance improvement.

Charmaine Kleiber, PhD, RN, CPNP, is an advanced practice nurse for research at the Children's Hospital of Iowa, The University of Iowa Hospitals and Clinics. Her research interests include techniques to reduce children's distress during medical procedures, informational needs of siblings of critically ill children, and symptom management for chronically ill children.

Kathleen A. Knafl, PhD, is Professor in the School of Nursing, Yale University, where she teaches courses in Family, Concept Development, and Qualitative Research. Her research interests focus on family response to childhood illness. She is especially interested in the concept of normalization and has written extensively on the topic. She serves on the editorial boards of the *Journal of Family Nursing* and the *Journal of Child and Family Health*. Her current research, a study on computer-assisted management of diabetes in children, explores how families incorporate a telemedicine network to manage a child's illness.

Carol Loan, MA, RN, CPNP, is an advanced registered nurse practitioner in the Newborn & Intermediate Care Nurseries at The University of Iowa Hospitals & Clinics.

Marie L. Lobo, PhD, RN, FAAN, is Associate Professor in the College of Nursing, Medical University of South Carolina. Currently, she is evaluating the effect of a home-visiting program during the first year of life. She has also worked with children and families across the health-illness continuum primarily in the community.

Colette Lothe, MSN, RN, completed a master's thesis at The University of Iowa College of Nursing on the immunization status of 2-year-olds. She is a second-year medical student at The University of Iowa College of Medicine. She has clinical experience in pediatrics, neonatal nursing, and trauma nursing.

Ann Marie McCarthy, PhD, RN, PNP, is Associate Professor in the Parent, Child, and Family Area of study at The University of Iowa College of Nursing. She is also a licensed pediatric psychologist who maintains a clinical practice for children and families coping with diabetes. Her research focuses on children with chronic health conditions and school-based health care. Her current research focuses on the academic achievement of children with diabetes, and the use of medications in schools, and cognitive behavioral interventions for procedural pain in children.

Lou Ann Montgomery, MA, RN, CCRN, is Director of Nursing Education at The University of Iowa Hospitals and Clinics. A former advance practice nurse in the Neonatal ICU/Transport Team, her research interests include family support of critically ill newborns, with a special emphasis on sibling support and educational interventions. She has published in these areas in several journals, both individually and as a member of the Family Interventions Research Team at The University of Iowa Hospitals and Clinics.

Barbara Neitzel-Schneider, MA, RN, CPNP, is a pediatric nurse practitioner at Integra Health Pediatric Clinic in Cedar Rapids, Iowa. Her roles include health maintenance examination of pediatric patients, diagnosis and treatment of acutely ill children, and family education. She is also a preceptor for nurse practitioner students from The University of Iowa College of Nursing.

Anita Nicholson, MA, RN, is Lecturer and Undergraduate Clinical Instructor at The University of Iowa College of Nursing. Her research interests involve families of the critically ill. She has been involved in two studies focusing on child visitation in the critical care units, and she has presented continuing education conferences on interventions for families of the critically ill.

Julie Osterhaus, MA, ARNP, RN, CPNP, is an advanced practice nurse/pediatric nurse practitioner in Pediatric Endocrinology at The University of Iowa Hospitals and Clinics working with pediatric endocrine and diabetes patients. She has experience in pediatric nursing administration in a pediatric outpatient setting, staff nursing in pediatric critical care, and general pediatrics.

Leonie Pallikkathayil, DNS, RN, is a tenured associate professor with dissertation privileges at the University of Kansas School of Nursing. Her teaching, research, publication, and organizational affiliations include areas such as mental health, suicide, fatigue, and ethics.

Shelley-Rae Pehler, MSN, RN, is a maternal-child/pediatric clinical nurse specialist at Genesis Medical Center in Davenport, Iowa. Her clinical experiences have been in the obstetrical and pediatric areas. Her research interests include spirituality in children. She is also a member of the Physiologic Focus Group of the Nursing Outcomes Classification Research Team.

Rita H. Pickler, PhD, RN, is Associate Professor of Maternal-Child Nursing at Virginia Commonwealth University. Her research and clinical interests are focused on children at risk, with particular interest in improving developmental and growth outcomes. She has conducted several studies involving nonnutritive sucking and is currently developing and studying a model of feeding readiness in preterm infants.

Susan Poulton, MSN, RN, PNP, is a school nurse consultant for the Grant Wood Area Education Agency in Cedar Rapids/Coralville, Iowa. Her primary interests are in the areas of school nursing and developmental disabilities.

Sandra Rae Powell, PhD, RN, is Associate Professor in the College of Nursing at The University of Iowa. Her research is focused on vulnerable populations, such as the mentally ill and homeless. She has long had an interest in the area of substance abuse and, as a result, has developed an interest in prevention.

Julie L. Ritland, MSN, RN, PNP, is Assistant Professor at Allen College. She has practiced in a variety of clinical settings and currently teaches in the areas of pediatrics and mental health. Her research interests include adolescent nutrition and exercise, techniques to reduce children's anxiety during medical procedures, and the pediatric grief process.

Kathleen Ross-Alaolmolki, PhD, RN, is Associate Professor at the University of Akron, College of Nursing, and teaches in the graduate and undergraduate programs. Her area of expertise is child and adolescent health nursing. Research interests include families who have a child with a chronic illness, adolescent parental attachment relationships and their relationship to adolescent well-being, and children's and adolescent's attitudes toward and use of conflict resolution skills.

Kathleen A. Simon, DNSc, RN, is Assistant Professor, College of Nursing, Medical University of South Carolina. Her research focuses on child coping with stressful life events, specifically acute and chronic illnesses. She has been involved in research related to the use of therapeutic play as an intervention to alter anxiety and to the use of drawings as an assessment of the anxiety of hospitalized children.

Mary E. Tiedeman, PhD, RN, is Assistant Professor, College of Nursing, Brigham Young University. Her research interest focuses on children's responses to stressful events from their perspective. She has done research examining the anxiety and fear responses of children to hospitalization and to ambulatory surgery. She is interested in identifying interventions that help children cope effectively with stressful situations and has conducted therapeutic play with hospitalized children.

Jane E. Wilkins, BSN, RN, is Coordinator of the Touching Hearts Perinatal Bereavement Program at The University of Iowa Hospitals and Clinics. She is an obstetric nurse specializing in maternal-fetal medicine and prenatal genetics. She was instrumental in the founding of the Touching Hearts Bereavement Program. In collaboration with The University of Iowa Department of Family Therapy, she assisted with research investigating the parental grieving process of a perinatal loss.

Janet K. Williams, PhD, RN, CPNP, CGC, is Associate Professor of Nursing at The University of Iowa. She is the director of the advanced practice genetic nursing program in the master's nursing program at The University of Iowa. She conducts research on the psychosocial aspects of genetic conditions for children and their families. She has published on behavioral aspects of Turner syndrome, the impact of this condition on parenting, and considerations when nurses participate in genetic testing of adults or children.

Tammie L. Willis, MS, RN, is a faculty member in the Department of Nursing at Penn Valley Community College. Her research interests include the development of critical thinking skills and child-related mental health issues.

Catherine Willoughby, MA, RN, is Nurse Manager for the Child and Adolescent Psychiatry Service at The University of Iowa Hospitals and Clinics. She has a special interest in mental health care for adolescents.

LEEDS BECKETT UNIVERSITY
LIBRARY
DISCARDED

Leeds Metropolitan University

17 0354685 0

Nursing Interventions for Infants, Children, and Families